STREET WORKOUT

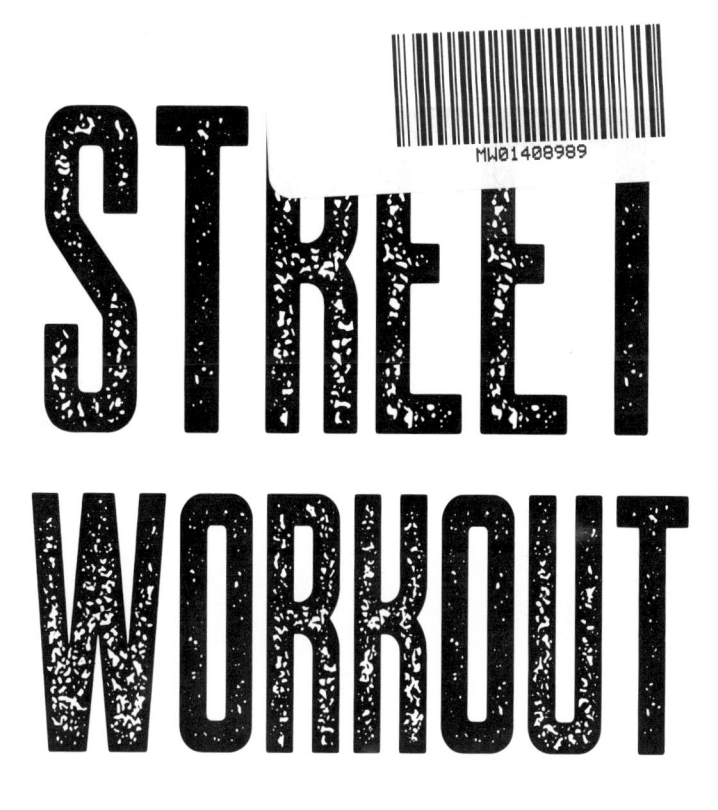

A WORLDWIDE ANTHOLOGY OF URBAN CALISTHENICS
—— HOW TO SCULPT A GOD-LIKE PHYSIQUE USING NOTHING BUT YOUR ENVIRONMENT

Al Kavadlo & Danny Kavadlo

STREET WORKOUT

Al Kavadlo & Danny Kavadlo

© Copyright 2016, Al Kavadlo & Danny Kavadlo
A Dragon Door Publications, Inc. production
All rights under International and Pan-American Copyright conventions.
Published in the United States by: Dragon Door Publications, Inc.
5 East County Rd B, #3 • Little Canada, MN 55117
Tel: (651) 487-2180 • Fax: (651) 487-3954
Credit card orders: 1-800-899-5111 • Email: support@dragondoor.com • Website: www.dragondoor.com

ISBN 10: 1-942812-06-X   ISBN 13: 978-1-942812-06-7
This edition first published in September 2016
Printed in China

No part of this book may be reproduced in any form or by any means without the prior written consent of the Publisher, excepting brief quotes used in reviews.

BOOK DESIGN: Derek Brigham • www.dbrigham.com • bigd@dbrigham.com

PHOTO CREDITS: Michael Alago, Martijn Bos, Mary Carol Fitzgerald, Neil Gavin, Adrienne Harvey, David Holbrook, Al Kavadlo, Danny Kavadlo, Grace Kavadlo, Wilson Cash Kavadlo, Kenny Lombardi, Rachel Phillips, Michael Polito & Annie Vo

The Kavadlo brothers are contributors to Bodybuilding.com, where portions of this work have appeared.

DISCLAIMER: The authors and publisher of this material are not responsible in any manner whatsoever for any injury that may occur through following the instructions contained in this material. The activities, physical and otherwise, described herein for informational purposes only, may be too strenuous or dangerous for some people and the reader(s) should consult a physician before engaging in them. The content of this book is for informational and educational purposes only and should not be considered medical advice, diagnosis, or treatment. Readers should not disregard, or delay in obtaining, medical advice for any medical condition they may have, and should seek the assistance of their health care professionals for any such conditions because of information contained within this publication.

— Table of Contents —

FOREWORD
By John DuCane V

AUTHORS' NOTE 1

I - WHAT IS STREET WORKOUT?
Chapter 1. Street Workout At Dawn 5

Chapter 2. Street Workout Culture 9

Chapter 3. Street Workout Training 13

II - FOUNDATIONAL PROGRESSIONS
Chapter 4. Push 19

Chapter 5. Pull 59

Chapter 6. Squat 91

Chapter 7. Flex 125

Chapter 8. Bridge 149

III - SKILLS & "TRICKS"
Chapter 9. Floor Holds 171

Chapter 10. Bar Moves 215

Chapter 11. Human Flag 245

IV - PROGRAMMING

Chapter 12. Assessments 283

Chapter 13. Street Workouts 287

Chapter 14. Training Templates 313

V - BONUS SECTION

Chapter 15. Ask Al 321

Chapter 16. Danny's Dos & Don'ts 335

Chapter 17. Building A Backyard Pull-Up Bar 347

Chapter 18. Taking It To The Streets 353

ACKNOWLEDGMENTS 364

ABOUT THE AUTHORS 365

INDEX OF EXERCISES 366

FOREWORD

Life is mysterious. Small acts blaze up into wild firestorms. The glimmer of a slight desire transforms into an incandescent passion that seems to light the world. A single thought triggers a raging torrent of ideas. A casual encounter leads to the deepest of bonds. The force of creation sparks new patterns of beauty and insight. Webs of interconnection form beneath the surface of our understanding.

We wonder why we do what we do, from where we came and to where we go…

Of such stuff has been my friendship with two remarkable men, the brothers **Al Kavadlo** and **Danny Kavadlo**…

It was **Paul Wade** who nudged the Kavadlos into my consciousness for the first time. A couple of rangy, flamboyant, tat-drenched, muscular misfits who decked out ***Convict Conditioning 2*** with their calisthenic stylings. Their Human Flag—set in the same Alcatraz rec yard once haunted by Al Capone and The Birdman—signaled that a new band had crashed the stage…

And it was Paul Wade again who made the next nudge—recommending Al's writing to me and suggesting that I consider publishing him. So I checked Al out…

What I discovered was not just Al himself, but a whole nother world…

I discovered that Al was an artist whose preferred medium is his own body. Calisthenics means "beautiful movement" and Al re-creates himself daily, on that basis, as on ongoing artwork. Now, artworks need a setting in which to best display themselves—and that setting becomes an extension of the artwork. In his case, Al chooses to display himself against the gritty graffiti, scaffolding and distressed brick of down-and-dirty, "street" NYC. Al's favorite workout spot? Tompkins Square Park—where the doors have been ripped off the toilets to cut down on the fix-traffic of local junkies…

As part of his art, Al cultivates a smiling, happy Zen-guy look—even when performing some of the toughest moves on the planet, like the one-arm pull-up or the front lever. Yet simmering beneath that Zen smile is a fierce will, a formidable drive and a fanatical commitment to doing things just right. As with almost all great performers, Al's rust never sleeps...

That other world that Al is a portal to? That would be the culture and international network called "Street Workout". If Al's immediate setting is New York, his global context can be defined by those two words...He and his brother Danny represent the street workout ethos to the max. Their book, Street Workout, is not only a paean to this movement but is sure to become that movement's Bible...

As a publisher with a passion to share the best-of-the-best when it comes to the realm of physical cultivation, I like to work with authors who are the "complete package". The author as "complete package" combines many, many attributes: they bring innovation and insight to the table. They are creative, thorough and inquisitive. They walk their talk and look the part. They are natural leaders. They are relentless and skilled self-promoters. Their writing style scintillates with their individual, distinct, differentiated voice. They have a strong and loyal following. They know their stuff inside out, but remain open to new ideas and input. They are passionate about every aspect of their craft and their physical practice. And finally, they are a joy to work with.

Rare to find? Yes. Very. Tall order? Yes. Very. Got some such "complete packages"? Why...yes, yes, I do...and Al Kavadlo is one of them...

So I both applaud myself and feel fortunate to have taken Paul's hint and signed on Al as a Dragon Door author. Talk about small acts that blaze up into firestorms... We have gone on to publish a series of wonderful titles with Al: **Raising the Bar, Pushing the Limits, Stretching Your Boundaries** and **Zen Mind, Strong Body**. And now, the monumental **Street Workout** he has co-authored with brother Danny...

It's not much of a surprise, then, that when Paul Wade and I were looking for a natural born leader for our **Progressive Calisthenics Certification (PCC)** program, we chose Al... who in turn recruited Danny to fellow-preach the new bodyweight exercise gospel.

Right from the get-go Al and Danny knocked the PCC ball out of the park. From its launch in June 2013, the PCC has become the undisputed gold standard for calisthenics training—nothing else comes close. And there is no question in my mind that it will remain THE place to go for the finest bodyweight exercise instruction, globally. Al and Danny's deep passion, humility, care, graciousness, kindness, knowledge and skill have inspired hundreds upon hundreds of practitioners to go forth and spread the good word about the wonders of calisthenic cultivation. It's a great thing to behold...

Street Workout is saturated with the vibe and brilliant teachings I have experienced from Al and Danny at every workshop I have attended. And you'll see phenomenal photographs taken in almost all the countries they've taught in, be it Italy, Germany, Sweden, Ireland, England, Australia, China, Holland or the USA... "Rich" doesn't begin to describe the breadth and depth of the creative artistry of the illustrations—off the charts.

Now, one of the best things that has happened in my life is to count Mister Danny Kavadlo as a good friend—and to watch the rise and rise of this great man within the Dragon Door community. And how remarkable is it to have two brothers who can both live up to my "complete package" descriptor? Because Danny is most certainly also the "complete package".

A perfect foil for Grandmaster Al, Danny's menacing scowl, bristling musculature, stacked intensity and punkoid posturing belie a heart of gold and a deep-felt love for his fellow humans. When Danny does smile, he lights up the room. When Danny's booming cadence penetrates the room with his urgent inflections, it's an outright delight to watch the fire of his passion ignite his students. So good...so good...

And like brother Al, what a coach! Danny celebrates every achievement of every student with an infectious, ecstatic roar that rings with authentic excitement and happiness for their accomplishment. Like Al, Danny squeezes greatness from his clients with his care-infused observations and skillful cueing. No one interacts with Danny without leaving enriched...

Yes, Danny has his demons—don't we all—but he is the ultimate celebrator of life. I have joked that Danny would see the worst situation as a "glass one-tenth full"—but mostly his glass appears to be more like "nine-tenths full". Love it!

Danny is also a multifaceted artist, a creator, an instigator of transformation and a very literate gentleman. All three of his previous titles with Dragon Door, **Everybody Needs Training, Diamond-Cut Abs** and **Strength Rules** have shone with his distinct, flamboyant creativity. Danny knows how to plunge to the nitty-gritty of what's really real in the fraud-filled fitness biz. He savages the flimflam of the supplement and packaged foods industry, in a way that is to-the-point, convincing and simultaneously amusing. He nails what you really need to do in your workouts to get real, lasting results—and keep on getting them.

And talk about "walking the walk"... Danny is a striding billboard for what the physical cultivation artist can achieve with calisthenics alone. Danny's a specimen all right—but he radiates "hard-earned". Brutally honest about all the training and diet follies he's fallen for in his earlier years, Danny's own body is his own best proof he's got this training thing figured out finally!

Many years in gestation and many years in the making, **Street Workout** is the brothers' first collaboration in print. The two of them are a rock star act at the PCC workshops. But a book is a whole nother kettle of fish... Each brother has their very distinct personality, writing style and presentation method. To successfully merge two great artistic talents into one cohesive text is a major feat.

Well, I'm here to report that the brothers have pulled it off...

Street Workout is one of those landmark titles that define a genre—the treasured lodestone and must-have reference for hardcore fans and raw beginners alike. The brothers bring it—and then some. I can tell that their trenchwork teaching at the dozens of worldwide PCCs, their previous experience authoring Dragon Door titles, their consistent engagement through blogs and articles with their constituency, and their constant absorption of new perspectives has elevated both their games to dizzying heights.

Al and Danny have listened well and grown accordingly. They have given and given so much—and have received back in equal measure. **Street Workout** is the fruit of that splendid dynamic.

Whether it be the section on foundational progressions for push, pull, squat, flex and bridge... Whether it be the section on the skills and "tricks" you need to achieve floor holds, bar moves and the human flag... Whether it be the section on programming that covers assessments, street workout and training templates...—all is systematically revealed, with a mix of clarity, precision, intelligence, creativity, humor and pizzazz that have become the brothers' hallmark.

Congratulations on your masterpiece, Al and Danny—and thank you for being in my life...

John Du Cane

John Du Cane
Founder and CEO, Dragon Door Publications

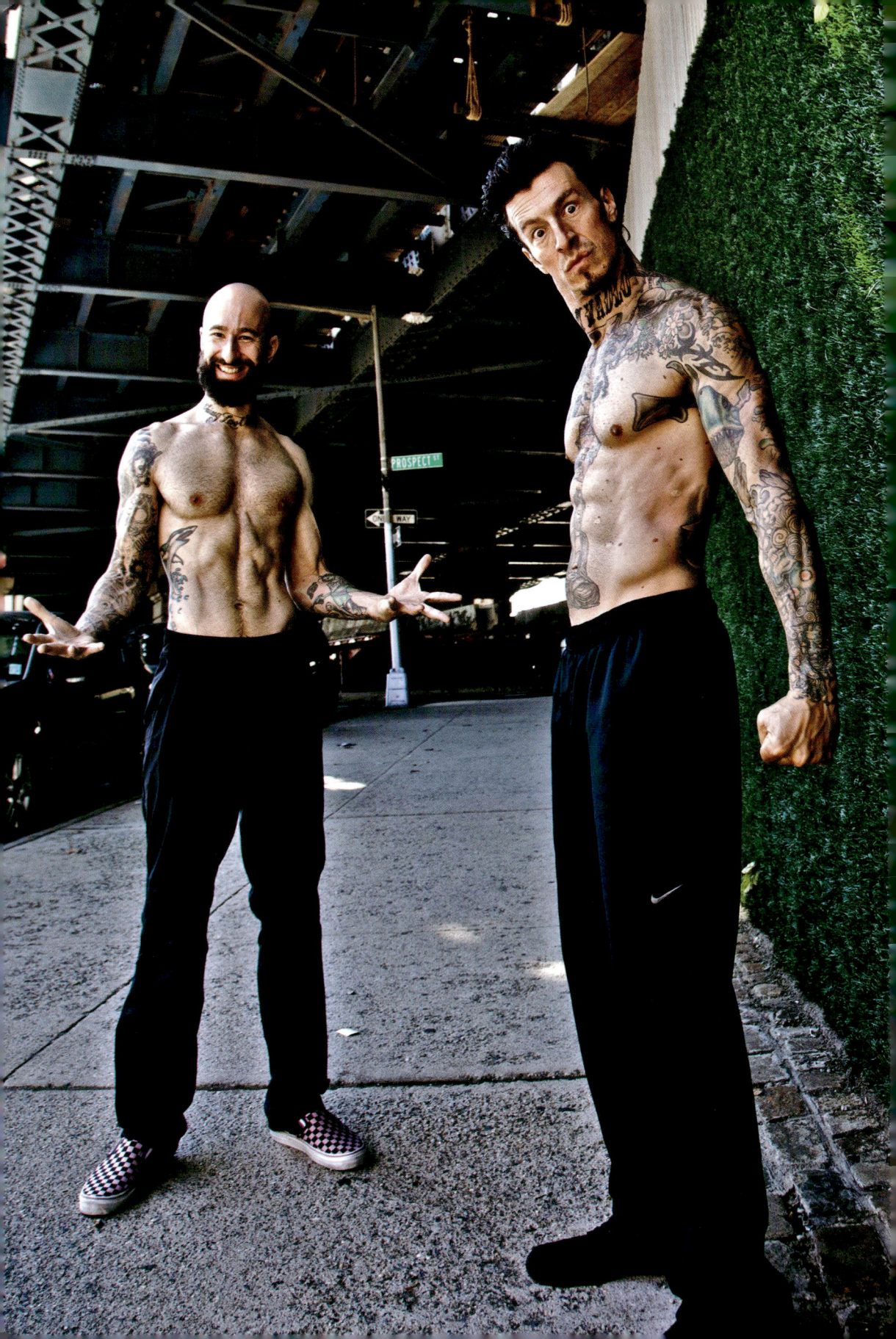

AUTHORS' NOTE

Dear Reader,

There is no doubt that the Street Workout movement has taken over the world. From the back alleys of New York, to the cobblestone streets of Europe, to the Australian outback, this modern explosion of urban calisthenics is simply undeniable. We consider ourselves extremely lucky and grateful to have played a role in its ascendancy. Even more so, we are thankful to have had the amazing opportunity to connect with so many calisthenics enthusiasts from all over the planet, whether via social media, at your local pull-up bar or at Dragon Door's acclaimed Progressive Calisthenics Certification. There is an instant camaraderie between those of us who train bodyweight. Calisthenics practitioners are known for supporting each other and spreading a positive attitude.

Over the last few years, we've had the privilege of teaching in dozens of cities and over ten countries, spanning across four continents. Street Workout has taken us places we never thought we would go and introduced us to many amazing people who we otherwise may never have met. The book you are holding is not only the most comprehensive compilation of urban calisthenics exercises and progressions ever assembled, it is also an anthology of our experiences.

The photographs in this manual span the course of several years. They were compiled from our extensive travels, our interactive workouts, our going to your hometowns and our getting to know you. The thrill and joy of working out in the Street Workout style is trumped only by the experiences we've shared relating with you guys.

We've both written books on calisthenics before, but never have either of us been involved in a project of this magnitude. While some of these exercises will seem familiar (there's always more to say about the basics), others will be brand new to you. We've refined our teachings over the years, and we've got some new tricks up our sleeve. Until we're dead in the ground, our work is not over.

Please enjoy this book. Apply it. Challenge it. Expand it and make its contents your own. Our only hope is that you love using it as much as we loved making it.

Your friends,

Al Kavadlo   *Danny Kavadlo*

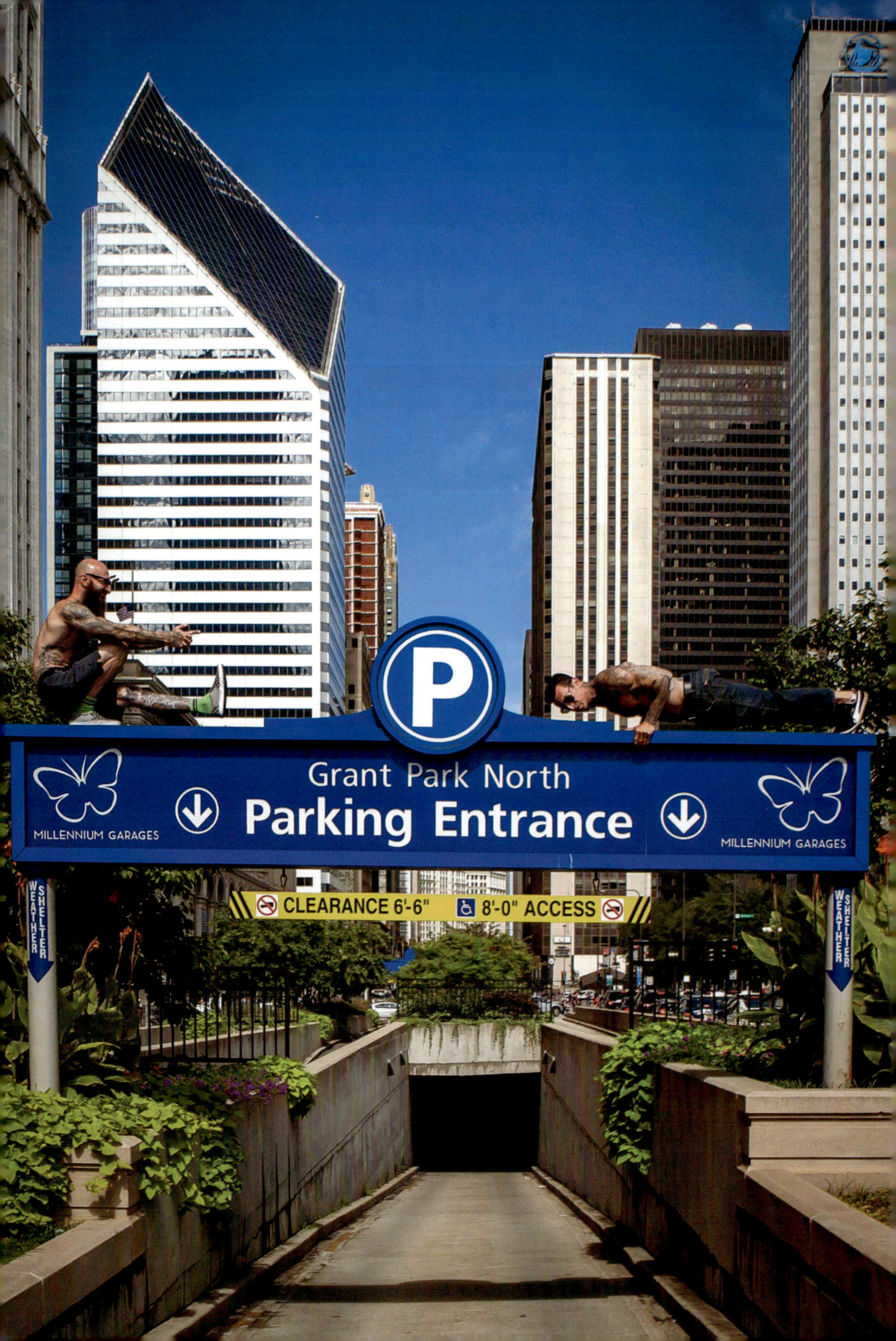
P
Grant Park North
Parking Entrance
MILLENNIUM GARAGES
MILLENNIUM GARAGES
CLEARANCE 6'-6"
8'-0" ACCESS
WEATHER SHELTER
WEATHER SHELTER

I

What Is Street Workout?

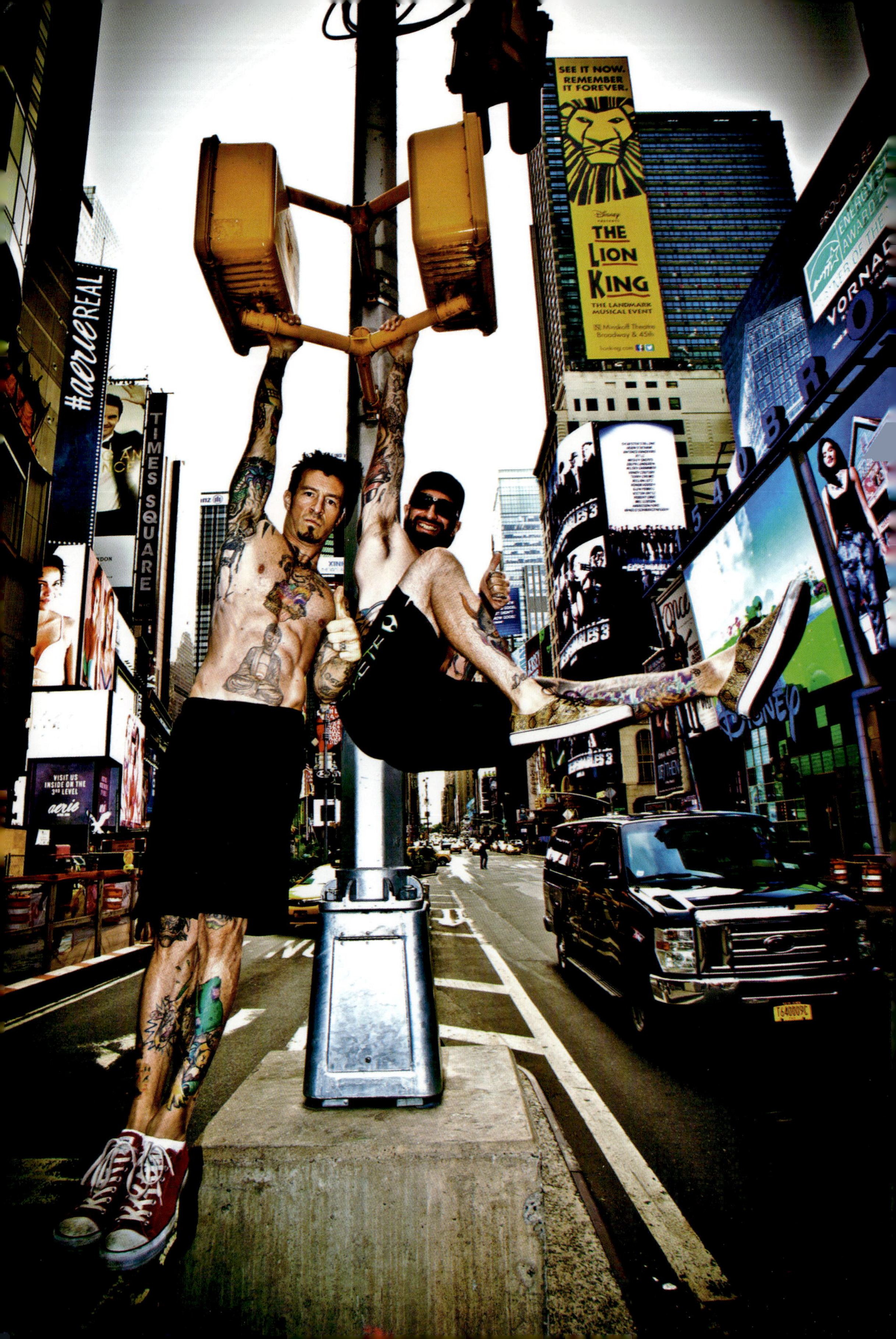
SEE IT NOW. REMEMBER IT FOREVER.
THE LION KING
THE LANDMARK MUSICAL EVENT
#aerieREAL
TIMES SQUARE
VISIT US INSIDE ON THE 3rd LEVEL
aerie

Chapter 1

Street Workout At Dawn

In the beginning, we crawled. We hunted. We climbed. We played.

We did a lot of things.

Early man used his arms, legs and entire body every time he pulled himself up a tree to pick fruit or hoisted up a mammoth carcass for the weekly feast. He didn't isolate body parts when he fought to survive. He didn't jump or sprint because it was "leg day." He did it because a saber-toothed tiger was gonna rip him apart if he didn't.

Fast forward a few millennia and we find mankind erecting the Egyptian Sphinx, Stonehenge and the Great Wall of China. It takes a great deal of raw, physical strength to move mountain-sized boulders, but we had it. There was no isolation there, friends, just the full body working together in harmony. Trust me, these architects were not at the gym doing three sets of ten hammer curls.

The Acropolis. The Great Buddha of Kamakura. The Brooklyn Bridge. Our ancestors didn't use any modern gym equipment to get in shape for masterfully designing and building these incredible structures. In fact, they built these amazing structures because they understood (from an architectural perspective) that leverage, one of the key principles of calisthenics, could help create something incredible, whether it's a majestic pyramid or a sculpted human body.

Training the body without the use of external resistance equipment is known as calisthenics. It has been around since the dawn of humanity. Calisthenics, or bodyweight training, is the oldest and noblest form of exercise. Pressing, pulling and squatting are hard-wired into our DNA. Way before the invention of the modern gym, using only our bodies for resistance was not just the *best* way to train... it was the *only* way. It's no wonder so many of us get excited, inspired and motivated by this phenomenon! In fact, the modern gym (sometimes called "globo-gym"), with all its fancy, bi-angular lat pull-down machines, shiny cable crossovers and digitized, fake bicycles is a recent invention of the 20th century. Calisthenics is timeless.

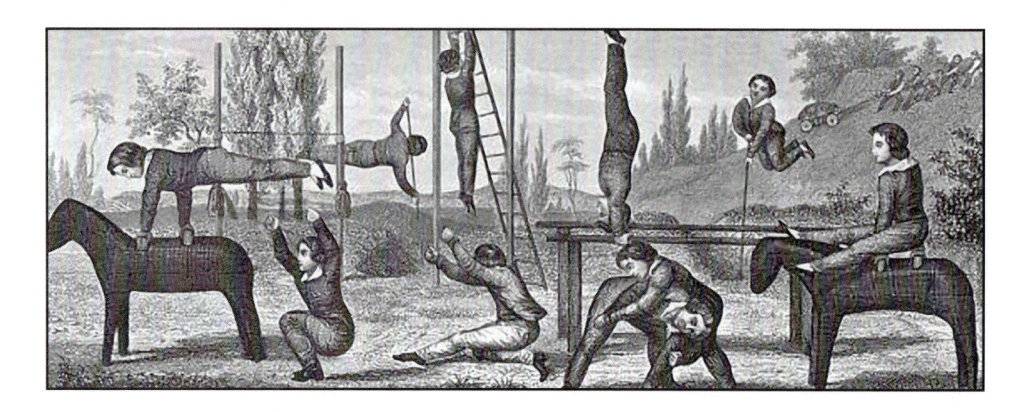

That's not to say that gyms did not previously exist. They did, but not in the modern sense. The very first gyms (or "gymnasia") of ancient Greece consisted of exclusively bodyweight exercise. The minimalist equipment used, for example, were parallel bars, climbing ropes and running paths. In fact the word "calisthenics" has its roots in Greek and translates approximately to "beautiful strength." It's interesting to note that these gyms also taught wisdom, philosophy and linguistics.

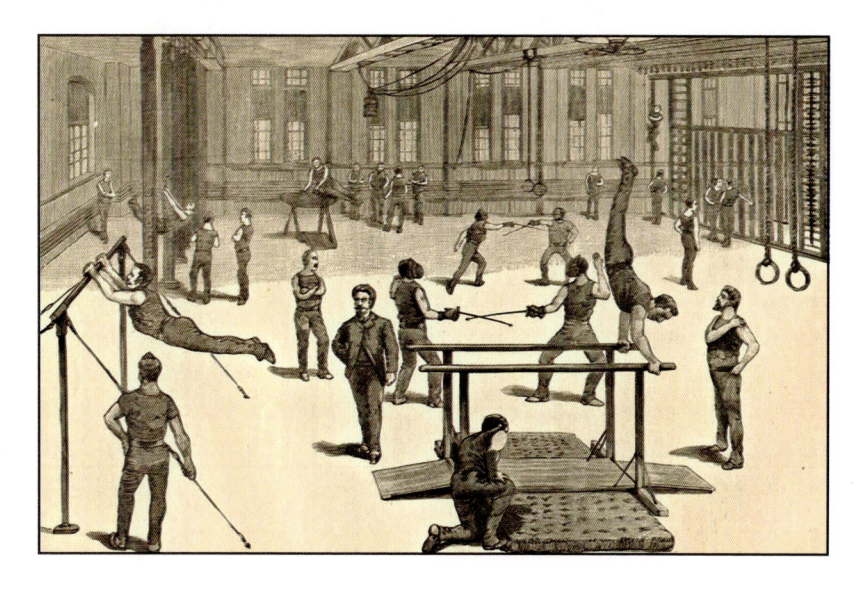

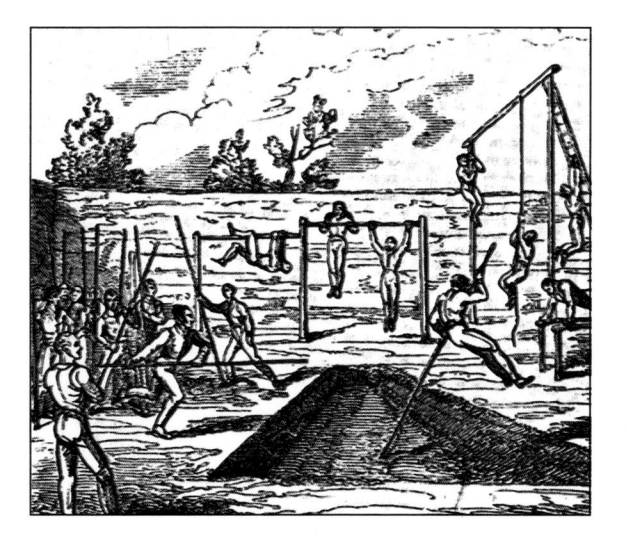

In the era in which we grew up, the aforementioned globo-gyms had become the standard. Strange but true. Thank goodness that in the 1980's New York of our youth, we were too young and too broke to visit them. I guess we were lucky in that when we were kids, minimalism wasn't a trend; it was our only choice. Our fitness journey started out with push-up and pull-up contests. In fact, the only equipment we owned at the start of our odyssey was a doorframe pull-up bar. (It was a piece of pipe, for the record, unlike the pre-fabricated ergonomic ones manufactured today and sold at retail conglomerates.) Man, we loved that thing!

For many years we've observed numerous big box fitness chains opening up all over the place. We even worked at a few of them. (Hey, hey, hey—everybody's gotta make a living somehow.) But now on a global scale, it appears that fitness culture is returning to its roots. It's nice to see. This resurgence, referred to as the Street Workout movement, taps into so many elements you simply can't find in the contemporary big box gym. These include the elegant minimalism of bodyweight training, the splendor of the great outdoors and the empowerment of owning a body that's truly self-made. Not to mention the bad-ass feats of strength associated with extreme calisthenics.

The improvisational element of Street Workout is equally appealing. When you use what the world has provided around you, rather than what you've been told to use by the corporate equipment manufacturers, you awaken a creative, even artistic, part of your mind. Whereas commercial gym members use multiple thousand-pound machines to train one muscle at a time, we can look at a pole, fence or street sign and come up with a dozen full-body exercises on the spot. It's no wonder that so many have abandoned the gym entirely.

The ability to observe and use your surroundings is a human trait that's dying these days. With our eyes constantly buried in GPS navigators and our hands crippled from text messaging people who aren't there, it's nice to actually get in touch with what's physically around you. People go to the gym, get on a treadmill and watch a TV screen. It seems that no one lives in the present anymore. But when you're using your grip on your actual *environment*, you're living right here, right now. And it feels good. When it seems as though the fitness world is nothing more than a bloated bastion of isolated movements and impractical applications, Street Workout is a breath of fresh air. Stop the oppression and free your minds, brothers and sisters!

We know it can be intimidating for a beginner to go to the local park to train, but fear not: this community is very inviting. Unlike a gym, there's no fee for this club. We welcome all comers.

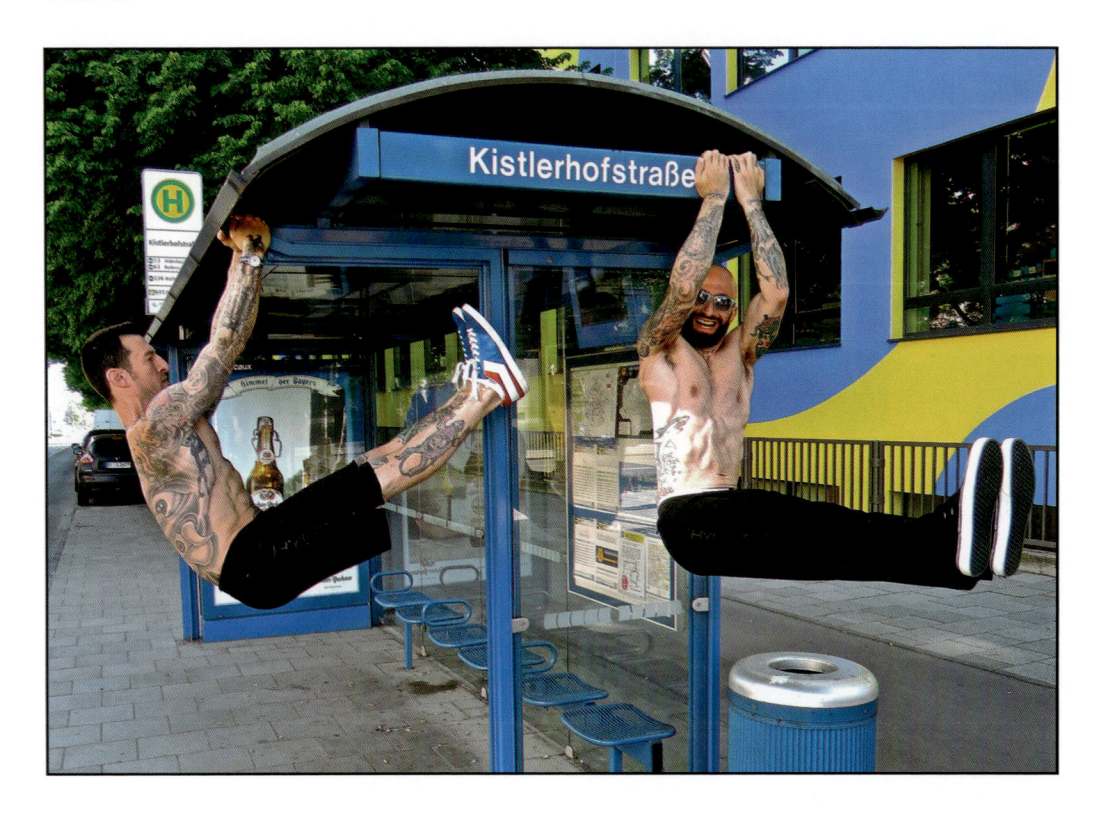

CHAPTER 2

Street Workout Culture

Around the turn of the millennium, calisthenics crews convened in New York City and trained on construction sites and scaffolding, as well as in parks, playgrounds and other public pull-up stations. As more and more people identified with the new breed and moved further away from the gym, the culture grew. New groups emerged, including teams, meet-ups, boot camps and pull-up jams. We've personally witnessed the legendary Tompkins Square Park in New York City go from a little known gym alternative far from the common path (early 2000's), to being a global destination, enticing tourists from all over the planet to visit and get their reps in. On another note, as native New Yorkers, we cannot help but *love* the fact that a place like Tompkins Square Park which used to be known for its riots and homeless junkies, is now a renowned fitness mecca. You can't make this stuff up!

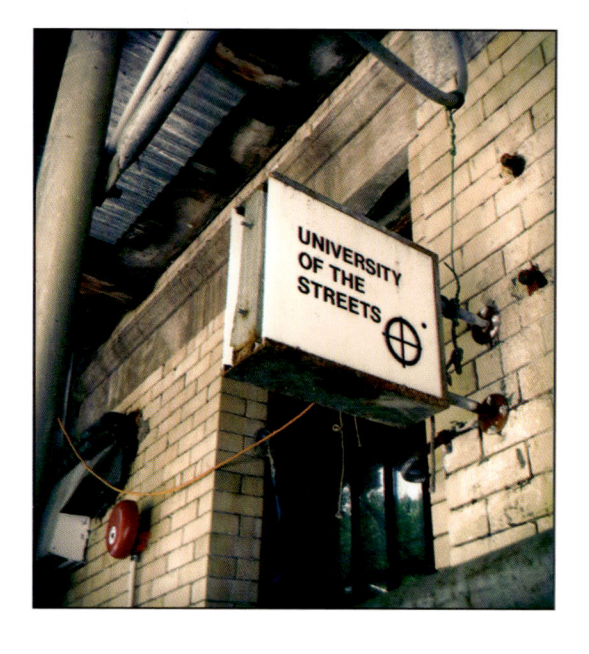

Ironically, while calisthenics is as ancient as humankind itself, a revolution of this magnitude could only exist in our current age of modern communication. While the planet has not changed in regard to its physical mass, there's no denying that the world is getting smaller (figuratively not literally). The internet and its many resources such as YouTube, Instagram and Facebook have all played a huge role in spreading the word. Now a kid in a small village in the Far East can learn pull-ups from a tutorial shot in New York City's East Village!

Yes, outdoor calisthenics has been around as long as humanity itself. But what's happening right now is on another level.

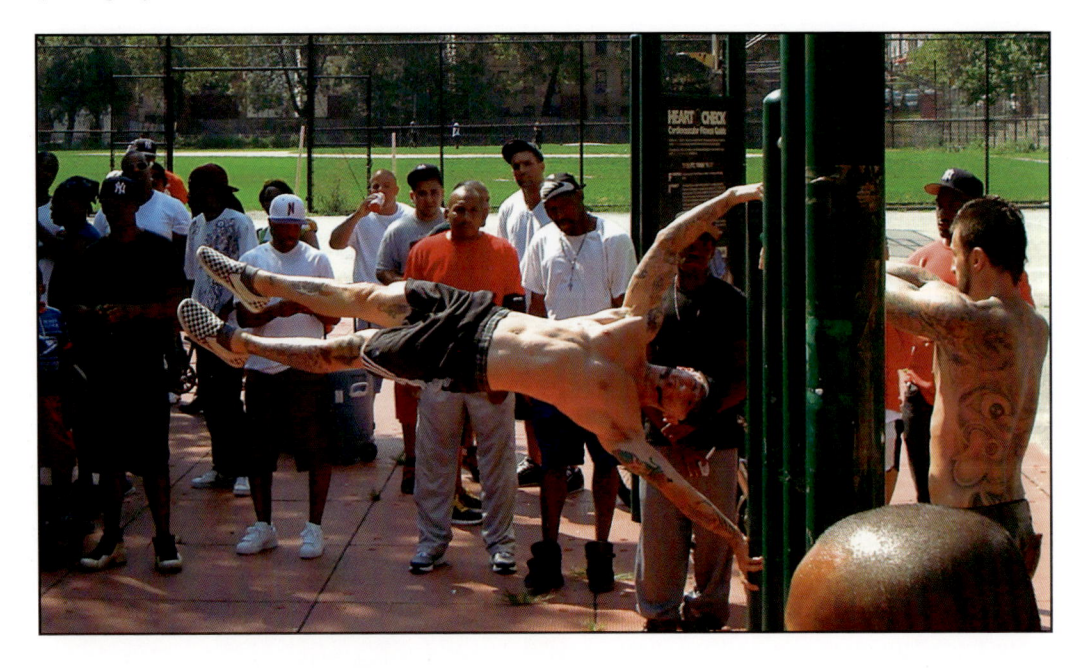

Over the years, the Street Workout phenomenon has spread all over these great States and across the ocean. Street Workout is now all over the planet. Europe has some of the fiercest calisthenics beasts we've seen. Asia, South America and Australia also boast some of the best. There are organized Street Workout competitions all over the world attended by thousands of fans, followers, friends and practitioners.

On a cultural level, Street Workout is revolutionary. The great anthropological equalizer if you will. Our community comes from different backgrounds and origins, assorted borders and parts of the world. We are united for a common cause: a love of fitness, form and function, a passion for self-improvement and a need to inspire others. Young and old, male and female, black and white, gay and straight: we are all represented.

But sociology aside, Street Workout is also the great equalizer of body types. Because calisthenics focuses on your pound-for-pound strength, the big guys and little guys have the same relative resistance: themselves. Allow us to elaborate; a muscular guy who's 6' 2" and weighs 250 lbs. will naturally have a higher bench press than an equally muscled individual of 5'6" and 150 lbs. Assuming the same body composition, it's simply a matter of physics. The heavier guy can lift more external weight. But if you put them both in a push-up contest, it's an even playing field. Street Workout is an equal opportunity employer. If your body mass is going up and your reps in push-ups are going down, are you really getting stronger?

While still far from the mainstream, one need look no further than a local park or the internet to see that the popularity of Street Workout grows every single day. In fact, there is a whole new generation of fitness freaks who have never even been to a gym. All they know is Street Workout! We are the past, the present and the future. The posse's getting bigger.

WE ARE NOT GYMNASTS

Yes, gymnasts and practitioners of Street Workout have a lot in common: We are both strong, we both use our bodyweight to train and we don't care much for high-tech equipment. But make no mistake; we are not gymnasts. There is no doubt that gymnasts are some of the strongest athletes in the world. In fact, the finest gymnasts make some of our advanced moves look easy. But gymnastics is a specified discipline encompassing a very particular set of rules for scoring, using very strict judgment.

We aren't really into judgment; it's not our thing. We don't like formal structure... that's why we do pull-ups off of scaffolding! We celebrate improvisation instead of punishing it. In fact, we love spontaneity. This team of misfits doesn't care to adhere to formal structure. For us, working out and having fun aren't distinguished from one another. Our training is our playtime.

The fact that we are NOT gymnasts is part of what makes us special.

We didn't have National Team coaches. We are born from the streets. We don't use smooth rings, adjustable straps or even chalk. We use a truck, a street sign or a mailbox. We are not gymnasts.

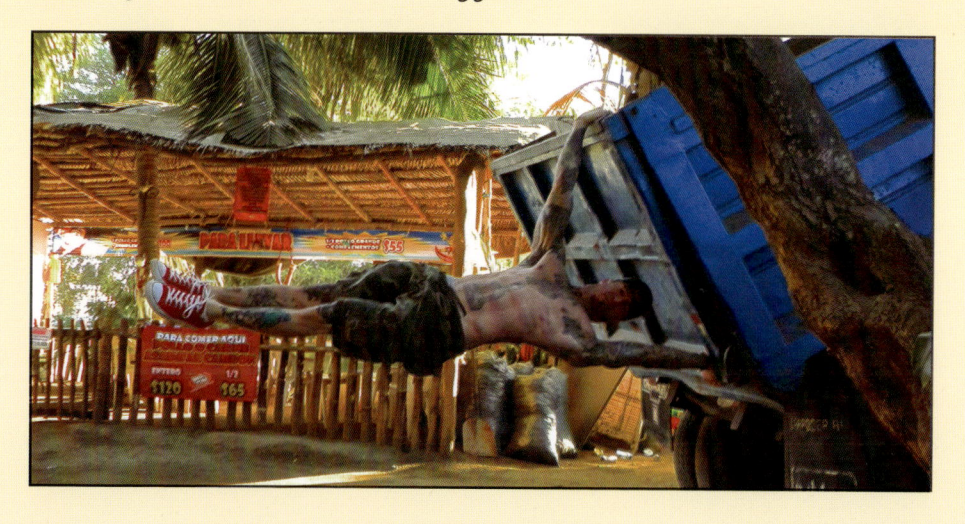

KAVADLO BROS.

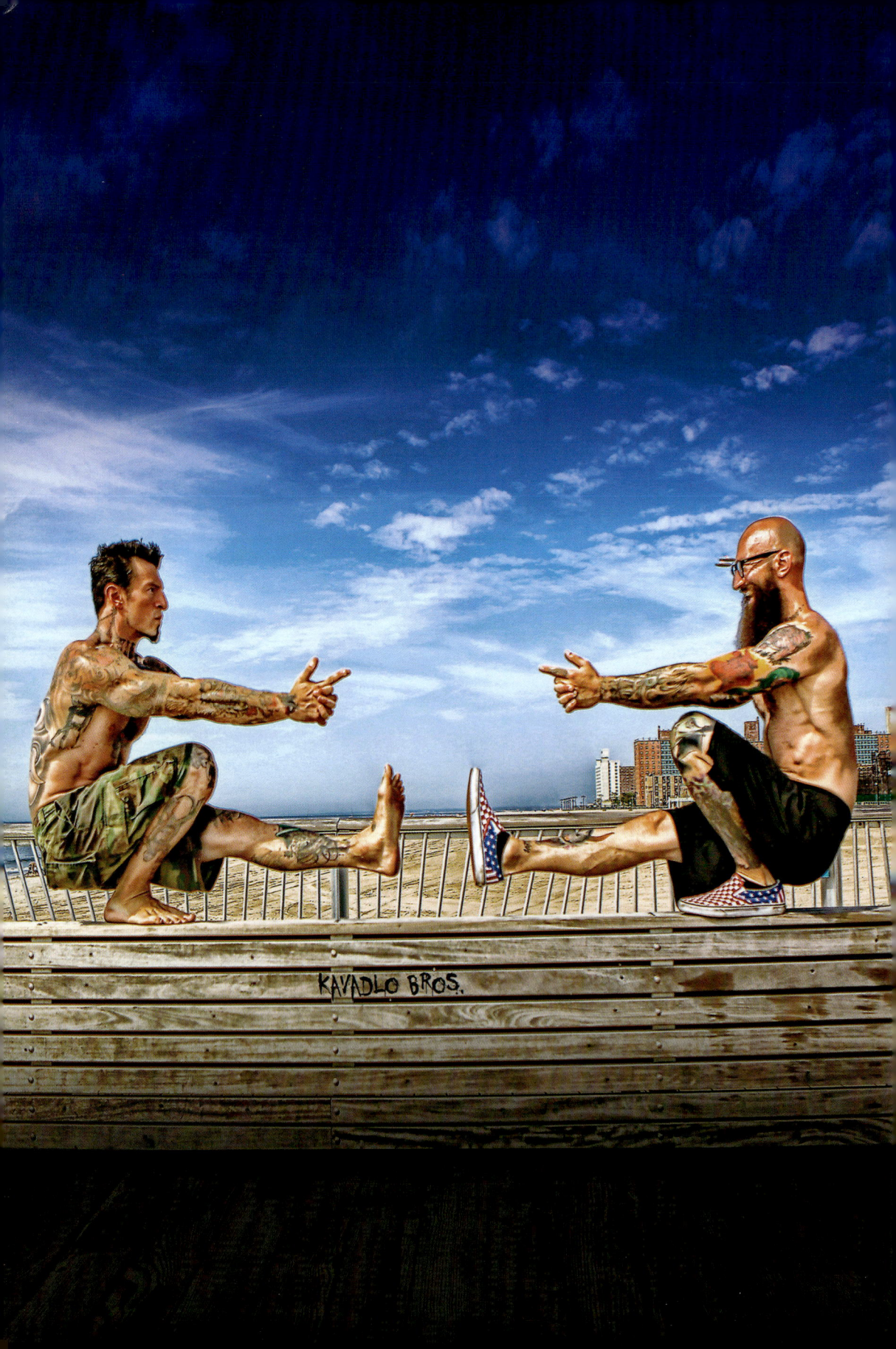

CHAPTER 3

Street Workout Training

We are born with a primal urge to be outside. We're animals, not built to sit under florescent lights in a climate controlled, window-less room. It's bad enough that so many good people have to do this at their jobs. Let's not do it during our workouts.

Working out, like life, should be fun, adventurous, primal and pure. No training style embodies these elements quite like Street Workout does. Give us a traffic light and we'll show you pull-ups, hand balancing, hanging knee raises and bar levers! We don't need anything fancy. To the Street Workout enthusiast, a well-equipped gym consists of two things: you and your environment. You can train in a park or off a ledge. Anything is fair game.

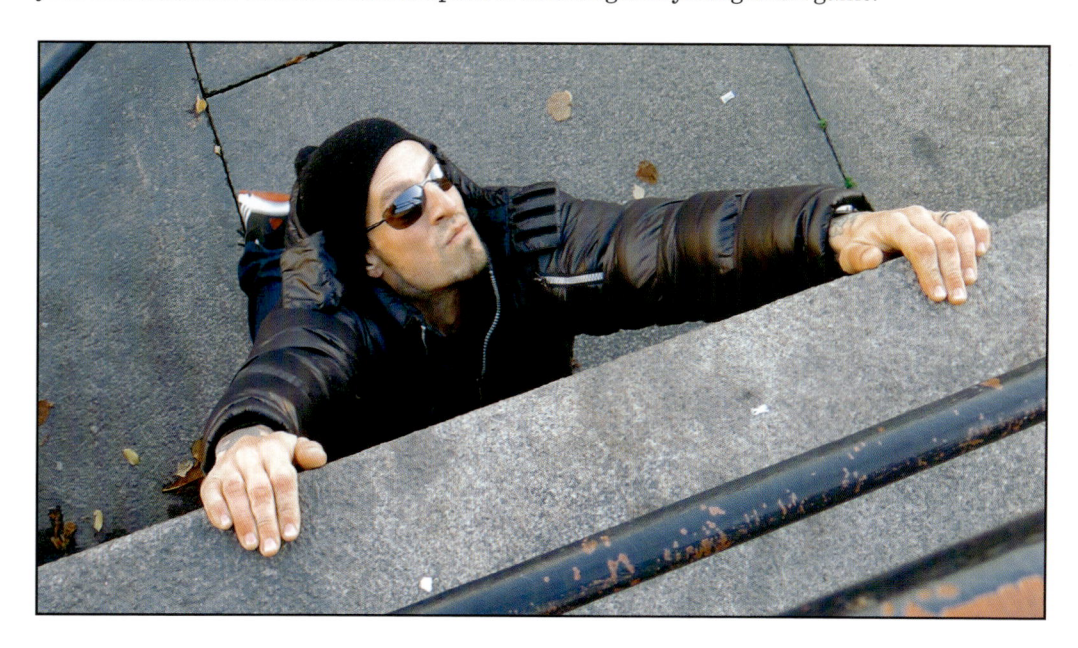

Street Workout celebrates the use of our whole body cohesively, rather than attempting to isolate small body parts one-at-a-time. And while there is no doubt that different exercises emphasize certain muscles more than others, we'd like to be crystal clear that 100% isolation in any modality is impossible. The human body was built to be used as a whole. Further, employing numerous muscle groups promotes greater overall strength. Pull-ups, for example use the biceps, lats, abs, shoulders and more. There are no machines in a gym that come close to simulating the overall effect and strength gains. Someone who can confidently pull his or her body up and over a real object is a lot more impressive than somebody who moves a weight stack straight up and down a machine.

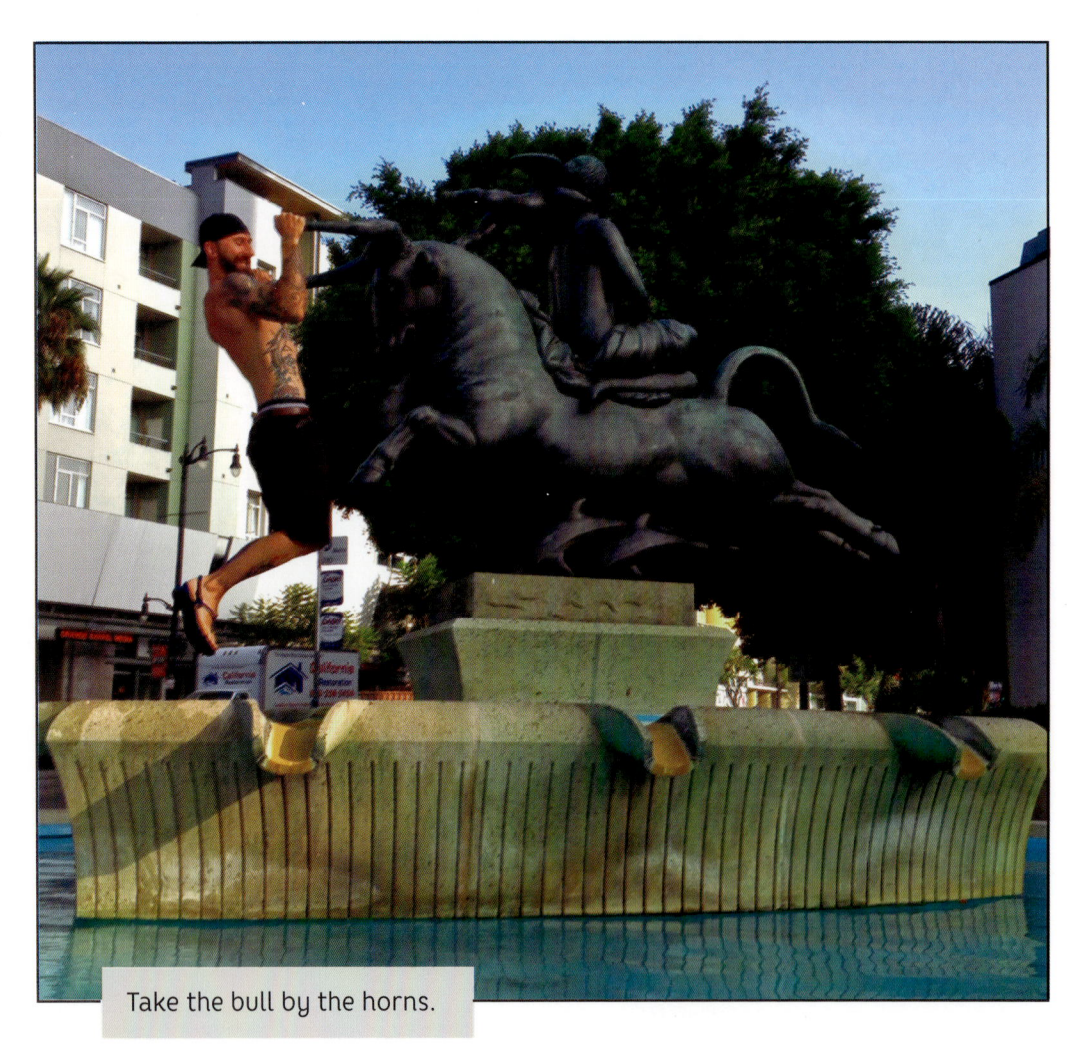

Take the bull by the horns.

Street Workout moves signify the perfect marriage of strength, flexibility and balance, as all of those elements are necessary. Furthermore, there is an additional proprioceptive demand to many of these exercises, as they confuse the nervous system and challenge us to work on our spatial awareness within this world. Exercises such as the pistol squat, back lever, handstand and many others are perfect examples of this fusion.

Street Workout builds real world, universal strength.

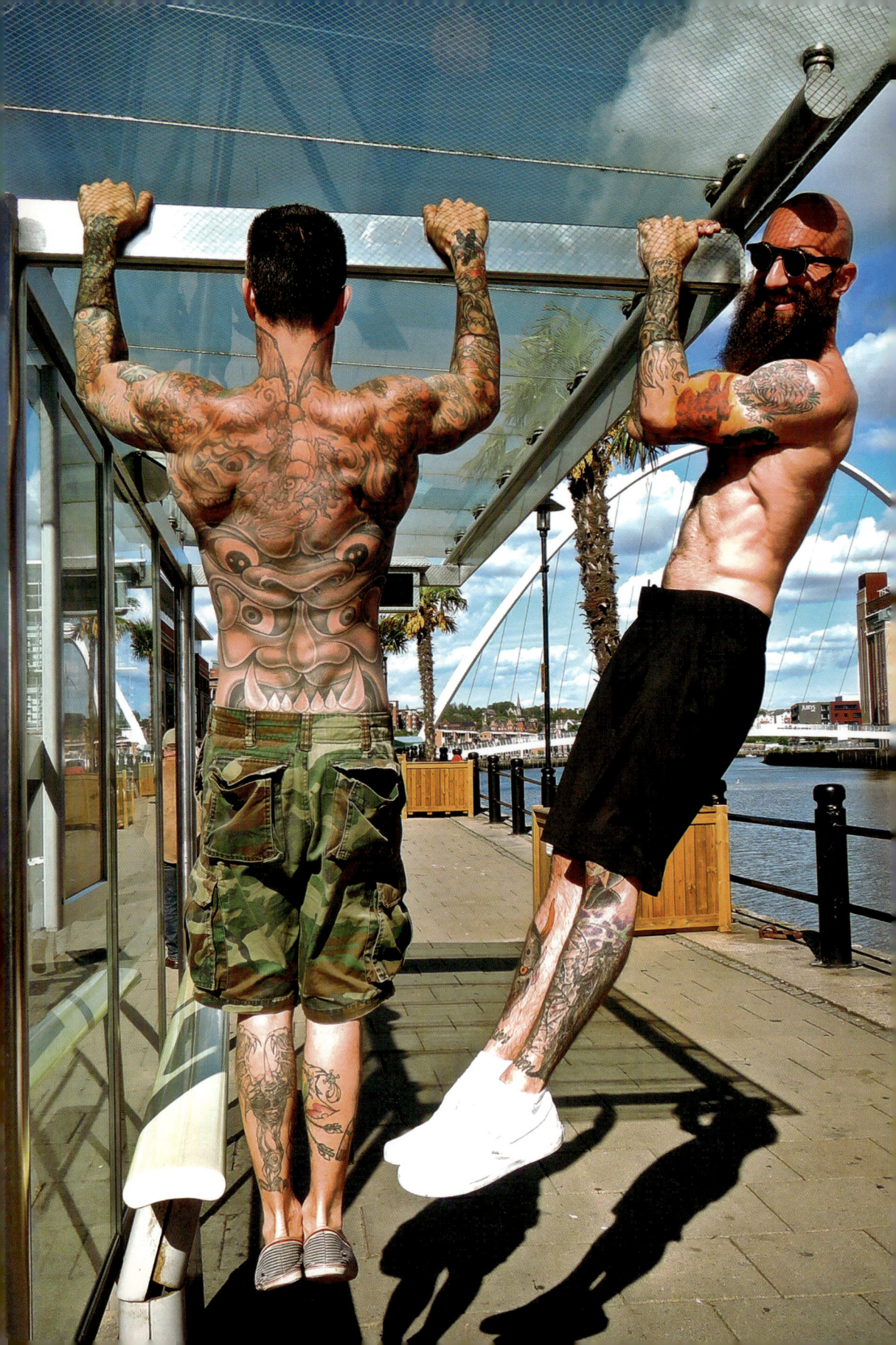

II
Foundational Progressions

Pushing, pulling and squatting your own bodyweight along with forward flexion and back bridging represent the basics of getting brutally strong, solid and unbreakable. Detractors often argue that you need to incorporate external resistance to progress in your training. That assertion is completely false. In fact, one could spend a lifetime pursuing only the exercises in this section and constantly make gains. By utilizing basic principles of progression such as the manipulation of leverage, adding or removing points of contact and/or increasing the range of motion, you can continue to get stronger without ever having to pick up a weight.

If you're new to the world of Street Workout, you'll need to spend a lot of time working on these foundational progressions. It's important to be well rounded and have a solid base in these essentials before moving ahead. Within each section, the exercises are shown in approximate order of difficulty. Despite the simplicity of each basic movement pattern, the later progressions get extremely intense. Progress will not be the same for everyone. Trust your own first hand experience.

The nobility, virtue and integrity of these movement patterns are undeniable. In fact, the lucid, broad strokes contained herein represent the heart and soul of Street Workout.

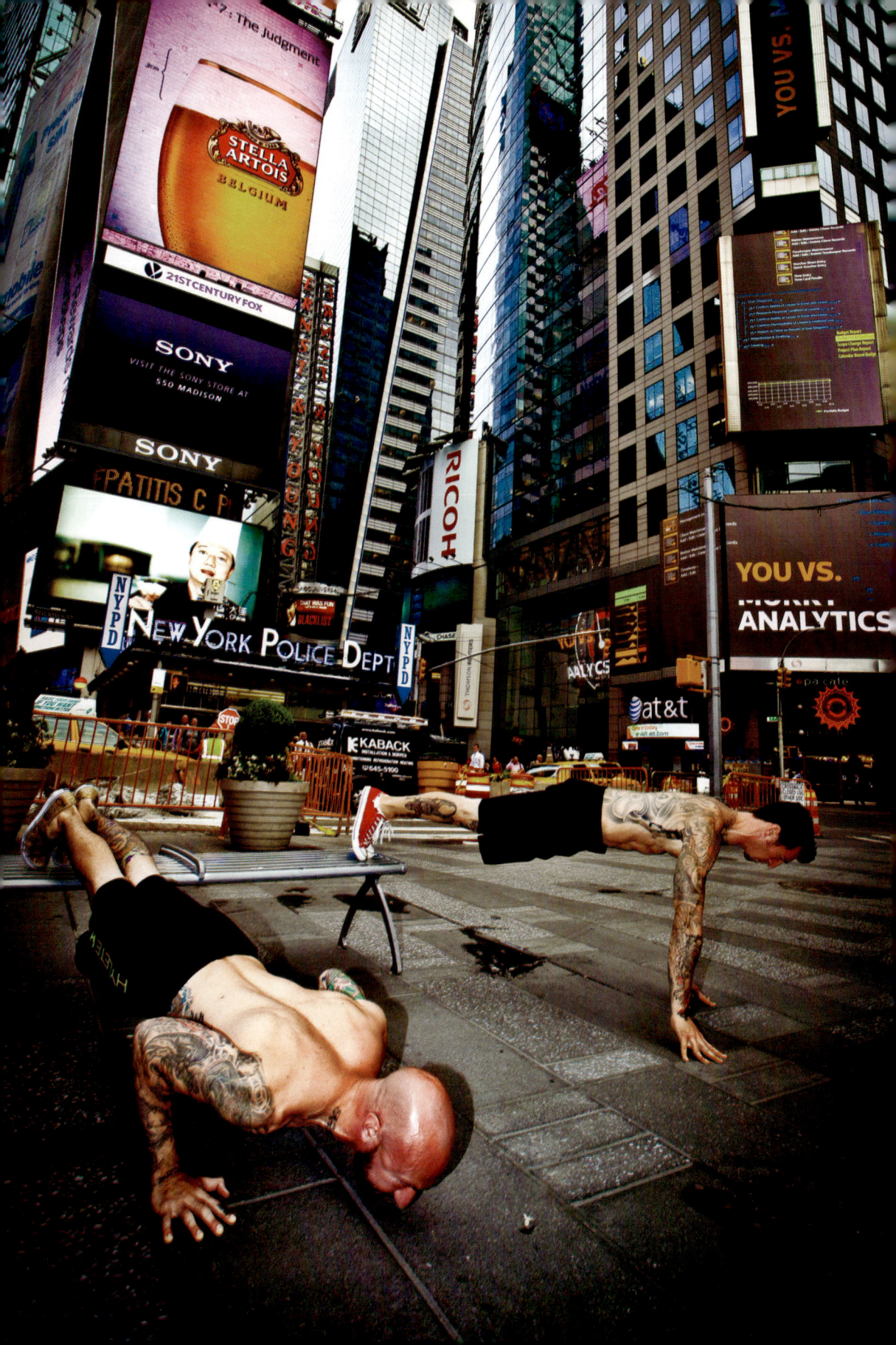

Chapter 4

Push

Upper body pushing is an essential element in every modality of strength training. Without a strong push, we couldn't amply care for ourselves, carry out daily tasks or move heavy objects. When push comes to shove, this stuff is important!

The exercises in this section are divided in three categories: Horizontal Push, Overhead Press and Dip, depending on the spatial plane of motion and which muscles are primarily employed. Horizontal Push refers to any exercise in which you push your arm(s) out in front of your chest and away from your body. Overhead Press involves pressing your hands above your shoulders, which is typically done by inverting the body when training calisthenics. Dips involve pushing your hands down toward your hips while your torso is in an upright position. But make no mistake; there is a great deal of overlap as all of these exercises utilize the chest, shoulders, arms (particularly the triceps) and abs.

HORIZONTAL PUSH PROGRESSIONS

The noble push-up. Honest. Strong. True. The push-up is one of our all-around favorite exercises: it requires no equipment, it's adaptable to any fitness level and it can be varied in an infinite number of ways to suit a vast array of goals. The push-up is such a simple move, but that's where its beauty lies. As you will see, there are so many push-up modifications and progressions that no matter your needs, you can—and should—be incorporating several variations into your routine. Whether for joint health, increased mobility, or simply to build spectacular strength, everybody can utilize some form of the push-up to help them improve. Though the push-up works the entire body, the main muscles emphasized are the chest, which acts primarily at the shoulder joint, and the triceps, which act at the elbow.

PLANK

The plank involves holding yourself horizontally in a straight line on just your forearms and your toes. Maintain tension throughout all of your muscles, including your abs, glutes and legs. Pull your shoulder-blades down and spread them apart while pressing into the ground with your elbows. Don't let your shoulders shrug up by your ears.

You can also perform a plank on your palms, which is the same as the top position of a push-up. People who lack shoulder and arm strength may find it harder to hold the plank on their hands, while those who lack core strength will likely find the elbow plank to be more challenging.

As the angle of the body gets closer to being parallel with the ground, it becomes harder for the trunk muscles to stabilize and maintain form, though having the elbows bent takes some stress off the shoulders and arms. Experiment with both versions.

If the full plank is too difficult, you can modify it by lowering from your toes down to your knees, maintaining a straight line from the shoulders to the knees. By shortening the length of your body, the leverage changes, making the exercise less difficult. To make it harder, you can elevate your feet.

When holding the plank, be mindful not to let your hips sag. Watch out that they don't wind up too high in the air either. You want a nice, straight line from your heels to the back of your head.

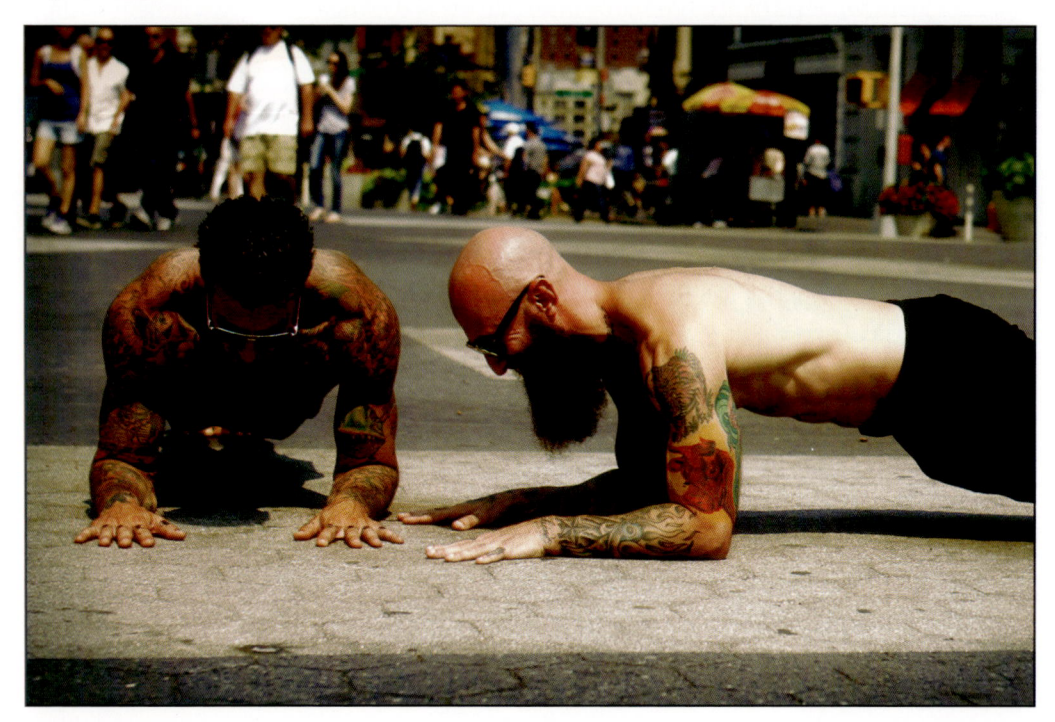

STREET WORKOUT

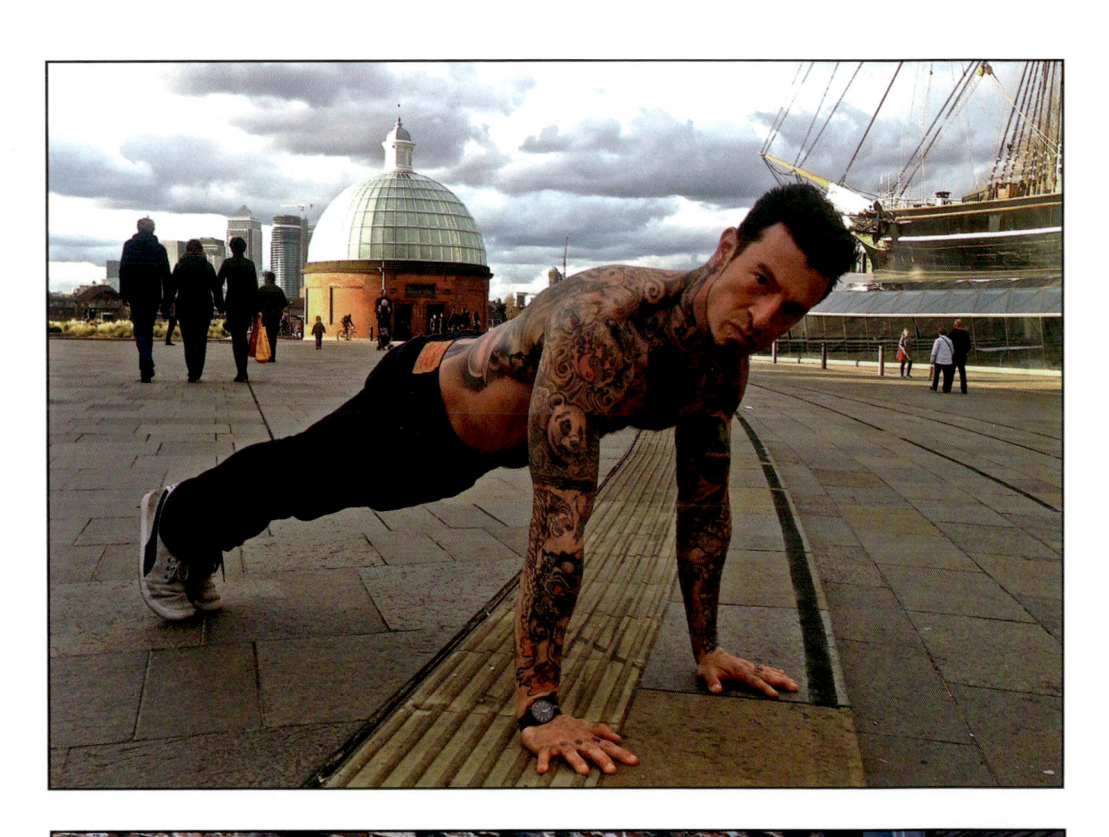

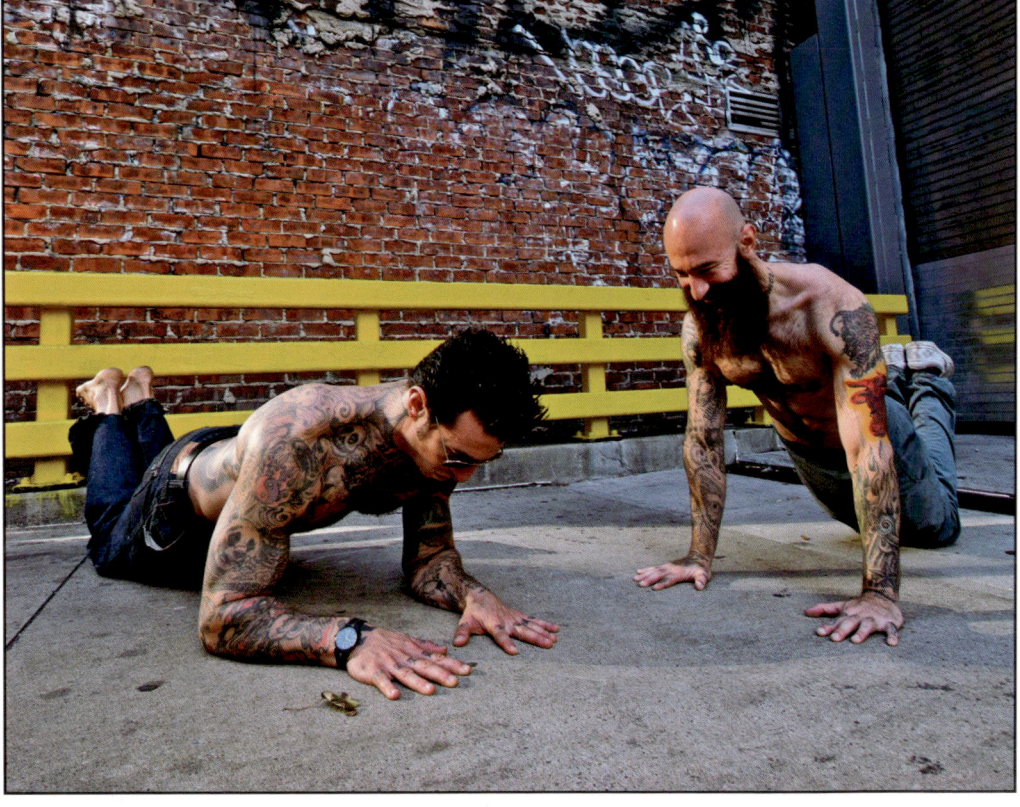

PUSH-UP

Assume a plank position on your palms with your hands slightly wider than your shoulders. Your thumbs should wind up right beneath your armpits. Keeping your heels together and your body straight, lower until your chest is just above the floor, pause for a moment and then press yourself back up. Point your elbows back and keep them relatively close to your body; do not flare them out to the sides. Be sure to maintain a straight plank from your heels to the back of your head.

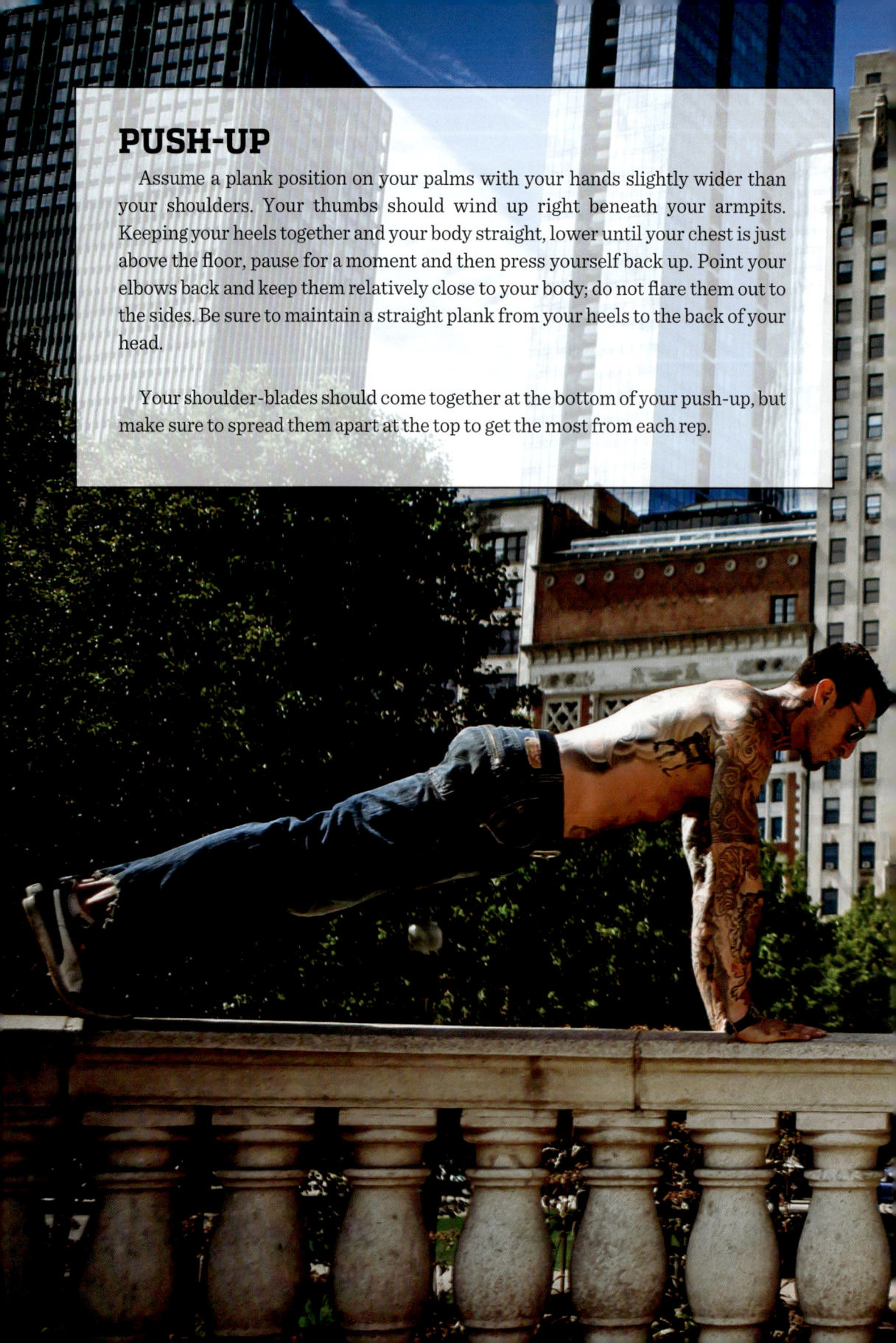

Your shoulder-blades should come together at the bottom of your push-up, but make sure to spread them apart at the top to get the most from each rep.

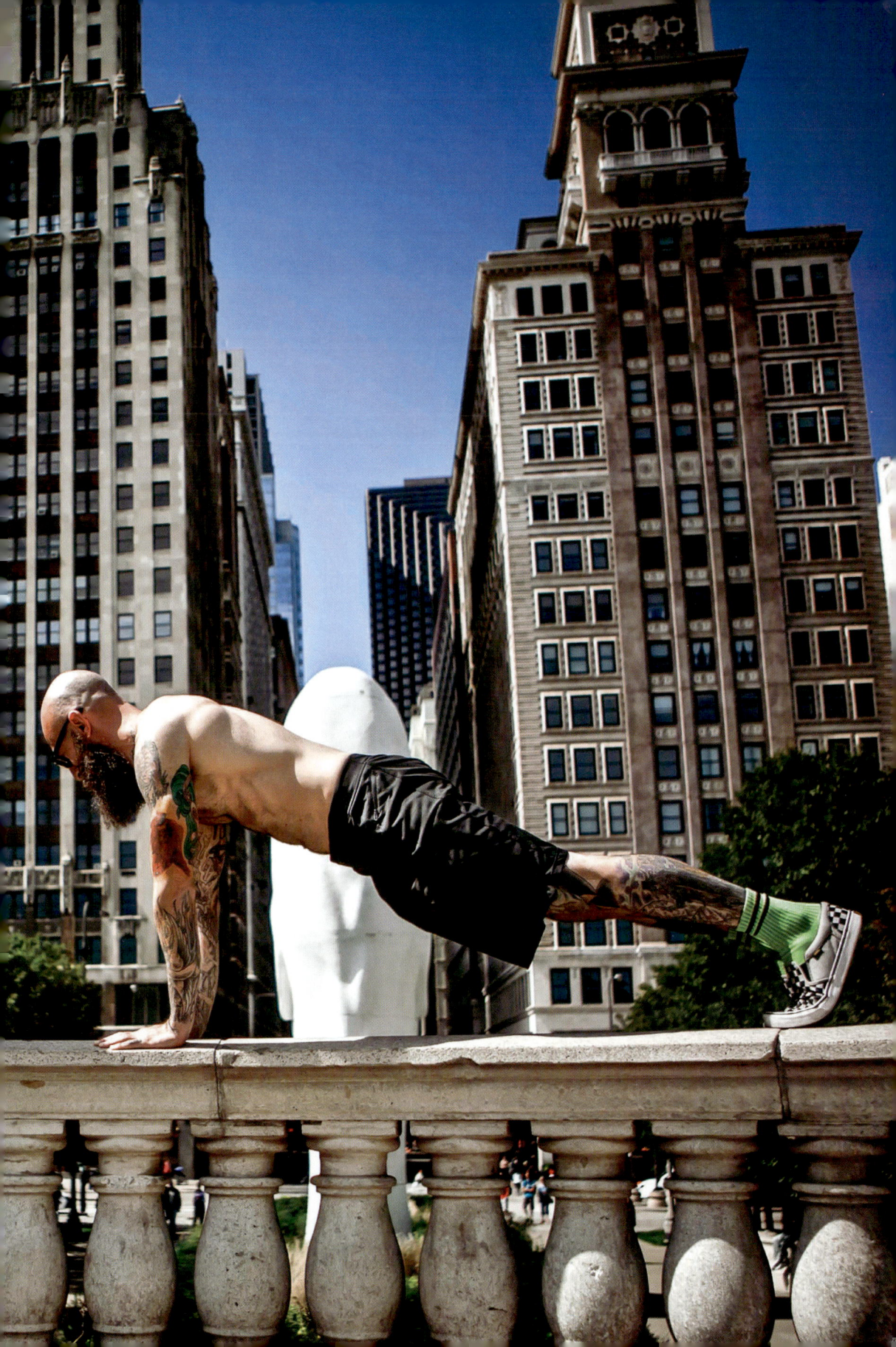

KNEELING PUSH-UP

Kneeling push-ups involve bending your knees and resting them on the floor instead of your toes. Like the kneeling plank, shortening the length of your body changes the leverage, making the exercise less difficult. Note that for this variation you will hinge from your knees instead of your feet.

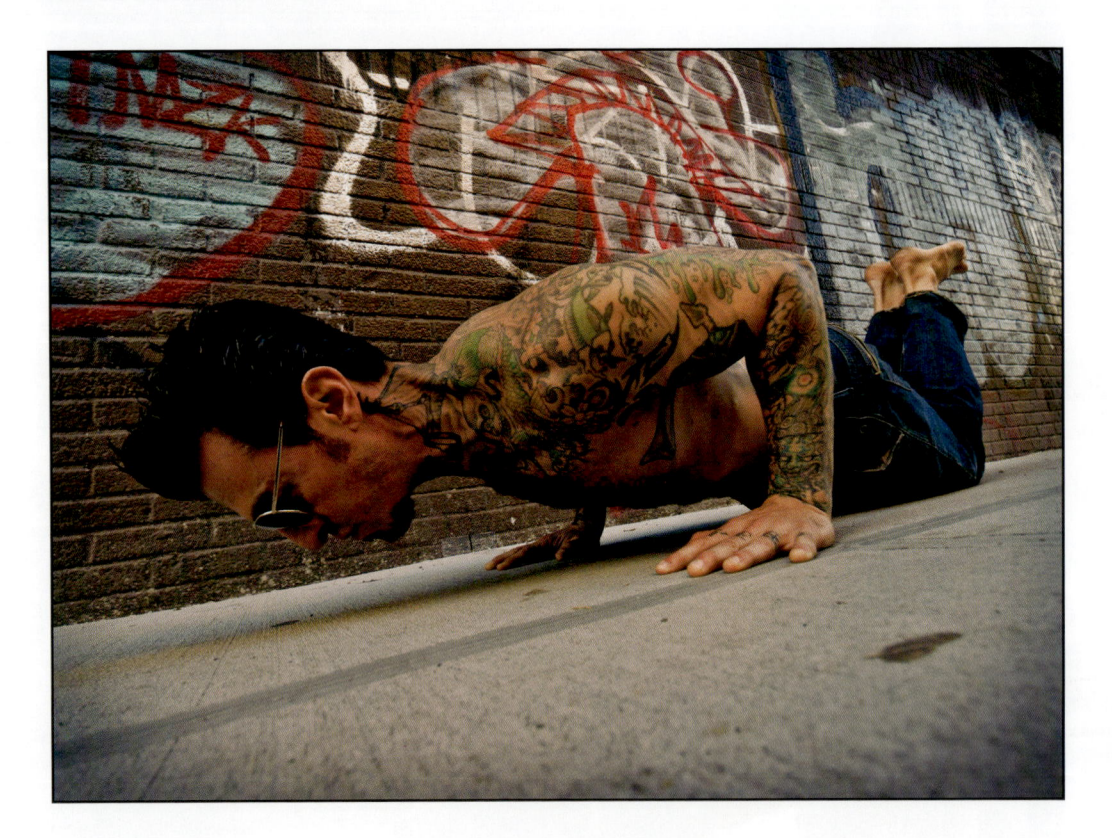

STRADDLE PUSH-UP

Spreading your feet wide is a great way to make push-ups slightly more forgiving. In a standard push-up, the heels are together, but in a straddle push-up, they are apart. The wider stance provides a larger base of support, while keeping your legs straddled shortens the length of your body by several inches.

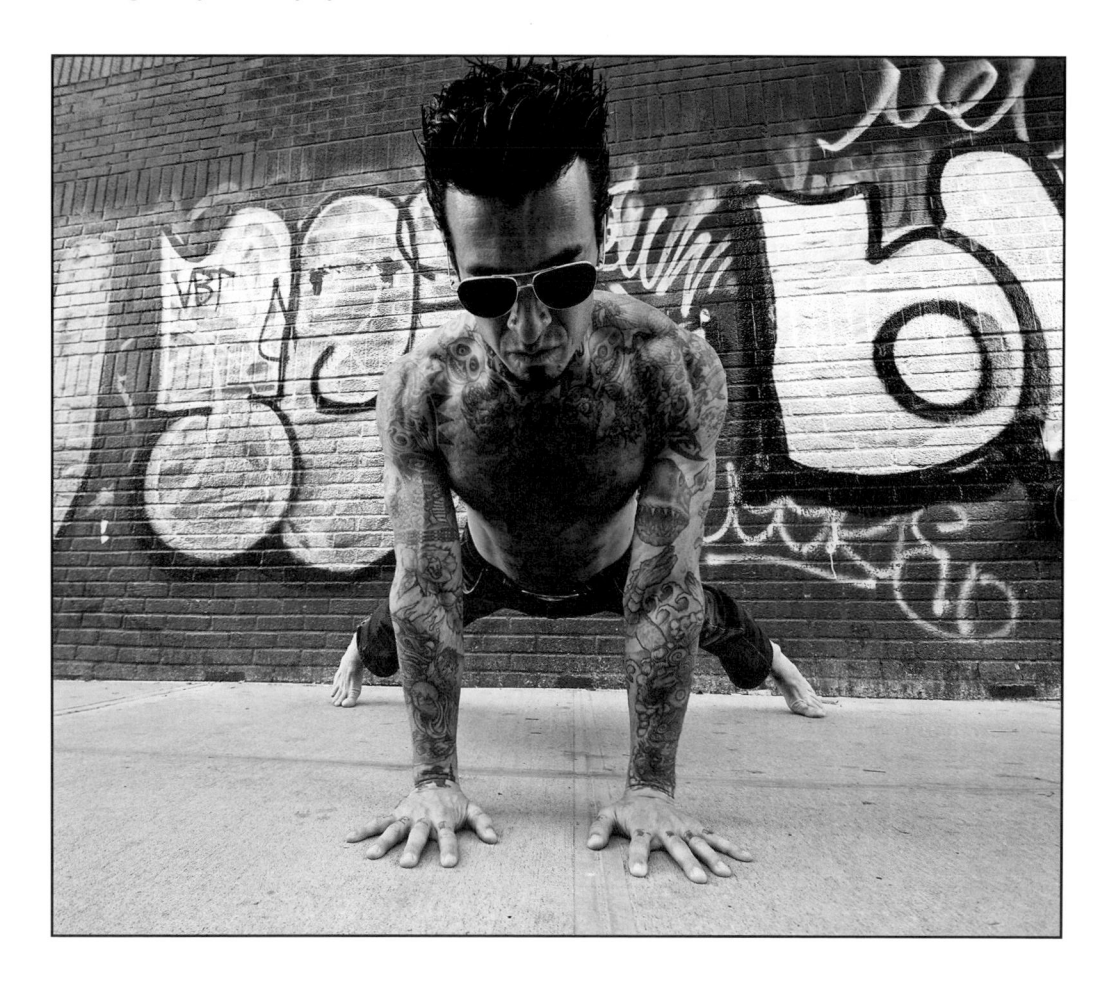

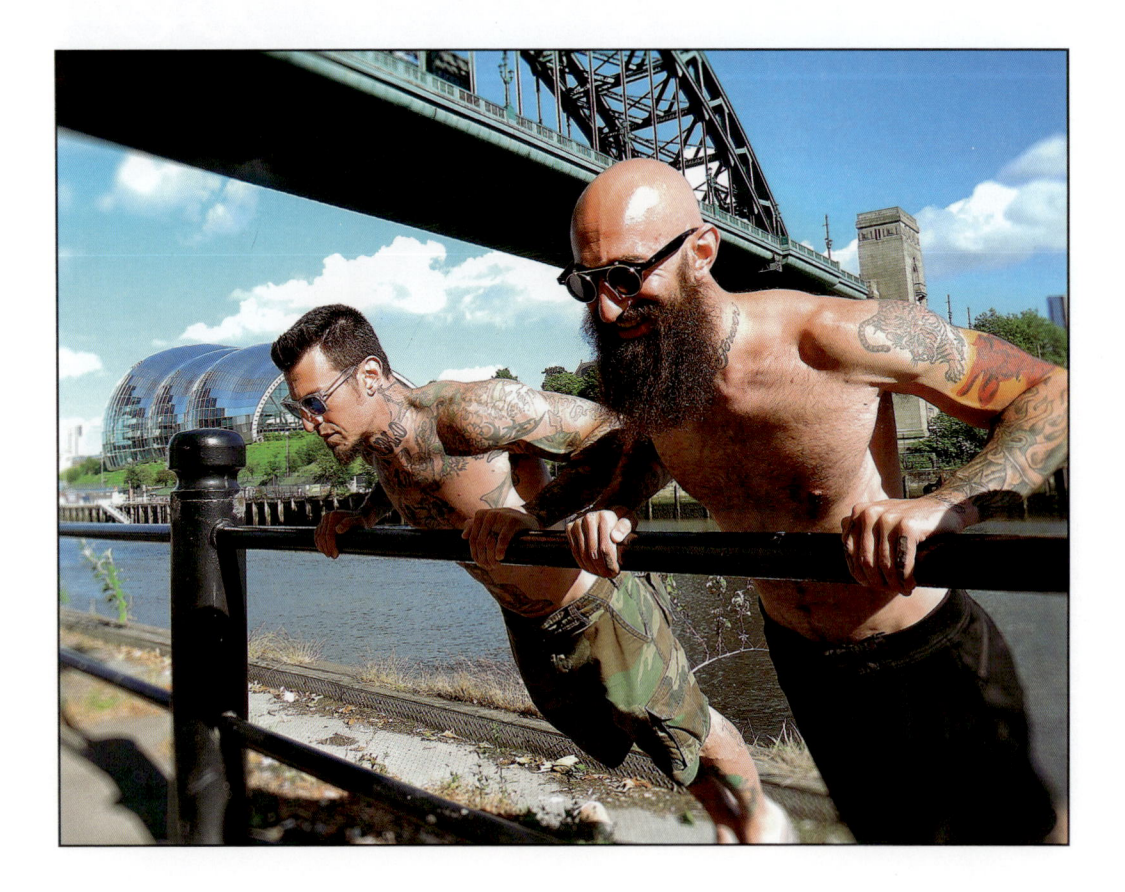

HANDS ELEVATED PUSH-UP

Elevating your hands is another great way to make standard push-ups a bit less difficult. By positioning your body on an incline, you put more of your weight in your feet, making less work for your arms.

The higher the incline, the less difficult the push-up will be. Start with a high incline at first and work your way toward a lower one over time.

FEET ELEVATED PUSH-UP

Just as placing your hands on an elevated surface can make the push-up less difficult, placing your feet on an elevated surface will have the opposite effect. The higher your feet, the more weight winds up in your hands and the more difficult the exercise becomes.

You can experiment with elevating your hands as well in order to allow room for your head to go all the way down.

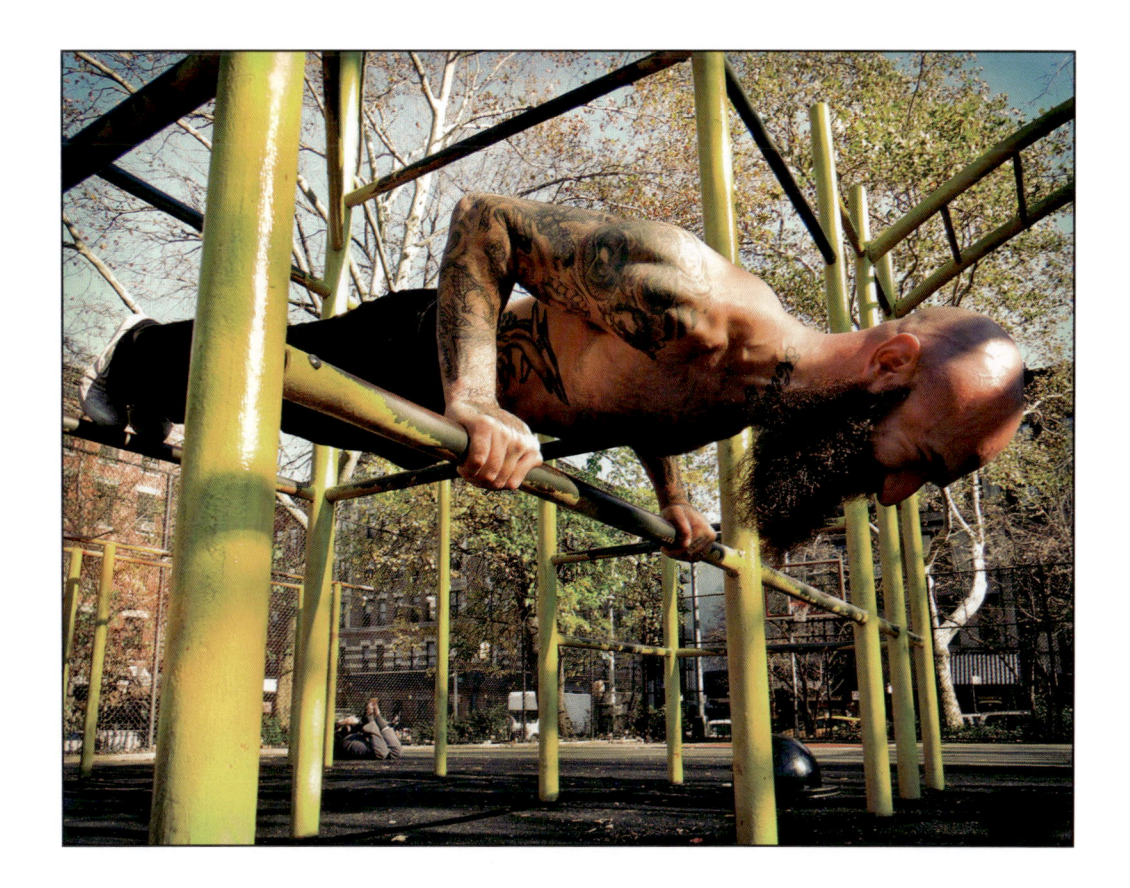

NARROW PUSH-UP

Bringing your hands closer together during push-ups will make the exercise more difficult and also shift more emphasis onto your triceps.

By decreasing the distance between your hands, you create less favorable leverage, thereby adding a new challenge—as well as multiplying the muscle-building potential of the classic push-up. The closer your hands get to each other, the more difficult the move becomes.

When performing narrow push-ups, keep your hands beneath your chest and your elbows tight by your sides, rather than flaring them out. This will protect your joints and help you get the most from your triceps on every rep.

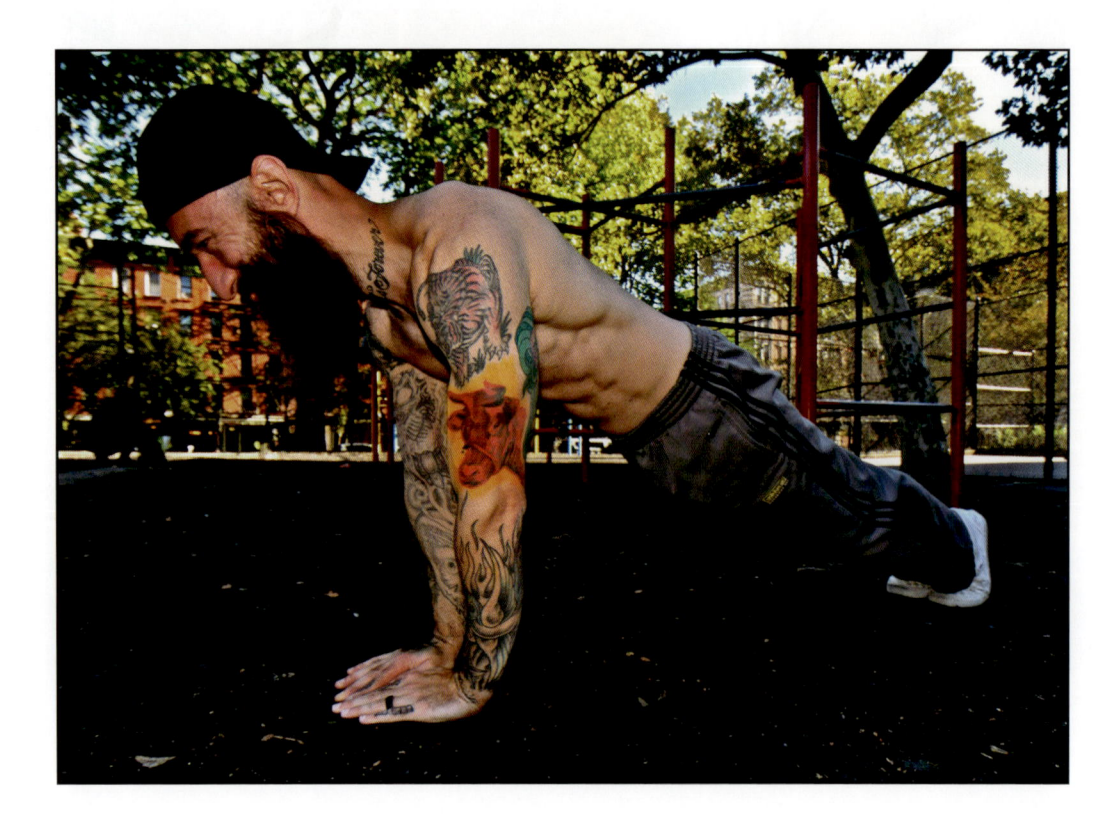

WIDE PUSH-UP

Like the narrow push-up, most people will find that using a wide hand placement on push-ups will also add a degree of difficulty. Keeping your hands farther apart will put a bit more emphasis on your chest and can make the leverage more difficult. You may find that turning your hands out slightly works best for wide push-ups.

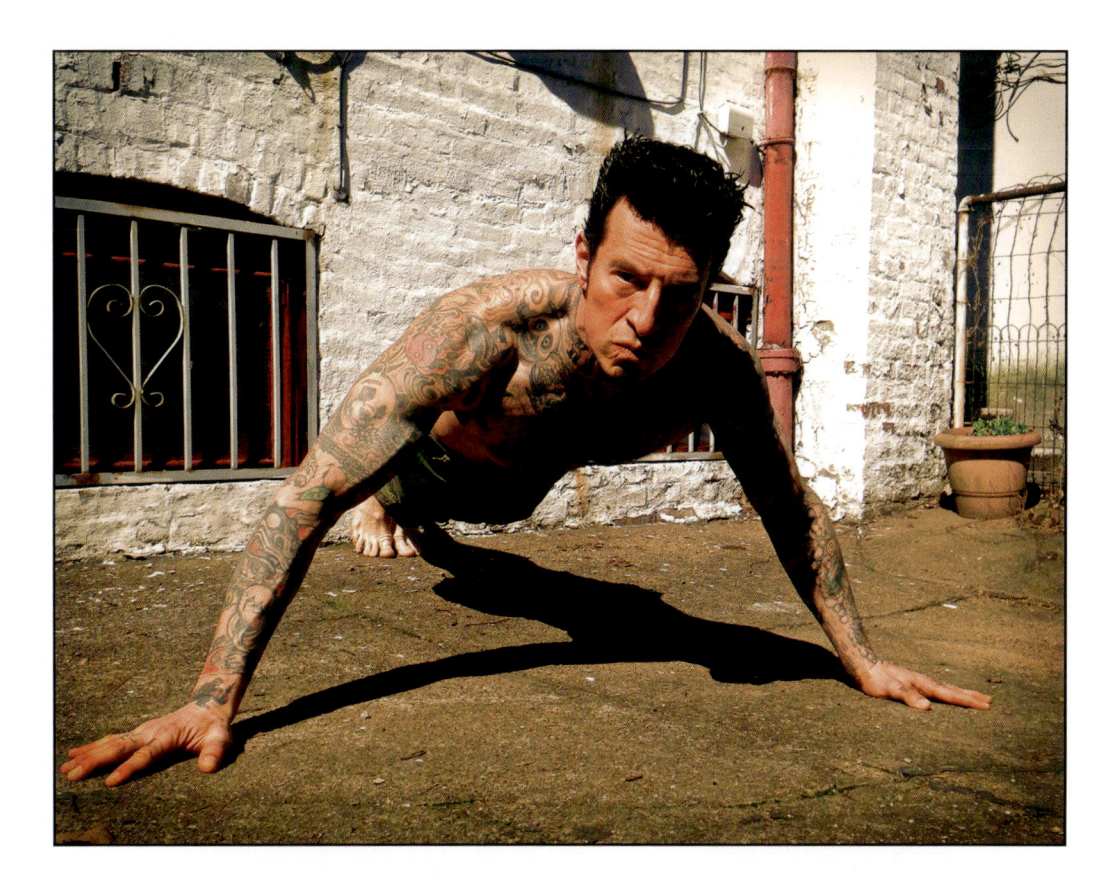

HOLLOW BODY

The hollow body drill is a fantastic way to learn how to fully engage your core. This skill will have massive carryover into planks, push-ups and many other bodyweight exercises.

Lie on your back with your knees tucked close to your chest and hands at your sides. Brace your abs and press your lower back into the ground. Slowly begin extending your legs straight with your heels just a few inches from the floor, while still maintaining the flat-back (hollow) position.

If you are able to fully extend your legs without losing contact between the ground and your lower back, try tucking your chin and reaching your arms overhead to progress the difficulty. The longer you make your body, the harder it will become to hold the position. As such, your trunk muscles will have to do more work to maintain form, which will cause you to get stronger.

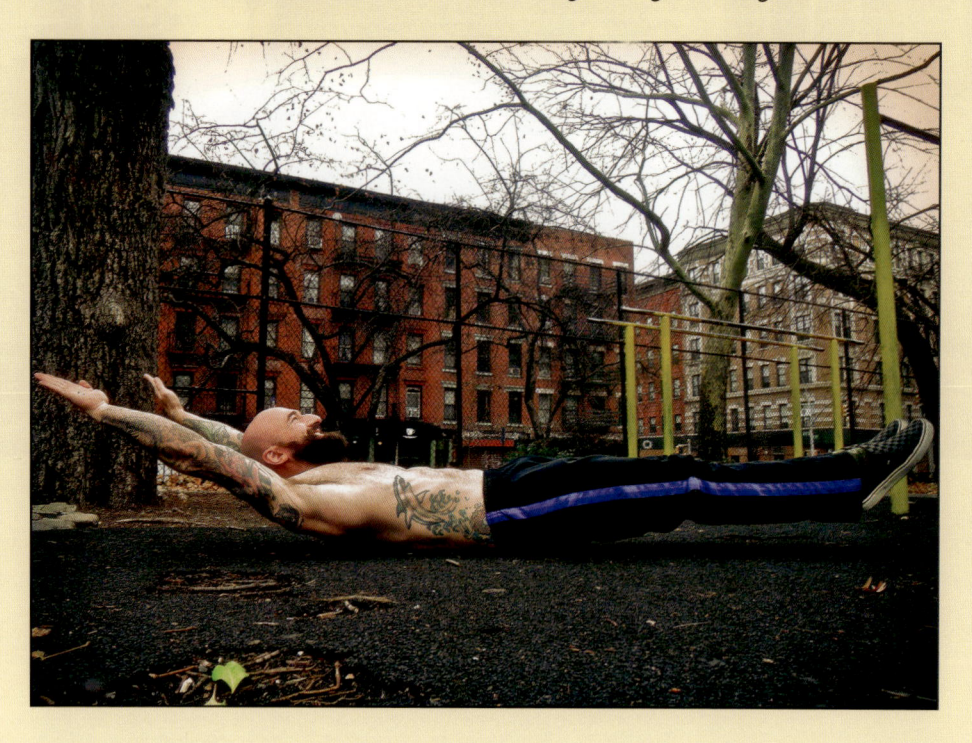

KNUCKLE PUSH-UP

Push-ups performed on the tops of your closed fists are called knuckle push-ups. They allow for a bigger range of motion by creating space for you to go lower than flat palm push-ups. They also pose a unique stability challenge due to the reduced surface contact between your body and the ground.

For people with wrist flexibility issues, however, the knuckle push-up can actually be more accessible than placing the palms flat with the wrists bent back for the standard variety.

Additionally, the skin on your hands may be sensitive when starting out, so the simple discomfort of supporting your weight on your knuckles may be an obstacle.

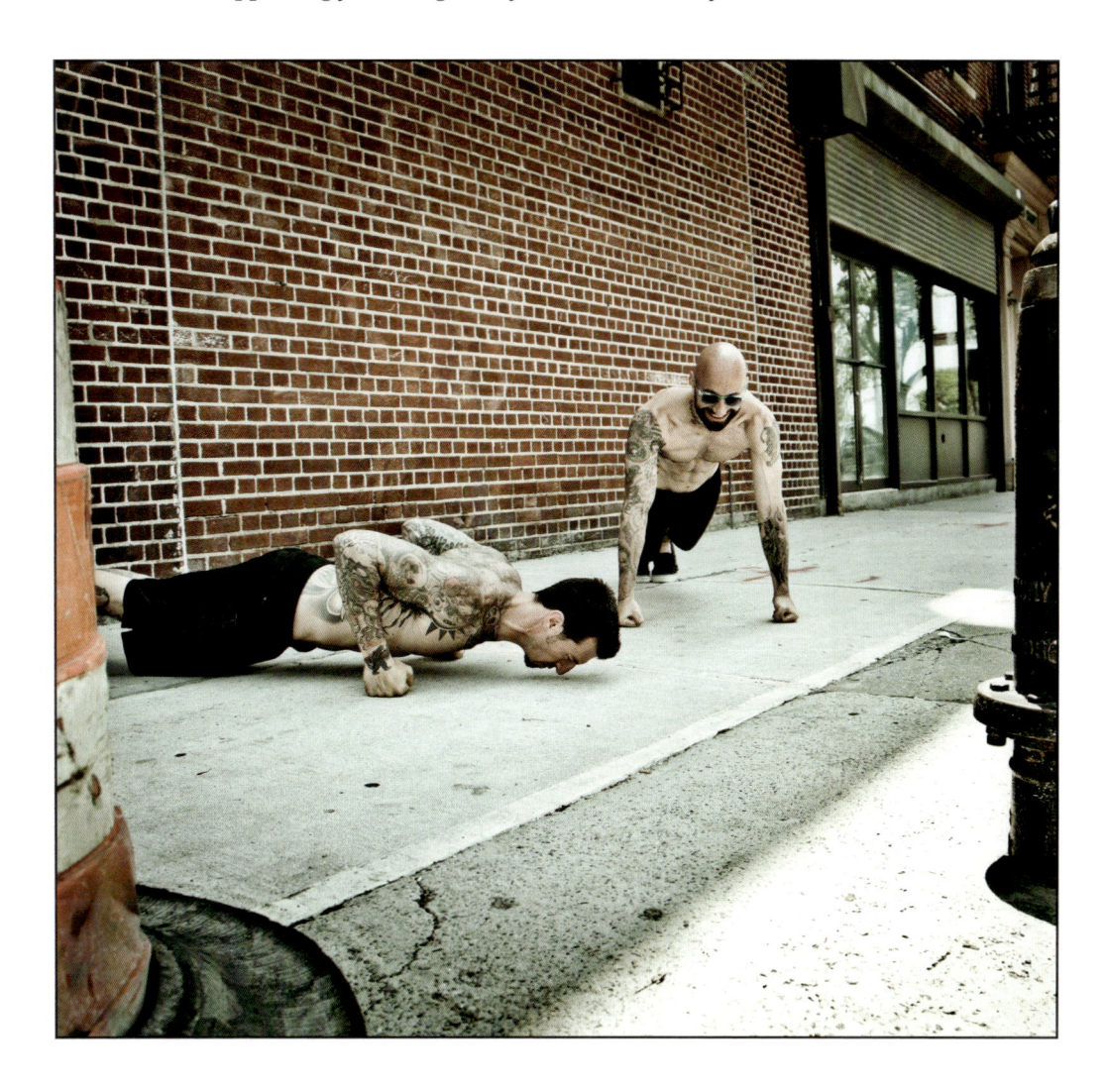

FINGERTIP PUSH-UP

Raising yourself up on your fingers adds a whole new element to your push-up training. In addition to involving a slew of often-neglected muscles, doing push-ups on your fingertips allows you to increase your range of motion by elevating you farther from the ground. As the hands are a key component of so many exercises, practicing fingertip push-ups will help your training across the board.

It's important to note that the term "fingertip push-up" can be misleading. You don't actually want to be all the way on the tips of your fingers, but rather on the pads of them with the tips slightly bent back. Some people's digits will wind up bending more than others. This is not a huge deal. Just don't allow any part of your palm to touch the ground.

It's also worth noting that practicing fingertip push-ups can be a nice way to counter all the hanging grip work that is such a large part of the Street Workout style of training.

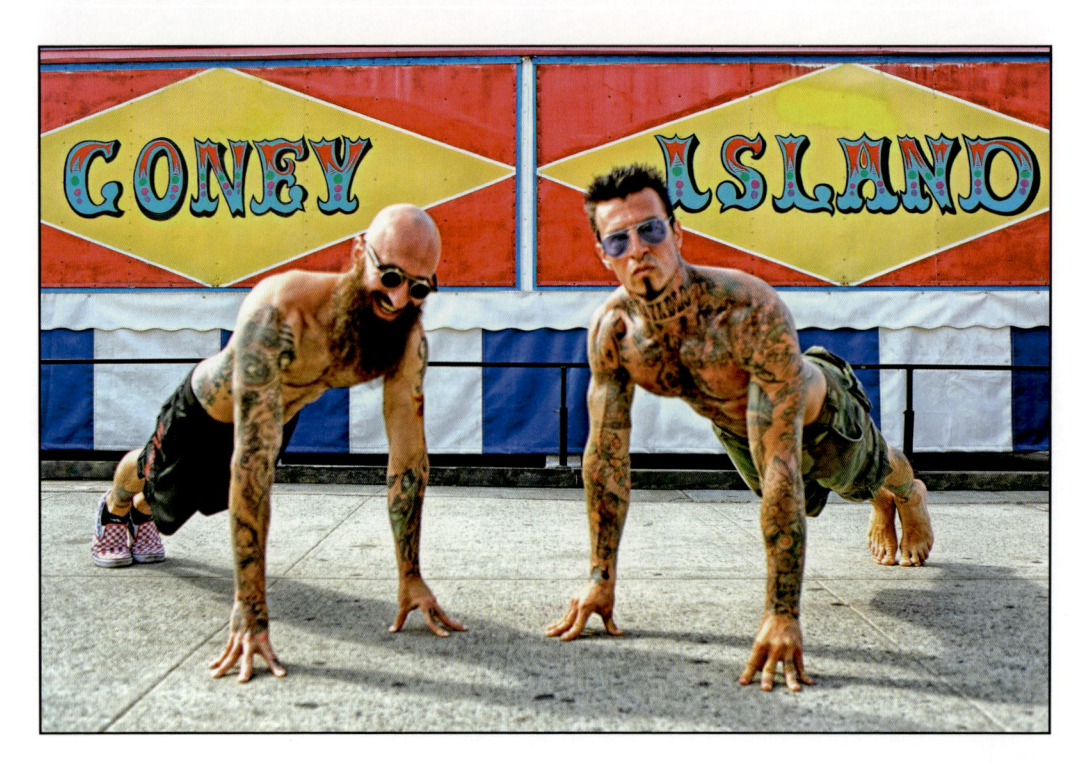

CLAW PUSH-UP

The claw push-up is an advanced variant on the fingertip push-up that has you all the way up on the very tips of your fingers with your hands resembling a claw-like position. Though some purists call this the "true fingertip push-up," the one mentioned previously is still the industry standard. Semantics aside, it is a useful tool for advanced grip trainees.

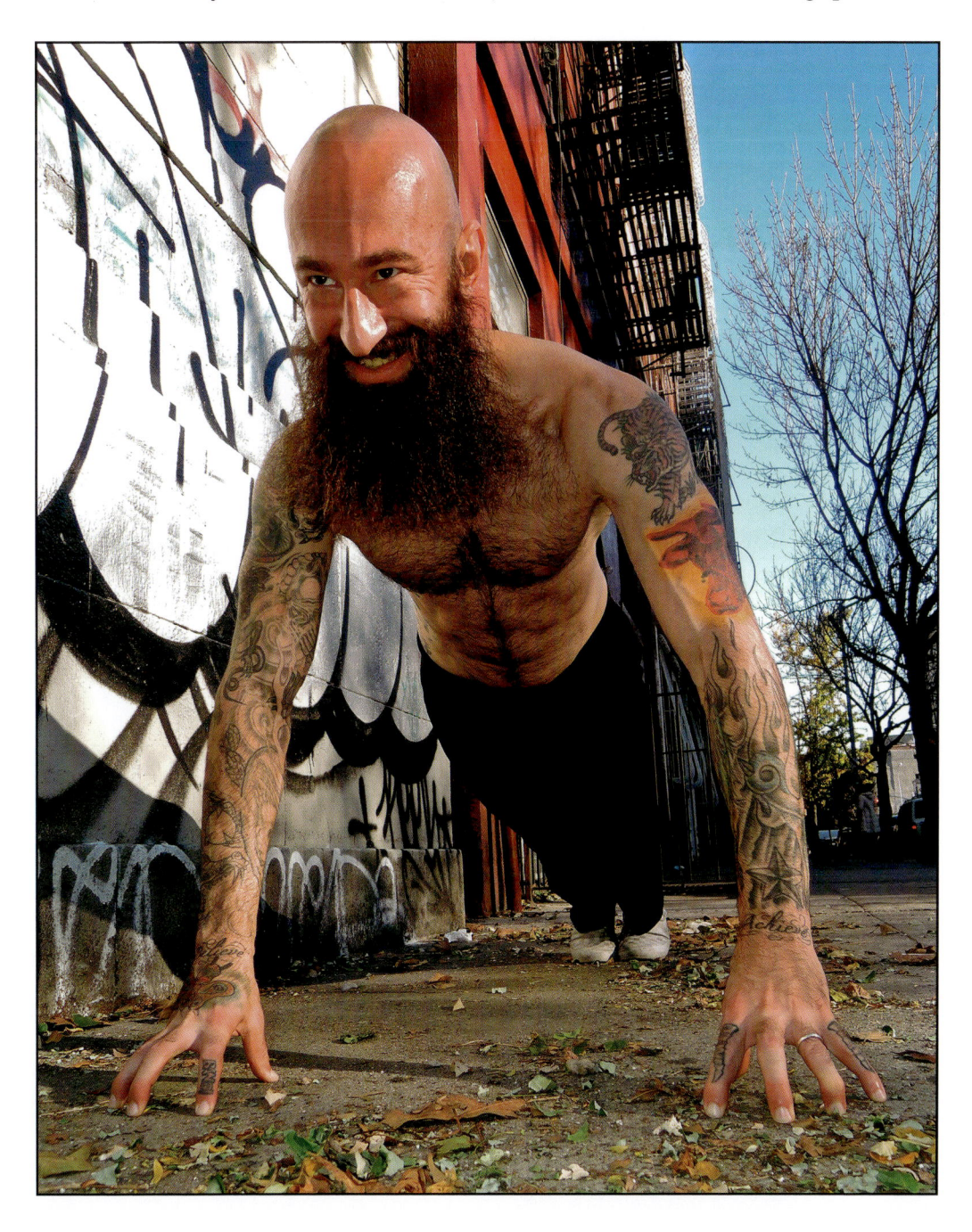

ONE LEG PUSH-UP

Removing a point of contact is one of the most universal ways to increase the intensity of almost any calisthenics exercise. In the case of the push-up, lifting one foot off the ground is a great way to introduce this concept. By reducing the number of contact points, your remaining limbs, as well as your core, are compelled to pick up the slack. You can even bring your knee toward your elbow for an added challenge.

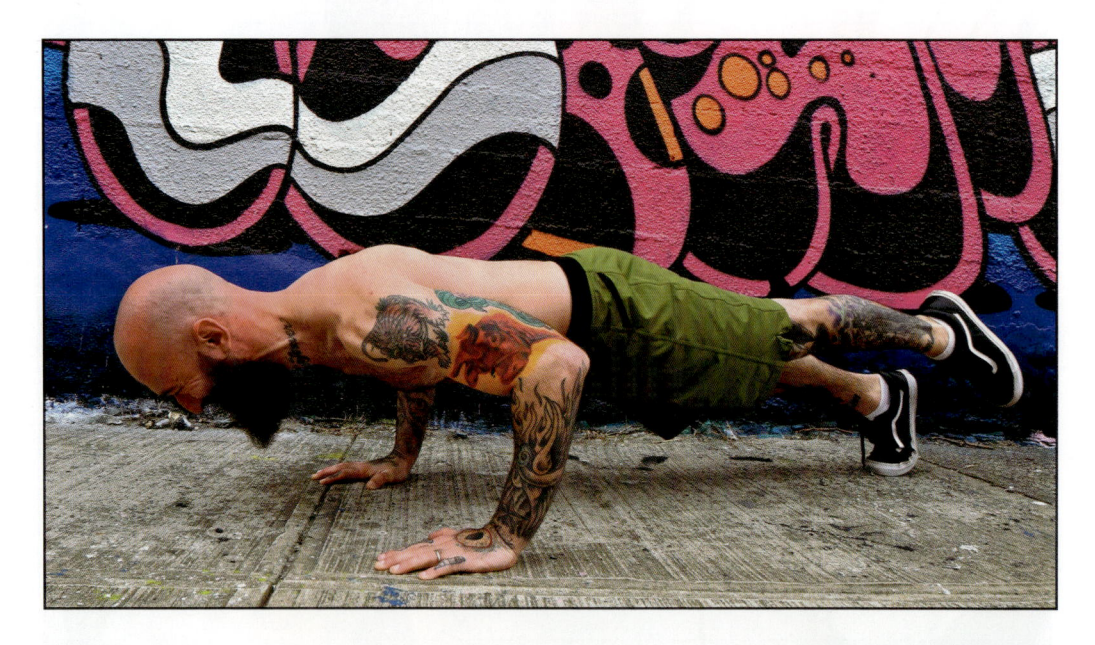

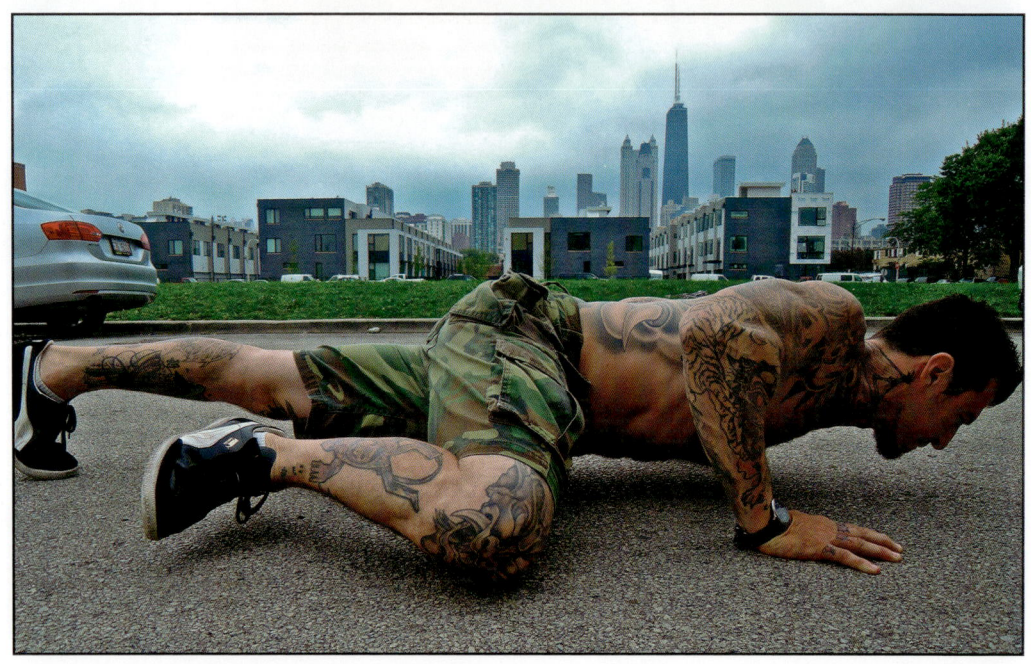

HINGE PUSH-UP

Begin in a standard push-up position, then lower yourself to the bottom. Instead of pressing yourself back up from there, however, shift your weight back onto your elbows. You'll wind up in a forearm plank with your palms flat on the floor in front of your shoulders. Pause here briefly, then slide forward, lift your elbows off the floor and press yourself back to the top.

Your toes and feet will need to flex back and forth as you slide in and out. The hinge push-up also requires a lot of trunk stability, so remember to keep your abs, back and glutes engaged throughout.

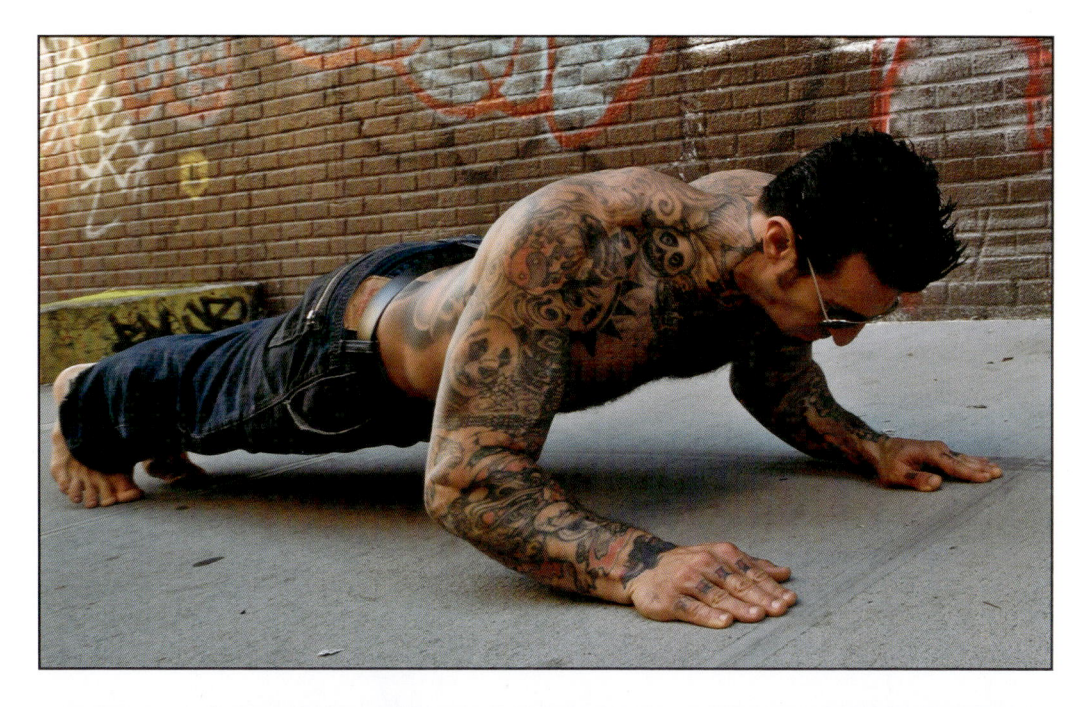

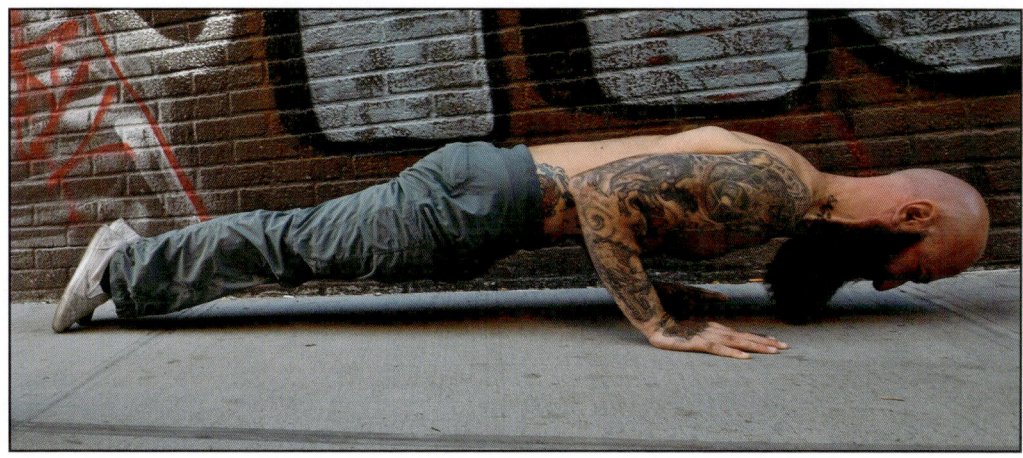

ARCHER PUSH-UP

For the archer push-up you will begin with a very wide hand placement—even wider than you would for a wide push-up. From there, keep one arm straight while you bend the other, so your body slides toward the side of the arm that bends. The archer push-up moves laterally as well as up and down.

To make the move more manageable, you can start with your hands a bit closer and allow your straight arm to have a small bend in the elbow. In time, aim to eliminate that bend. Play around with gradually moving your arms farther out to allow for a full range of motion.

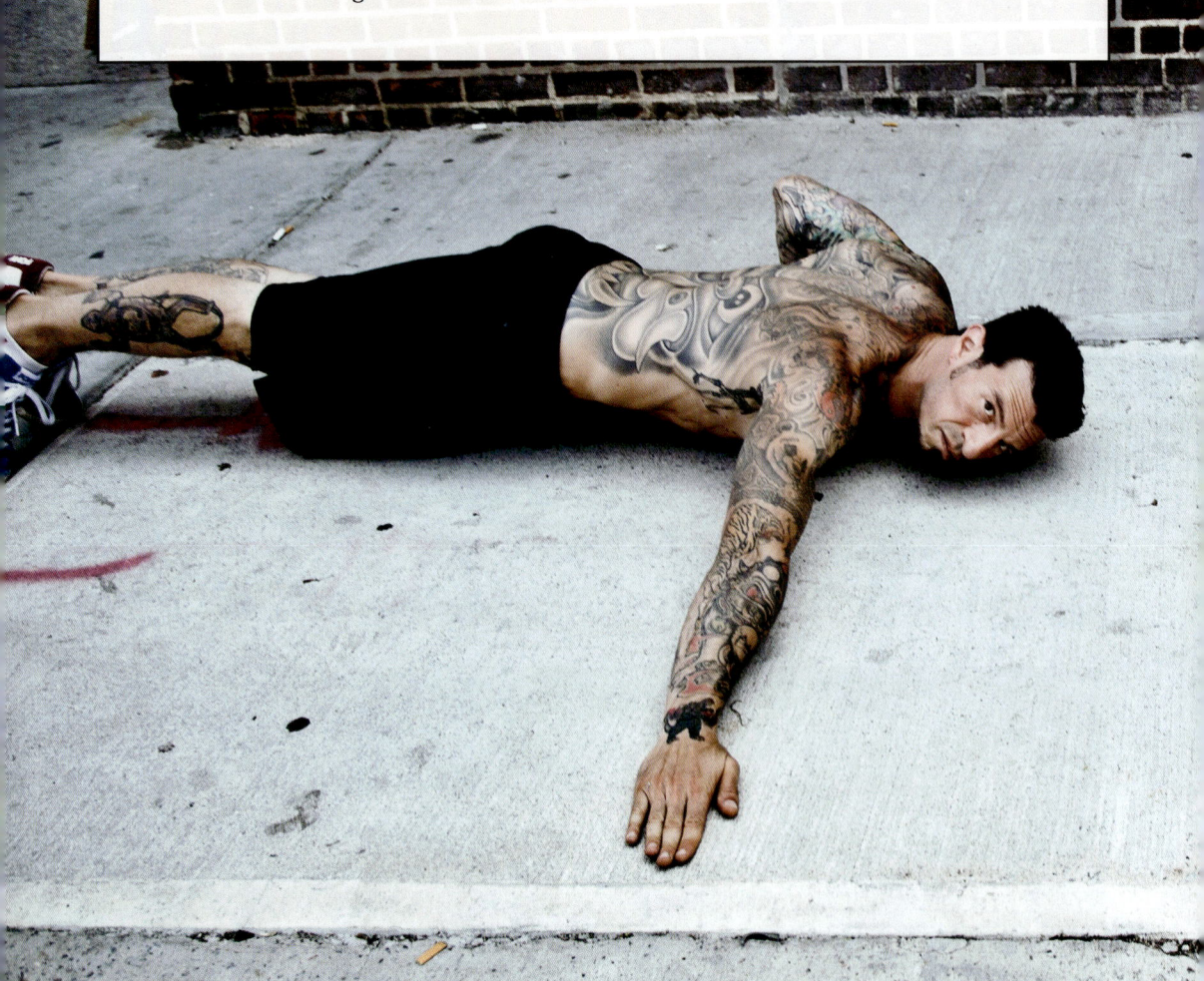

Do your best to avoid twisting sideways or "snaking" at your hips when performing archer push-ups. Like a standard push-up, you may want to start out practicing with your feet spread apart. As you gain strength and control, you can progress toward performing them with your heels touching.

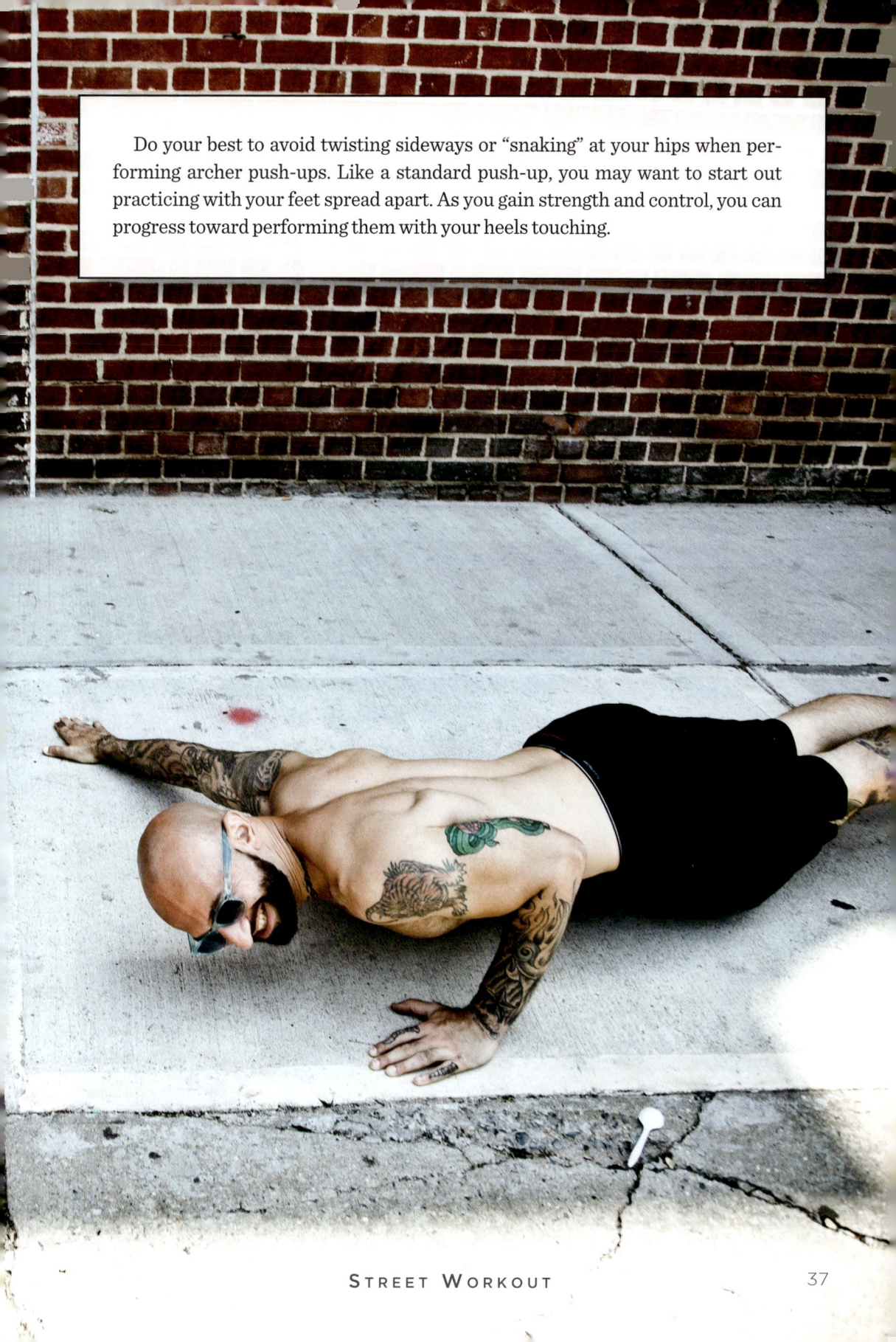

IGUANA PUSH-UP

To perform iguana push-ups, you'll need a rail or straight bar to position under your body. A single bar from a pair of parallel bars can work nicely. Grip the bar tightly with both hands while you cross one leg over the other and perform your push-ups from this position. You'll need to brace your core and go slowly in order to avoid tipping over. If you're looking for a push-up that will give you a balance and stability challenge, look no further than the iguana push-up.

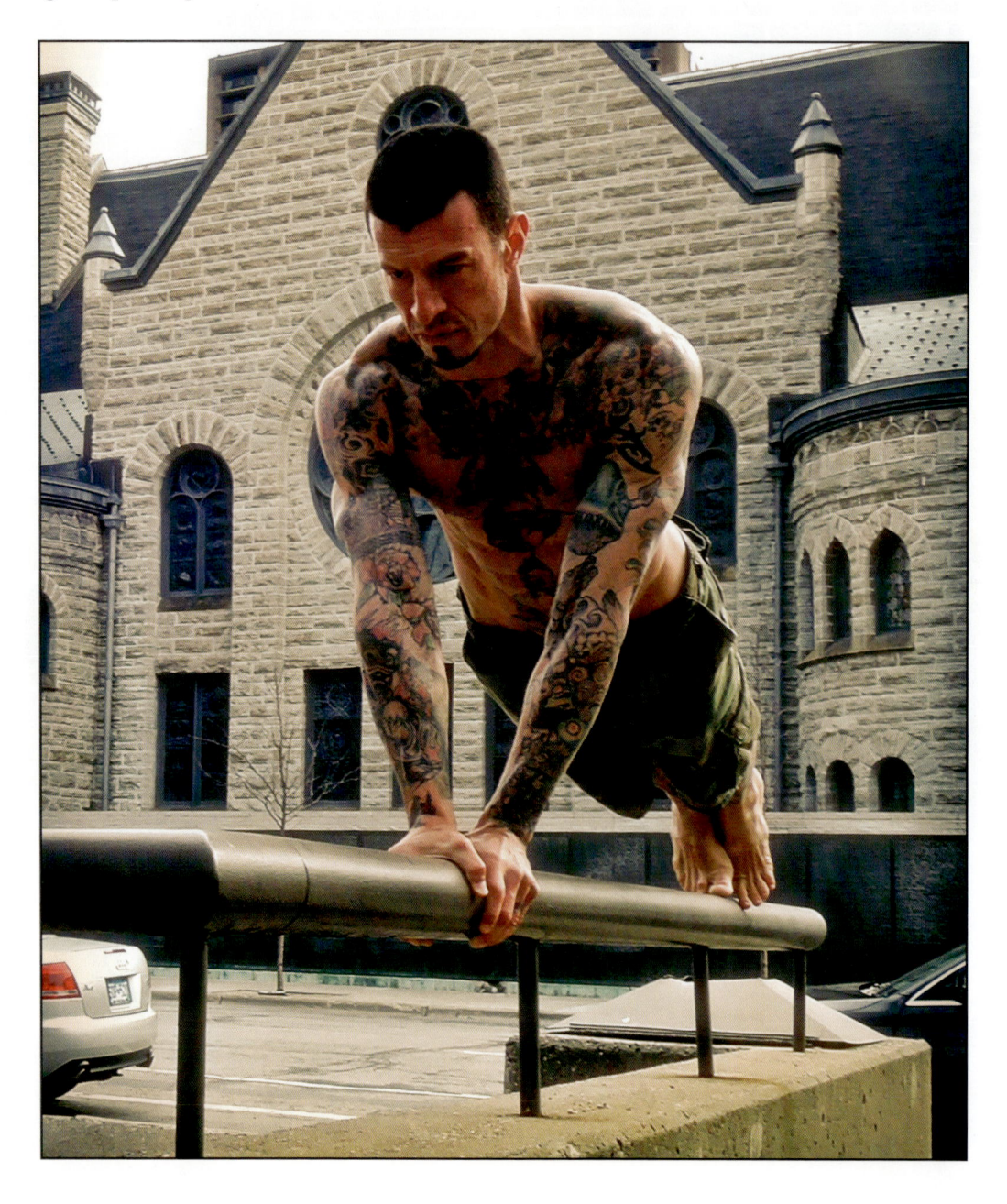

ONE ARM PUSH-UP

A lot of the techniques we recommend for learning the one arm push-up are the same that we suggest for beginners who are learning to do push-ups with both arms. That said, you can start out working toward a one arm push-up by simply holding a plank on one arm.

Once you've gotten a feel for that, try practicing a one arm push-up with your hand on an elevated surface. This will help you get a feel for the movement pattern without having to bear as much weight.

The higher the elevation, the less difficult the move becomes, so start with a fairly high surface and work your way down from there.

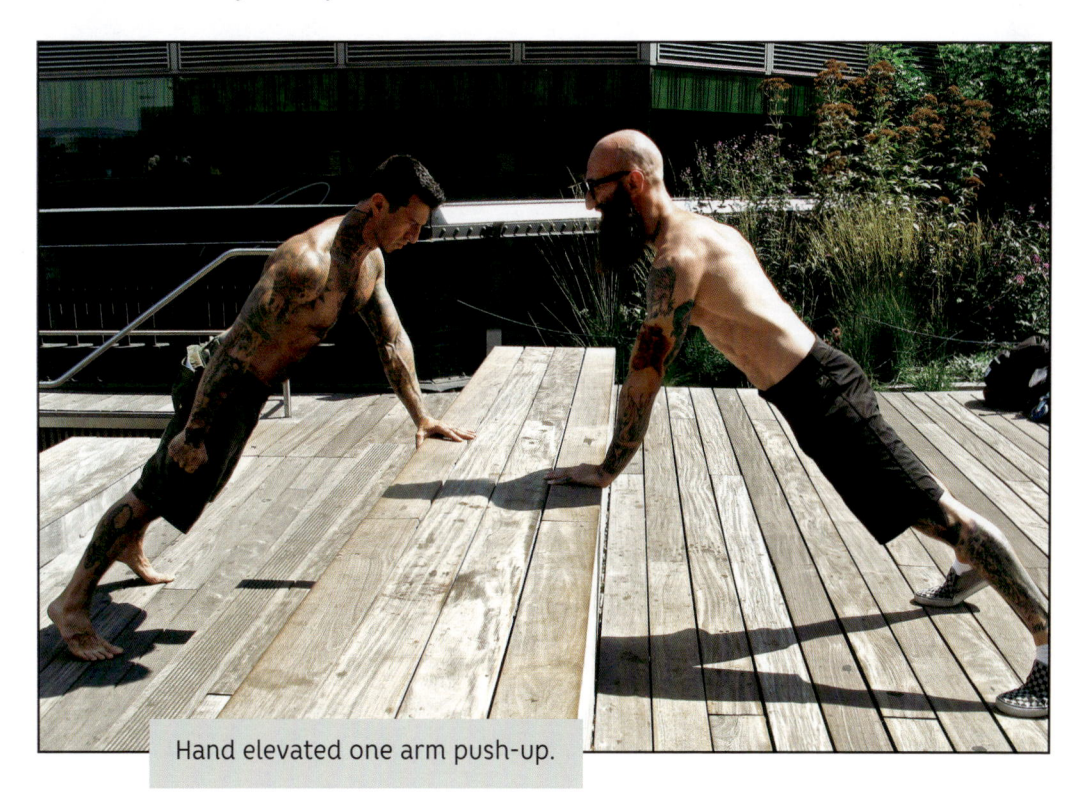

Hand elevated one arm push-up.

The form of a one arm push-up is a bit different from the standard two arm version. Your legs will need to be farther apart than in a classic push-up and your pushing hand should be almost centered beneath your body, rather than off to the side. More like where it would be positioned for a narrow push-up than a standard one.

As a general guideline, the closer your feet are positioned to each other, the harder the exercise becomes. Begin with your feet nice and wide to help get the feel for the movement pattern. Eventually you may try working toward narrowing your stance.

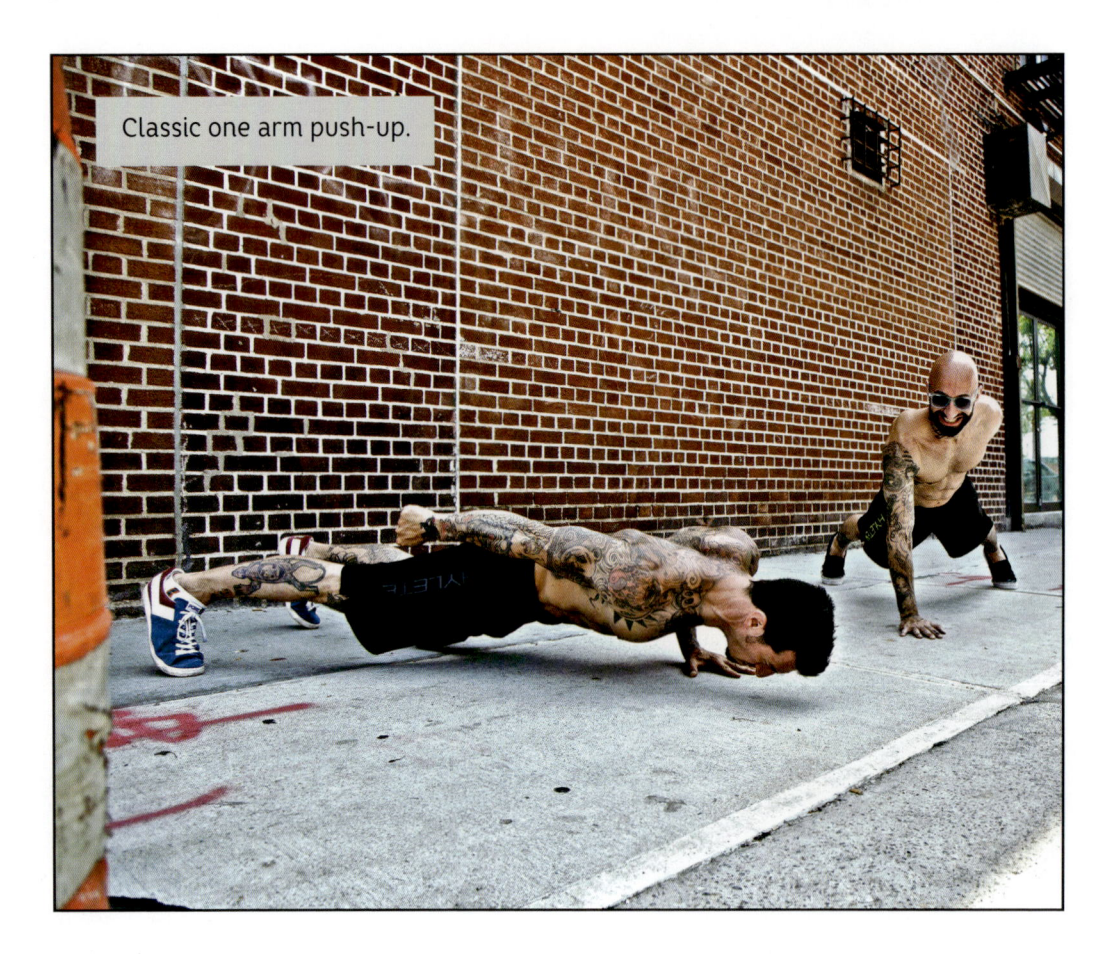

Classic one arm push-up.

Though it's true that only one arm is in contact with the ground, the phrase "one arm push-up" is a little misleading. If you don't contract your legs, abs, glutes—even your other arm—there's absolutely no way you can do a proper one arm push-up. There is also a great deal of cross-tension required between the pushing arm and the opposite leg. For example when performing a one arm push-up with your left arm, make sure to remain flexed, solid and unwavering all the way down to your right leg. To take it a step further, you can even remove the left leg completely and perform a one arm push-up using only one arm and one leg.

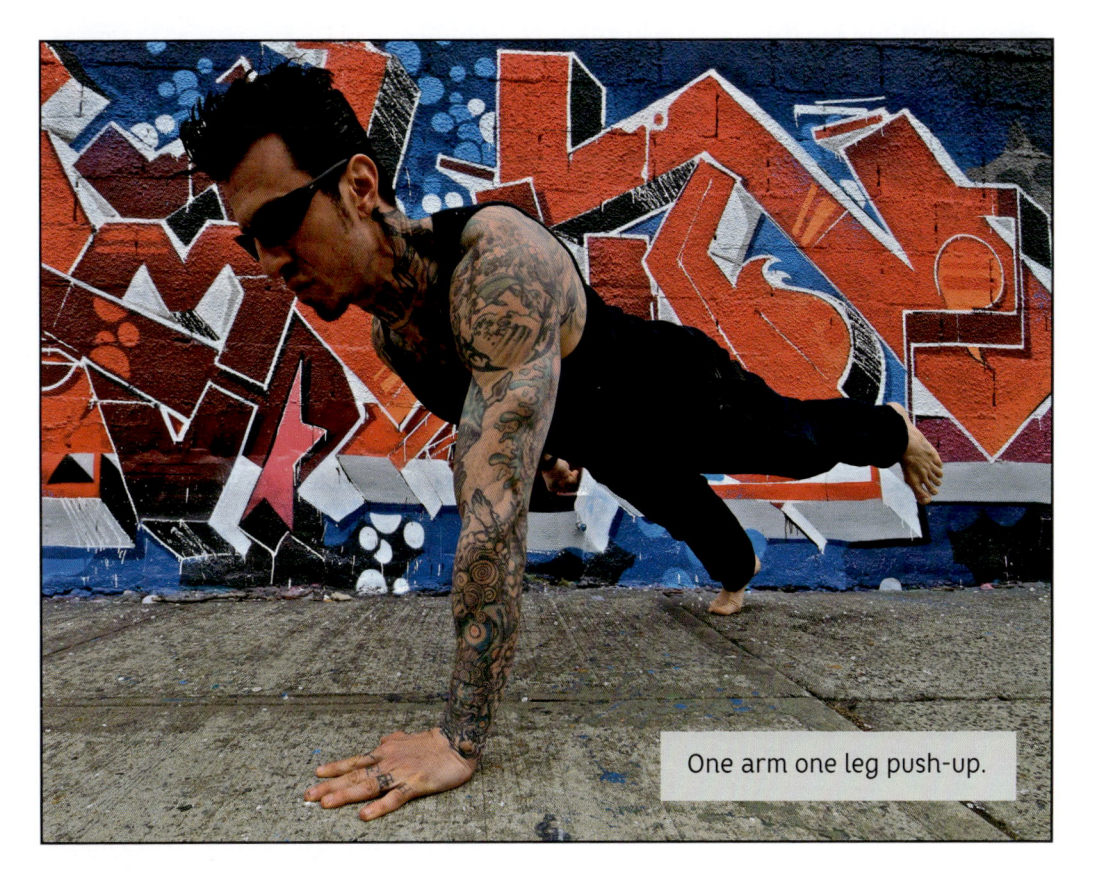

One arm one leg push-up.

As with a narrow push-up, your arm should remain close to your side on the way down as well as the way up. Your other arm can be held against your body, placed behind the back or extended out to the side. Experiment with different arm positions to find what works best for you.

The Plyo-Matrix Freestyle Push-ups

Any explosive push-up where the body (or part of it) gets airborne is referred to as a "plyometric" push-up. Although there are many variations in existence, they all require pushing into the ground fast and hard in order to generate the requisite force needed.

The most recognizable plyometric push-up is probably the "clapping" push-up, in which the practitioner gets his or her upper body high enough off the ground to clap their hands before returning to the starting position. Clapping push-ups can be performed with the hands behind the back as well, or even with multiple claps, where the subject switches from the front to the back of the body.

It is of note, however, that there are many types of plyometric push-ups that do not involve a clap at all. If you are new to plyometrics, simply getting your hands off the ground for any distance or duration is a great place to start.

By the same token, there are variations that involve getting both your hands and feet off the ground, and push-ups where you touch your fingers to your toes in the top position.

Freestyling in the push-up arena is such an expansive genre that it is not uncommon to witness push-ups which explode up and land in an entirely different place than they started. Circling motions, transferring from hands to forearms and back, moving your hands to your head and even one-arm plyometric push-ups are all fair game in the world of freestyle push-ups!

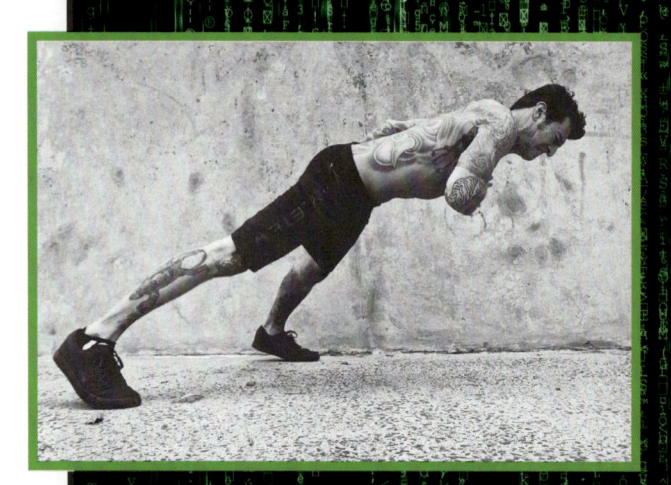

OVERHEAD PRESS PROGRESSIONS

Your shoulders get a substantial workout from all upper body calisthenics strength training and are used in every exercise mentioned thus far. But when we change from the horizontal (push) plane to the vertical (press) plane, we switch the main emphasis from the chest to the shoulders. While it's true that each of the following exercises still incorporates the chest (not to mention the arms, abs, glutes and back), the primary mover is now the shoulders.

Even those who can military press massive poundage in the weight room are often humbled when they attempt many of these exercises, but if they stick with it, they'll discover that there are astronomical gains to be had. Take these progressions slowly. Let's get strong!

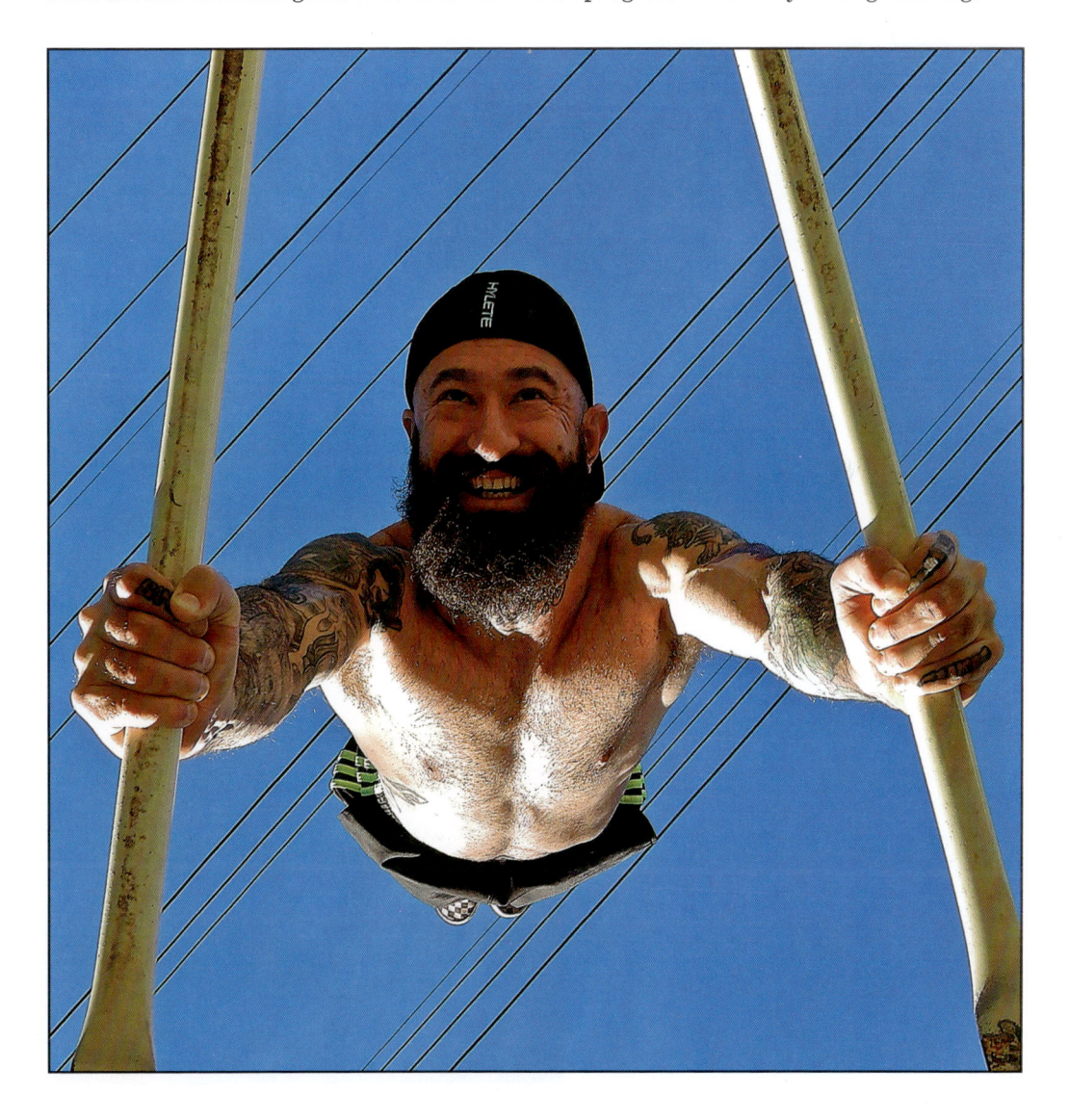

HINDU PRESS

Start in a plank, then lift your hips all the way in the air, positioning your shoulders in a straight line with your hips and hands. Keep your legs as straight as you can, but be aware that folks with tight hamstrings will need to bend the knees slightly.

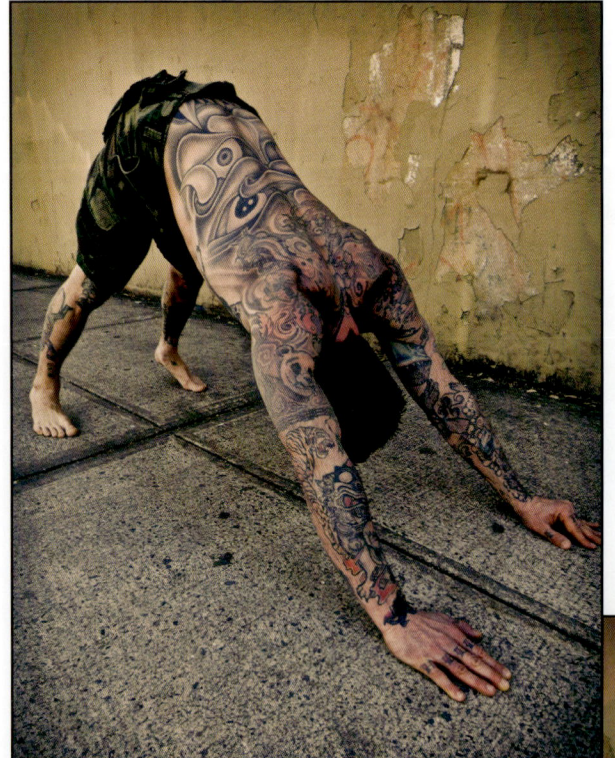

Lower the top of your head towards the ground, keeping your hips high, then quickly drop your hips, swoop your torso up and look in the air. Keep your arms straight as you press your hips back to the starting position to begin the next rep.

The Hindu press is a great lead-up step toward the pike press because it incorporates the intensity of the negative phase but has a relatively easy pressing phase.

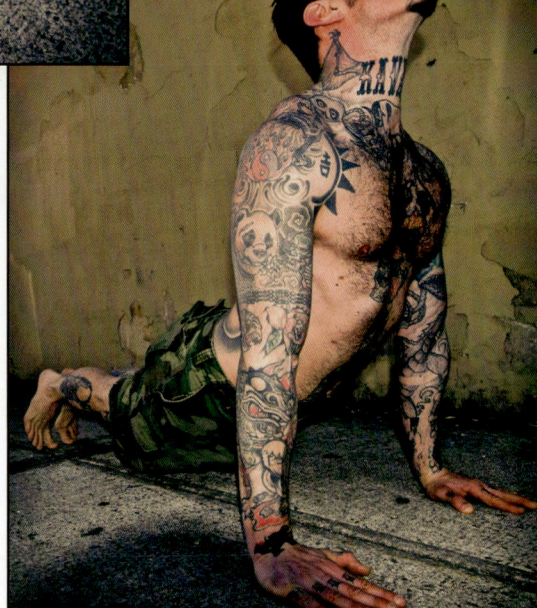

PIKE PRESS

The pike press begins like the Hindu press with your hips in the air and shoulders in line with your hands and hips. From here, lower your head toward the ground, keeping your hips in the air, then press yourself back to the top position. As with most other pushing exercises, be mindful that your elbows point back, rather than flaring out toward the sides.

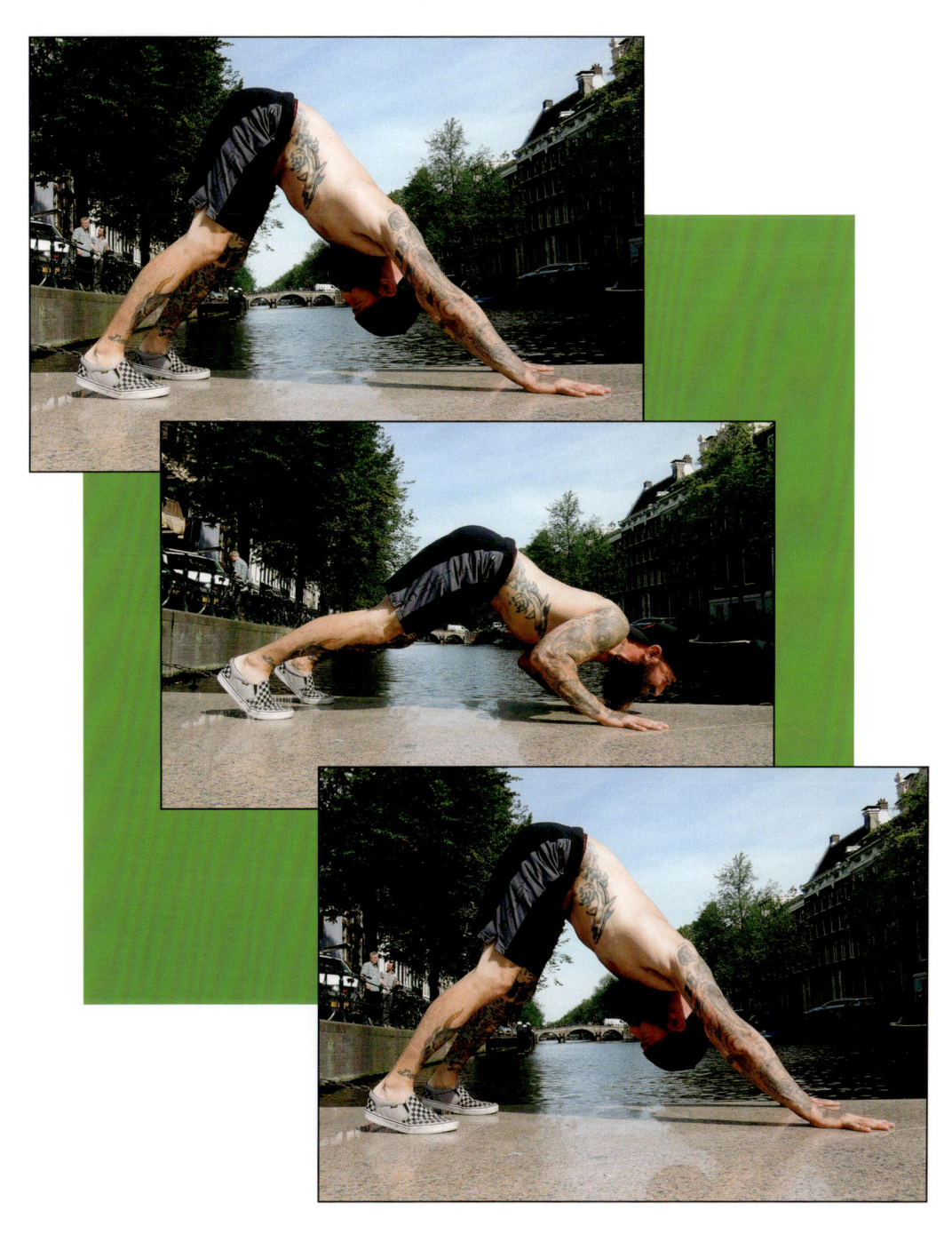

STREET WORKOUT

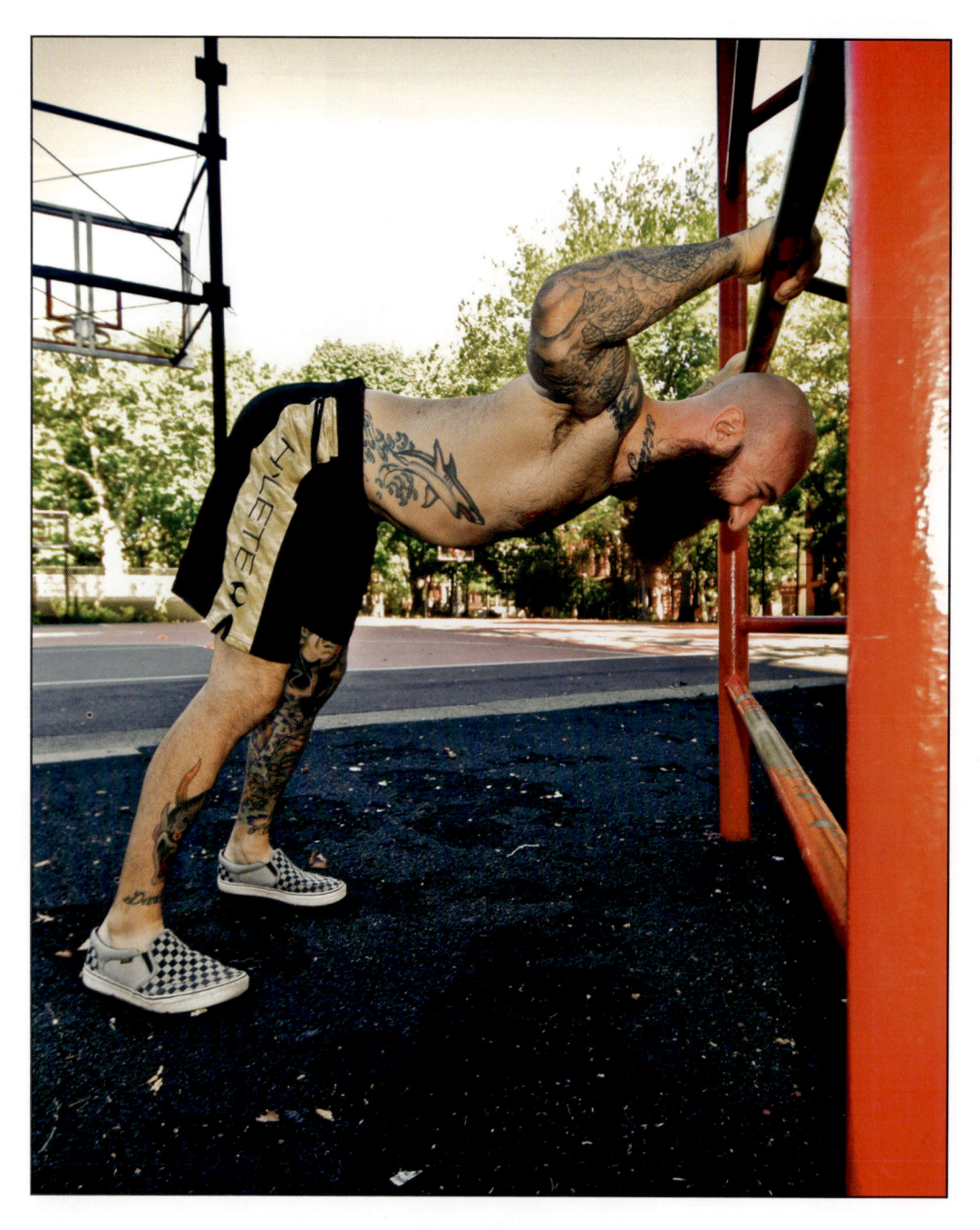

HANDS ELEVATED PIKE PRESS

Like the standard push-up, placing your hands higher than your feet when you perform a pike press is a good way to make the move less difficult. You can practice on any number of objects that you might encounter. Again, the higher the elevation, the less of your bodyweight you will need to press.

FEET ELEVATED PIKE PRESS

Elevating your feet makes the pike press more difficult, as it places more of your weight in your hands. As with all pike press variants, remember to make sure that your hips stay above your shoulders so that your pressing movement remains in a vertical plane.

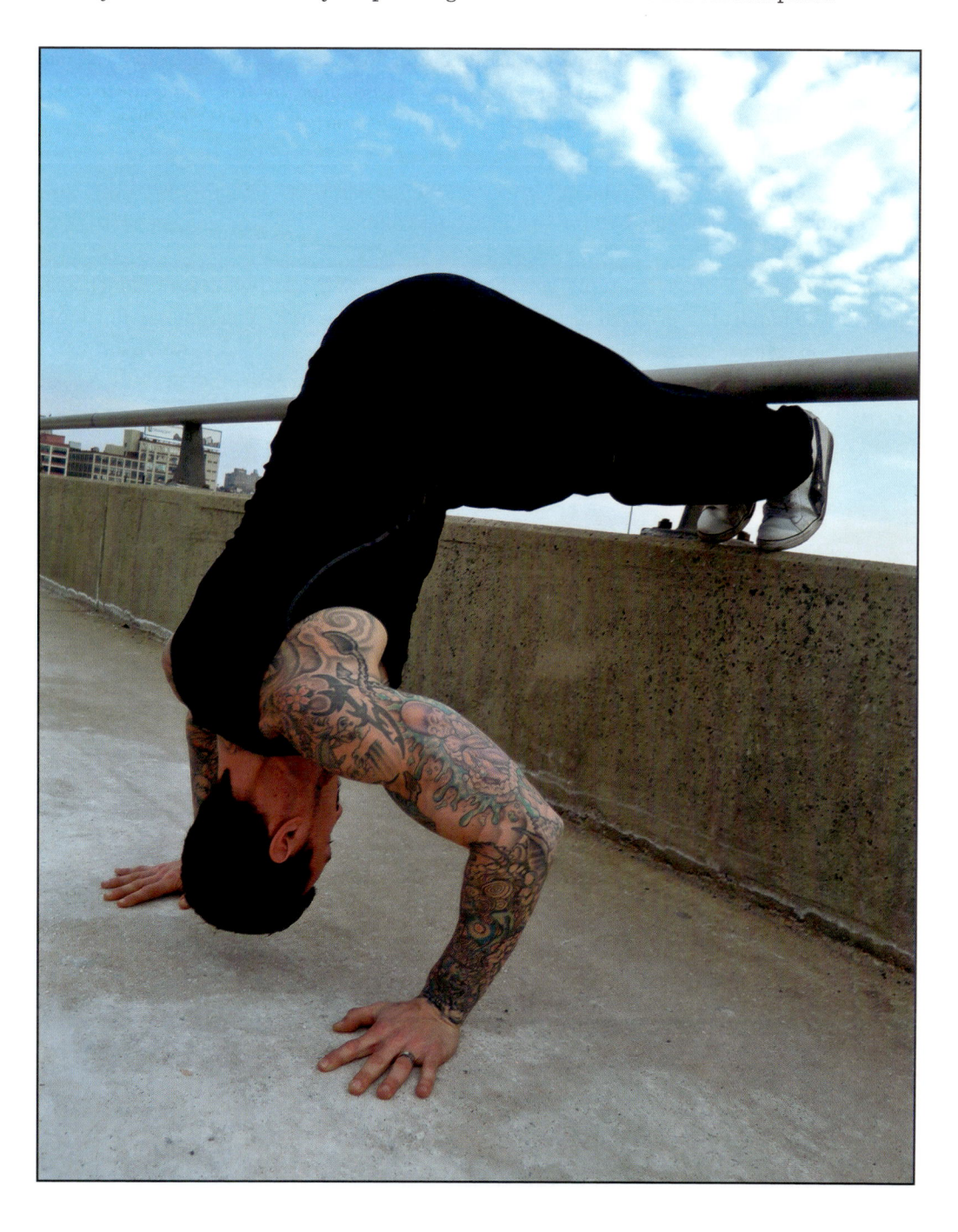

WALL HANDSTAND PRESS

The wall handstand press, aka handstand push-up, is among the best known advanced bodyweight exercises.

Kick up into a handstand with your back facing a wall, then lower your head to the ground and press yourself back to the start position. Just like regular push-ups, you can experiment with various hand-widths and placements. Engage your glutes and abs in order to avoid excessively bending your back.

Once you get a feel for handstand presses, you can try them facing toward the wall, rather than having your back to it for an added challenge.

Like the other pushing variations, you can experiment with narrowing your hand placement on the handstand press in order to make the exercise more challenging. For more information on handstands, see Section III, Part 9 "Floor Holds."

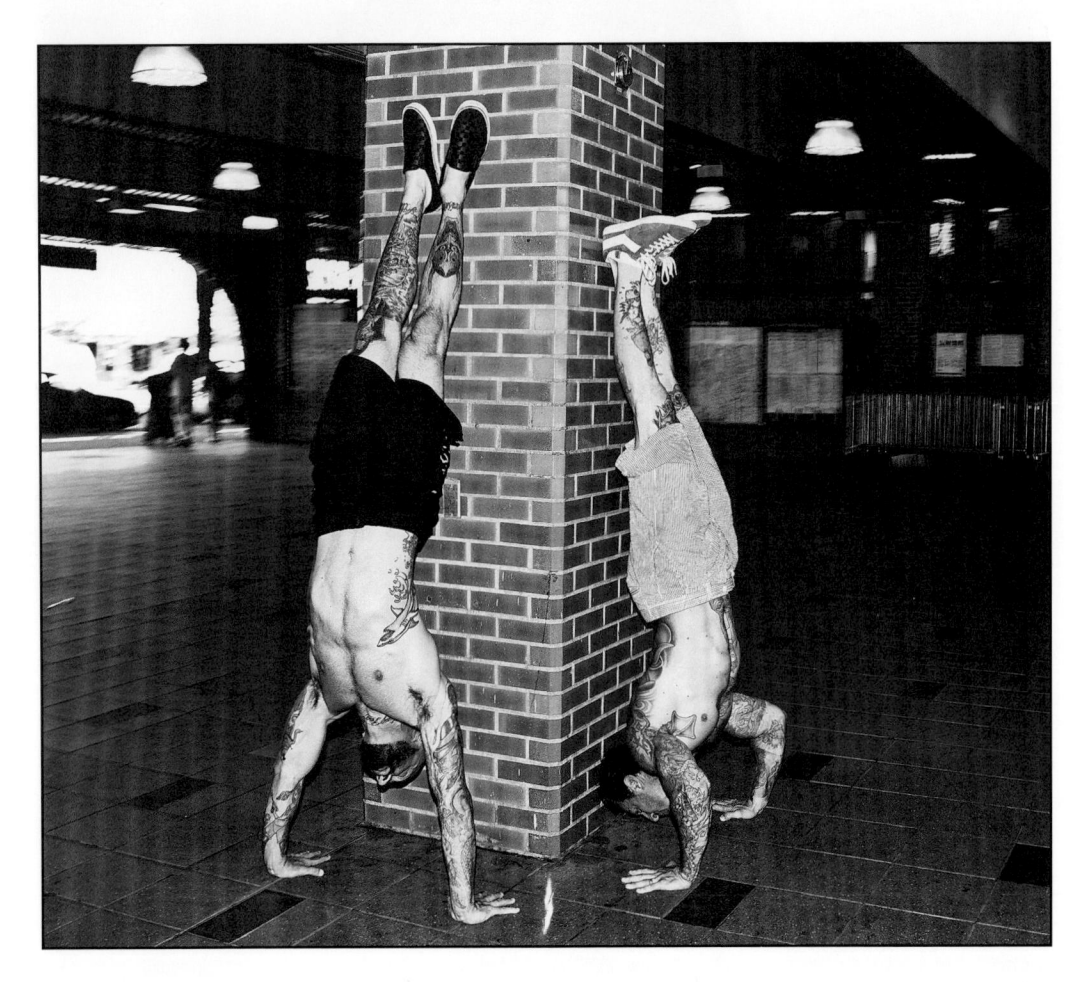

ULTIMATE HANDSTAND PRESS

When you perform a standard handstand press on the ground you can only go until the top of your head reaches the floor. You might be able to add an extra inch by tilting your head and going down to your nose. If you want to use a full range of motion for this exercise, however, you'll need to elevate your hands to create room for your head to drop below surface level. This is the ultimate handstand press!

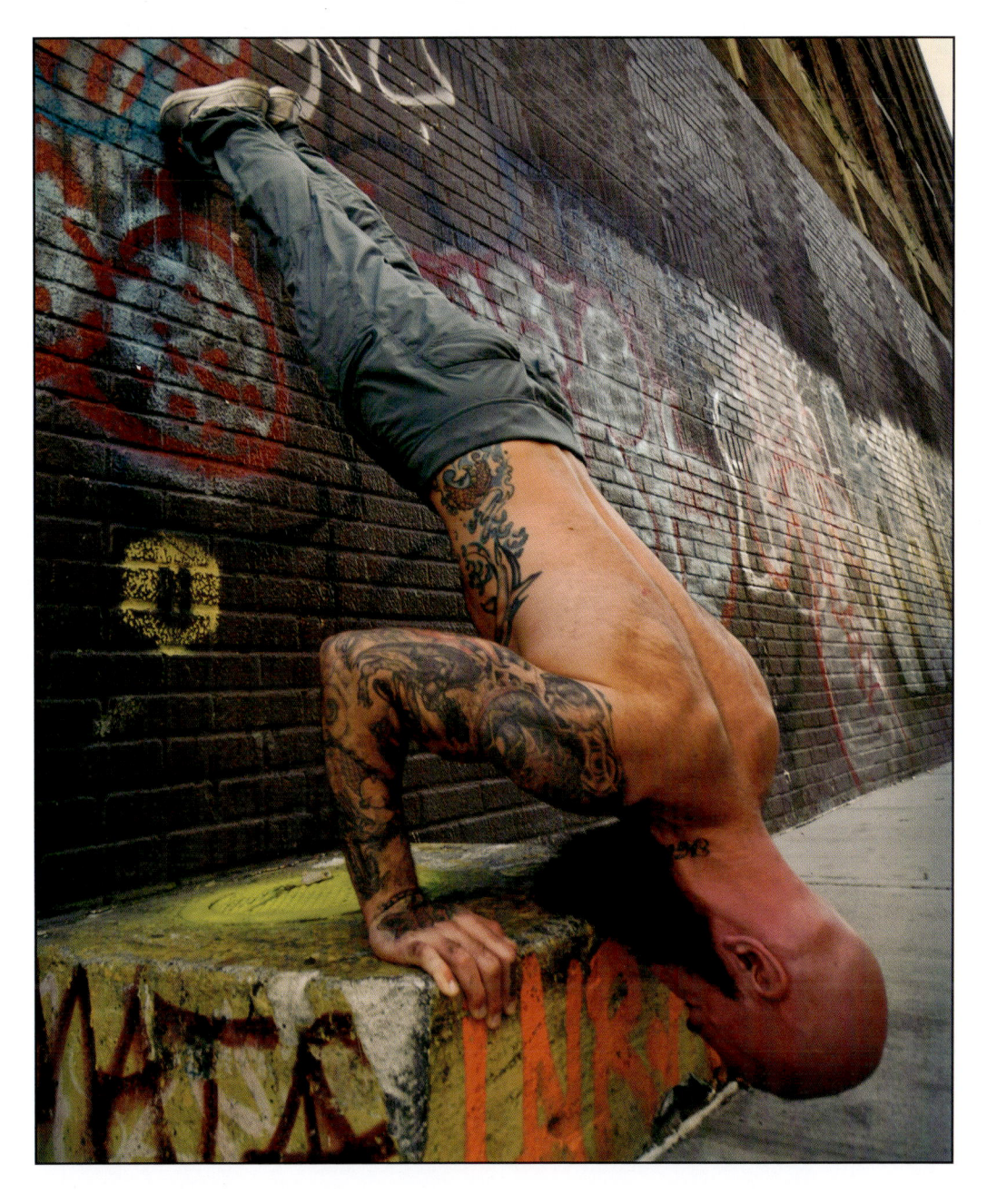

DIP PROGRESSIONS

The dip is the unsung hero of calisthenics strength training. In a universe of one-arm push-ups, handstand presses and other-worldly bodyweight feats of strength, do not forget that the humble dip is a key component in developing well-rounded pushing power.

Any time you are pushing your body weight while your torso is in an upright position, you are doing a dip. Because of this different angle, dips place a greater emphasis on the triceps than the horizontal push or overhead press. Often overlooked and underrated, dips are in a class all their own.

BENCH DIP

The bench variation is the best way for beginners to get started with dips. Place both hands behind your back, palms down on a bench or other object that's about 18-24 inches tall. Keep your back straight and bend from your elbows and shoulders to lower yourself down while keeping your torso upright, then press yourself back up to the top.

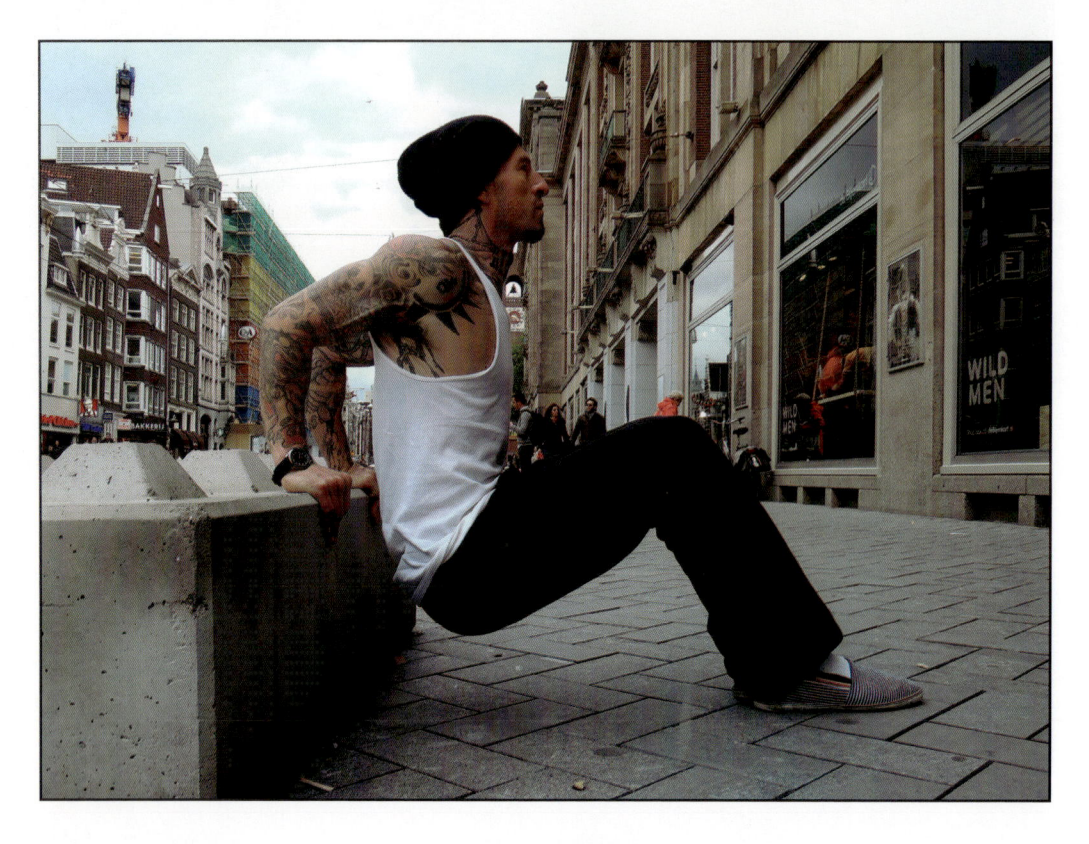

Beginners should start with knees bent and feet flat on the floor. This will allow you to push gently with your feet in order to give your arms some assistance if they need it. As that becomes easier, you can progress to doing dips with your legs straight and your toes pointed up. Let your legs relax and allow your hips to hang down right below your shoulders. Keep your chest up; don't hunch your back or shrug.

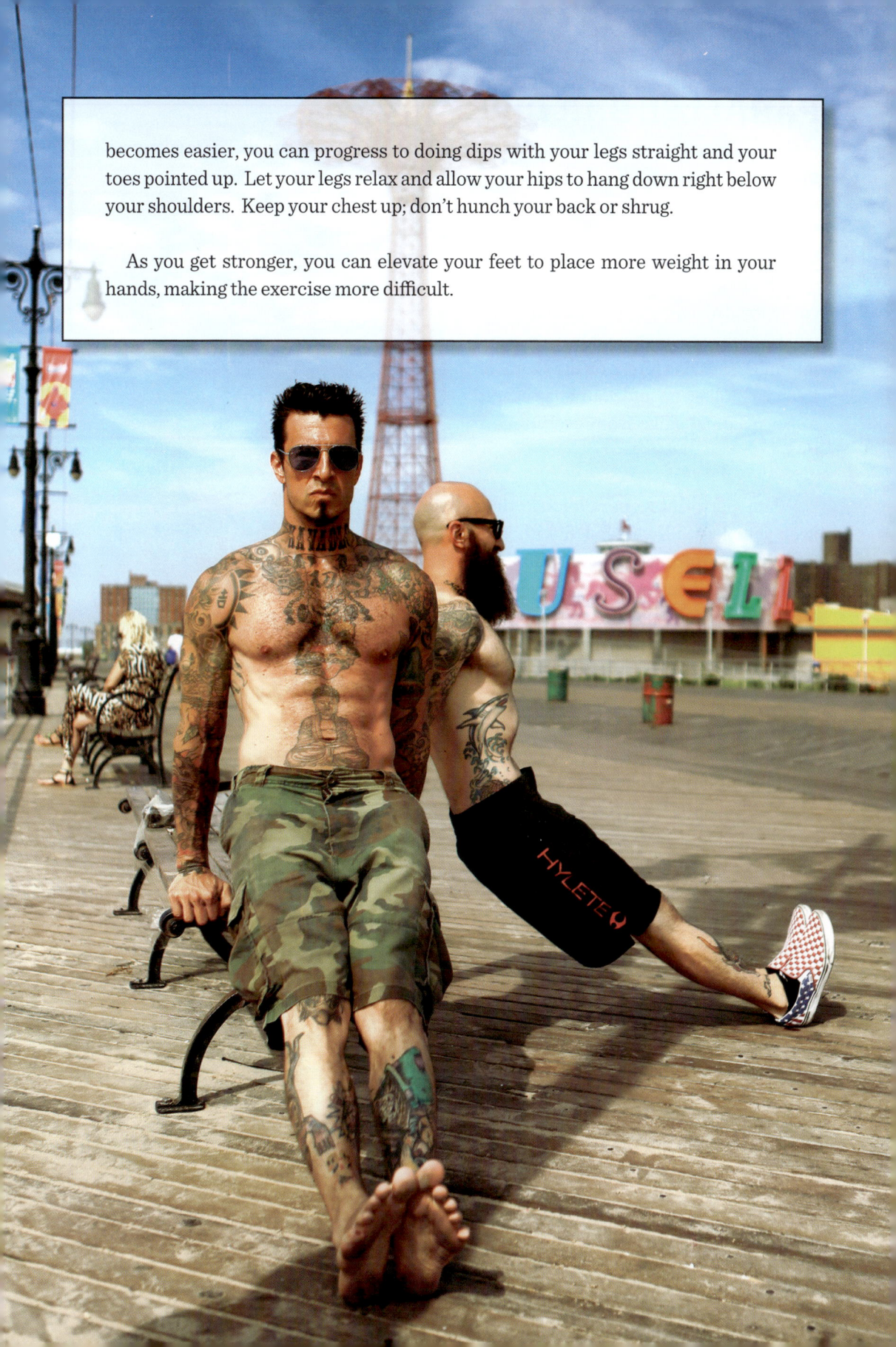

As you get stronger, you can elevate your feet to place more weight in your hands, making the exercise more difficult.

PARALLEL BAR DIP

For this variation you will hold yourself upright between two parallel bars with your feet in the air the entire time.

Grab the bars tightly and lower yourself down, bending at the elbows and shoulders. Make sure your elbows point behind you instead of flaring out to the sides. This will keep the tension on your triceps and minimize shearing forces on the shoulder. Keep your chest up and your abs engaged to get maximal gains from every repetition.

When performing parallel bar dips, keep your legs fully extended with your feet slightly in front of you. (Think back to that hollow-body position.) This places greater emphasis on your core, making your body tighter and keeping your body weight in front of you.

Conversely, bent knees and feet behind you can alter the leverage of the exercise, making it more mechanically advantageous and slightly more forgiving.

Beginners may feel more comfortable in the latter position, and may even choose to cross their ankles in order to generate more tension. Experiment to find what works best for you. It will not be the same for everybody.

You can also play with the nuances of elbow and shoulder flexion. The more you lean forward, the more you work your chest. The more upright you stay, the more you work your triceps and core.

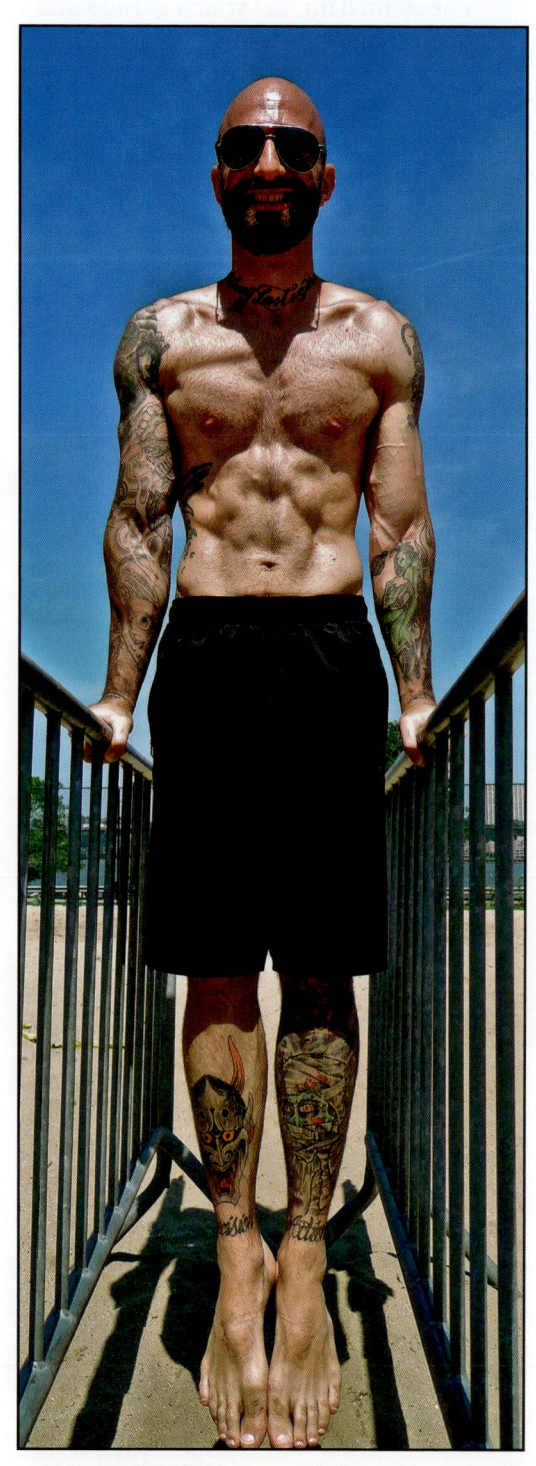

STRAIGHT BAR DIP

The straight bar dip is performed with both hands on a single bar positioned in front of the body. When you do a parallel bar dip, you lower yourself in between the bars, but when you dip on a straight bar, your body must move around the bar. As such, you'll need to reach your legs out in front during the descent in order to keep balanced.

The simple change of having a single bar in front of you puts you at a greater mechanical disadvantage. With it comes a chance of slipping around and off the bar that does not exist with parallel bars. To avoid this, in addition to reaching your legs forward, you'll need to pitch your upper body in front of the bar as well.

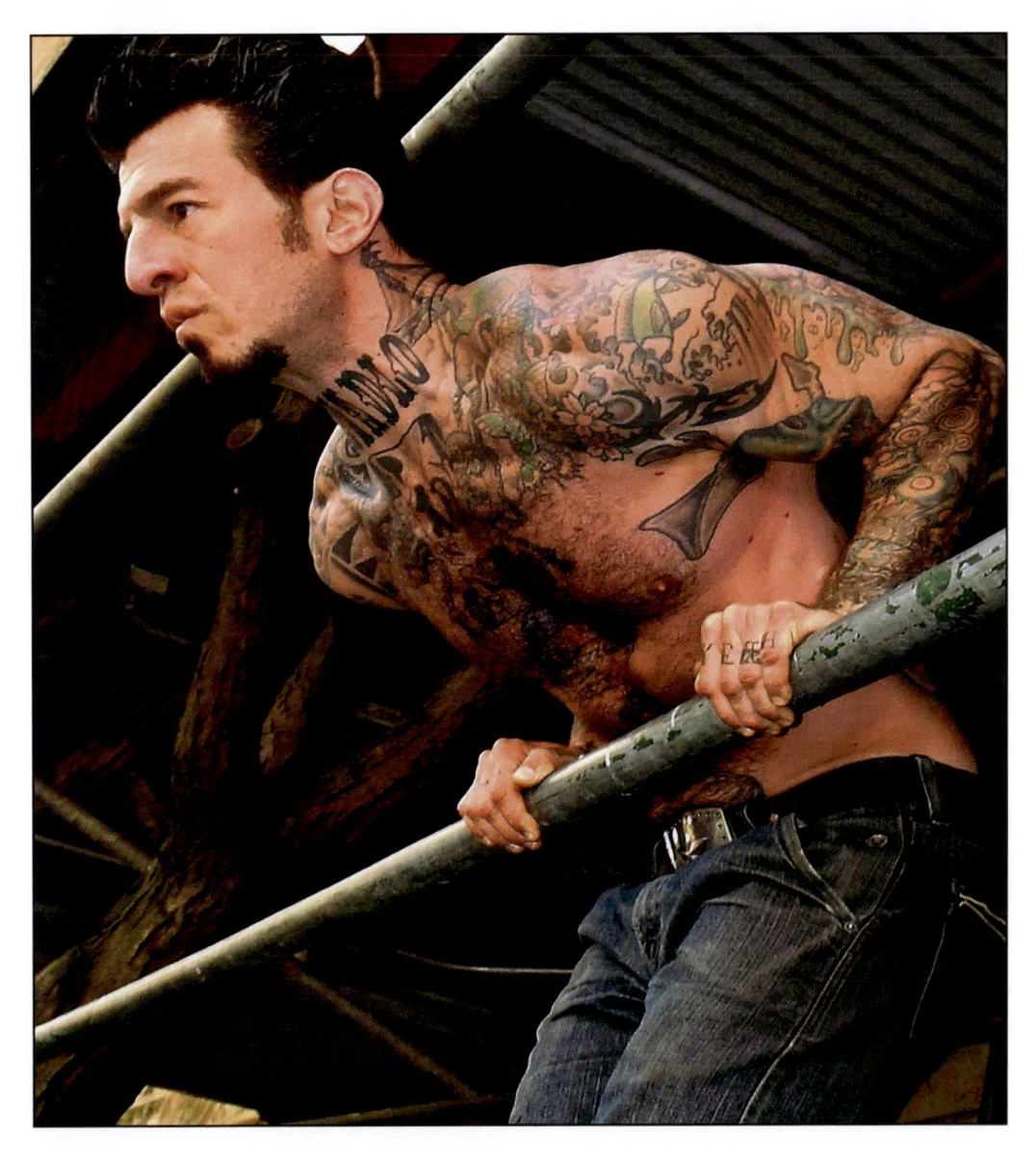

PERPENDICULAR BAR DIP

This is a dip performed in between two bars that form a perpendicular angle. You can think of it as the halfway point between a parallel bar dip and straight bar dip. In the world of Street Workout we encourage you to explore your surroundings and experiment with varied set-ups.

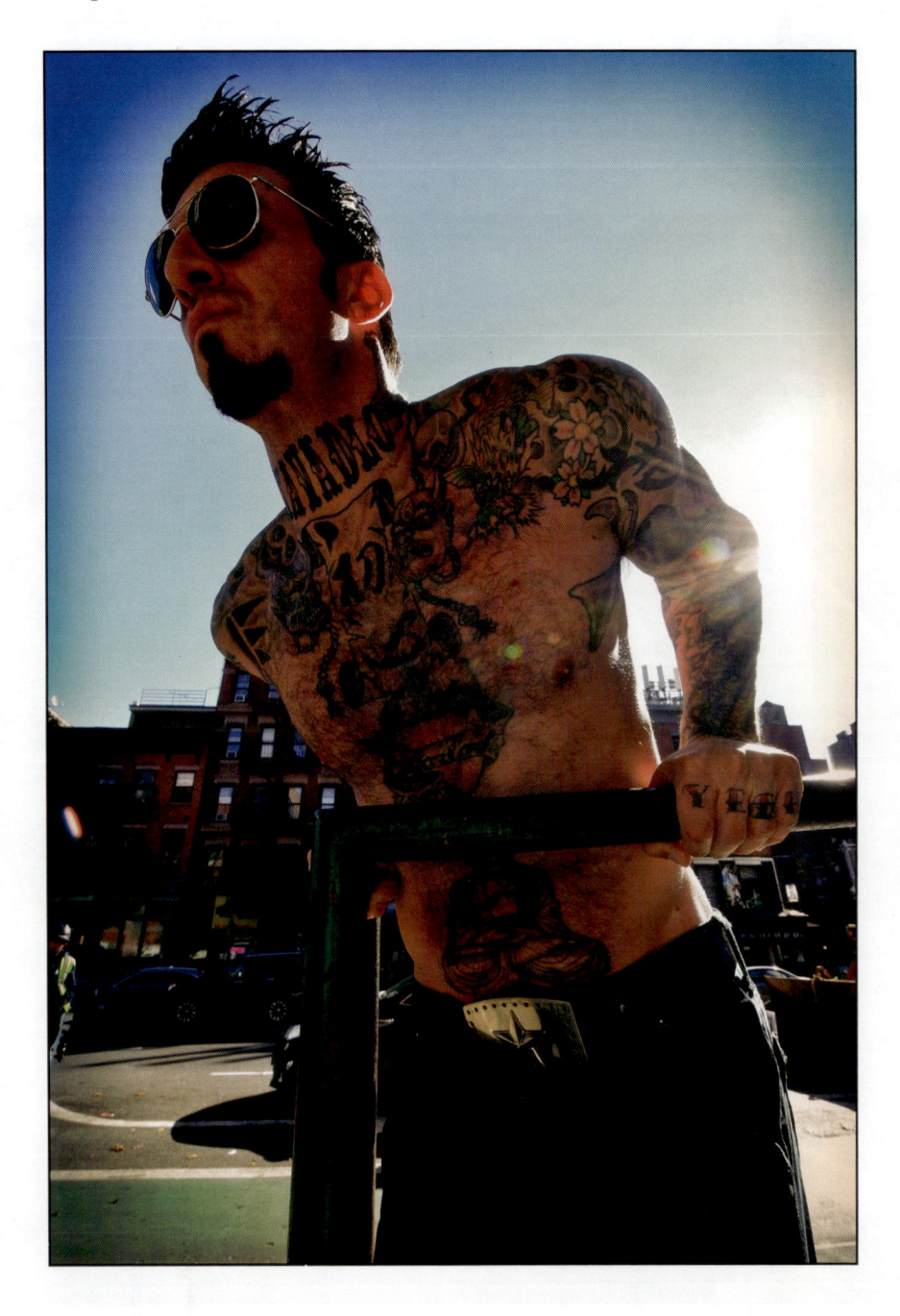

RUSSIAN DIP

Also known as a hinge dip, the Russian dip starts out like a standard parallel bar dip. When you reach the bottom of the normal range of motion, shift your weight back onto your elbows, putting your forearms in contact with the bars. Squeeze the bars tightly and contract your abs as you shift your weight back onto your hands, sliding your shoulders in front of your wrists, just before pressing yourself back to the start position.

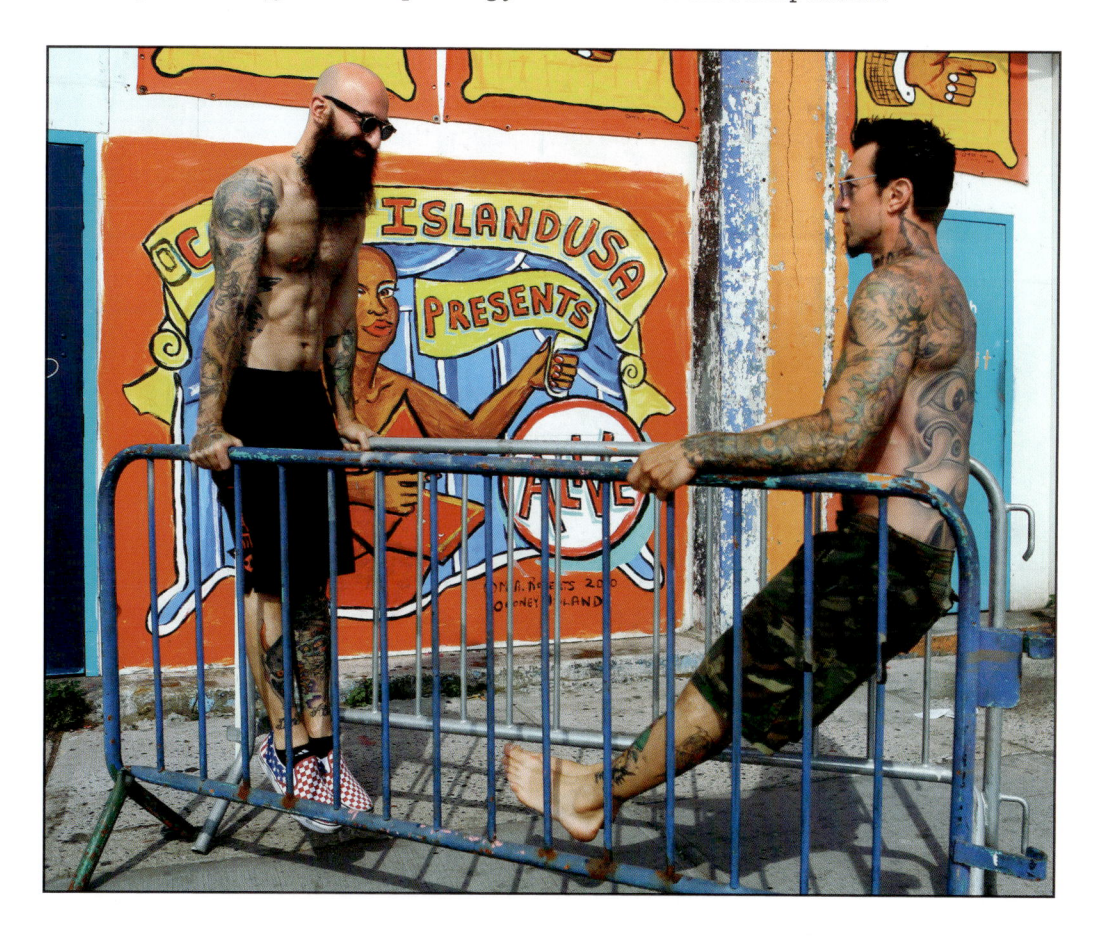

KOREAN DIP

A Korean dip is a behind-the-back dip that's performed on a pull-up bar. It's almost like a bench dip, except your legs and feet are in the air.

This is one of the hardest dip variations, so make sure you are comfortable with the previous progressions before attempting the Korean dip. As it is difficult to control your body from this angle, you'll really need to focus on engaging your abs and lower back muscles. You'll likely find that your legs will need to reach behind the bar as you lower down in order to remain stable. As such, it helps to keep your hamstrings and glutes contracted. There is also a mobility component to the Korean dip, as having the bar behind your back can give your shoulders a deep stretch as well. Feel free to experiment with both overhand as well as underhand grips when practicing Korean dips.

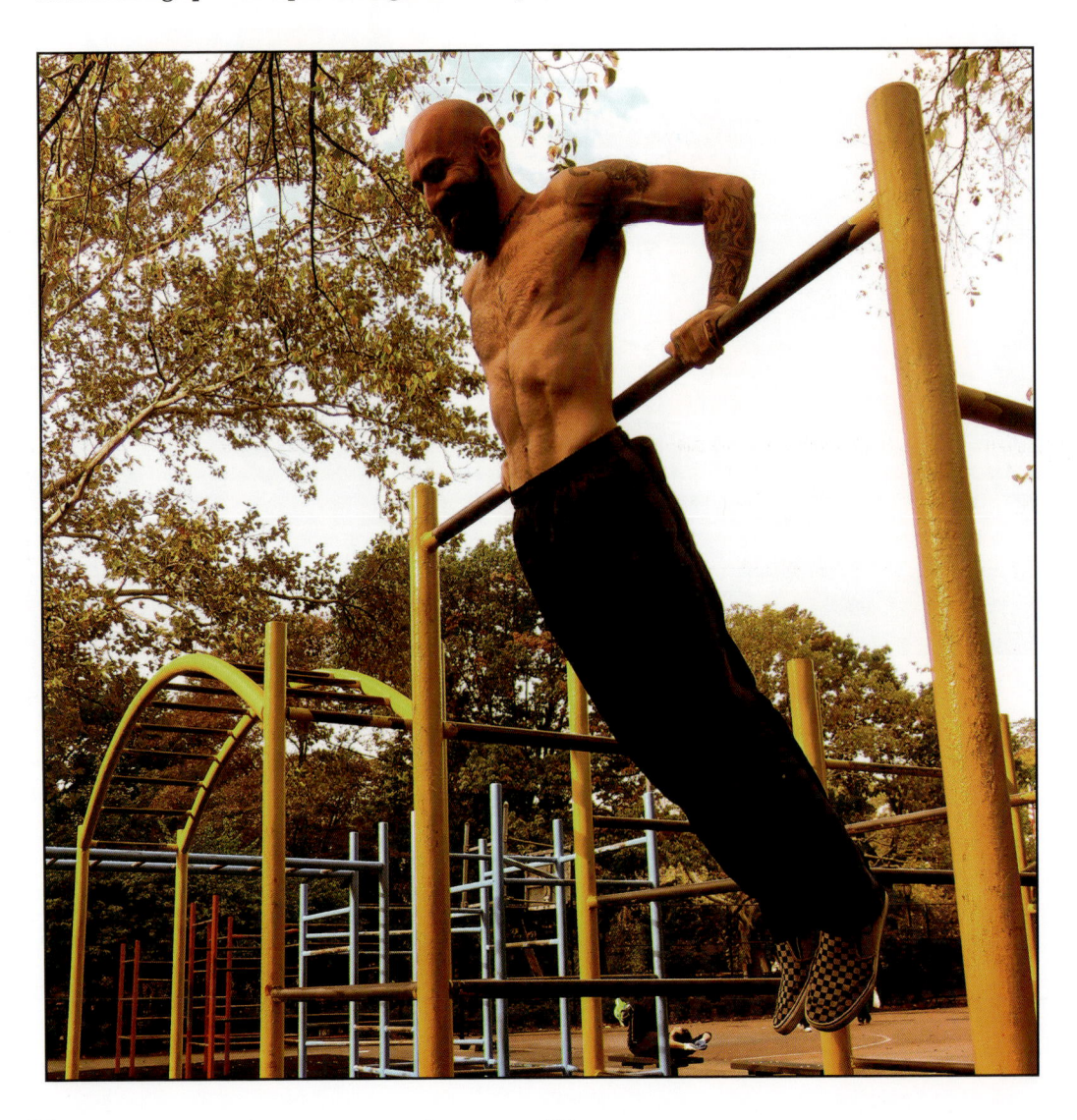

The Plyo-Matrix Explosive Dips

Like its cousin the push-up, the dip can also be done in an explosive fashion. Not only is it important to have a solid foundation in classic dips before embarking on plyometric dips, it's also recommended that you have strong, conditioned hands before taking this path. Usually, when someone tries a plyometric dip for the first time, they are shocked at how jarring it is, due to the amount of impact that has to be absorbed by the wrists and hands.

The basic plyometric dip simply involves lifting your hands off the dip bars at the top of the repetition, then placing them back down before the next rep. The difficulty (and yields) can be increased by lifting your hands higher in the air. This naturally will challenge you to get more height from your body so you will need to generate extra force. You can even include a clap at the top.

Beyond that, advanced variations include "hopping" across the dip bars on your hands, or even generating enough height and explosiveness to rotate your body 180 degrees, so that you wind up facing the opposite direction from which you started.

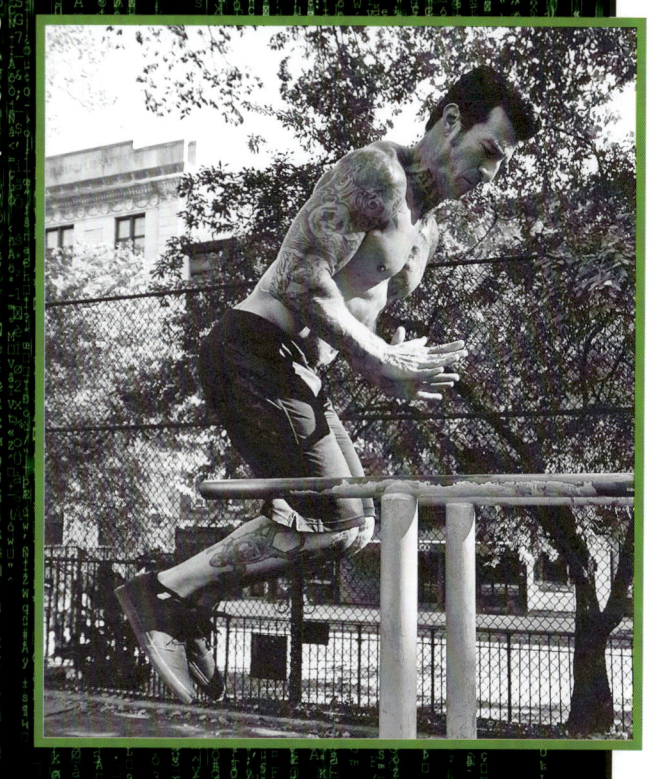

Street Workout

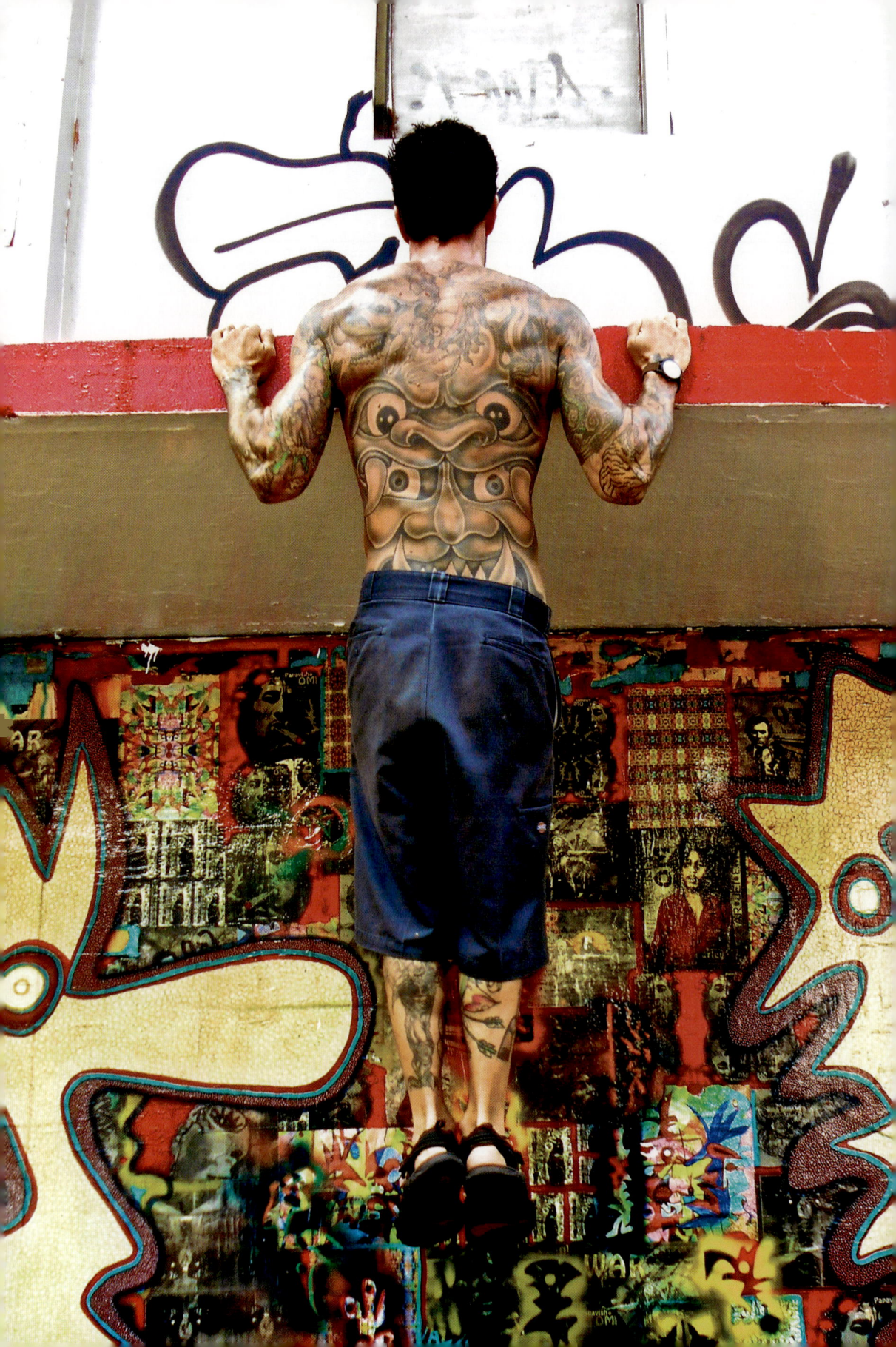

CHAPTER 5

Pull

When we were coming up, the question, "How much can you bench?" was very much en vogue, with little attention paid to the back muscles. You could say upper body pulling power is often underrated in traditional strength training. Even those in the gym who were focused on pulling used strange lat pull-down machines and cable rowing devices to work their backs. Quite the opposite of Street Workout, huh? Let's be perfectly clear about one thing: there is no substitute for the pull-up.

Beyond the realm of fitness, we as a culture spend a lot of time leaning forward at desks, on mobile communication devices or driving automobiles, causing our chests to sink in and our spines to curve. Balance is a key component of training and health. When we are constantly pushing forward, it becomes even more important to pull. Pull-ups help to restore and maintain this balance to your upper body.

The following exercises are divided into two categories: Horizontal Pull and Overhead Pull. Though we are dealing with two different planes of motion, all of the following pulling exercises use the biceps when you flex at the elbow and the muscles of the upper back (lats, traps and rhomboids) as you pull your elbows back behind you or toward your sides. Horizontal pulling is when you pull your hands toward your chest, without your arms ever going above your head. Overhead pulling is any pull that begins hanging from an overhead structure.

HORIZONTAL PULL PROGRESSIONS

Horizontal pulls are often touted as a progression leading up to the vertical. However, they also stand alone as viable exercises in their own right. Because it is a different plane of motion, this movement pattern works the muscles from a different angle. The following Australian (Aussie) pull-ups belong in everybody's program before, during and even after they are capable of performing overhead pull-ups.

AUSSIE PULL-UP

Get down under a bar that's about waist height with your legs extended so you form a straight line from your head to your heels. Grip tightly and brace your entire body as you pull your chest toward the bar. Lower yourself back to the bottom with control. Like the push-up, be careful not to bend your hips or shrug your shoulders. Dig your heels into the ground for traction if you are starting to slide.

To make the Aussie pull-up more accessible to beginners, use a bar that is chest height instead of waist height, which will allow for more favorable leverage.

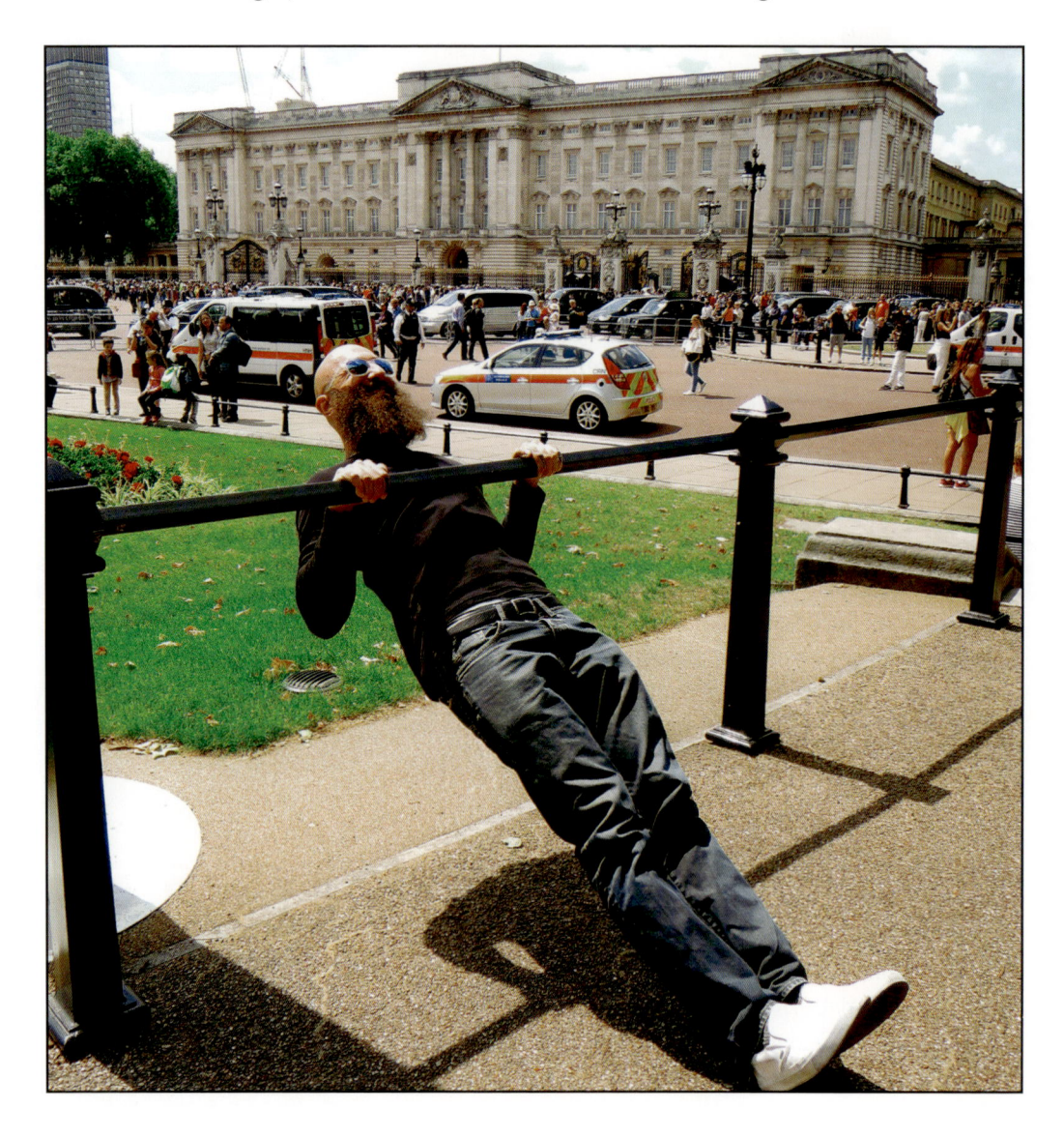

BENT KNEE AUSSIE

Just as bending your knees and shortening your body length makes a push-up less difficult, bending your knees during an Aussie pull-up will have the same effect. In addition to improving your leverage, bending your knees will also allow you to press with your feet if you need to assist your upper-body.

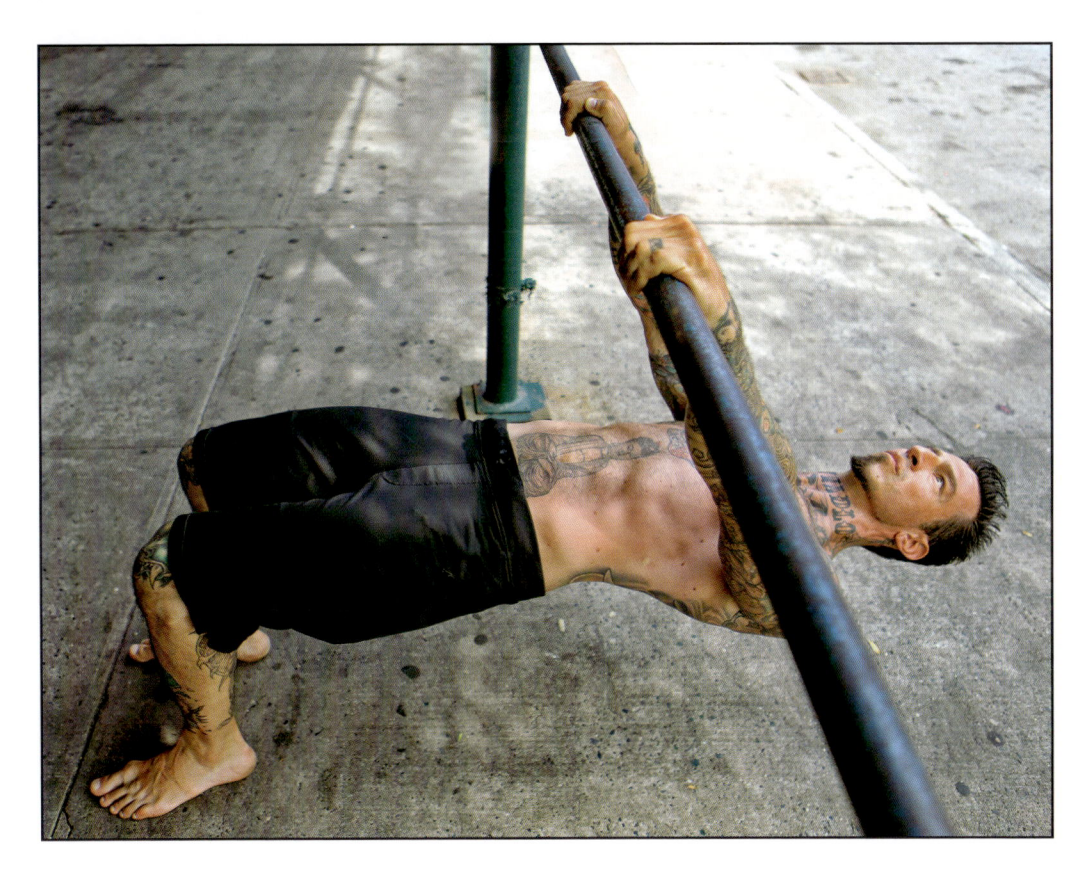

WIDE GRIP AUSSIE

A wide hand position will result in greater activation of your back muscles, with slightly less biceps recruitment. You can expect to feel this variation more in the rhomboids, lats and traps.

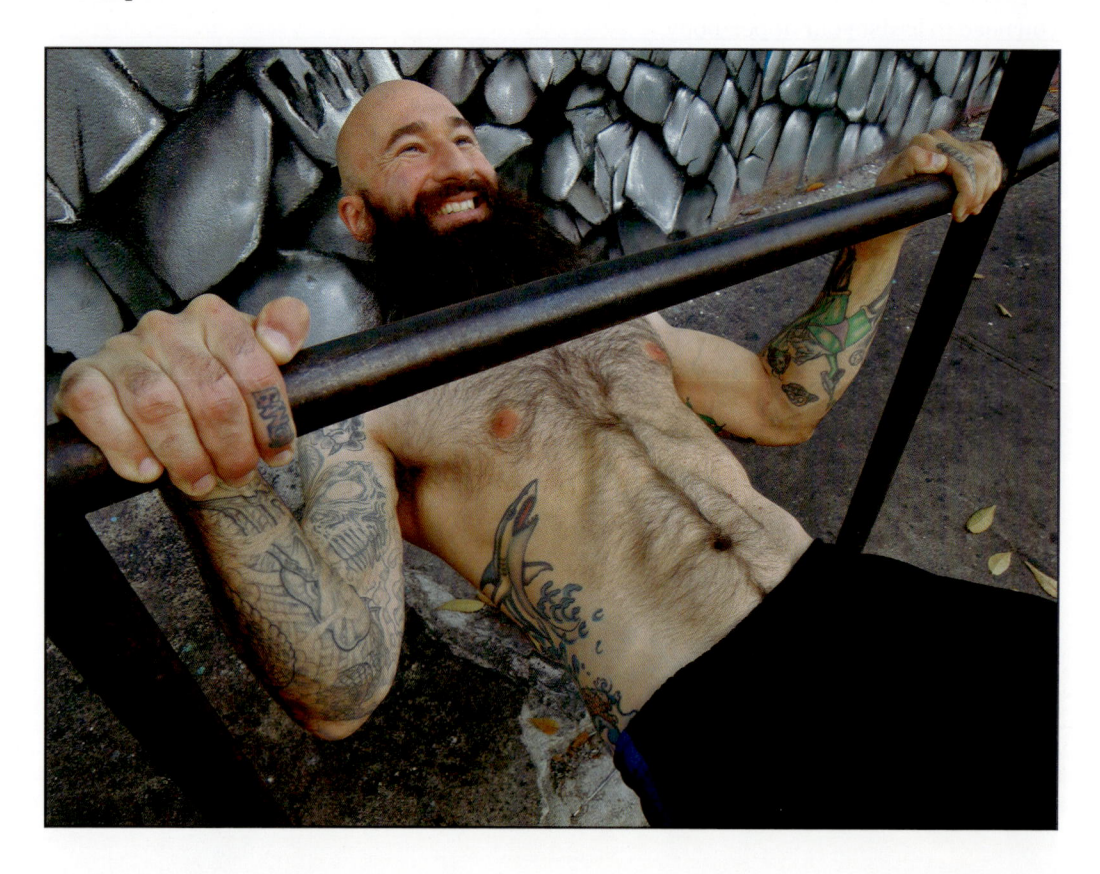

NARROW GRIP AUSSIE

Bringing your hands closer together during an Aussie pull-up will change the subtleties of muscle recruitment. You may feel more activation in your forearms and biceps. The narrow grip will also require some additional wrist mobility.

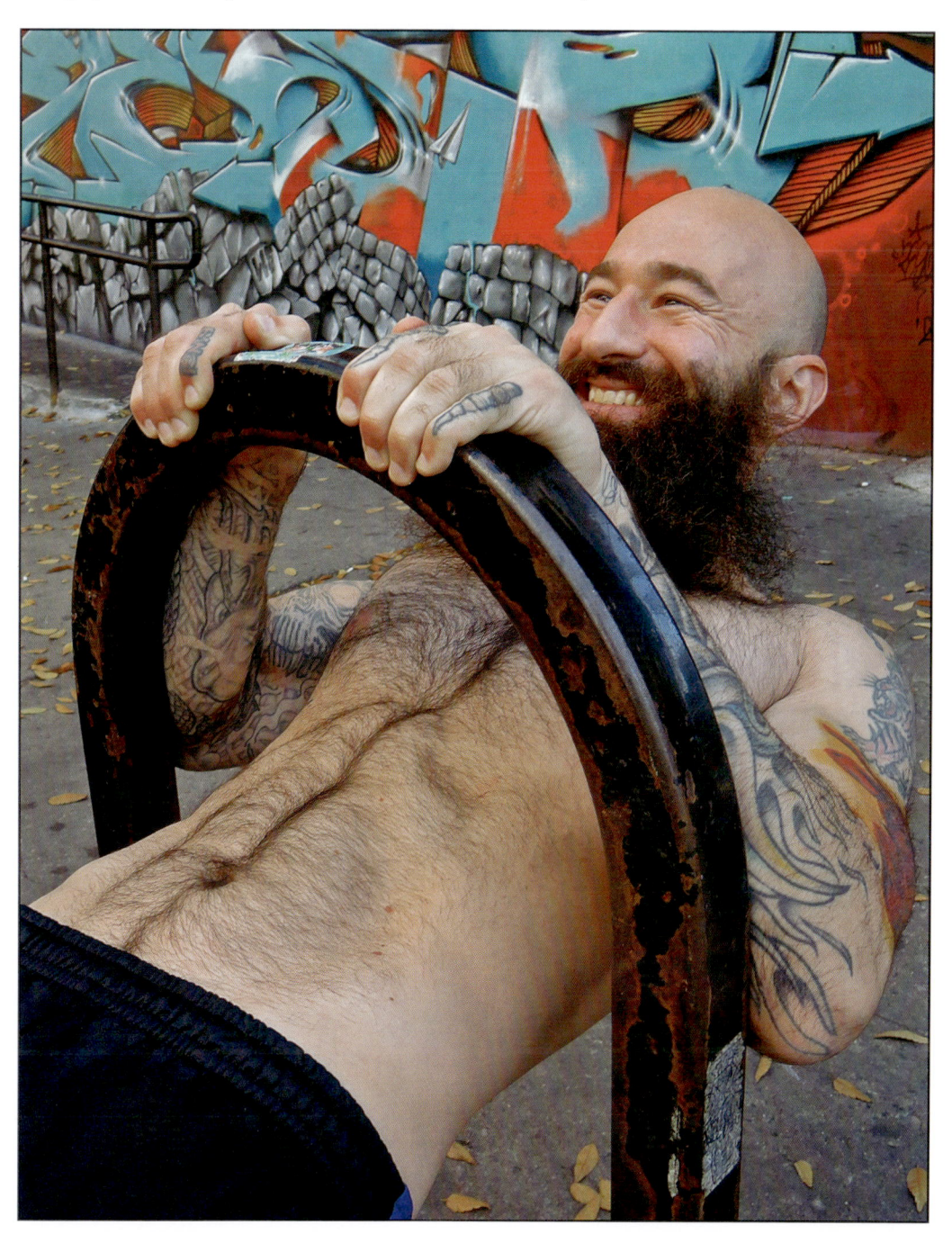

NEUTRAL GRIP AUSSIE

For some people, performing Aussie pull-ups with the hands facing each other can be more comfortable on the shoulder and elbow joints. You will need two parallel bars in order to perform this variation, which is known as a neutral grip Aussie pull-up. Dip bars work nicely. Even if you don't have any issues with standard Aussie pull-ups, give these a try to hit your muscles from a slightly different angle.

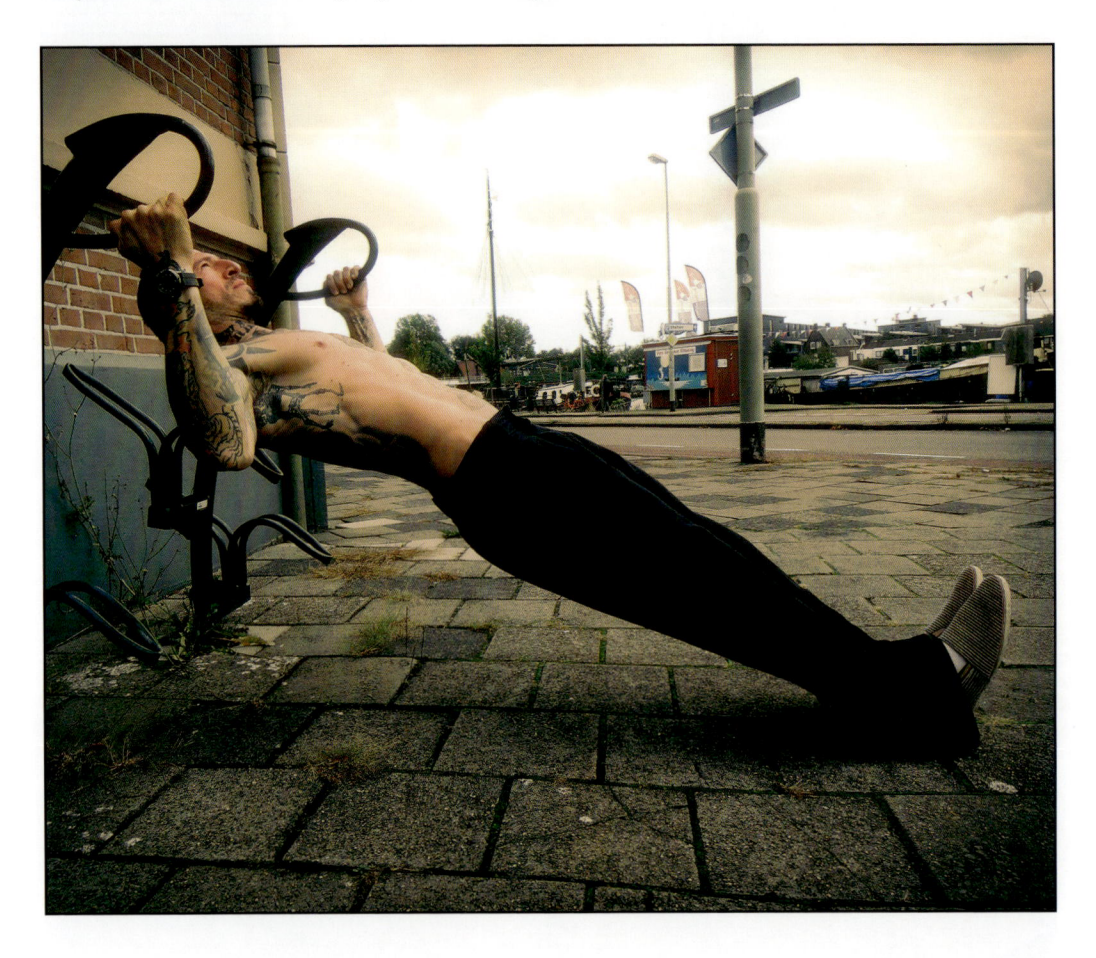

FEET ELEVATED AUSSIE

Just as a higher bar will make the Aussie pull-up easier, if you want to make your Aussie pull-up more difficult, you can use a lower bar. At a certain point, however, if the bar is too low then you'll wind up on the floor when you extend your arms. The fix for this is elevating your feet on a bench or another bar. The higher your feet get in relation to your hands, the more difficult the exercise becomes.

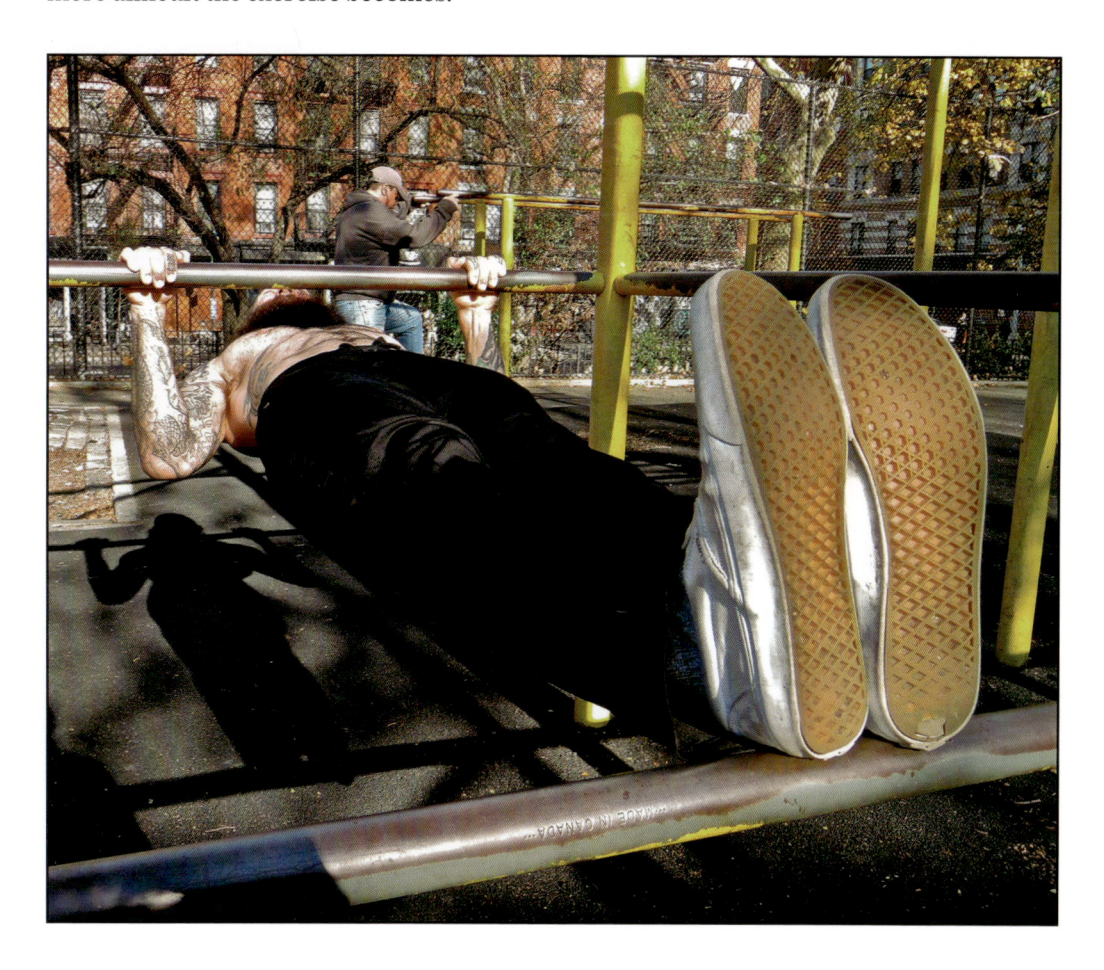

ARCHER AUSSIE

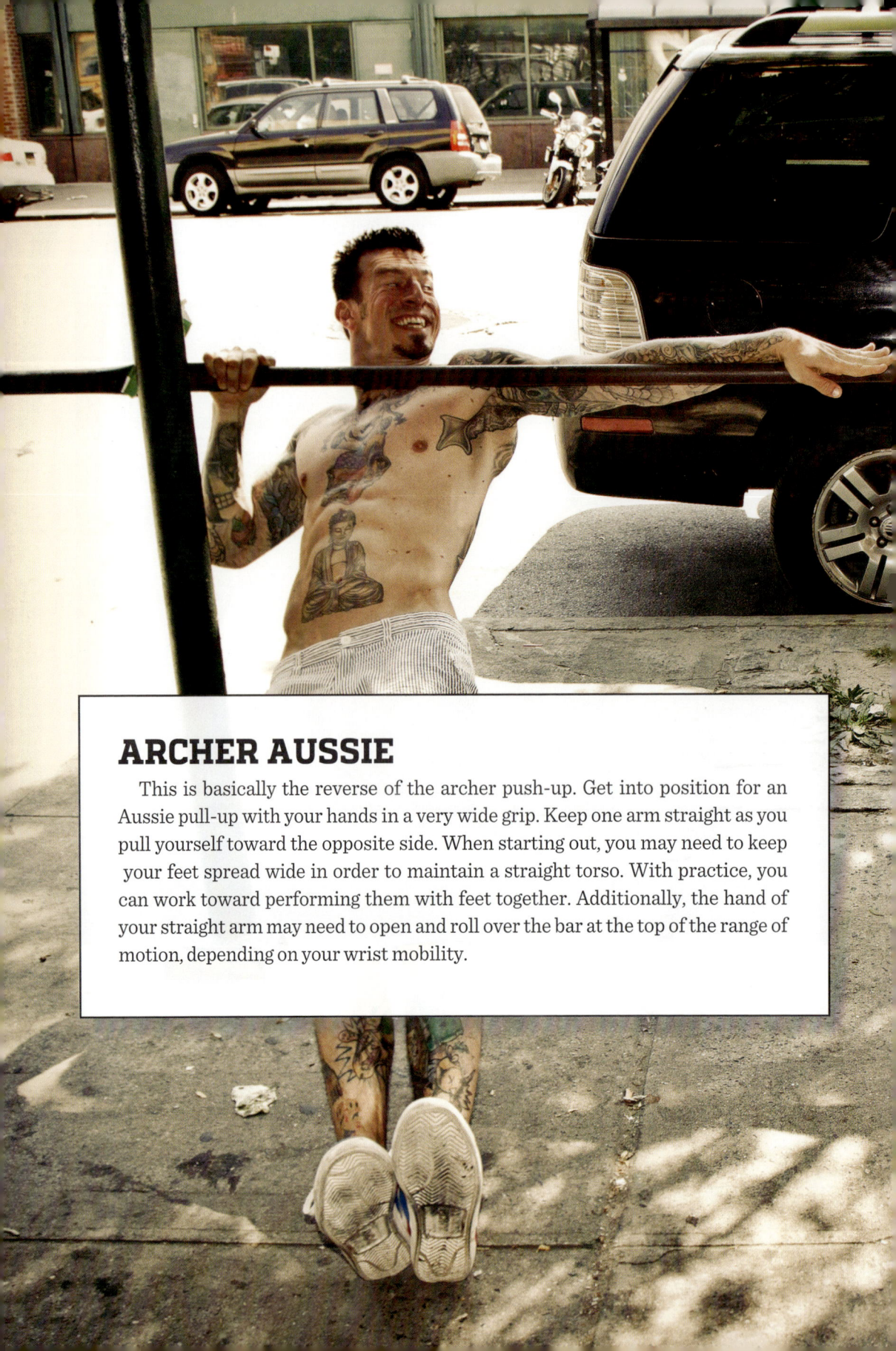

This is basically the reverse of the archer push-up. Get into position for an Aussie pull-up with your hands in a very wide grip. Keep one arm straight as you pull yourself toward the opposite side. When starting out, you may need to keep your feet spread wide in order to maintain a straight torso. With practice, you can work toward performing them with feet together. Additionally, the hand of your straight arm may need to open and roll over the bar at the top of the range of motion, depending on your wrist mobility.

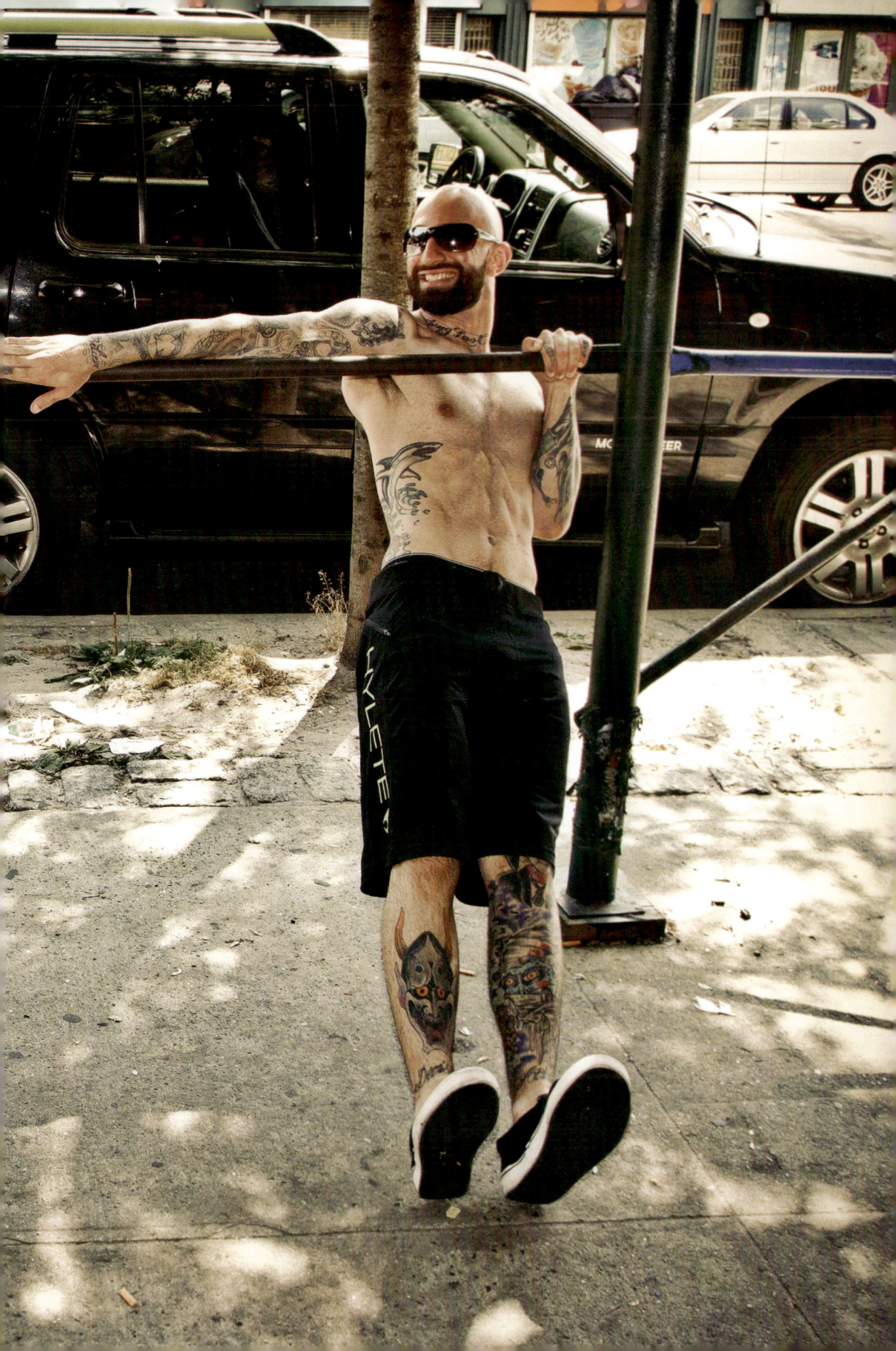

ONE ARM AUSSIE PULL-UP

Get into position for a narrow grip Aussie pull-up, then widen your legs into a straddle stance. Remove one arm and place it against your side. The pulling arm should be kept closer to the center of your body than in a two arm Aussie. Brace your entire body and begin pulling your chest toward the bar. As is often the case with single-limb exercises, do your best to avoid rotating your torso, but be prepared that a small amount of twisting at the trunk may be unavoidable.

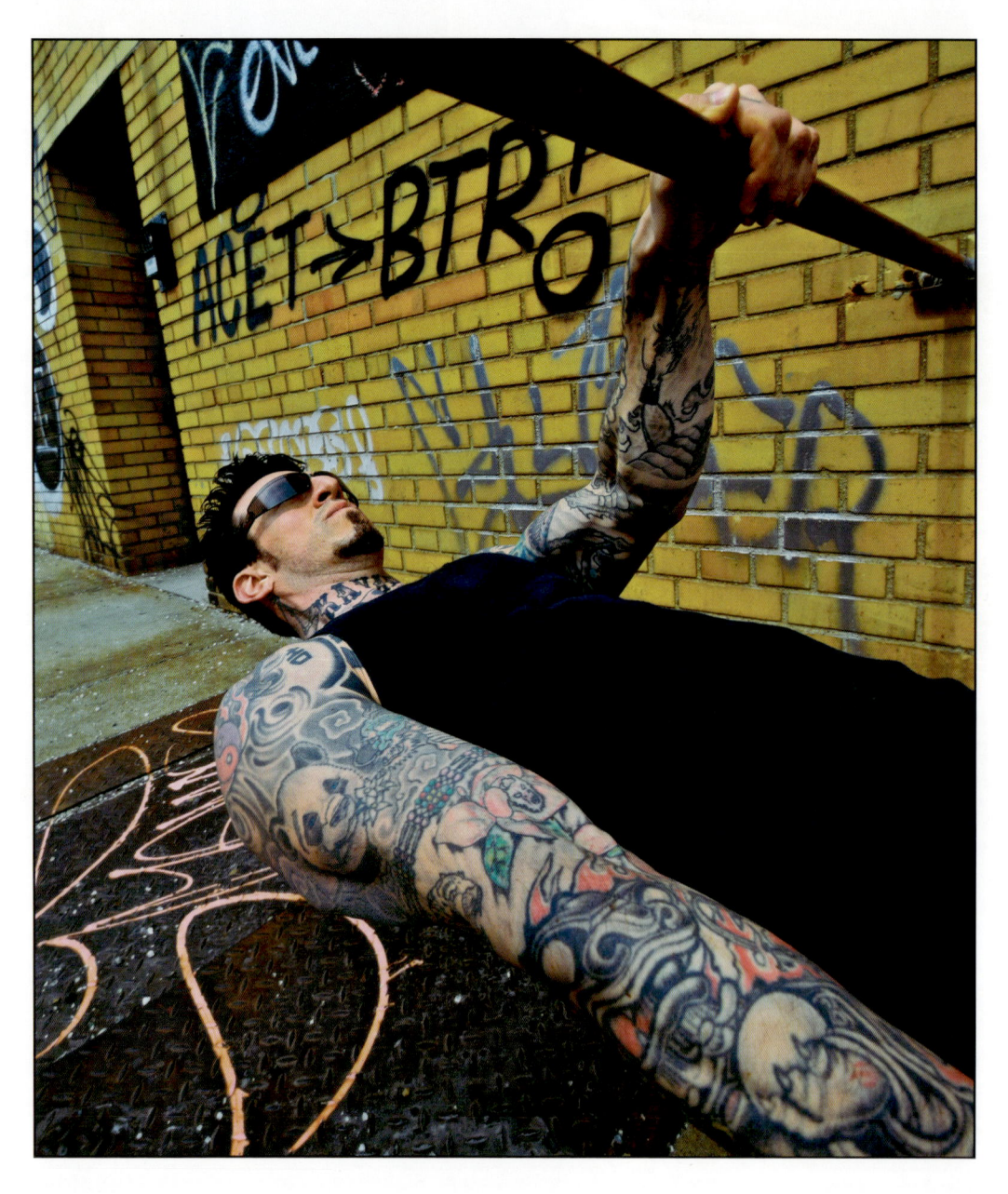

"CALLOUS-THENICS"

When you train Street Workout, you work way more than just your muscles. You strengthen your tendons, ligaments, bones and cartilage. And don't forget the largest organ of your body... the skin!

Your hands are going to toughen up when you hit the bars and you will develop callouses. This is a good thing. If you're worried about the appearance of your hands, just remind yourself how much better the rest of your body looks.

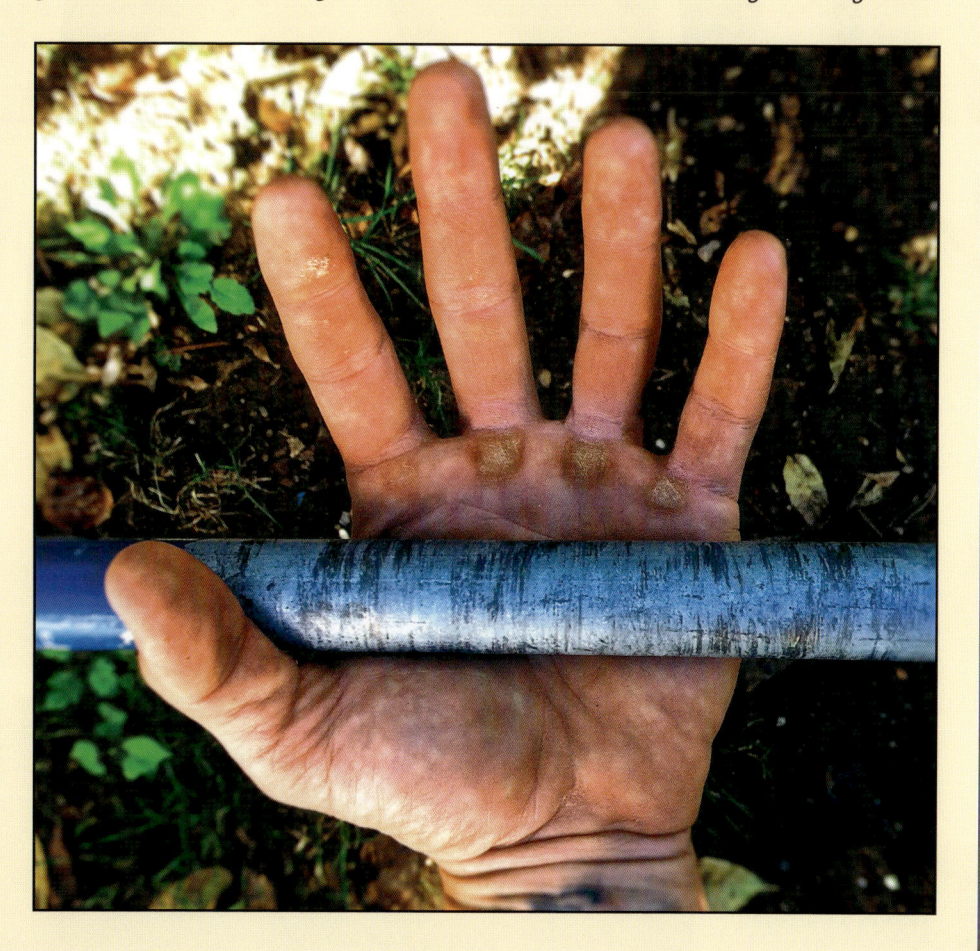

This is a bar hang.

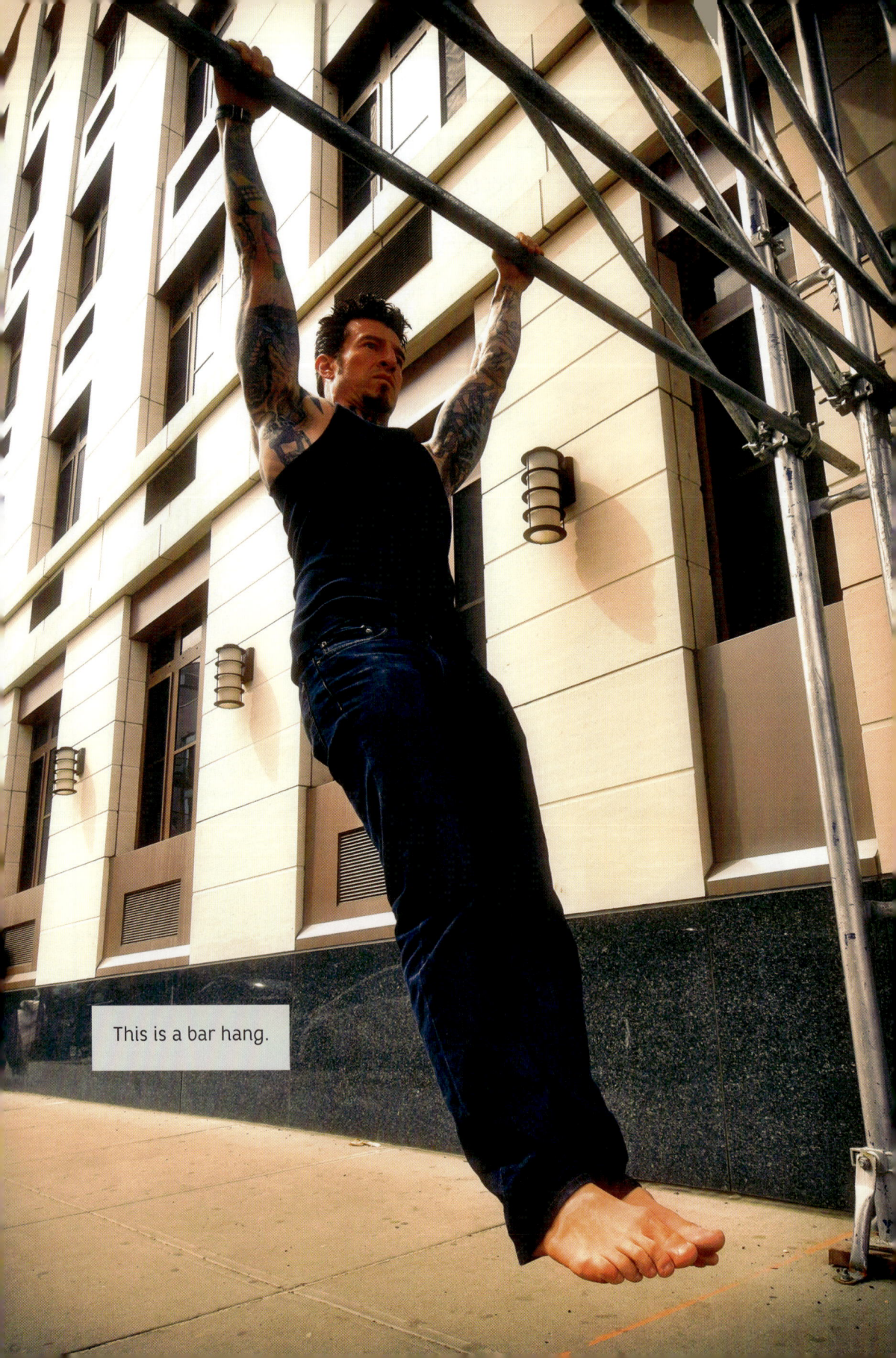

OVERHEAD PULL PROGRESSIONS

The overhead pull is the most universal exercise of the entire Street Workout movement. The pull-up and all its forms embody the true minimalistic spirit of calisthenics and employ the full body, not to mention the heart, soul and spirit. Any time you use your arms to pull yourself up while hanging from an overhead apparatus, you are doing a pull-up, the foundation of all advanced bar moves and one of the greatest exercises in the history of human movement. We're all here for the pull-ups!

BAR HANG

The most foundational move in bar calisthenics is the basic two-arm hang. Grasp an overhead bar tightly with an overhand grip while you keep your shoulder-blades pulled down and back. Engage your abs and think about tucking your pelvis forward, like you would in a plank or hollow body position. Just as the plank is a good starting point for learning to do a push-up, this is a great starting point for beginners who are working toward their first pull-up.

FLEX HANG

A flex hang (or flexed arm hang) involves holding yourself at the top of a pull-up with your chin over the bar. Once you get comfortable with straight arm bar hangs, this is the next step toward a full pull-up.

If you're new to the world of pull-up bar training, begin with an underhand grip. As you get stronger you can progress to an overhand grip, which most people will find more difficult.

Use a partner, a step or simply jump in order to get into position. Then hold your chin above the bar for time. If you can hold this position for even a few seconds, you are well on your way.

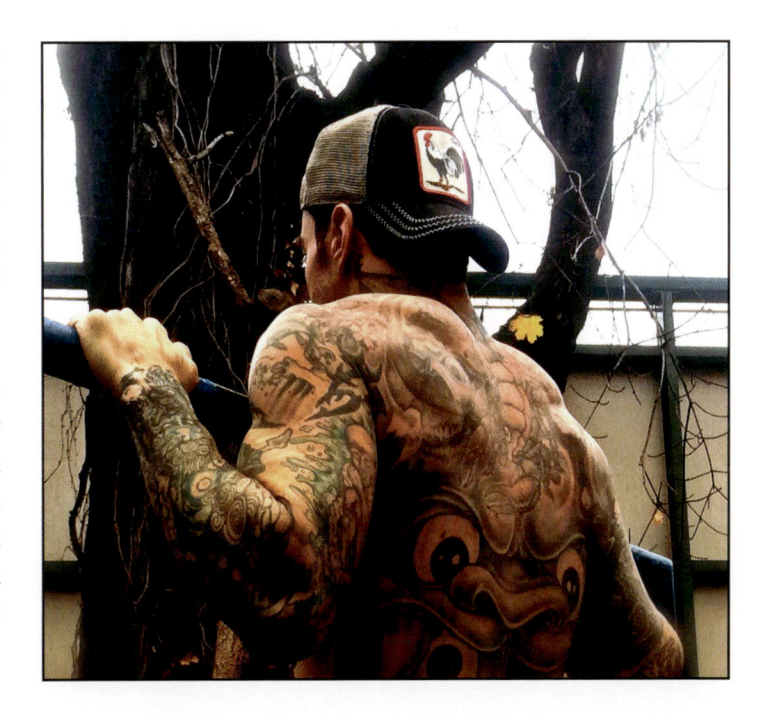

STREET WORKOUT

NEGATIVE PULL-UP

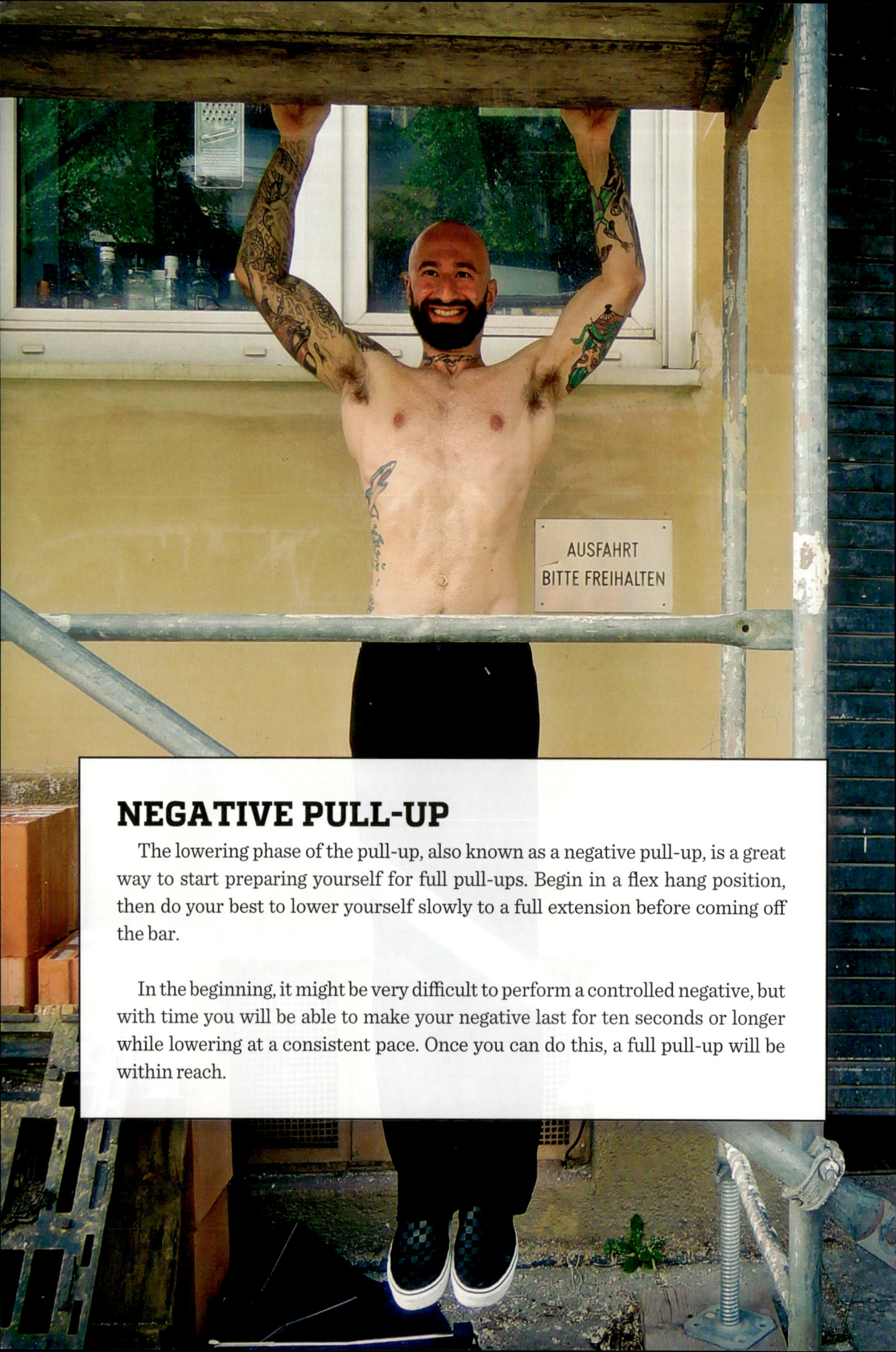

The lowering phase of the pull-up, also known as a negative pull-up, is a great way to start preparing yourself for full pull-ups. Begin in a flex hang position, then do your best to lower yourself slowly to a full extension before coming off the bar.

In the beginning, it might be very difficult to perform a controlled negative, but with time you will be able to make your negative last for ten seconds or longer while lowering at a consistent pace. Once you can do this, a full pull-up will be within reach.

PULL-UP/CHIN-UP

Grasp an overhead bar with your palms facing away from your body. Brace your trunk, pulling down and back through your scapulae as you bend your arms and pull your chest toward the bar. Lower yourself back down with control, being mindful to keep your abs engaged in order to avoid swinging. Your legs should remain straight and together throughout the entire range of motion, but beginners may want to cross their ankles in order to generate more tension. Though you obviously have to lean back a bit to avoid hitting your head on the bar, your torso shouldn't have to travel very far forward or backward.

As with the flex hang, most people will find starting out with an underhand grip (aka chin-up) to be less difficult. The disparity is due to the shift in muscle recruitment. The underhand grip allows you to use your arms more, while the overhand grip forces you to engage the muscles of your upper back to a greater degree (though both exercises work both muscle groups). Start with chin-ups, then begin to work on pull-ups after you can do several in a row, With time and practice, the disparity between the underhand and overhand grips will start to even out.

Also note that it's normal for your grip to be narrower in an underhand chin-up than in an overhand pull-up. For chin-ups, the hands should be placed just narrower than the shoulders; the standard overhand width is just wider than the shoulders.

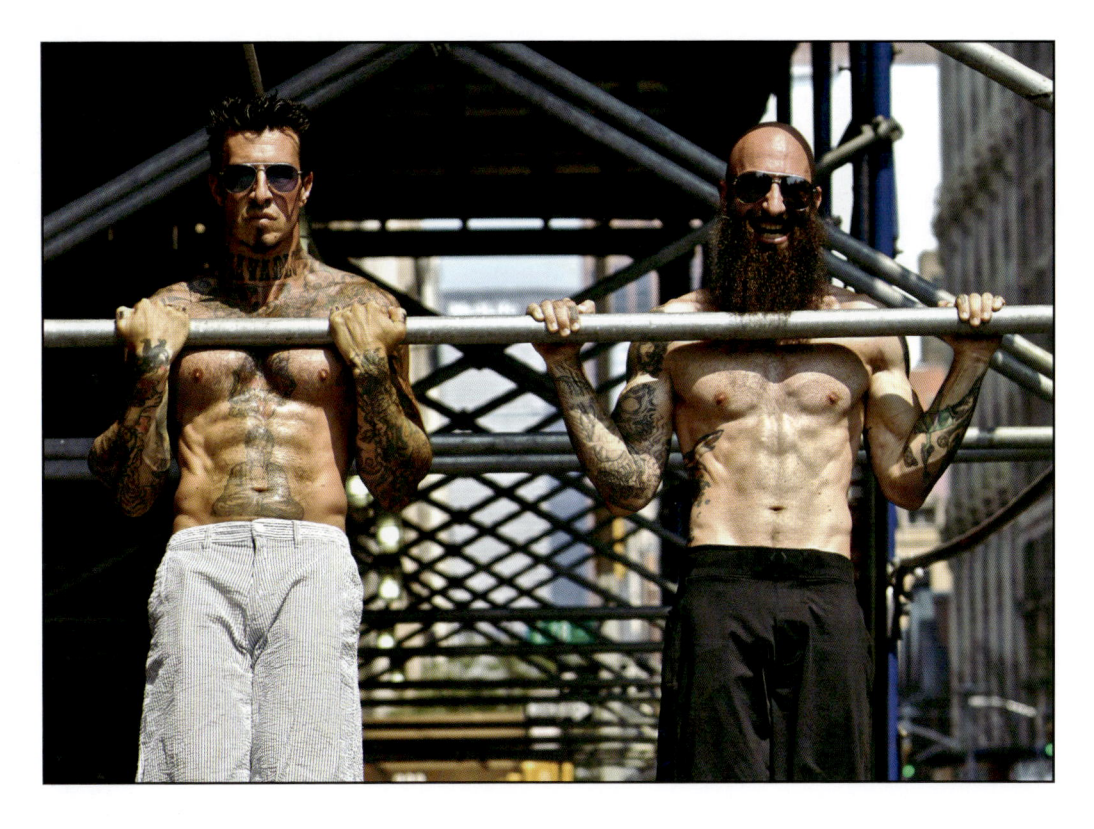

STREET WORKOUT

WIDE GRIP PULL-UP

As your grip gets wider, the amount of elbow flexion decreases, putting greater emphasis on the lats and other upper-back muscles. As such, most people will find wide pull-ups to be more difficult than the standard variety.

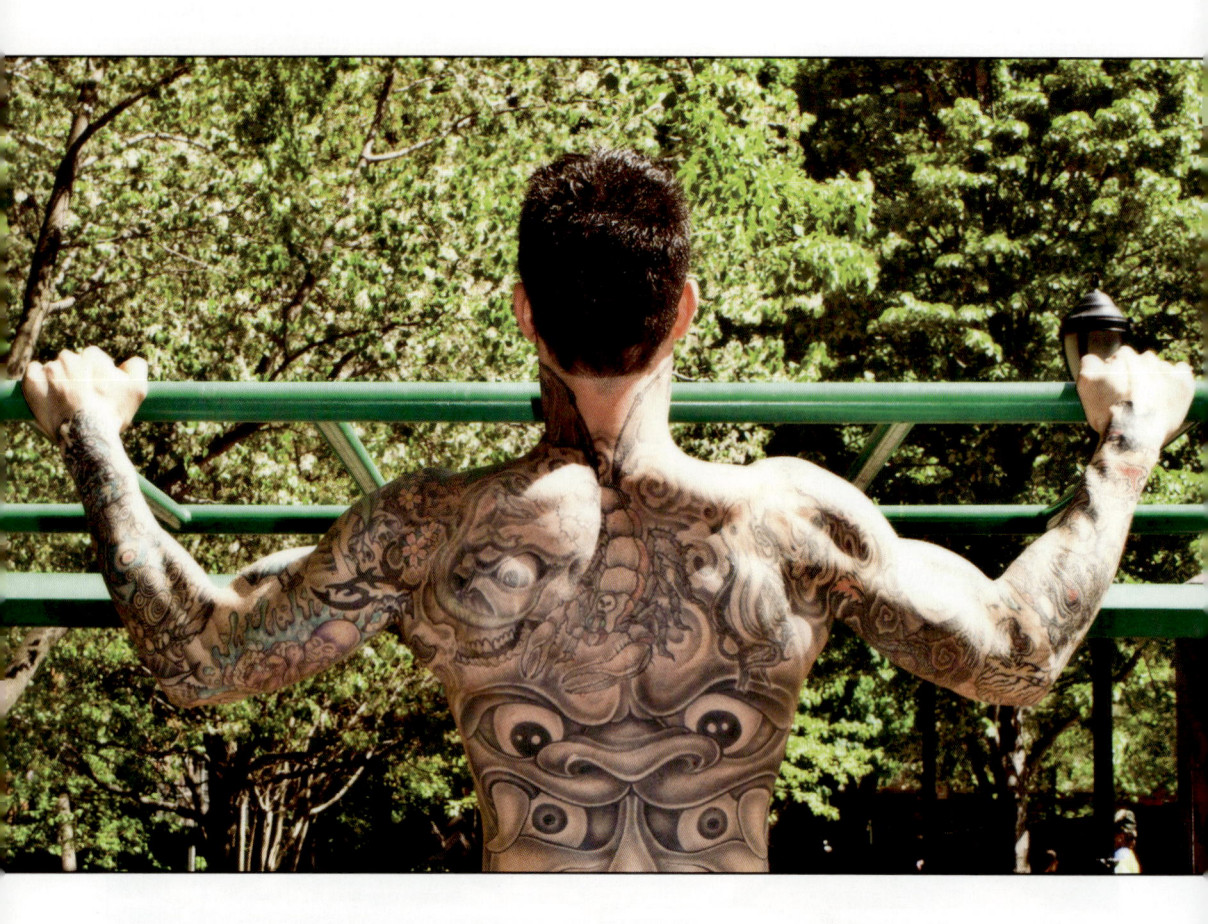

NARROW GRIP PULL-UP

Just like with push-ups, you are encouraged to play around with hand placement once you get comfortable with classic pull-ups and chin-ups. You will find that going narrower will place a bit more emphasis on the arms, particularly the biceps and forearms.

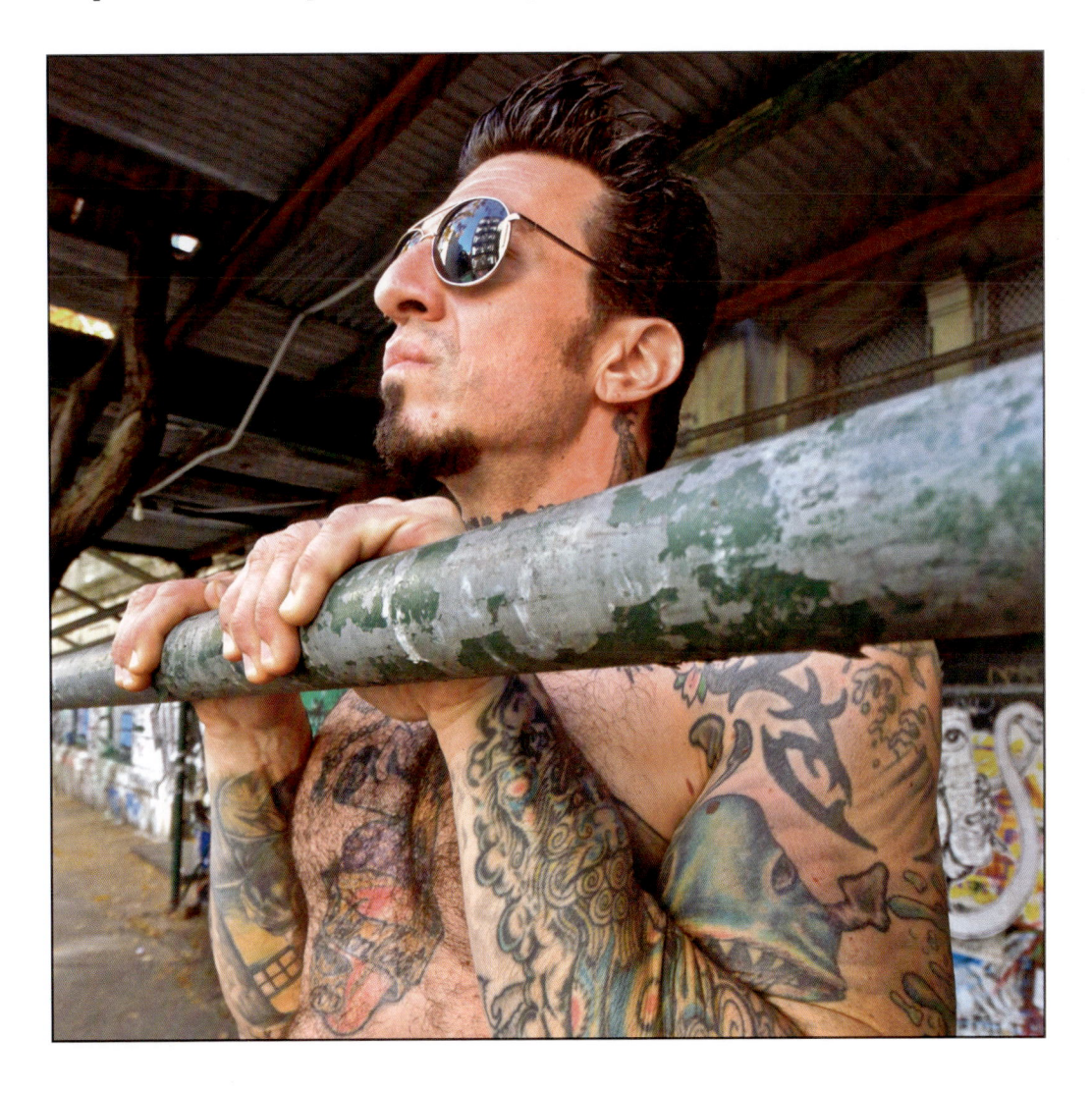

MIXED GRIP PULL-UP

A mixed grip pull-up involves one hand holding the bar with an overhand grip while the other hand is turned under. This variation can make for an interesting stability challenge as you try to keep your torso stable and facing forward. It can also be a useful tool for beginners who may be having a hard time transitioning from chin-ups to pull-ups.

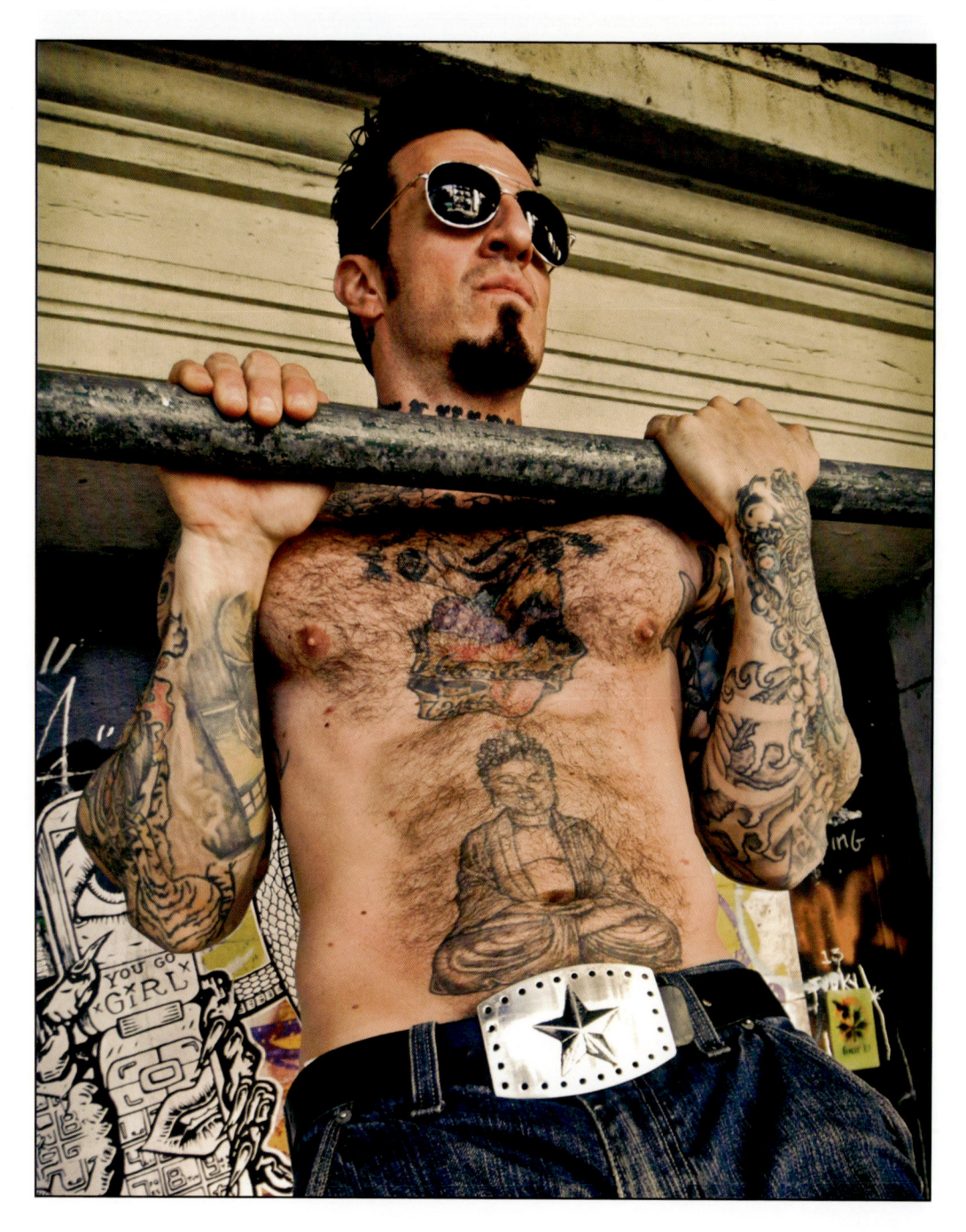

NEUTRAL GRIP PULL-UP

For some people, performing pull-ups with the hands facing each other can be more comfortable on the shoulder and elbow joints compared to either a palms-facing or palms-away grip. You will need two overhead bars that are parallel to each other in order to perform this variation, which is known as a neutral grip pull-up. Even if you don't have any issues with standard pull-ups, give neutral pull-ups a try to hit your muscles from a slightly different angle.

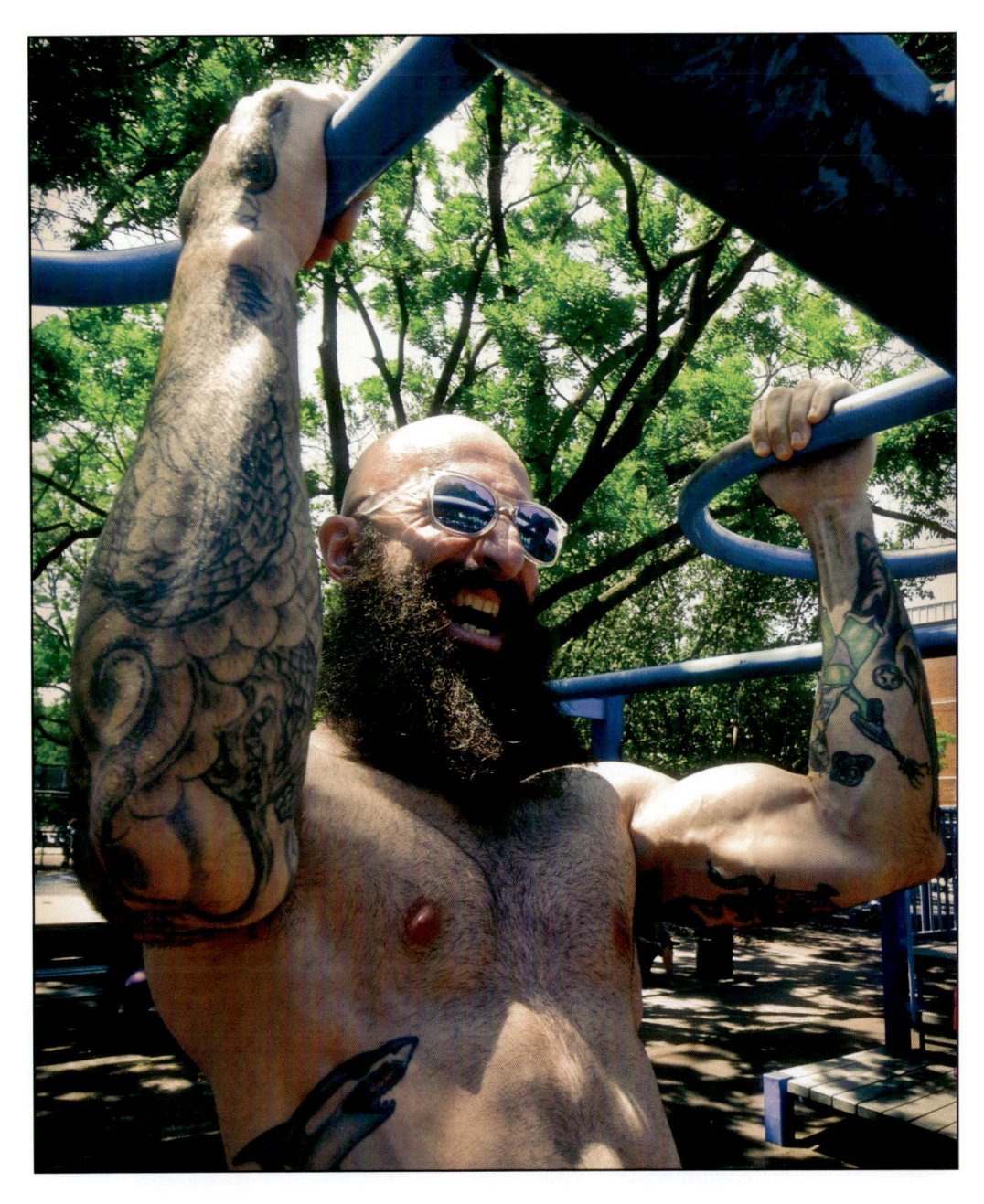

COMMANDO PULL-UP

A commando pull-up is similar to a neutral grip pull-up, except both hands are holding a single bar in a narrow grip. As such, your body will be in the same plane as the bar. This means you will have to pull yourself toward the side on the way up, which creates a unique challenge. Make sure to alternate which side of the bar your head passes with each rep.

It's also good to practice switching the position of your hands on alternating sets with variations like mixed grip and commando pull-ups. For example, if your right hand is closer to your face on the first set, keep your left hand closer on set number two. For this reason, aim to do an even number of sets if using this variation in your regimen.

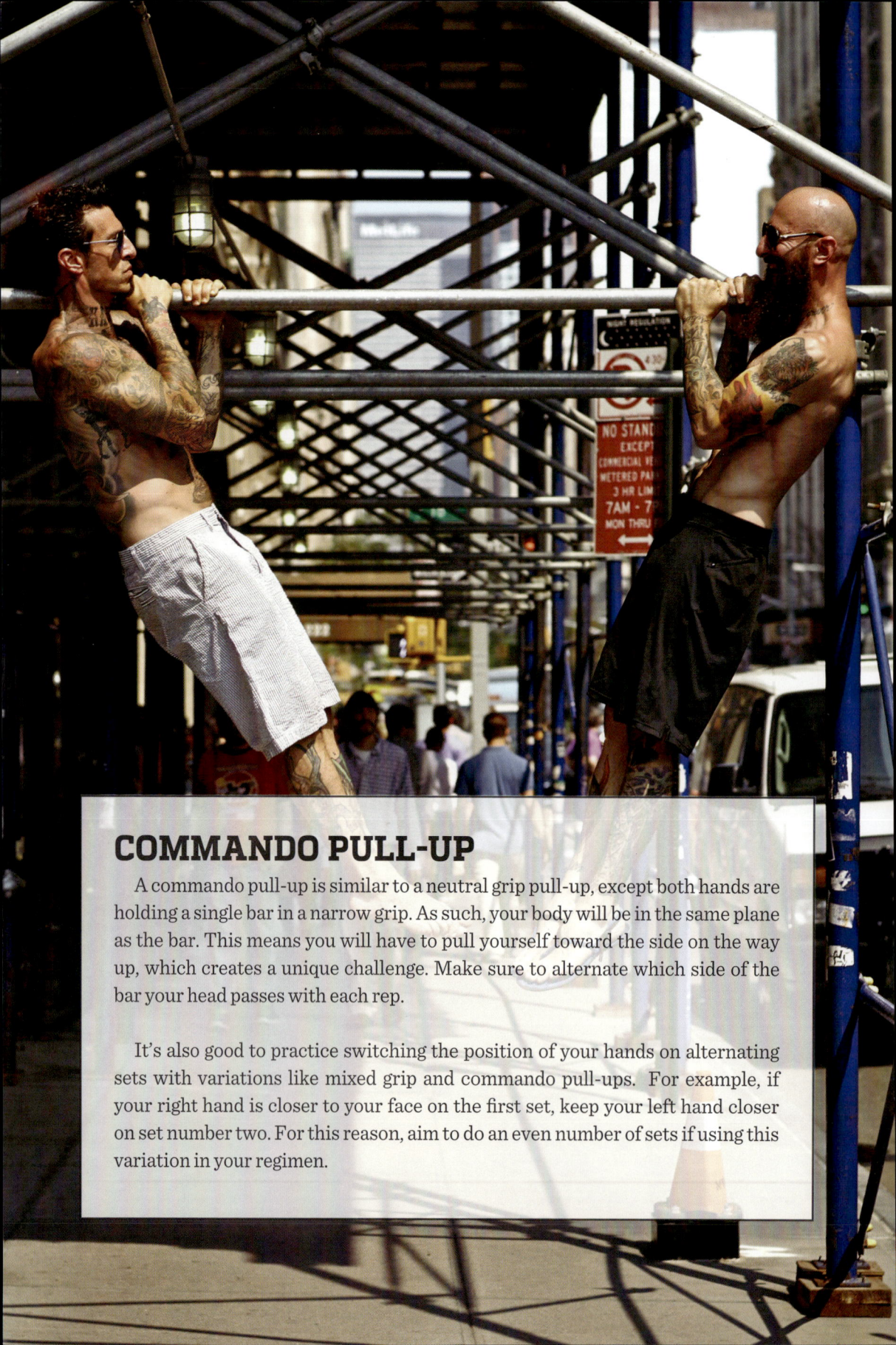

BUILD A MONSTER GRIP

As for pull-ups and all bar moves, there is no doubt that the surface from which you pull makes a difference. Fatter bars yield more grip strength. In the wild world of Street Workout, any surface is fair game so be prepared to also work your skin, bones and connective tissue, in addition to your muscles. You will find many objects unique unto themselves when you get creative!

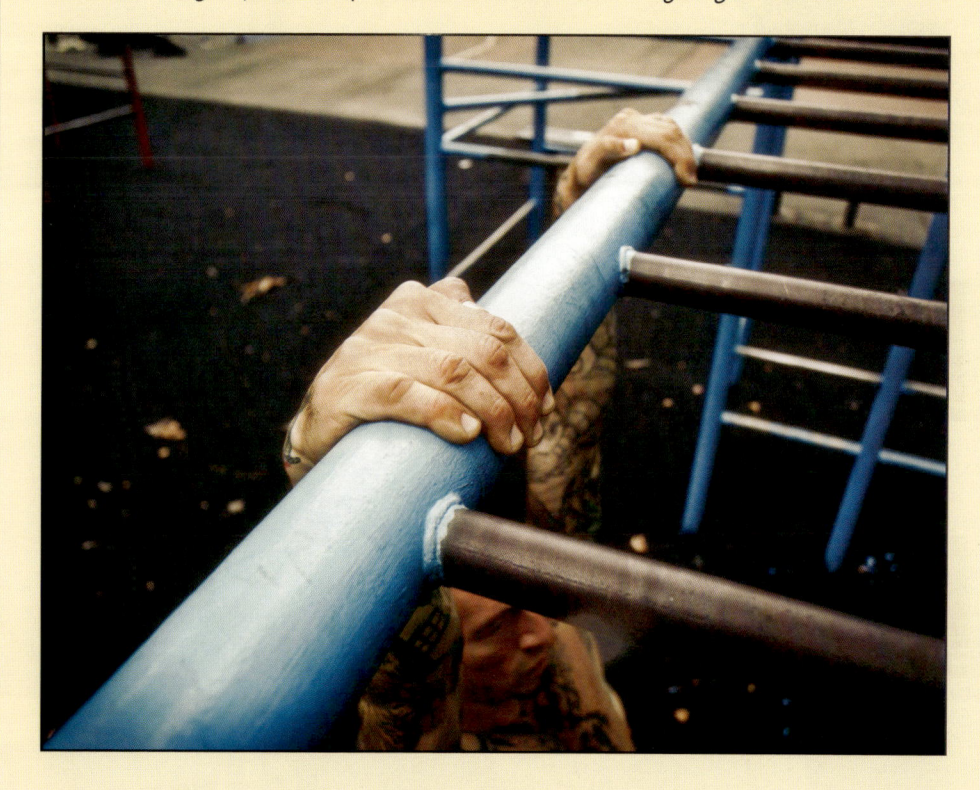

HEADBANGER PULL-UP

The headbanger pull-up begins with your chin just below the bar. From here the objective is to extend your body away from the bar while reaching your legs out to counterbalance. Almost like a bodyweight biceps curl, the headbanger pull-up is also a great core exercise.

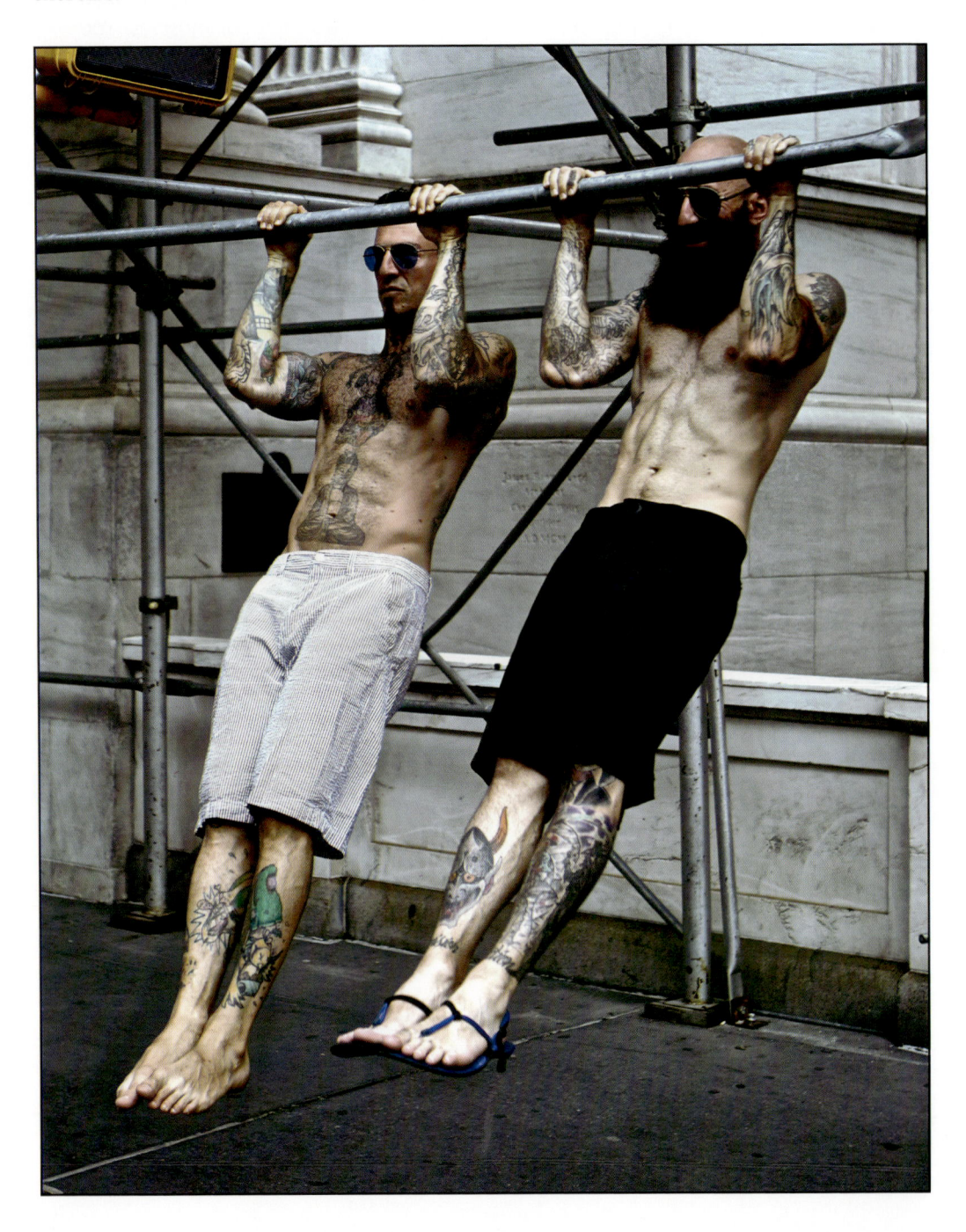

BEHIND THE NECK PULL-UP

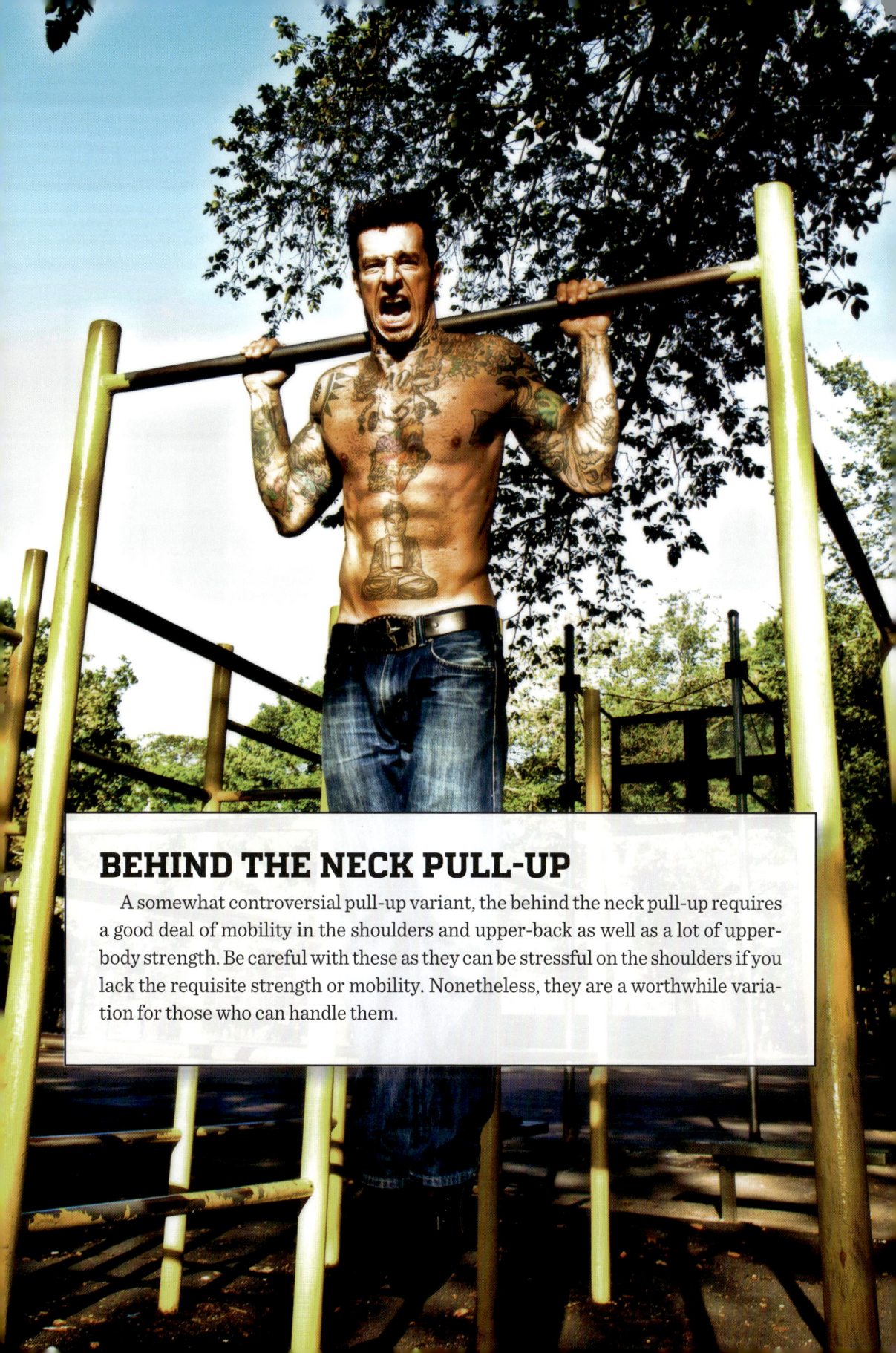

A somewhat controversial pull-up variant, the behind the neck pull-up requires a good deal of mobility in the shoulders and upper-back as well as a lot of upper-body strength. Be careful with these as they can be stressful on the shoulders if you lack the requisite strength or mobility. Nonetheless, they are a worthwhile variation for those who can handle them.

L PULL-UP

Keeping your legs at a 90 degree angle to your body while performing pull-ups adds a tremendous amount of difficulty to an already challenging exercise. Your abs, hip flexors and quadriceps will have to work extra hard to maintain this position as you pull yourself up. Additionally, the balance will change throughout the range of motion, forcing you to go slowly in order to maintain control.

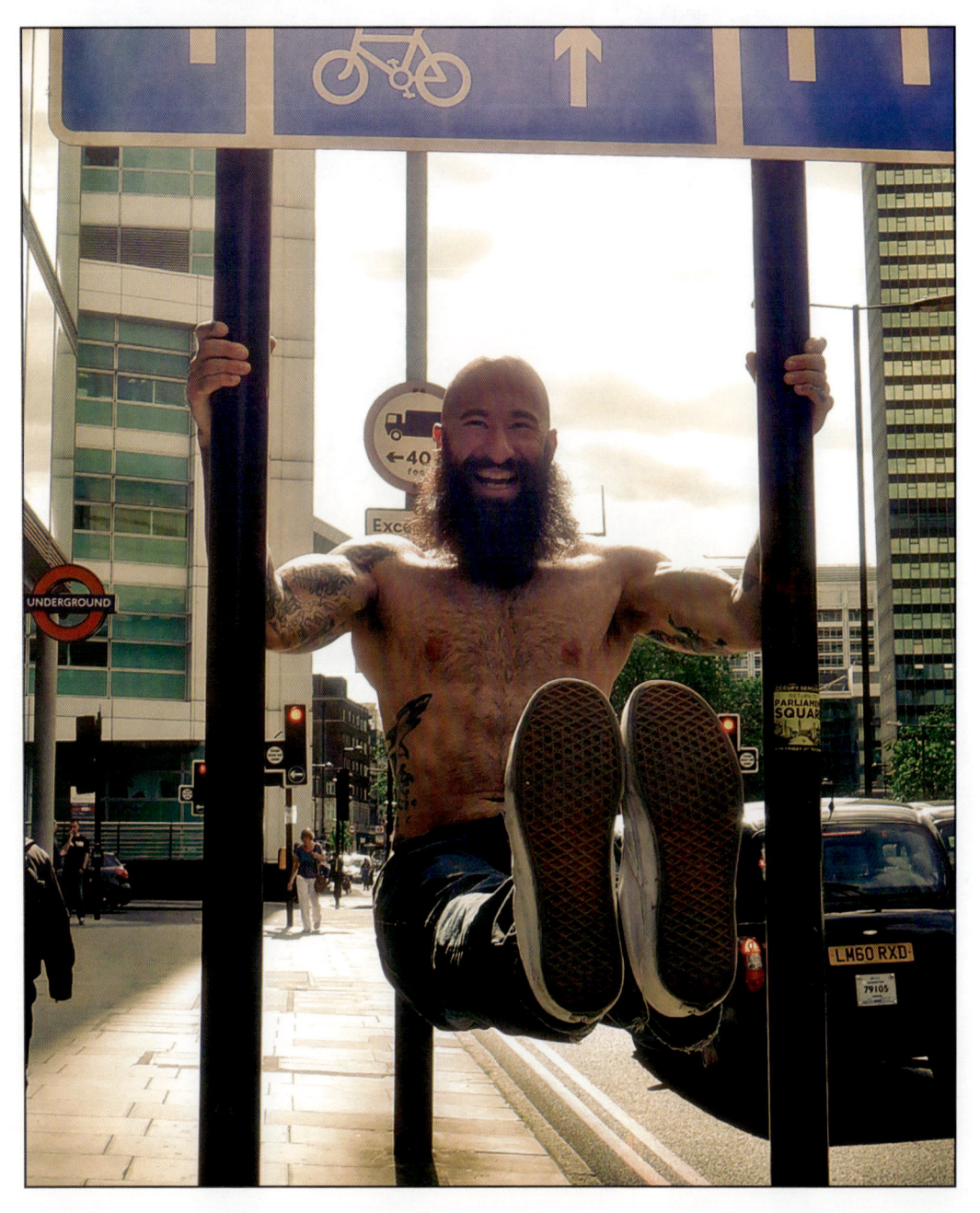

ARCHER PULL-UP

The archer pull-up is an advanced variation that involves keeping one arm straight while relying primarily on the opposite side to do the bulk of the pulling. Begin like you're performing a very wide pull-up, but bend only one of your arms as you pull your chin over the bar. This means your torso will shift toward that side while the opposite arm stays straight. You'll need to reach your legs slightly to the side to counterbalance. The hand of your straight arm may need to open and roll over the bar at the top of the range of motion, depending on your wrist mobility.

If you are unable to perform a full archer pull-up, you can allow your secondary arm to bend slightly in order to make the exercise less difficult. Once you get to the top, you can extend the arm fully and attempt a negative archer pull-up. In time, you shouldn't have to bend the secondary arm at all.

As with the other pull-up variants, most people will find it easier to begin with the primary pulling arm in an underhand grip.

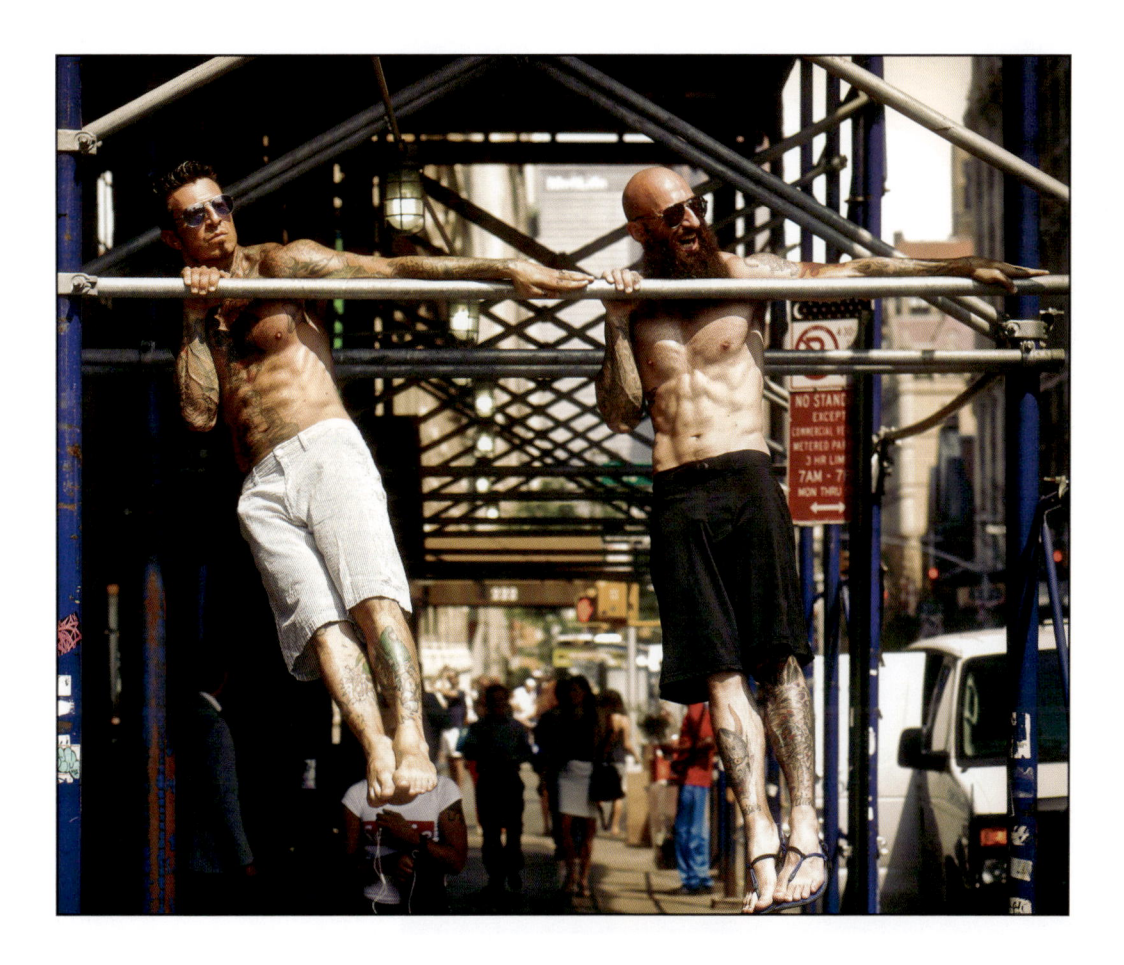

ONE ARM HANG

Hanging from one arm is great for building grip strength and shoulder stability. It is also an excellent starting point for training toward the one arm pull-up. Focus on keeping your lats and shoulders engaged while you hang. In the beginning, just holding on for a few seconds may be very challenging. Eventually, you can work toward longer one arm hangs. If you have access to monkey bars, we also recommend you practice swinging across them for additional single arm shoulder stability work.

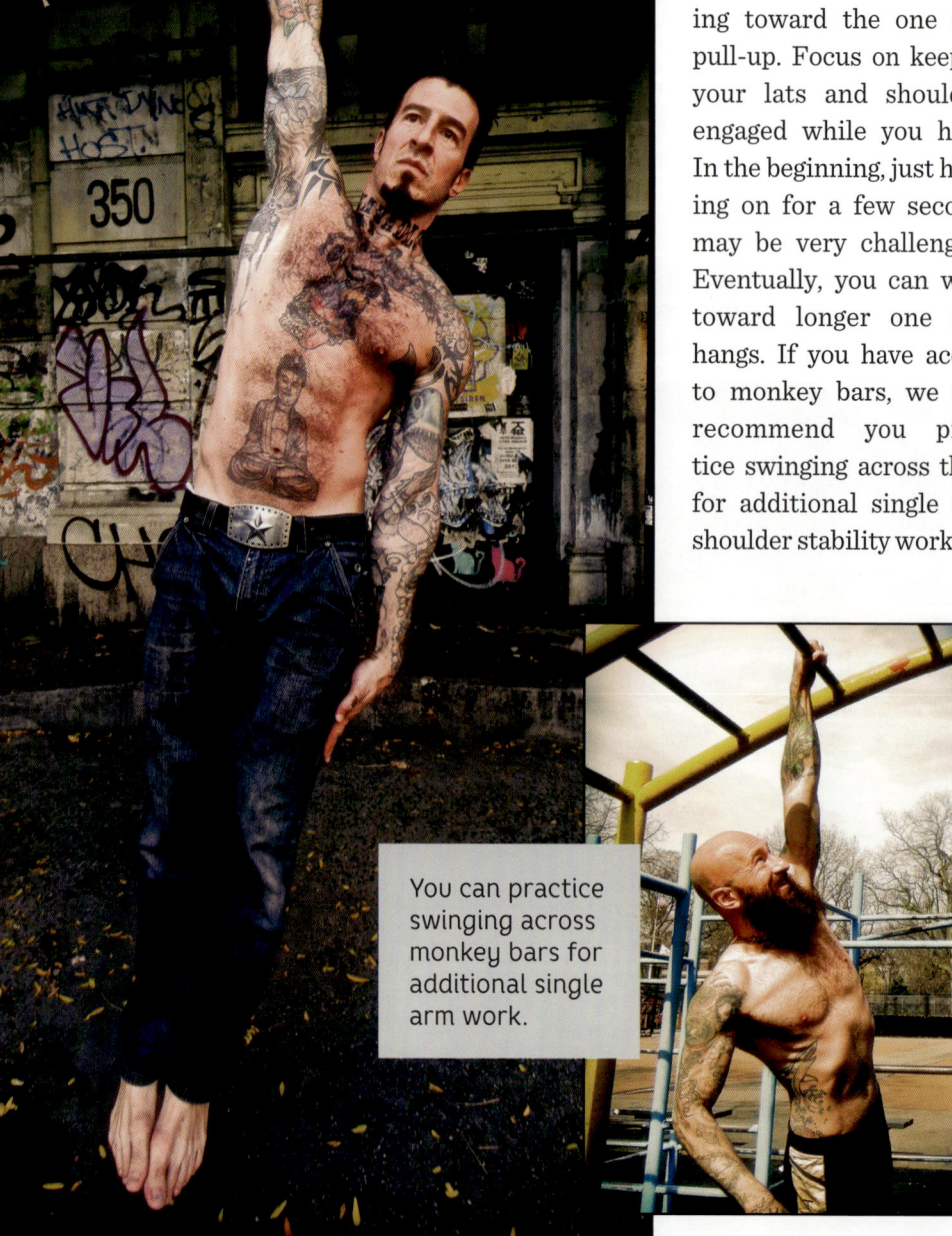

You can practice swinging across monkey bars for additional single arm work.

ONE ARM FLEX HANG

Starting at the top position of a pull-up with your chin above the bar, brace your entire body and carefully remove one hand. Begin with an underhand grip, as doing so allows you to keep the bar near the center of your body, making for better leverage. Though the burden of supporting your entire bodyweight appears to rest solely on one arm, your chest, lats, and abdominals are also an important part of the equation.

The first time most people try a one arm flex hang, they fall as soon as they take the other hand away. Don't be discouraged if that happens to you during your first few attempts. To help stay up, don't just think about your arm; focus on squeezing your whole body tight, especially your abs. You may find it helpful to keep your legs tucked close to your trunk when starting out. Eventually work toward holding the position with your legs extended.

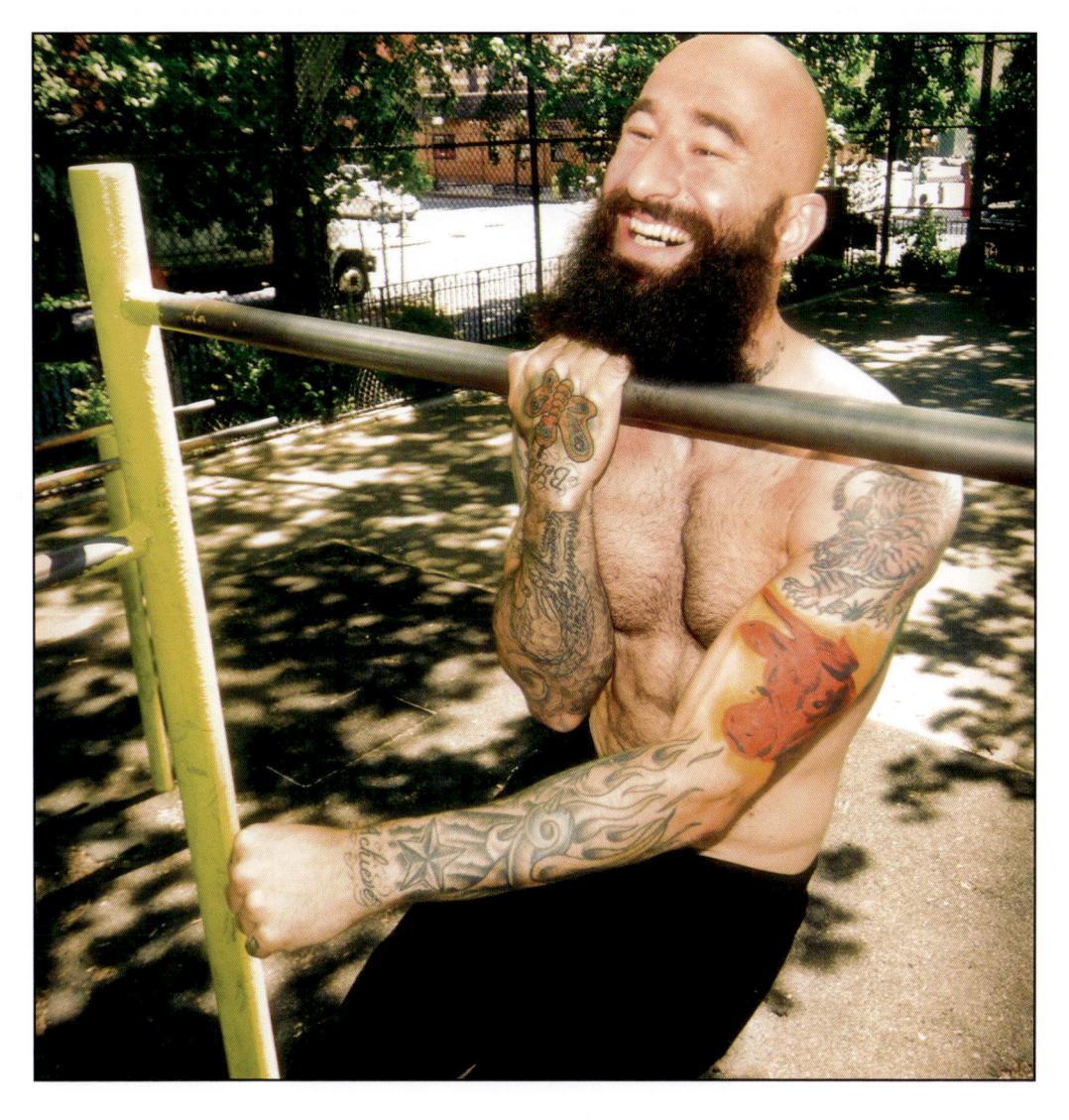

STREET WORKOUT

ONE HANDED PULL-UP

You can practice a self-assisted one arm pull-up by holding the wrist of your pulling arm with the hand of your secondary arm. This is known as a one handed pull-up. Your primary arm is the only one gripping the bar, but your secondary arm can still assist with pulling. Over time, you can work on progressively lowering your assisting hand down toward your elbow. The farther from your wrist you go, the more work your primary arm will have to do. Eventually, you won't need it at all.

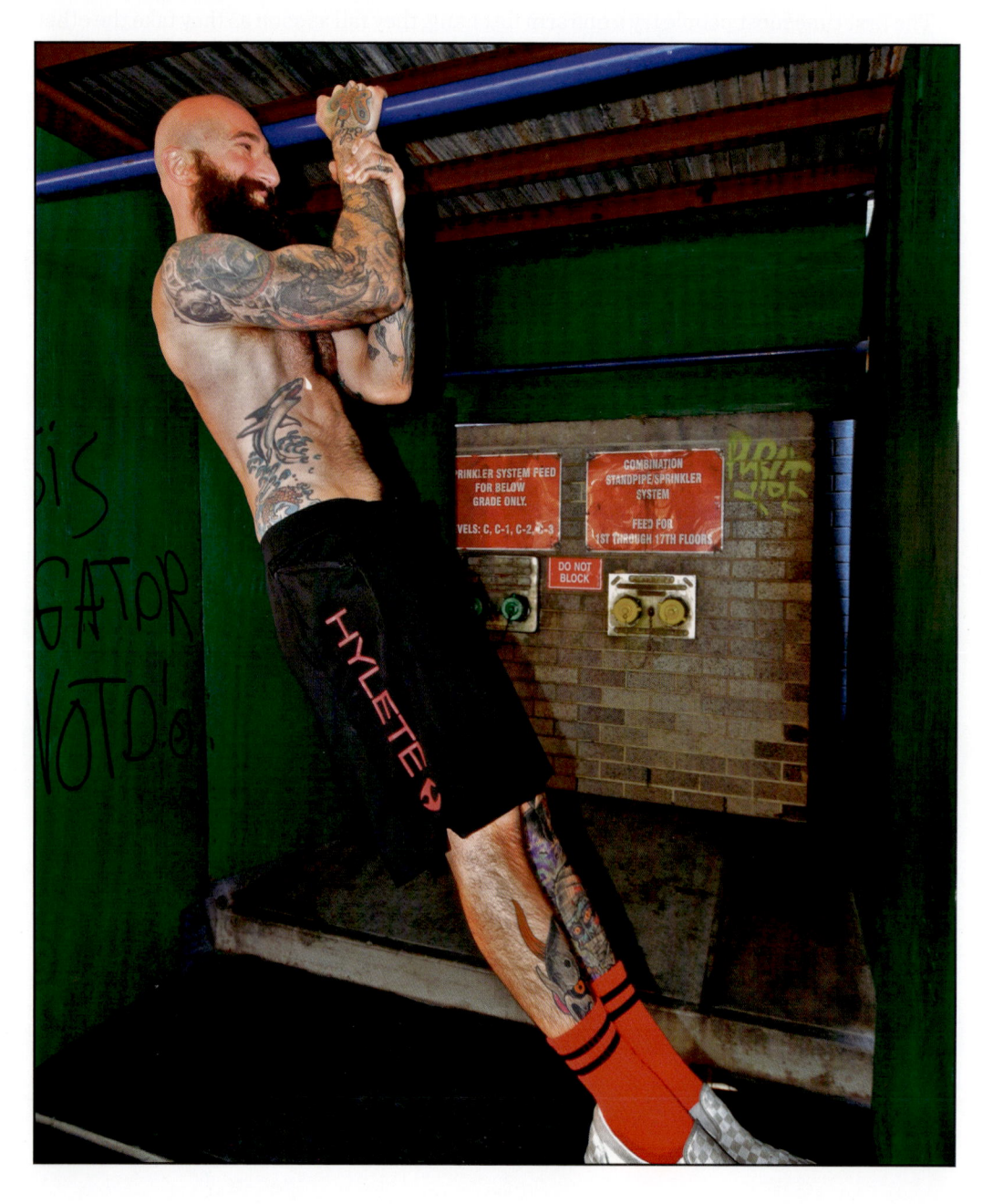

ONE ARM NEGATIVE

Once you can hold the top position of a one arm flex hang for several seconds, you can begin to work toward a controlled one arm negative. The idea is to start from a one-arm flexed hang position, then carefully lower yourself into a dead hang with as little momentum as possible. Performing the eccentric phase of the one arm pull-up is a great way to prepare your tendons and ligaments for the stress of the full move while simultaneously training your central nervous system to acclimate to the unusual movement pattern.

The first time you try to do a one-arm negative, you will probably drop like a stone. When starting out, it may help to not even think of it as a negative; just try to keep yourself up and let gravity take care of the rest. The closer you get to a full hang, the harder it becomes to maintain control during the descent. Be prepared to spend a lot of time on this step. You'll need to own every inch of the negative before you will be able to do a one arm pull-up.

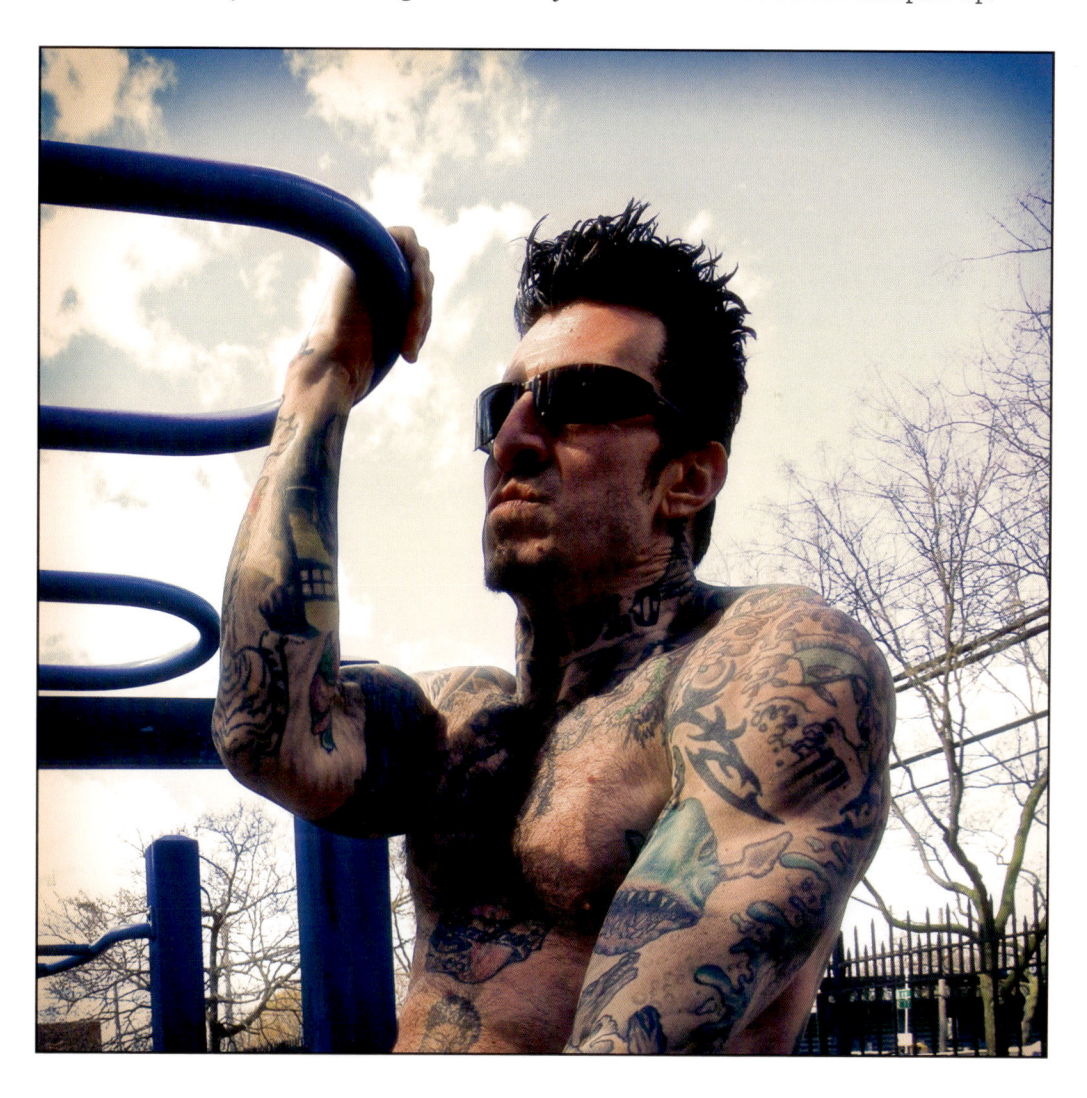

ONE ARM PULL-UP

The one arm pull-up is the granddaddy of them all! It is said that only 1 in 100,000 people will ever perform this exercise, but any able-bodied person who is willing to put in the time and effort can achieve a one arm pull-up in this lifetime.

Before you begin working toward a one-arm pull-up, make sure you spend plenty of time getting comfortable with all of the two arm varieties. Focus on getting to the point where you can perform at least 15 clean overhand pull-ups in one set without using momentum. Ideally, you should do closer to 20. This is the foundation for your one arm pull-up. Getting comfortable with archer pull-ups, one arm hangs and one arm negatives is also very helpful before embarking on the quest for the one arm pull-up.

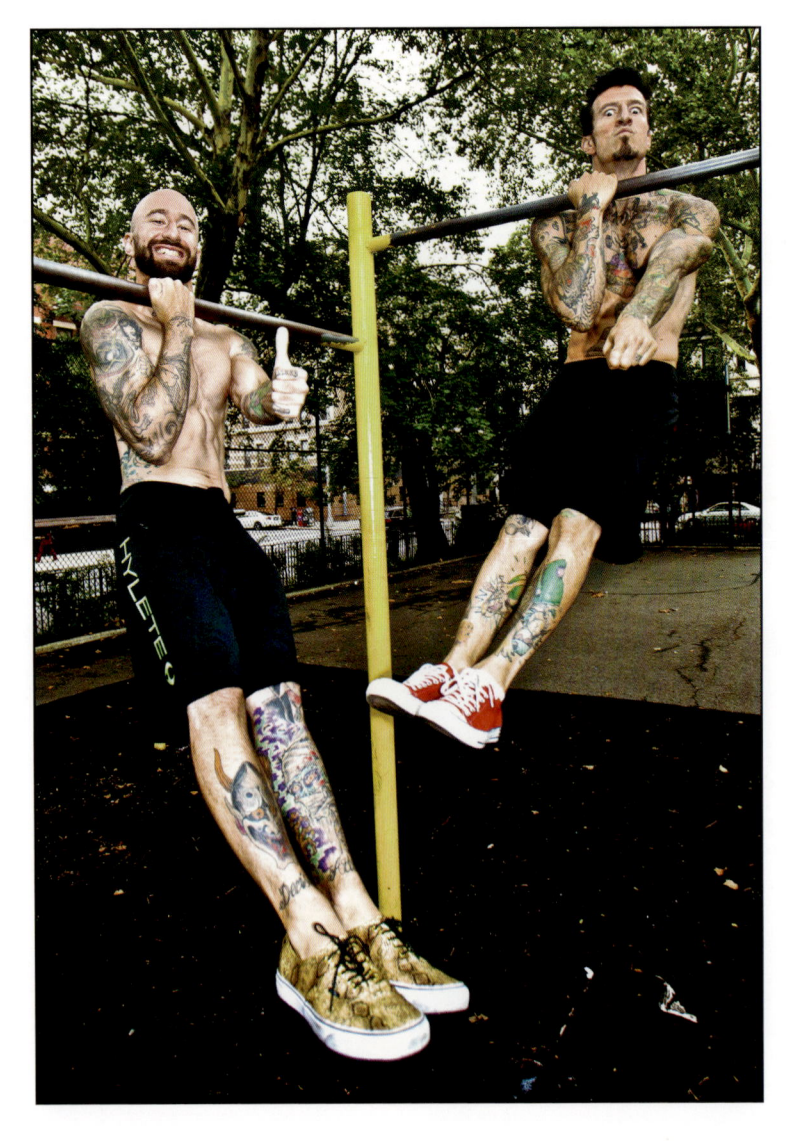

Due to the lopsided nature of using just one arm to pull yourself, some trunk rotation may be unavoidable. Your body will naturally twist as you go up. In the beginning, you should use this to your advantage, and practice turning in toward the bar as you pull. This will cause your grip to rotate from an overhand to an underhand position as you ascend. Eventually, you can work toward performing a one-arm pull-up with less rotation, keeping your hand in a pronated position throughout the whole range of motion.

Street Workout

Because the one-arm pull-up is a very intense move, you have to be careful not to overdo it. Not only will beginning your one-arm pull-up training give a shock to your muscles, it will also rock your connective tissue and central nervous system. This type of training can be very stressful on the elbow and shoulder joints in particular. Tendinitis is avoidable, but you've got to respect your body or you will pay the price.

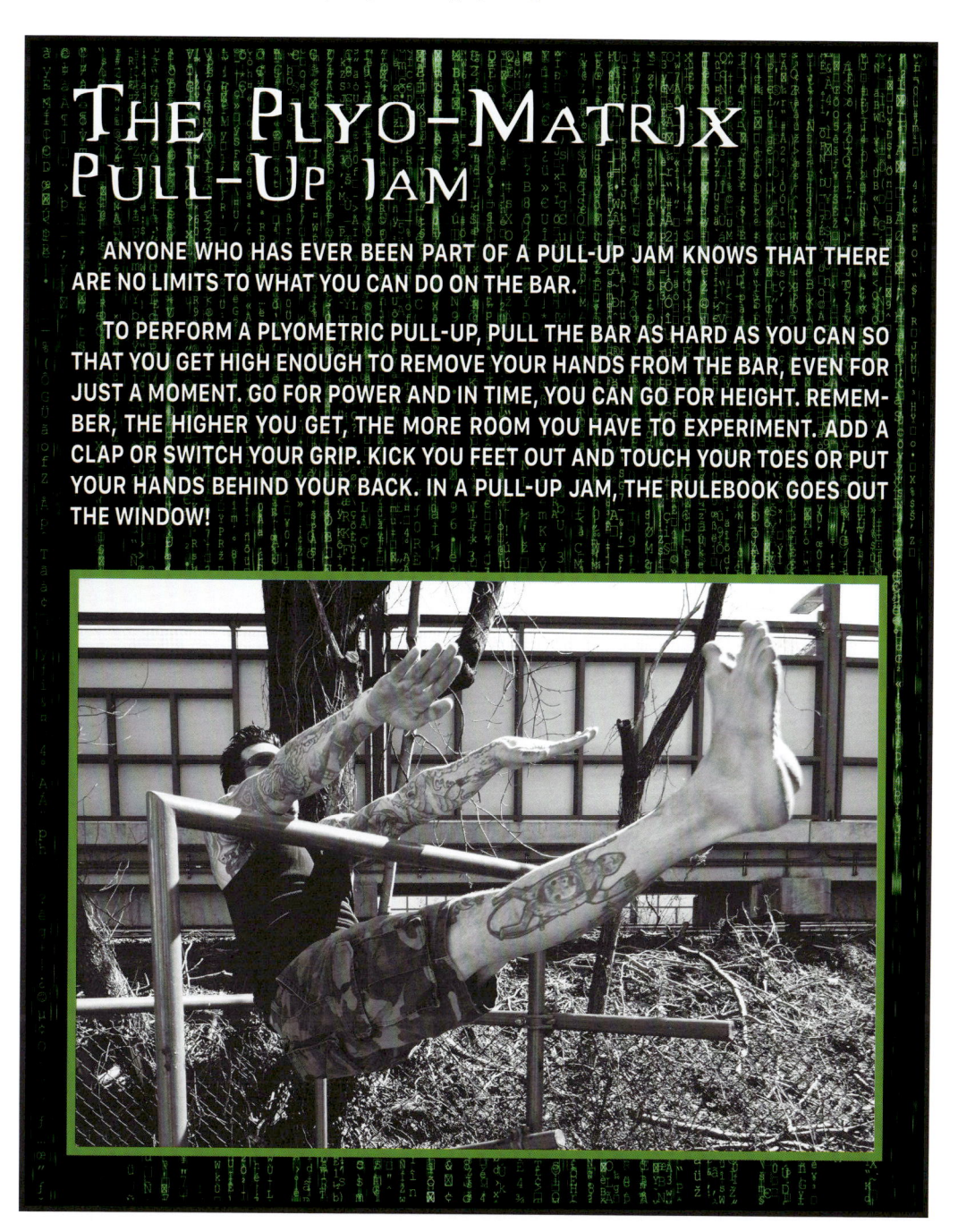

The Plyo-Matrix Pull-Up Jam

ANYONE WHO HAS EVER BEEN PART OF A PULL-UP JAM KNOWS THAT THERE ARE NO LIMITS TO WHAT YOU CAN DO ON THE BAR.

TO PERFORM A PLYOMETRIC PULL-UP, PULL THE BAR AS HARD AS YOU CAN SO THAT YOU GET HIGH ENOUGH TO REMOVE YOUR HANDS FROM THE BAR, EVEN FOR JUST A MOMENT. GO FOR POWER AND IN TIME, YOU CAN GO FOR HEIGHT. REMEMBER, THE HIGHER YOU GET, THE MORE ROOM YOU HAVE TO EXPERIMENT. ADD A CLAP OR SWITCH YOUR GRIP. KICK YOU FEET OUT AND TOUCH YOUR TOES OR PUT YOUR HANDS BEHIND YOUR BACK. IN A PULL-UP JAM, THE RULEBOOK GOES OUT THE WINDOW!

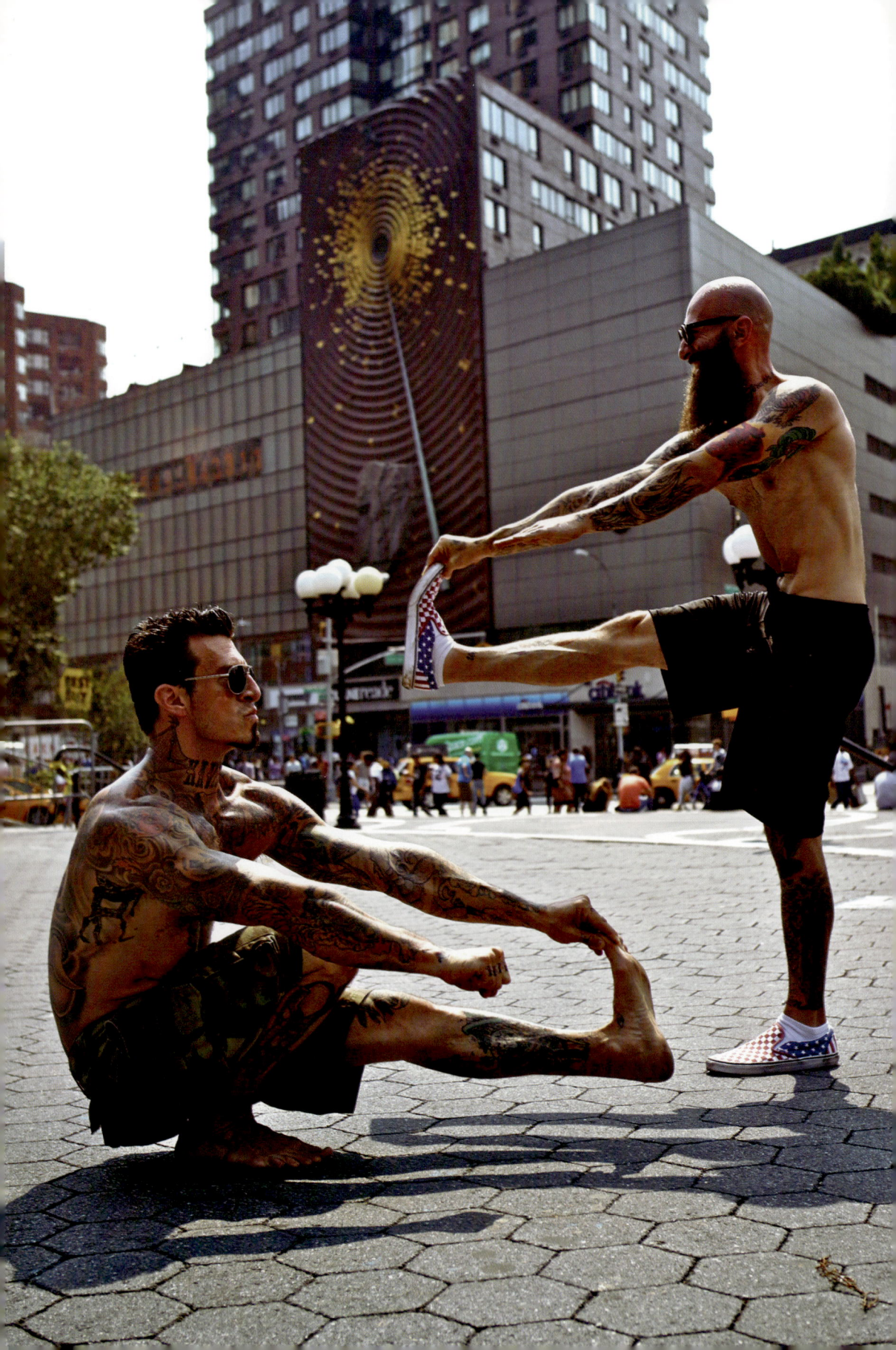

Chapter 6

Squat

You're not strong if you don't have strong legs. Period. Without powerful posts, you could not navigate with confidence throughout our world. Anyone would be able to knock you down. You couldn't stand tall.

Although the squat is the most foundational lower body calisthenics exercise, it is not the only one. As you will see, we will cover many moves here that are not squats at all. However, for organizational purposes, all movements that emphasize the legs are included in this section.

The squat is unique in that both the anterior (front) and posterior (back) of the legs are employed. Squats primarily utilize three joints: the hip, knee and ankle, with different muscles acting on each joint. The hamstrings and glutes facilitate the hip movement, the quadriceps extend at the knee and the calves are responsible for the ankles. Squats also recruit your tibialis, hip flexors, lower back, abdominals and more. That's right, squats hit every muscle in your lower body and then some. Further, they can be infinitely adjusted to suit any and all fitness levels.

These exercises are grouped into two categories: Two Leg and Single Leg. Get experience working with both legs before beginning on the single leg variants. Squats can be progressed or regressed infinitely to accommodate the most elite practitioner or the raw beginner.

TWO LEG PROGRESSIONS

Two-legged squats are as fundamental as you get. Every primate in the animal kingdom squats. In fact, human toddlers learn to squat before they learn to walk. For most squats, it is recommended that you keep your heels flat on the ground. This helps ensure that your glutes and hamstrings are fully involved, but as you will see, there are many incarnations of this bodyweight basic, and there are exceptions to every rule.

BENCH ASSISTED SQUAT

If you're new to squatting, you can use a step, bench or other sturdy object to assist yourself. Simply stand with your back to the object and sit down onto it, keeping both feet flat on the floor and reaching your arms forward to help with the balance. If you lose control, the object is there to catch you and prevent you from falling. With practice, you'll get better at controlling yourself on the way down. Eventually you can move to a lower object. In time, you'll be squatting all the way down without needing anything for support.

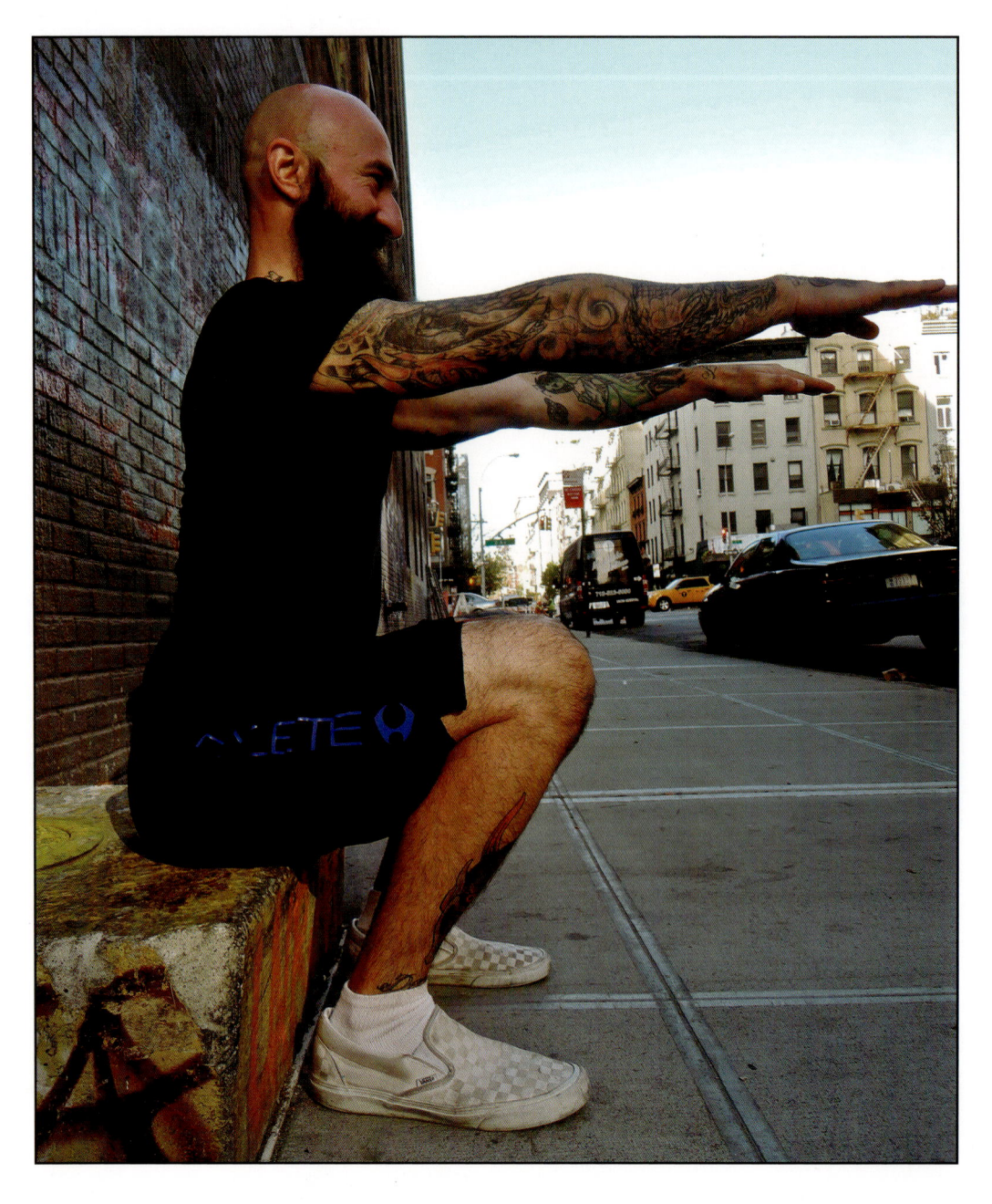

POLE ASSISTED SQUAT

Using a pole is another simple way to assist yourself if you're having a hard time with the balance and/or mobility aspects of the squat. Stand facing the pole (or doorframe or any other sturdy object you can hold onto for support). Grasp it gently as you squat, gradually lowering your hands down as you descend. Try to spend some time in the bottom position as it will provide a helpful stretch, then return to the top using your hands as needed.

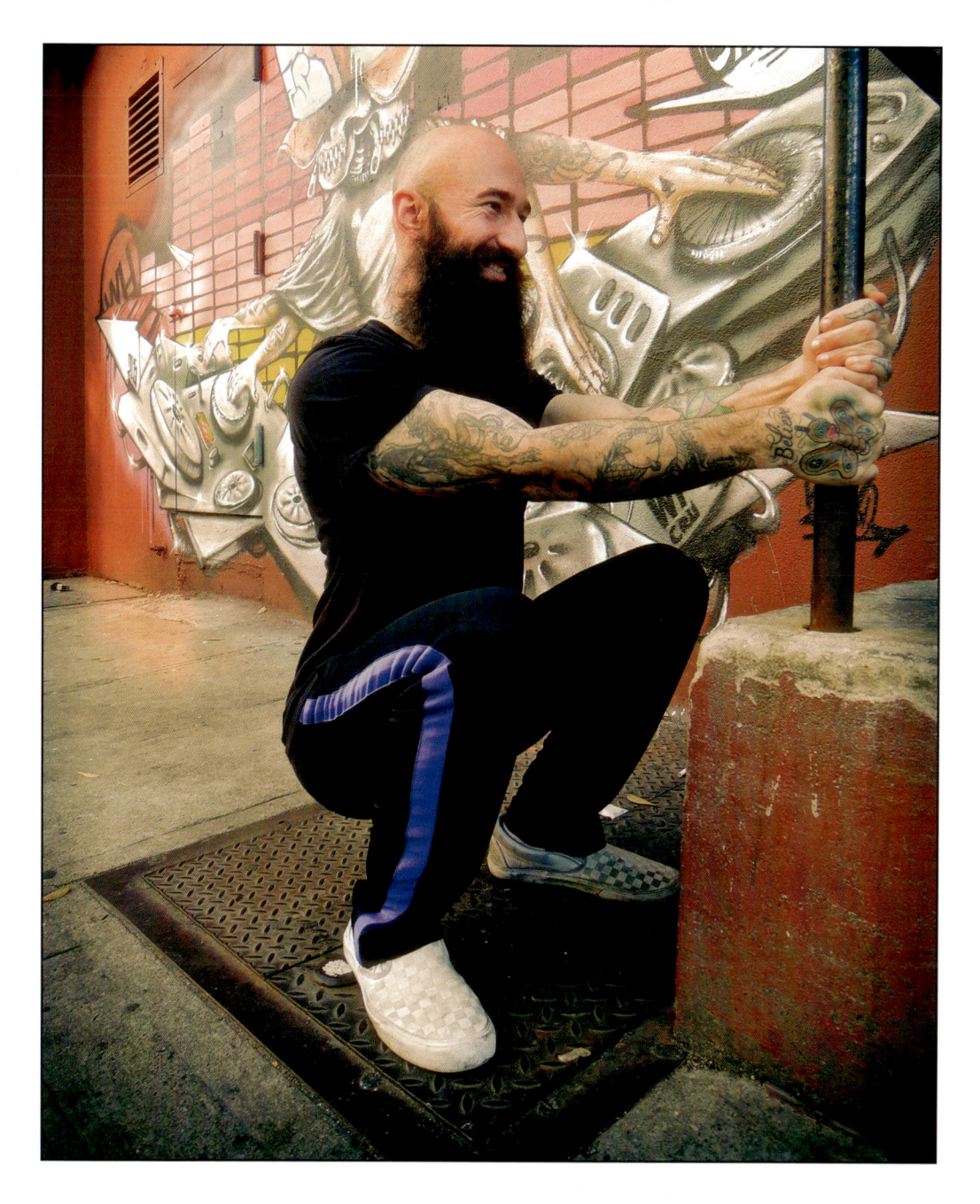

SQUAT

Stand tall with your feet shoulder width apart. Brace your trunk and sit back, bending your hips, knees and ankles to lower your butt towards your heels. It may help to raise your arms straight out in front of you on the way down to maintain balance, keeping your chin up and chest tall. Aim to get your hips below your knees before returning to the start position. Ideally, your calves will be pressed into your hamstrings in the bottom of your squat. Watch out for excessive rounding of the spine and be careful not to let your heels come off the floor.

Some people will feel best with their feet parallel and facing forward, others will find that turning the toes out slightly feels better. Either way, make sure your knees are tracking in the same plane as your toes. Don't let them bow inward or flare out.

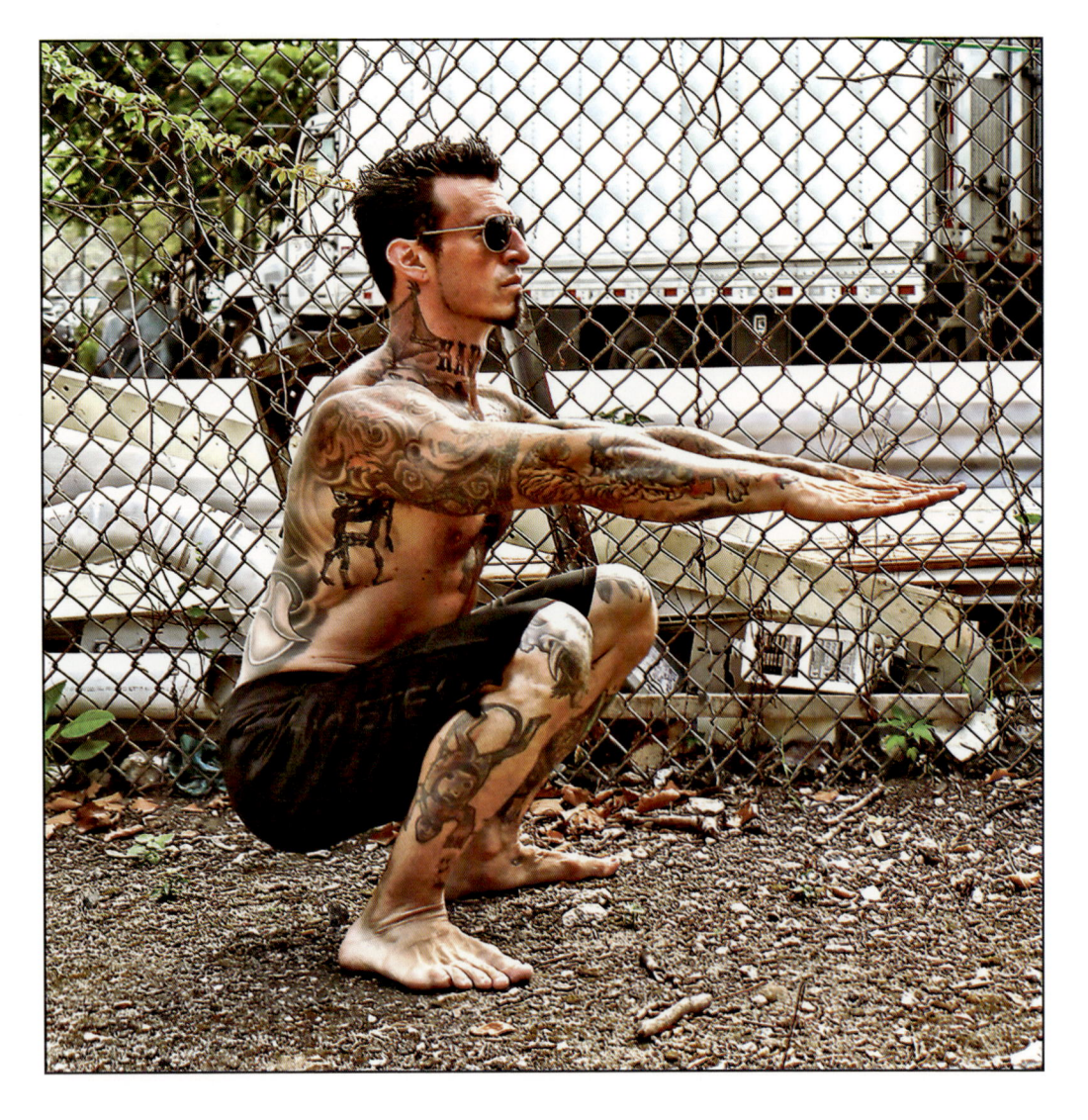

THE LOWDOWN

For many individuals, the mobility is the most difficult part of performing a full range of motion squat. If you're having issues getting low, we encourage you to spend extra time in the lowest position you can reasonably manage. It is helpful to press your elbows against the inside of your thighs for leverage. In time and with practice, your hips will learn to open up, allowing you to perform a deep squat.

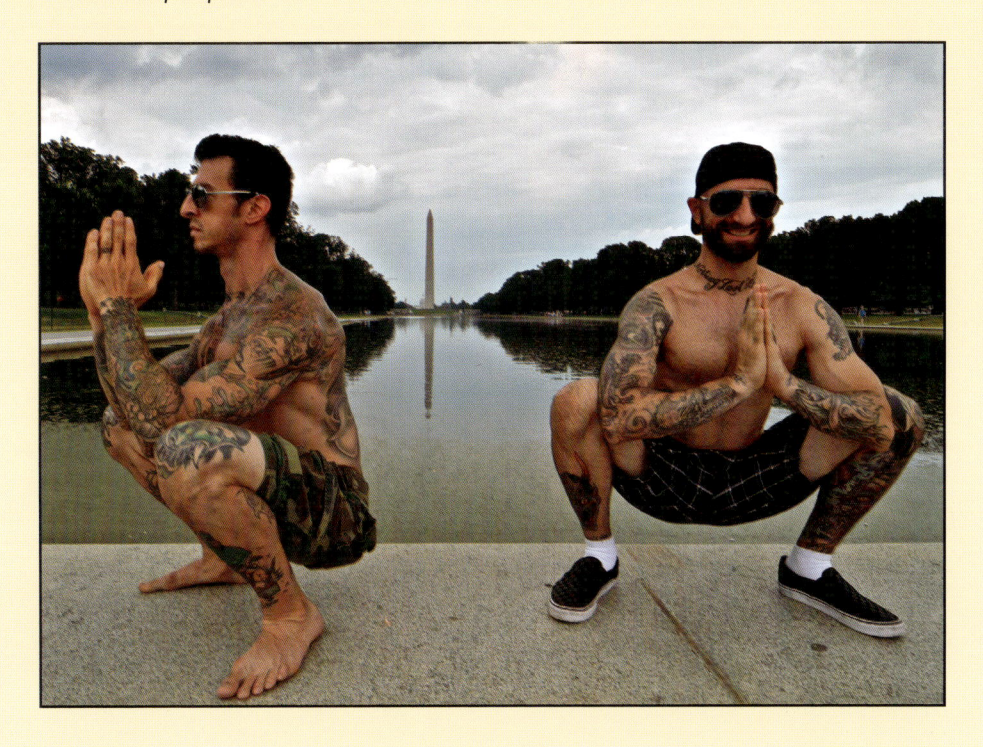

NARROW SQUAT

A narrow stance squat will place emphasis on the outer sweep of the thighs. The narrower you place your feet, the more flexibility is required in the hips, hamstrings and ankles to get into the bottom position. As such, getting all the down may be a mobility challenge for some.

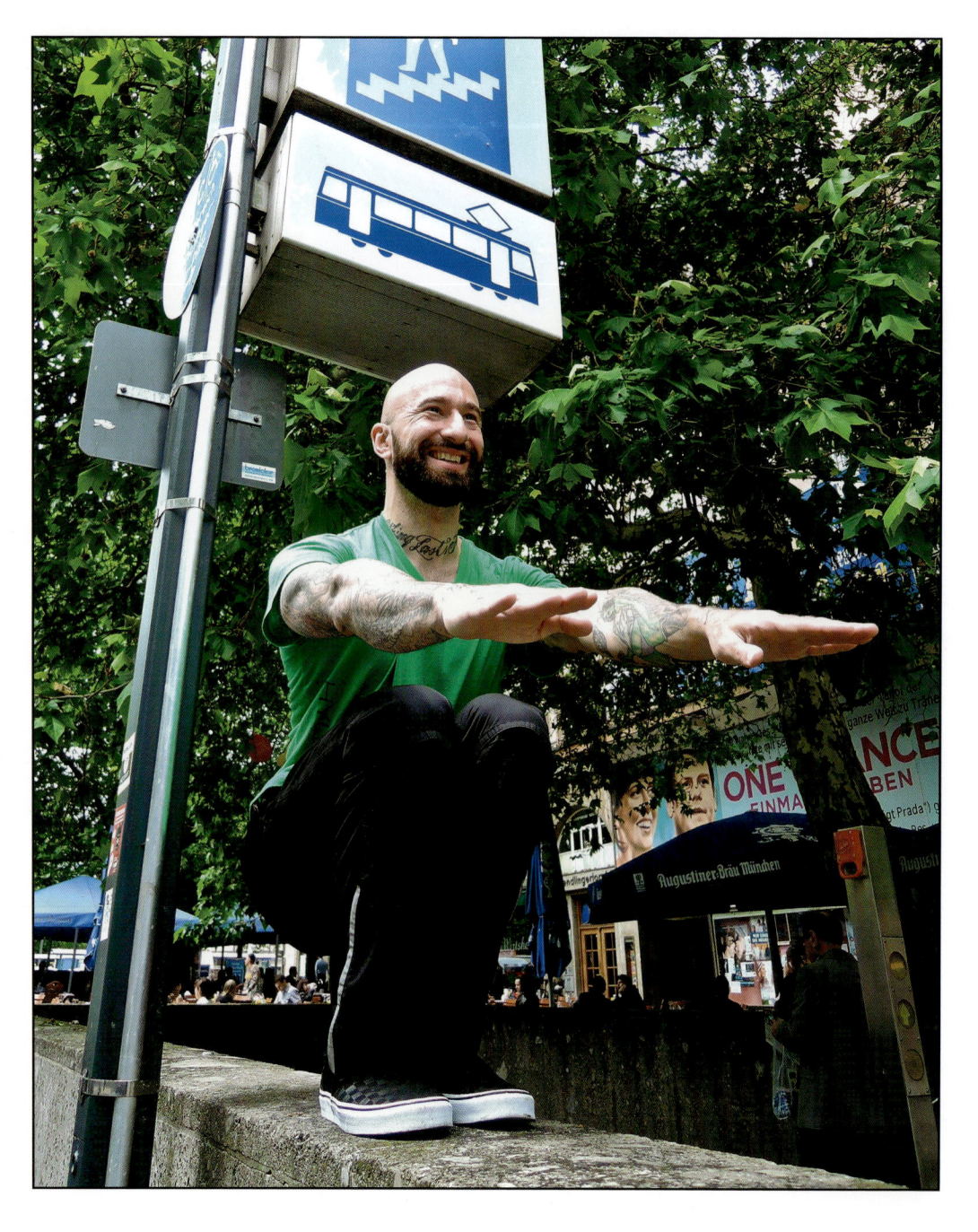

WIDE SQUAT

Varying your foot position will change the subtleties of muscle recruitment during a squat. A wide foot placement tends to emphasize the glutes and inner thighs. It may also provide a stretch for your hips. Experiment with different widths to see what feels right to you.

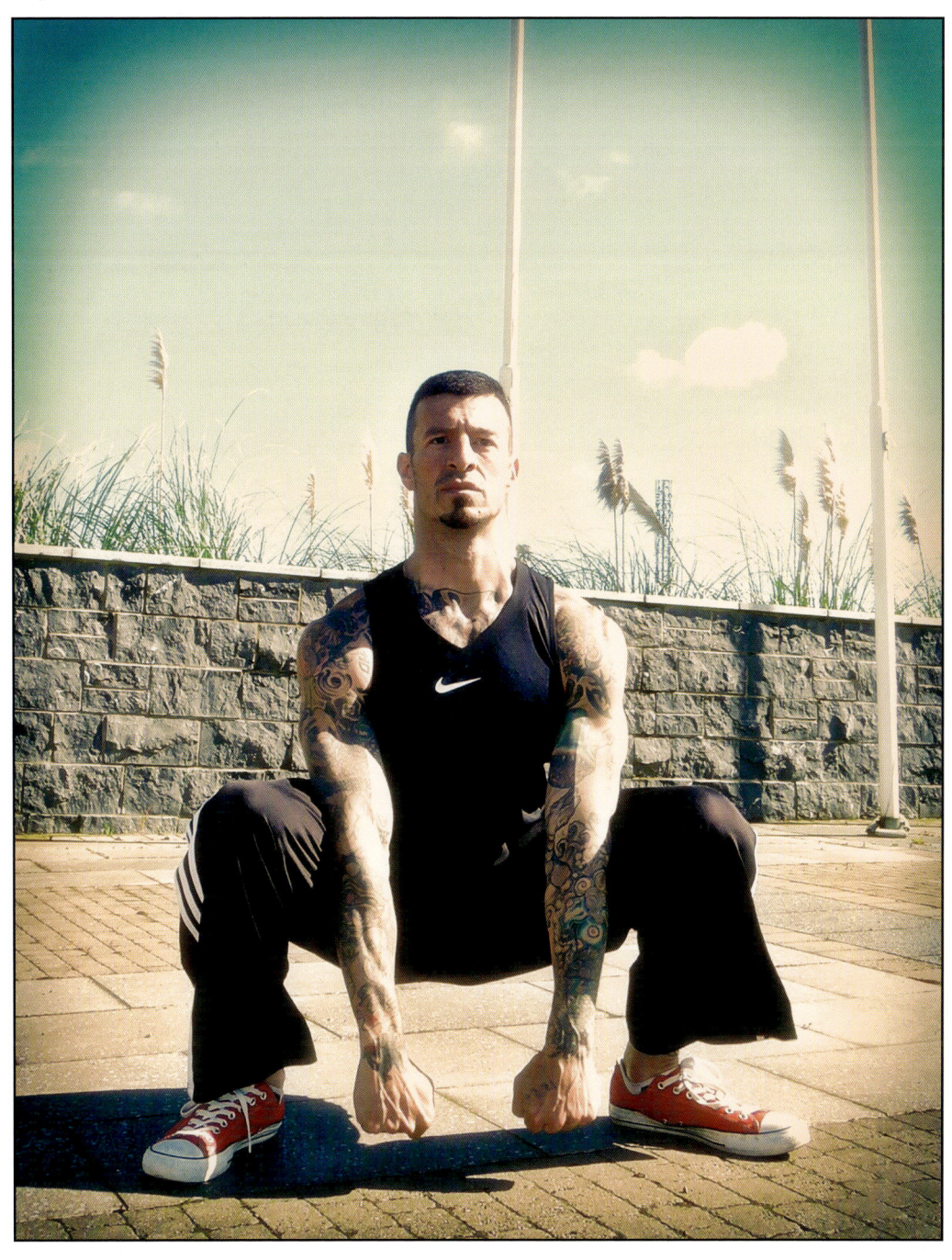

PRISONER SQUAT

The prisoner squat is a slightly more difficult variation of the standard squat that involves placing your hands behind your head with your fingers interlaced, rather than holding them in front or at your sides. As you begin descending into your squat, you will likely feel a stretch through your chest due to this change in arm position. Squeeze your shoulder blades down and back to help facilitate proper posture. You may be surprised by how much you feel this in your upper back. The balance may also be more difficult.

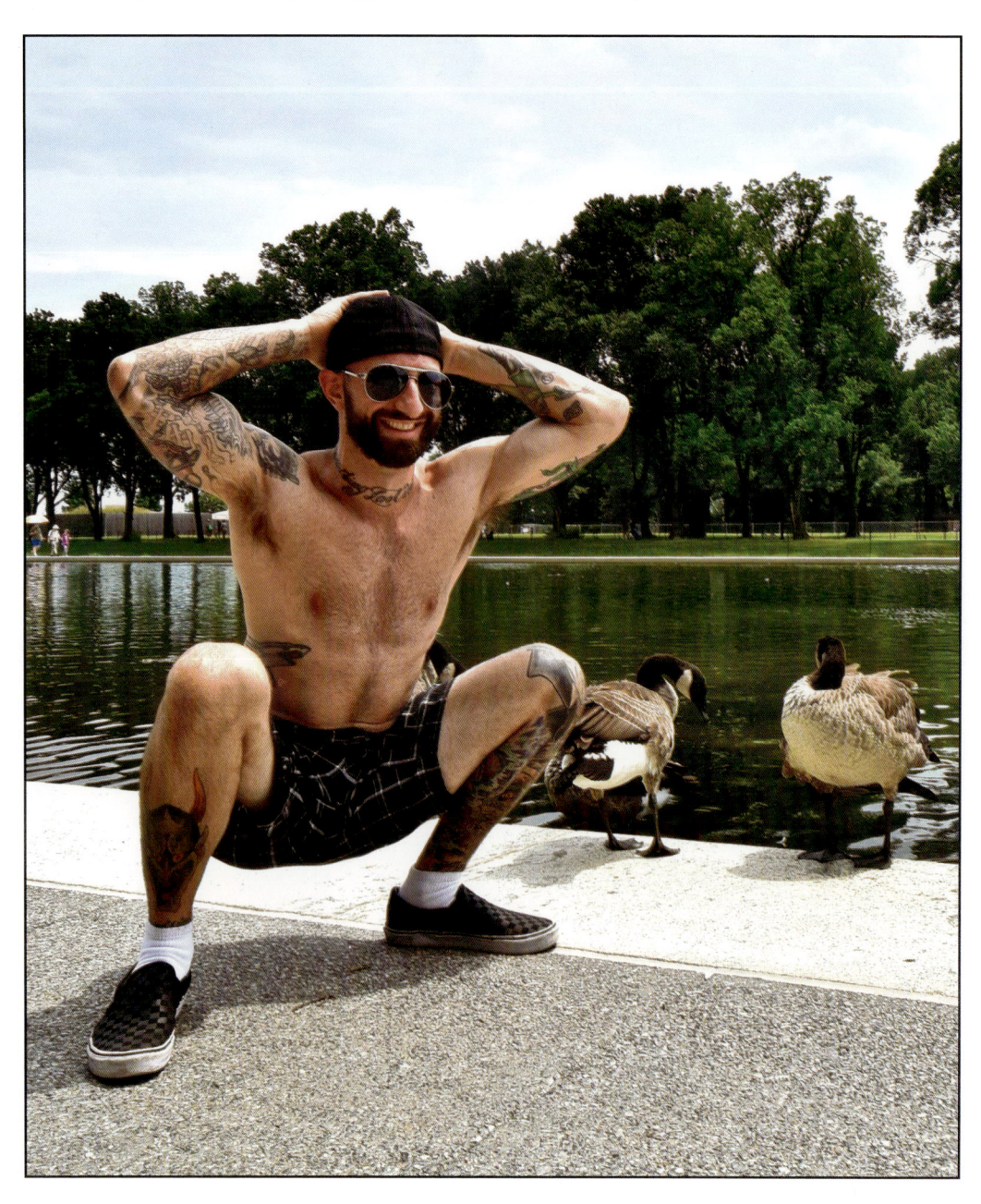

SPLIT SQUAT

For this variation you will begin in a split stance with one foot behind the body and the other in front. Your back foot will be bent so you're on your toes, while your front foot remains flat on the ground.

Keeping your torso upright, lower yourself down until both knees are bent to approximately 90 degrees, then return to the starting position.

It's helpful to think about initiating the movement from your back leg in order to avoid leaning too far forward. Your center of gravity should be about halfway between your two feet, with your weight evenly distributed on both legs.

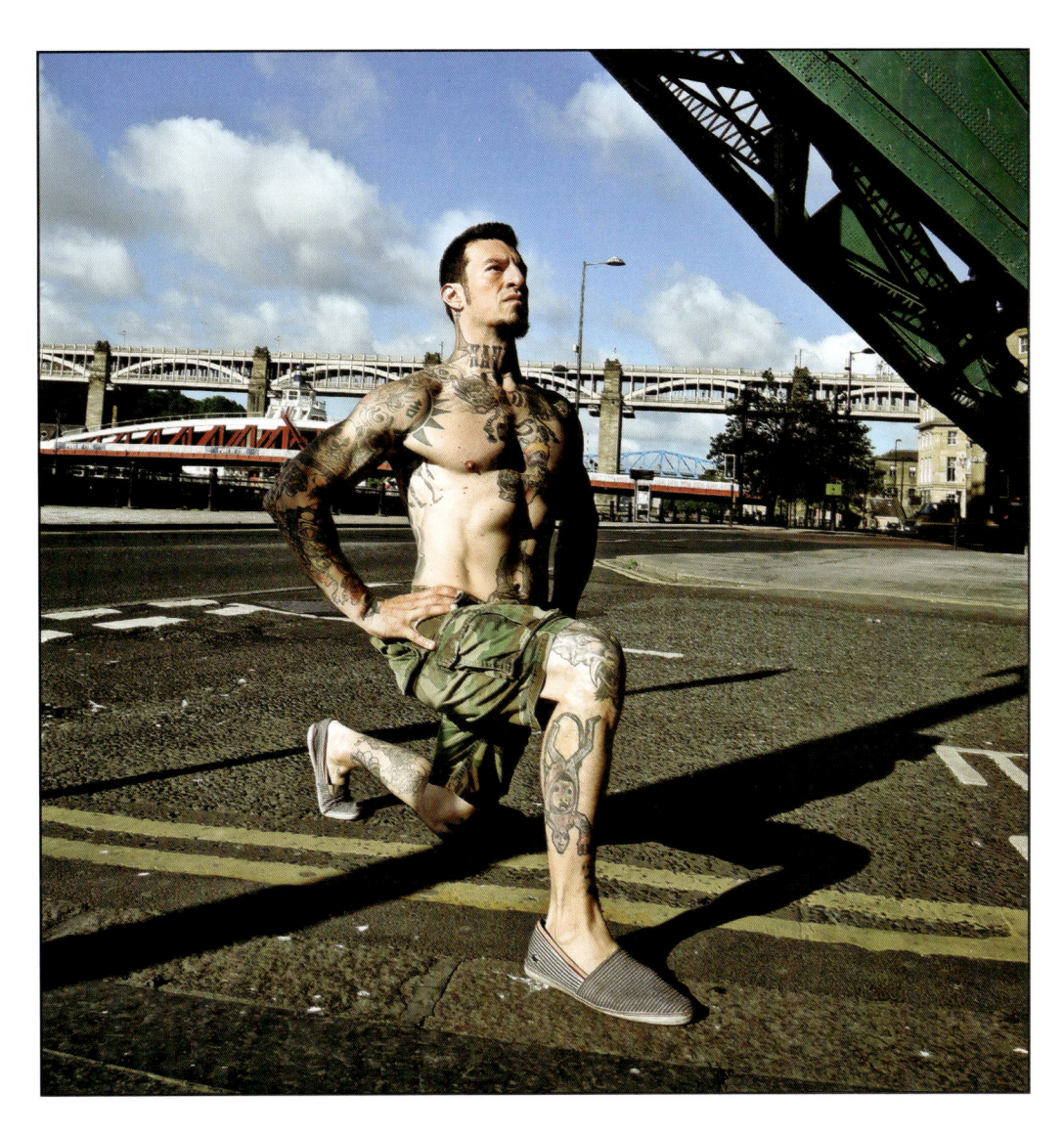

WALKING LUNGE

Beginning in a standing position, take a big step forward, then carefully lower your back knee until it's just above the ground. Your front foot should remain totally flat while your back foot bends, allowing the heel to come up—the same position as the bottom of a split squat. From here, stand up and take a step forward, bringing your feet together, then repeat on the opposite leg. Walking lunges can also be performed moving backwards for an added challenge.

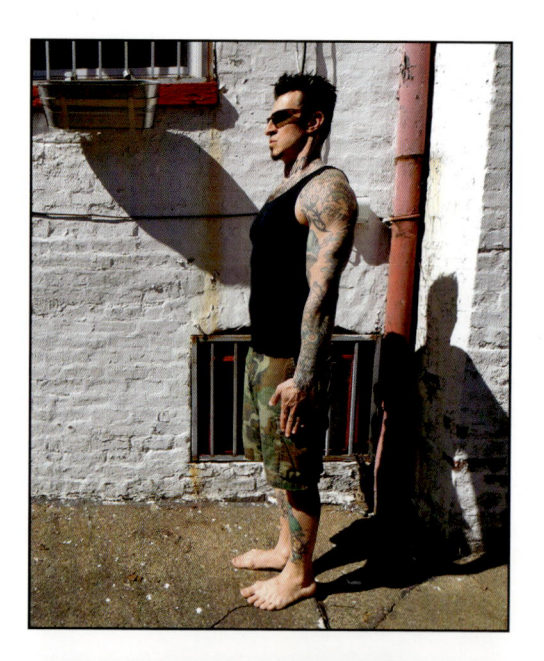

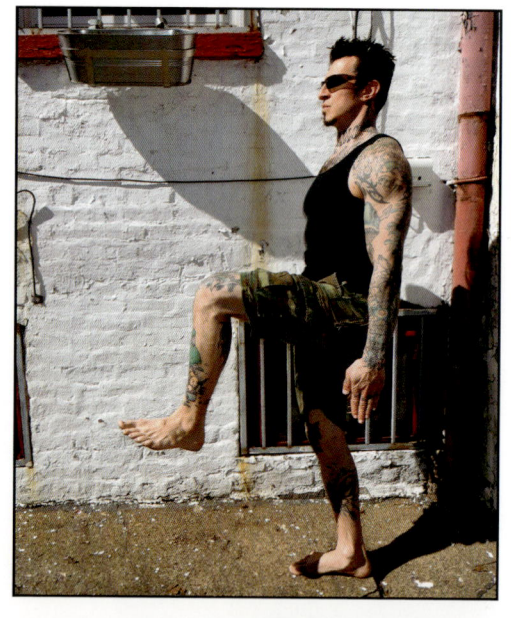

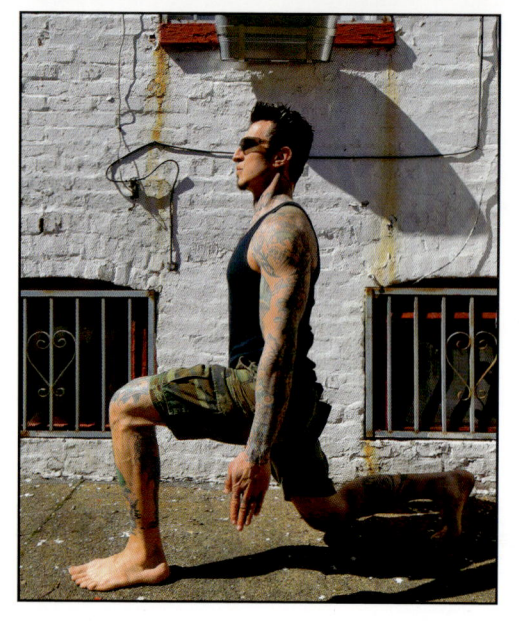

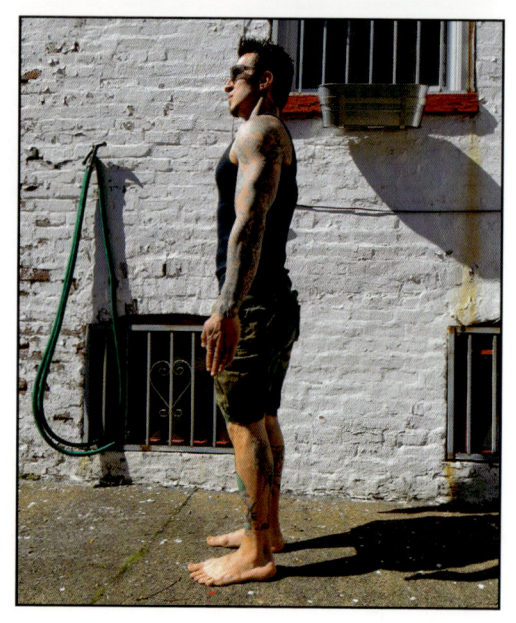

BULGARIAN SPLIT SQUAT

Get into a split stance with your rear foot elevated on a step, bench or other object. Place your front foot flat on the floor several inches in front of your hips. Bend both legs, lowering your back knee toward the ground, then return to the top position.

Elevating your rear foot during a split squat changes your weight-to-limb ratio, increasing the strength required from your front leg, while also giving you a stretch in the hip flexor of your rear leg. The higher the elevated object, the more intense the exercise becomes.

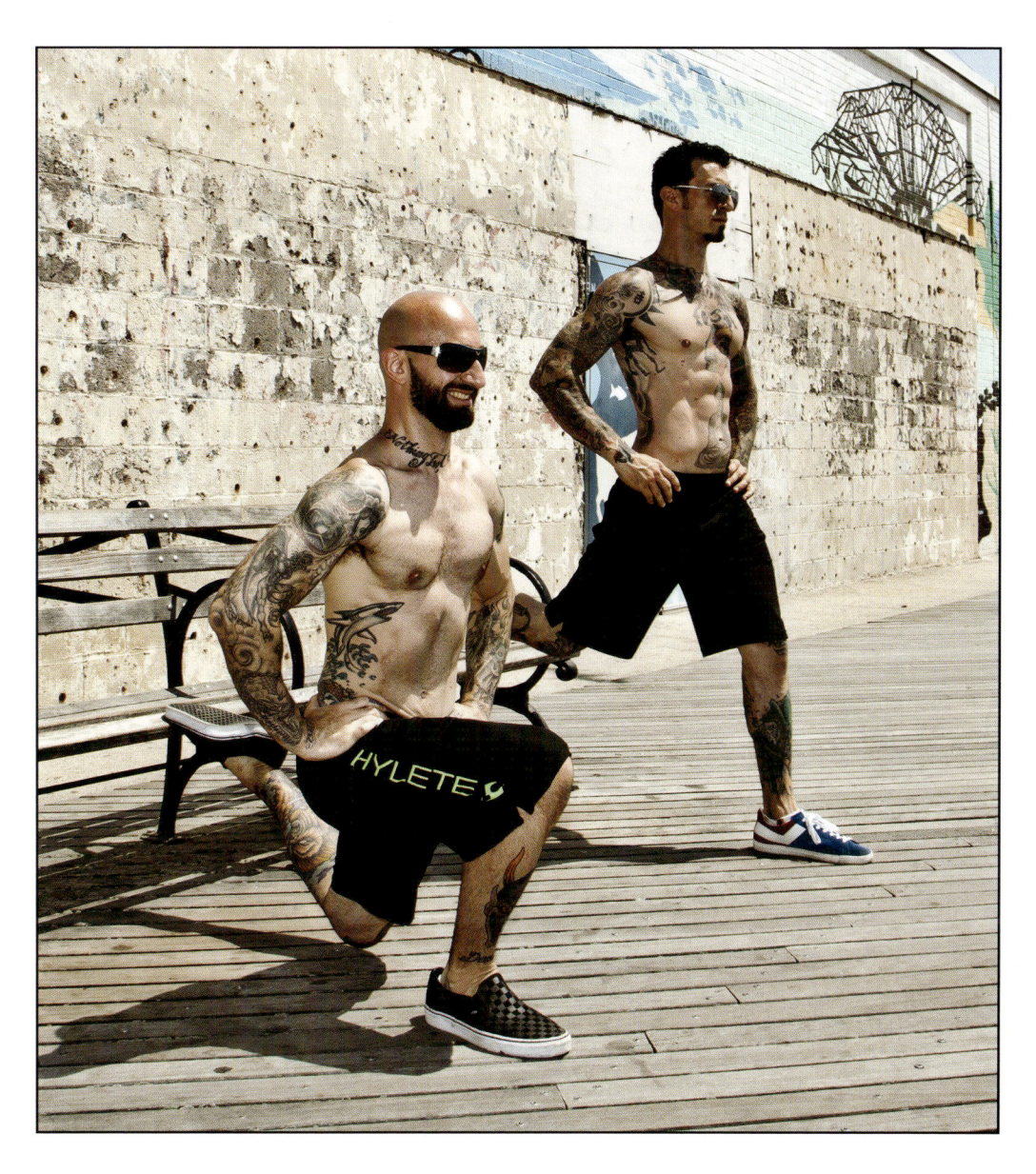

HINDU SQUAT

The Hindu squat is a squat that is intentionally performed on the tips of the toes. Though it is recommended to learn a standard squat with the heels down first, the Hindu squat can be a nice variant once you've established a solid foundation of leg strength. By lifting onto your toes, you can place more emphasis on the front of your thighs, as well as adding a unique balance component.

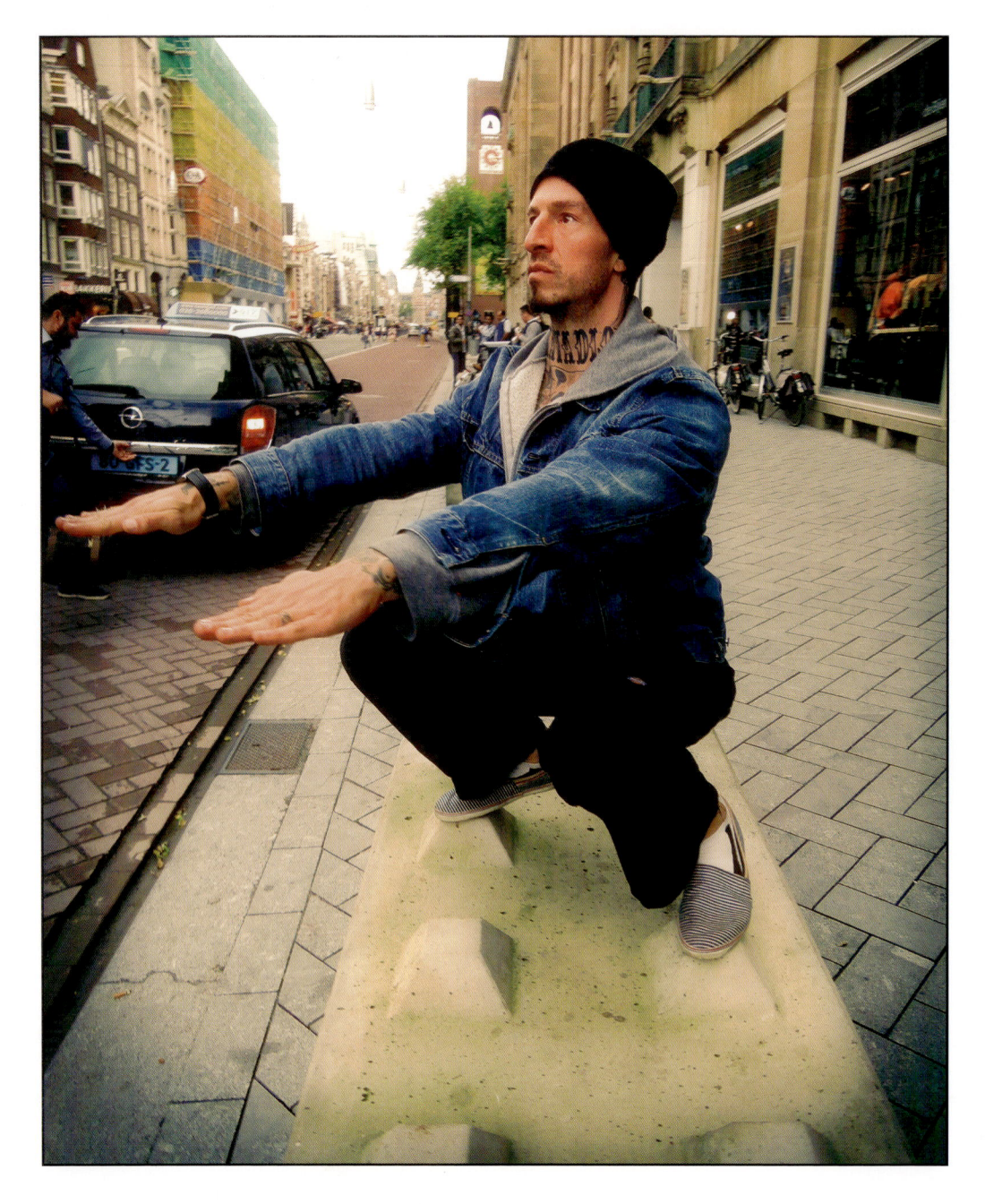

CALF RAISE

Stand on a step or other elevated surface with your heels hanging off the edge. Press your toes down and flex your calves to lift yourself all the way up onto the tips of your toes. Lower back down and repeat. Try it on one leg for an added challenge!

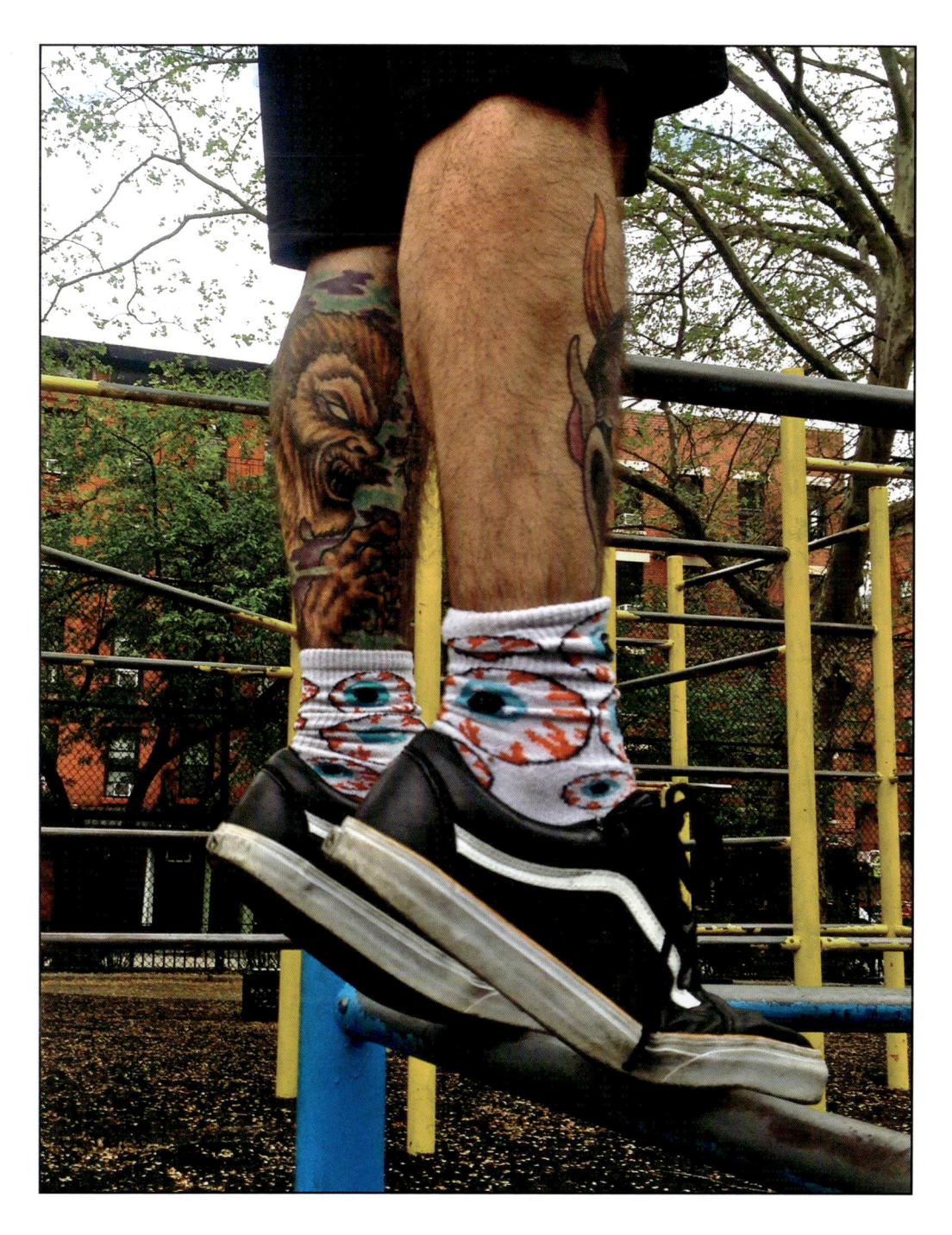

ARCHER SQUAT

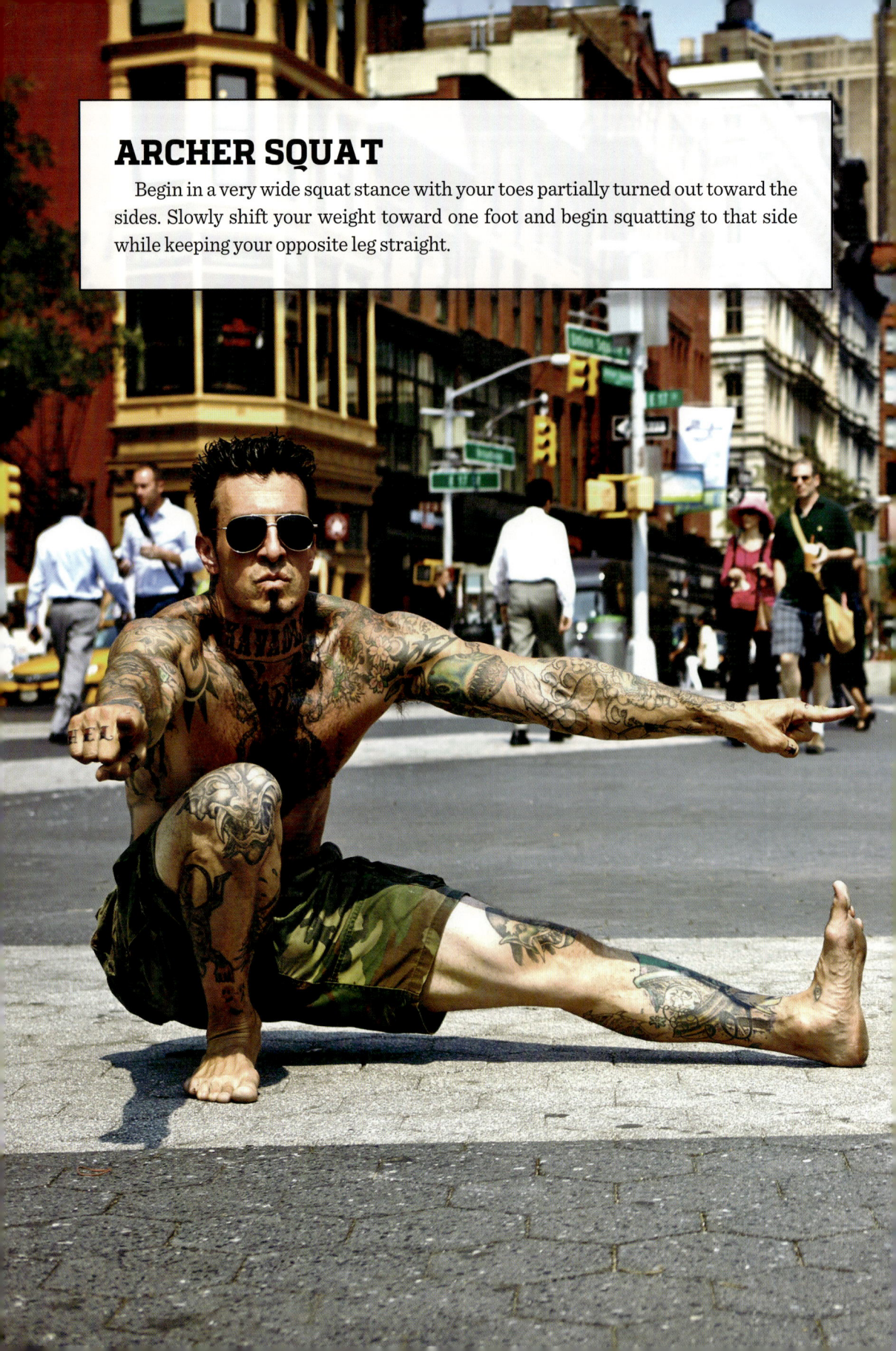

Begin in a very wide squat stance with your toes partially turned out toward the sides. Slowly shift your weight toward one foot and begin squatting to that side while keeping your opposite leg straight.

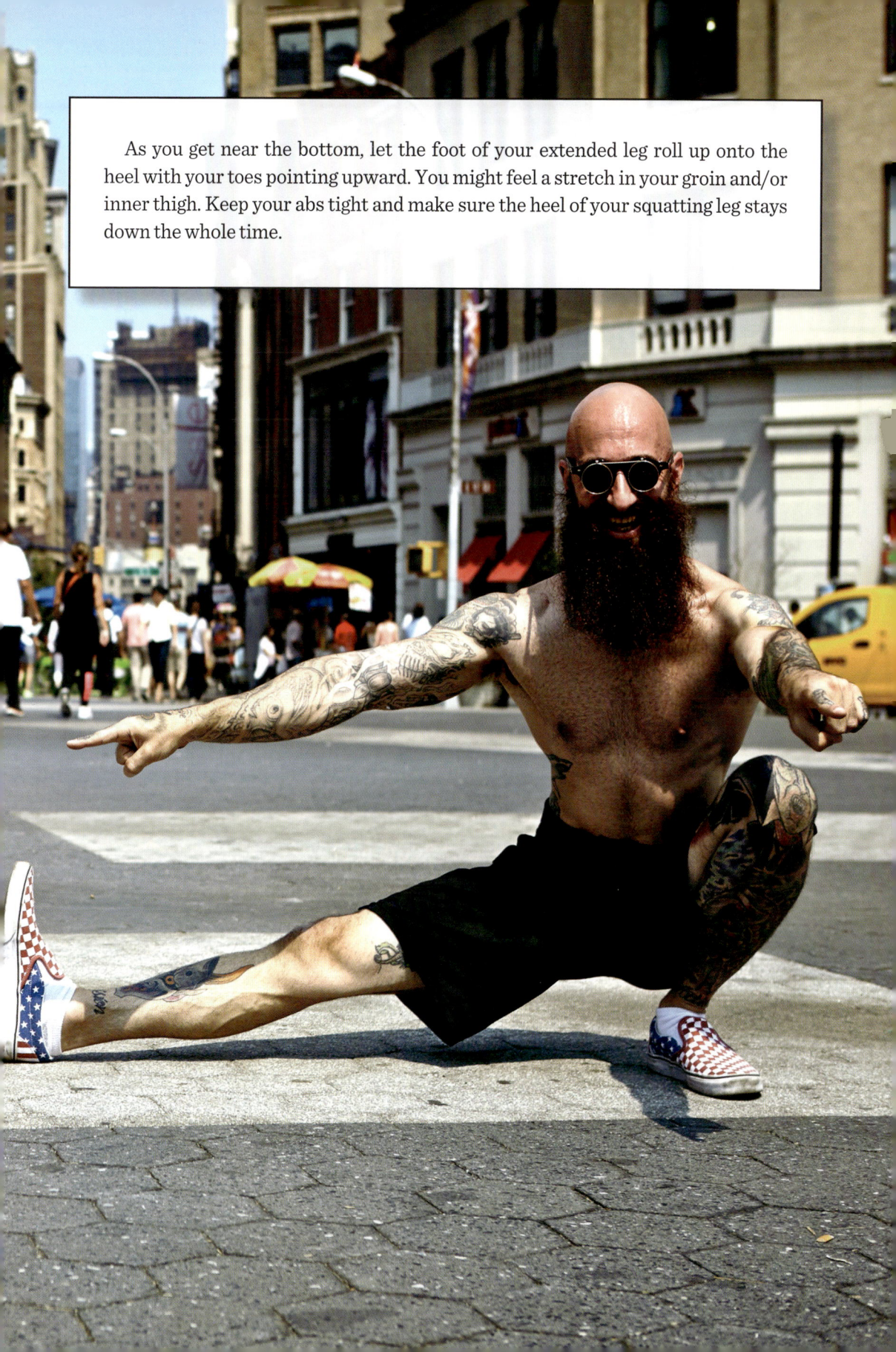

As you get near the bottom, let the foot of your extended leg roll up onto the heel with your toes pointing upward. You might feel a stretch in your groin and/or inner thigh. Keep your abs tight and make sure the heel of your squatting leg stays down the whole time.

SINGLE LEG PROGRESSIONS

One of the biggest misconceptions about calisthenics strength training is that you are limited in the capacity of how intensely you can train your legs. As you will see in this section, that is far from the truth.

As far as these variants go, it is important to train both legs evenly. One way to approach this is by alternating reps: right, left, right, left, etc. Another method is to perform a complete set on your less strong leg first. This way you can give it extra attention by training it while you're fresh, knowing that you'll be able to match it with the stronger leg.

SINGLE LEG STAND

It may not look like much, but simply standing on one leg can be a surprisingly difficult task if done for long enough. Start with ten seconds per leg and work your way up from there. The higher your hold your elevated leg, the more difficult it becomes.

Single leg stands can be challenging for the often overlooked muscles in your feet, as well as your legs.

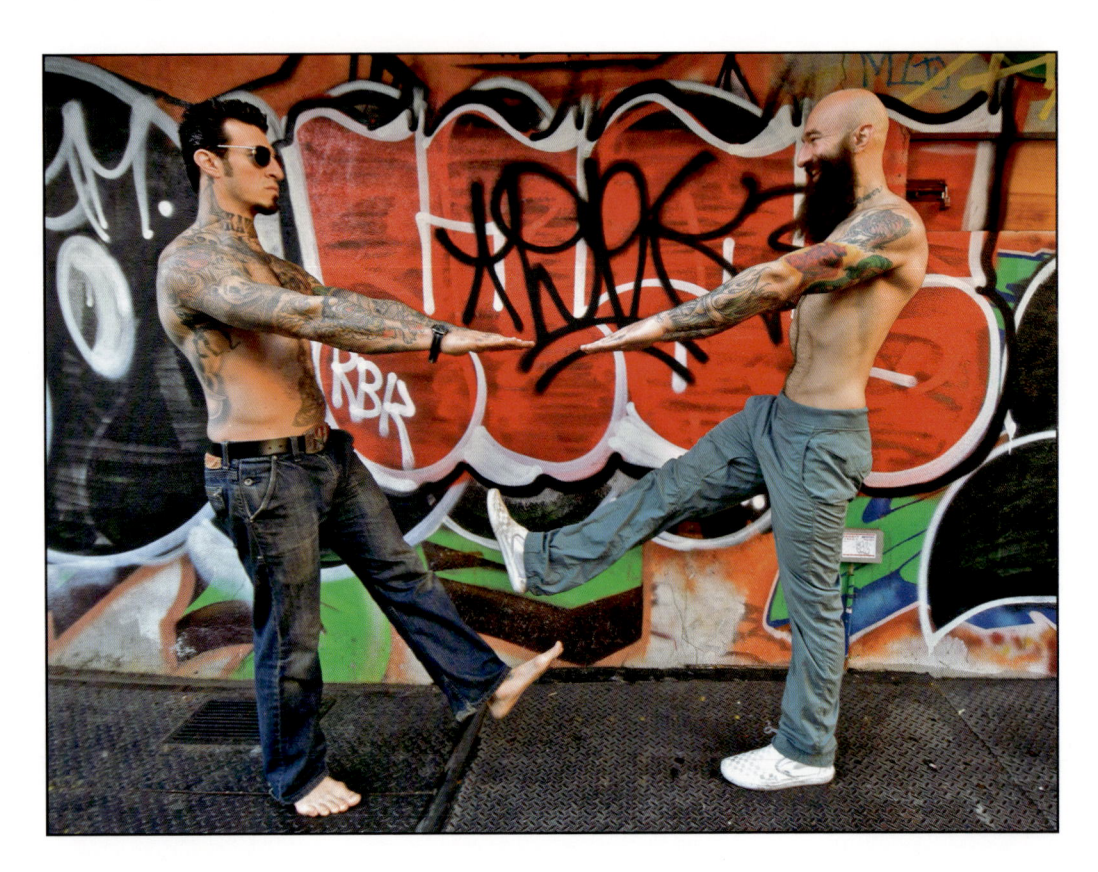

STEP-UP

Stand in front of a step, bench or other sturdy object that is about knee-height. Lift one knee and place your entire foot firmly on the object. Step yourself up by pressing down through your heel until your leg is fully extended. Lower back down and repeat.

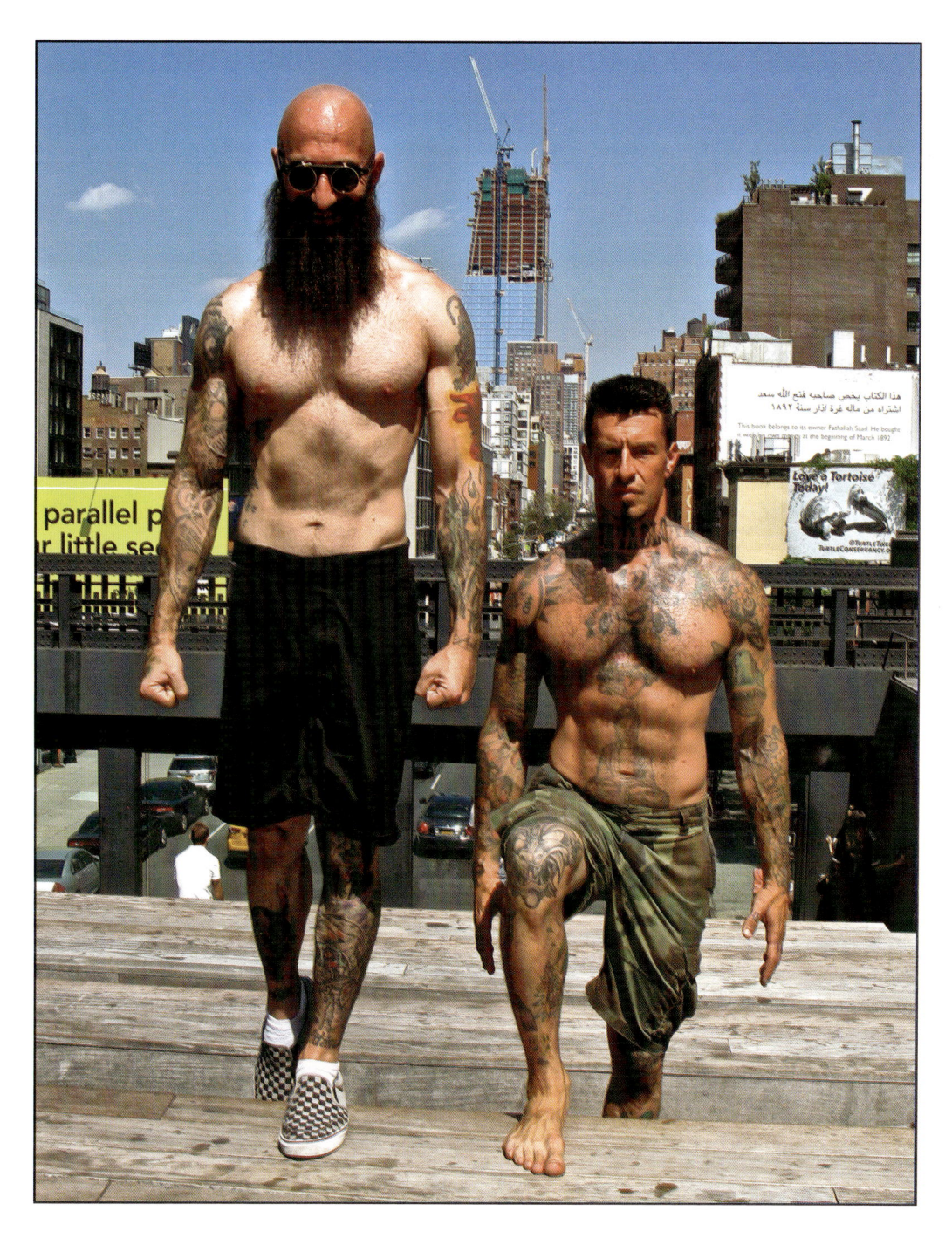

DRINKING BIRD

Stand on one foot with your opposite leg hovering just above the ground behind you. Begin bending forward at your hips while reaching your extended leg out, maintaining a straight line from your heel to the back of your head. You'll need to recruit the muscles of your lower back as you aim to get your trunk and extended leg parallel to the ground. You may feel a stretch in the hamstring of your standing leg. Brace your trunk as you return to the start position, being careful not to twist your body to the side on the way up. Your hands can be kept at your sides or placed overhead for an added challenge.

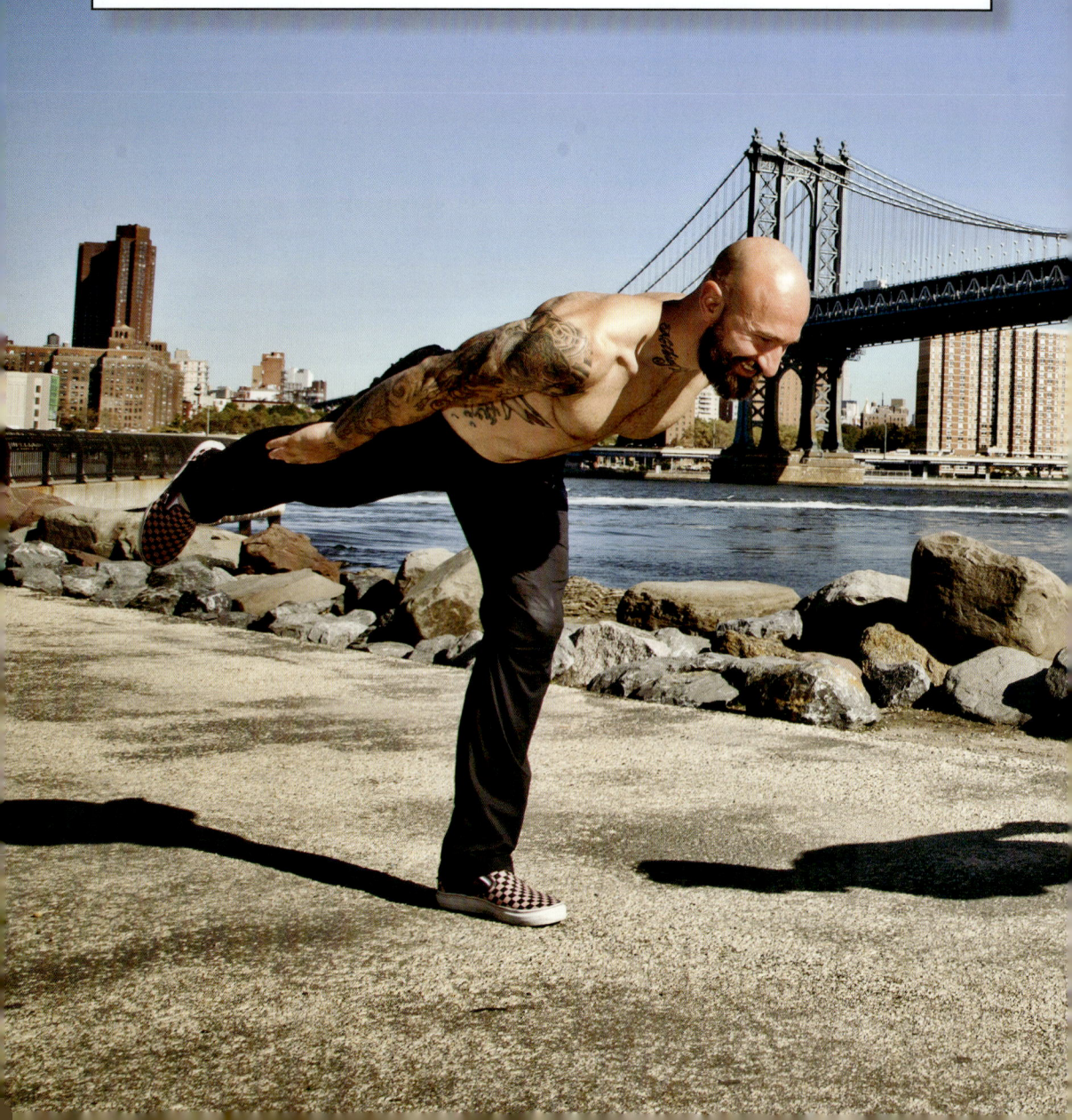

You may need to bend the knee of your standing leg in order to get low enough. With practice, you can work toward keeping it straighter.

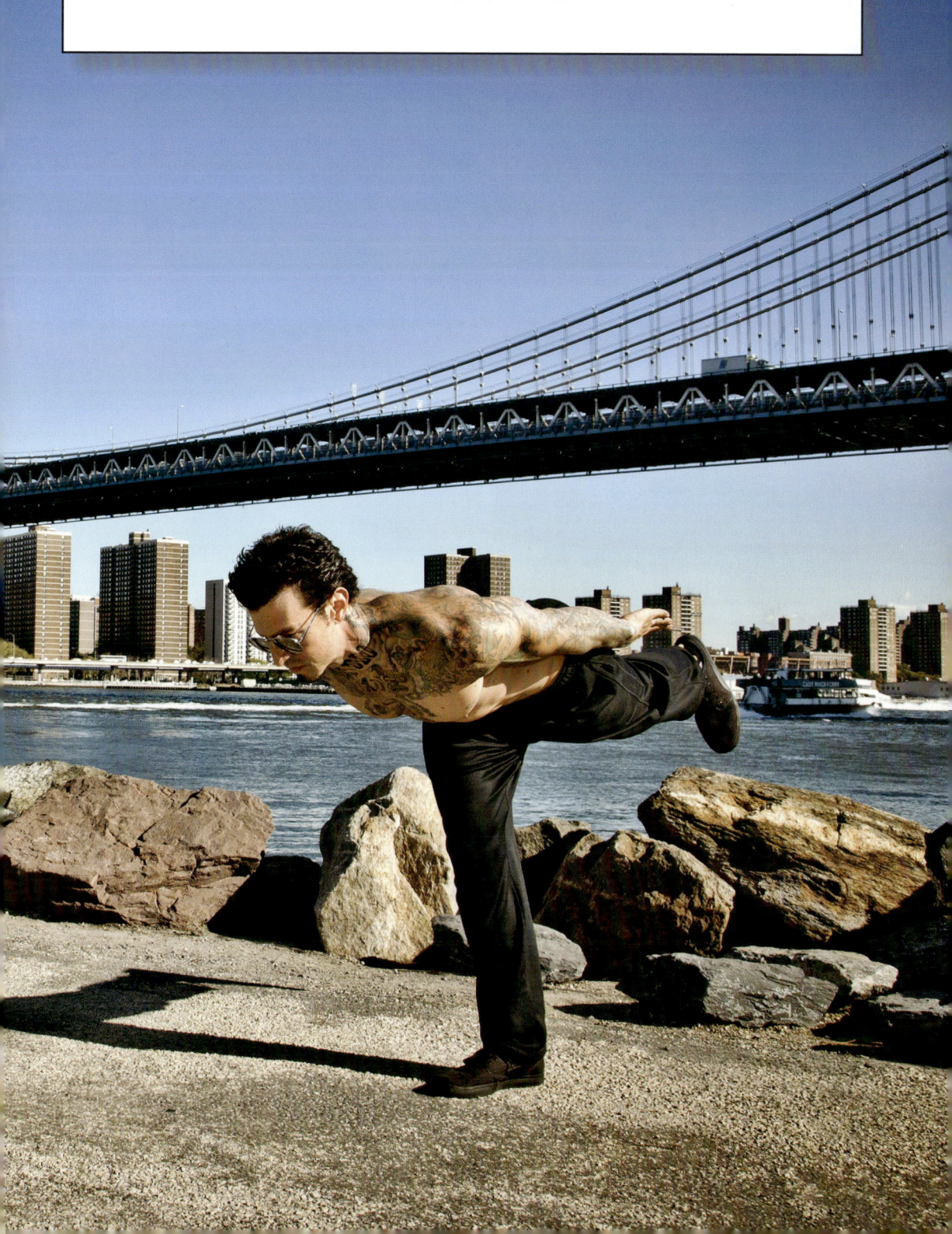

BENCH ASSISTED PISTOL

Stand with your back facing a bench or other object that's around knee-height. Lift one leg in the air, reach your arms in front of your body and carefully sit back onto the bench. (As with the two legged version of this exercise, it's okay if you lose your balance at first.) Pause briefly at the bottom, then drive your heel into the ground and brace your trunk by contracting your abs as you stand up in order to maintain control.

The bench assisted pistol is a helpful starting point for someone who is working toward a full pistol squat.

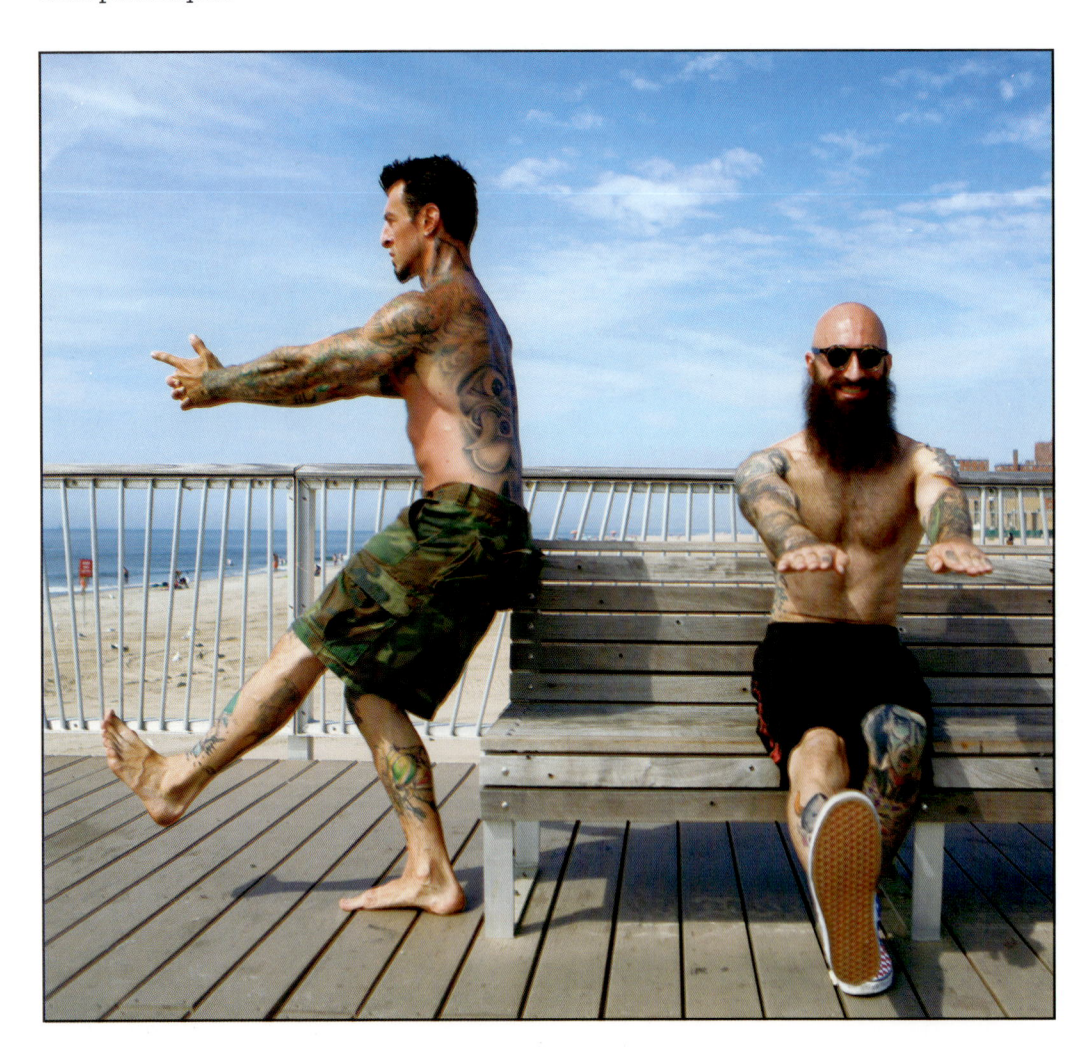

POLE ASSISTED PISTOL

Like the pole assisted two-legged squat, stand facing a pole (or doorframe or any other sturdy object you can hold onto for support). Grasp it gently and lift one leg into the air. With the other leg, lower yourself into the bottom of a single leg squat, gradually walking your hands down as you descend. Use your arms as much as you need to in order to control yourself on the way down and help get back to a standing position. With time you will learn to rely less on your arms. Eventually you won't need them at all anymore. The pole assisted pistol or "assistol" is another great way to ease yourself into the full pistol squat.

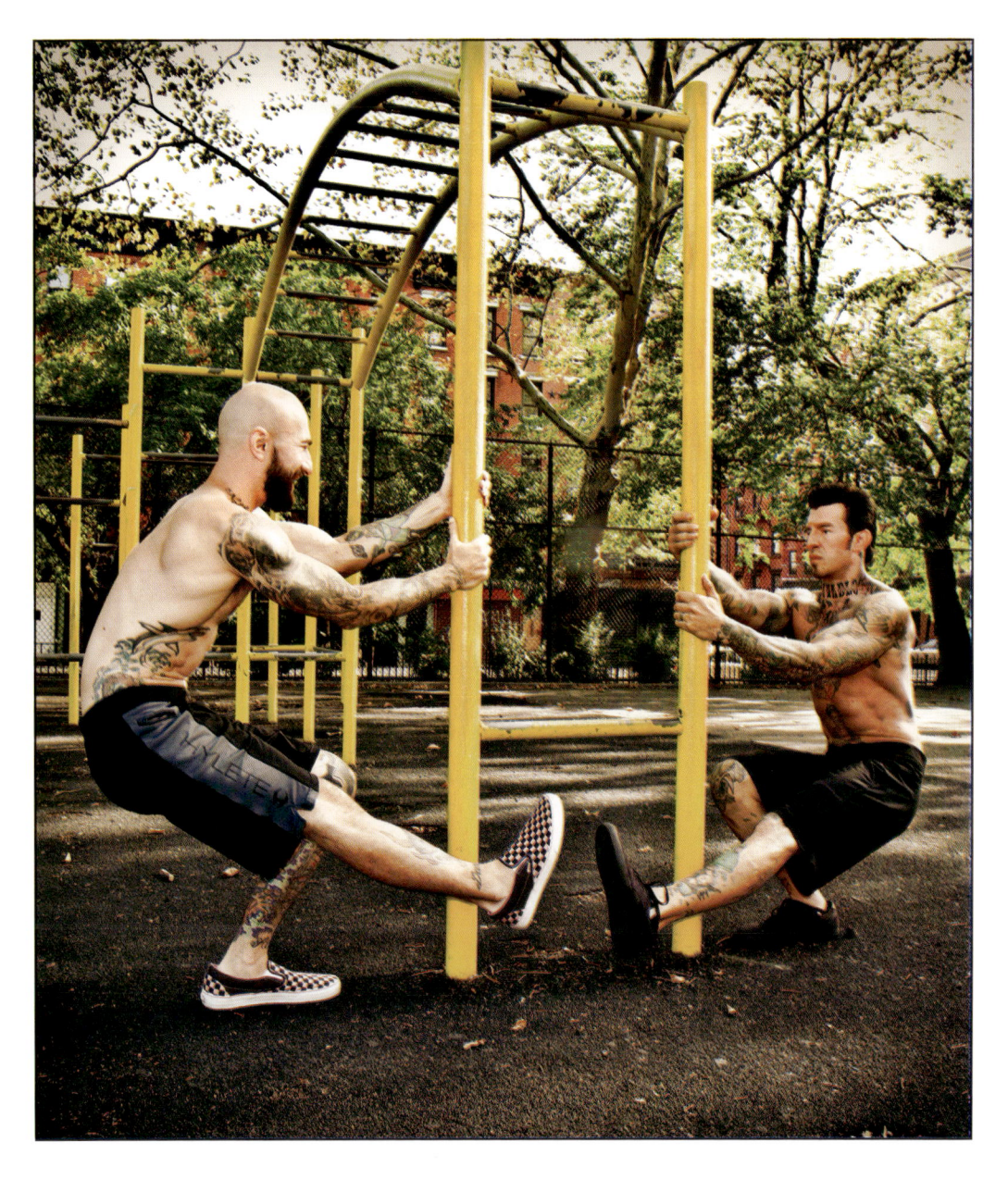

ELEVATED PISTOL

Stand on top of a bench or other object with one leg hanging off to the side. Reach your arms forward and slowly lower to the bottom of a one-legged squat while your opposite leg drops below the height of the bench.

Allowing your non-squatting leg to hang below parallel makes for more favorable leverage and balance than in a full pistol squat. It also requires less mobility in the hips and hamstrings. The lower you let your leg hang, the less mobility is required. When you've built up to a few good reps, try holding your extended leg a bit higher. Eventually you will be able to keep it high enough to perform a pistol on level ground.

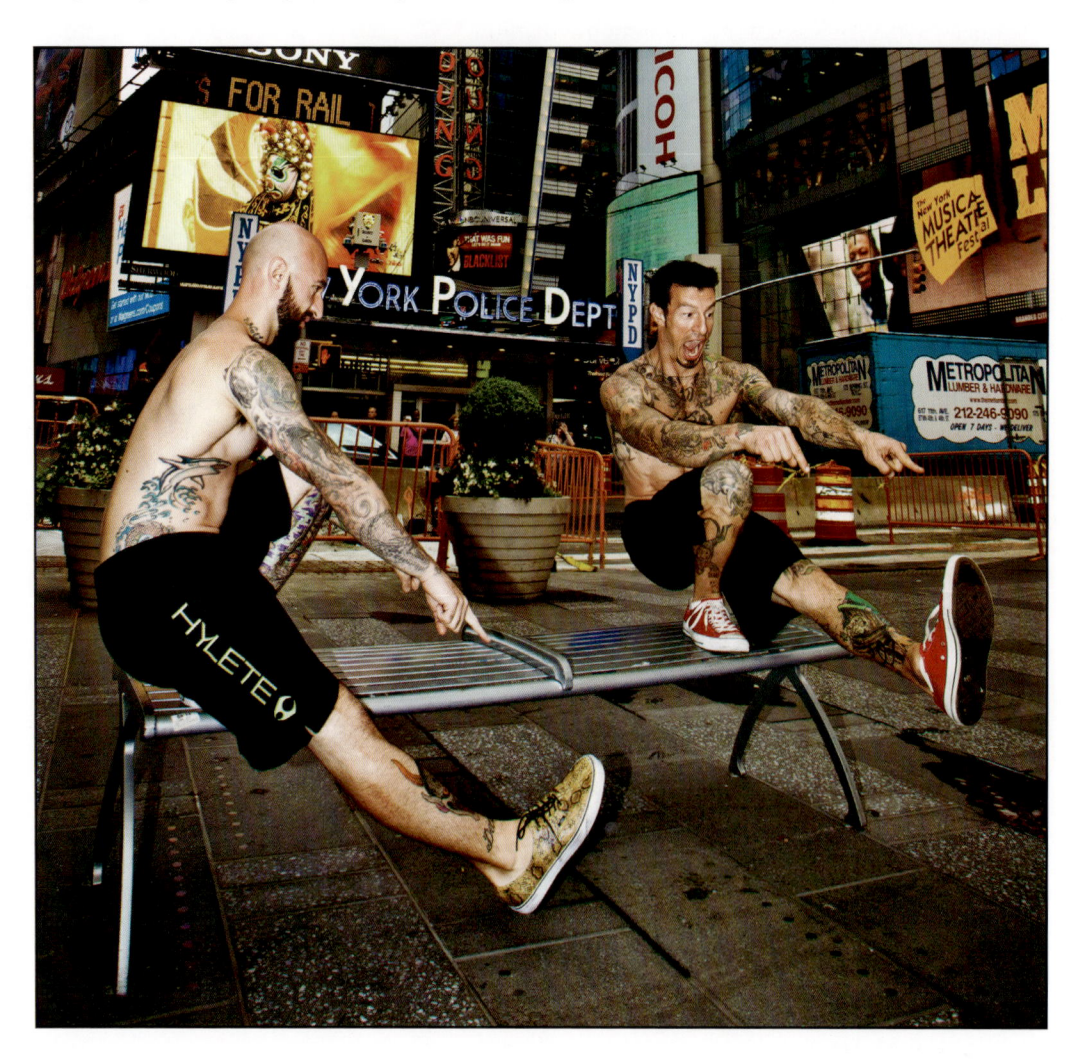

PISTOL SQUAT

There are many types of one legged squats, but the pistol is the gold standard. It's the perfect combination of strength, balance, flexibility and control.

From a standing position, reach one leg into the air with your knee straight, then squat down as low as possible on your standing leg. Pause briefly at the bottom, keeping tension in your abs, then return to the top position.

Don't be surprised if you feel your non-squatting leg working during a pistol. You will need to engage your hip flexors and quads on that side in order to keep your leg in the air. The term "one legged squat" can be a bit misleading.

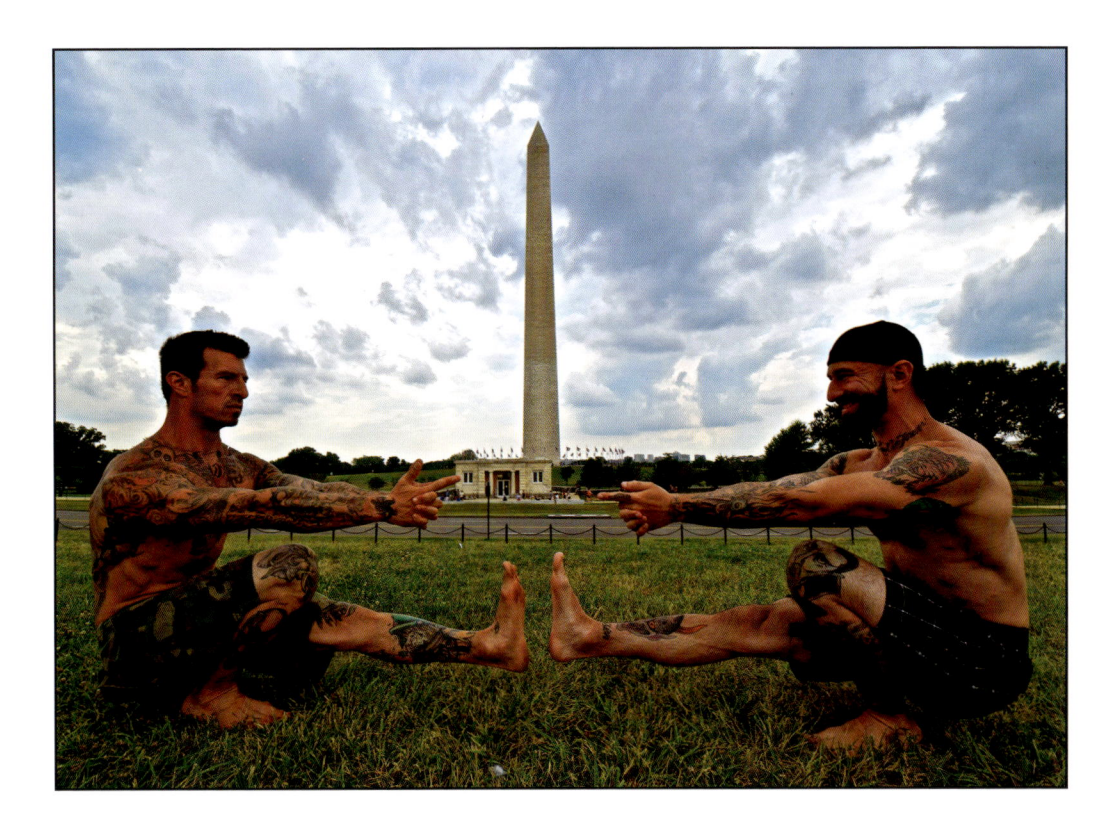

WUSHU PISTOL

If you've spent some time working on pistol squats, you may have at some point experienced a cramp in your non-squatting leg as you fought to keep it in the air. To minimize this issue, many people find holding the toe of their squatting leg to be helpful, particularly in the bottom position. This is also useful for those who have a hard time keeping the non-squatting leg straight. This variant is often referred to as a Wushu pistol. Holding your foot also helps facilitate full body tension.

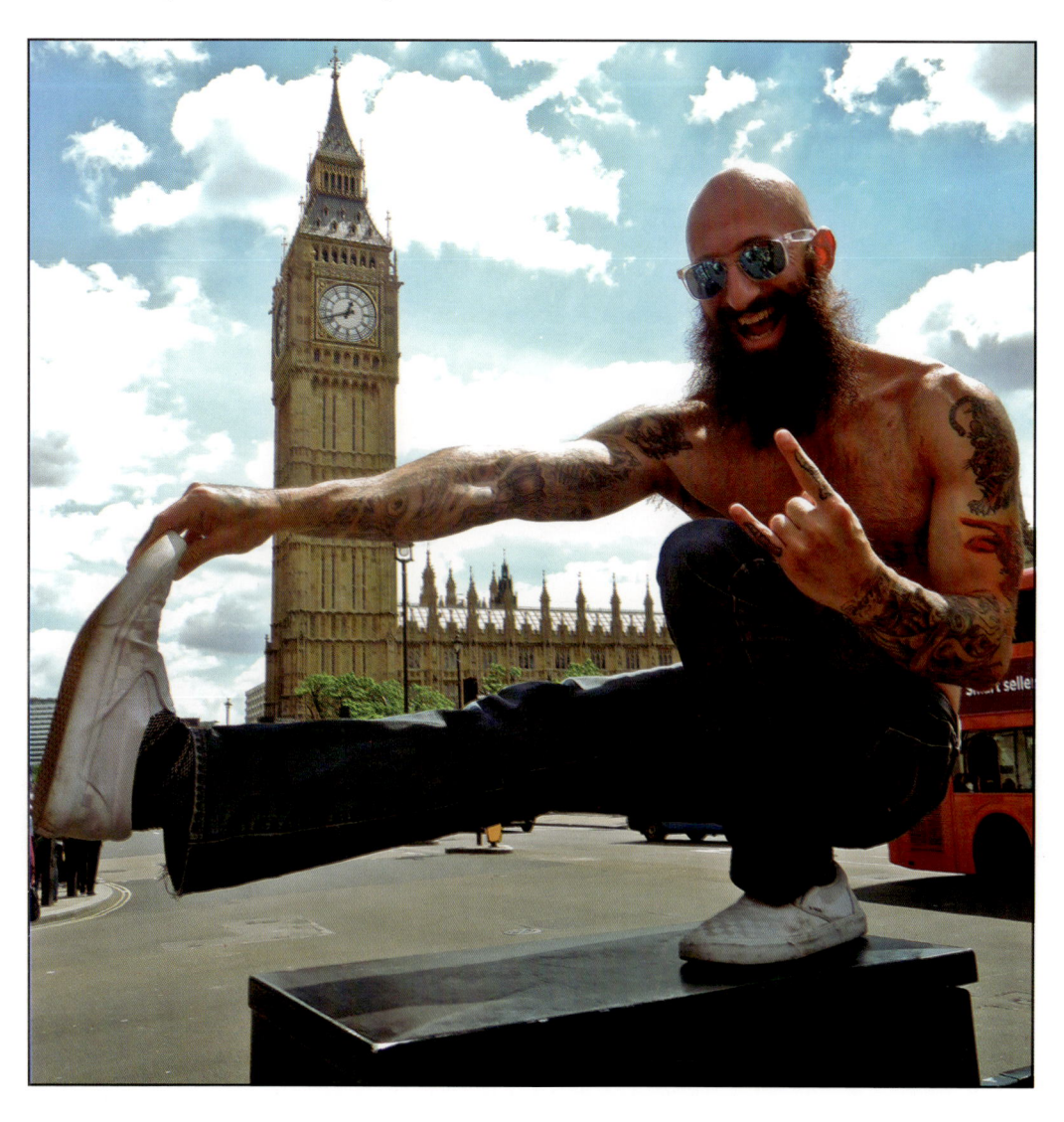

ADVANCED PISTOL

Once you've built the strength and control to perform lots of standard pistol squats, there is still room to continue to challenge yourself. If pistols with your arms held in front are becoming too easy, try placing your hands behind your head, like a prisoner squat. Once that is no longer a challenge, try holding your hands behind your back. This simple change in leverage will make the move significantly more difficult.

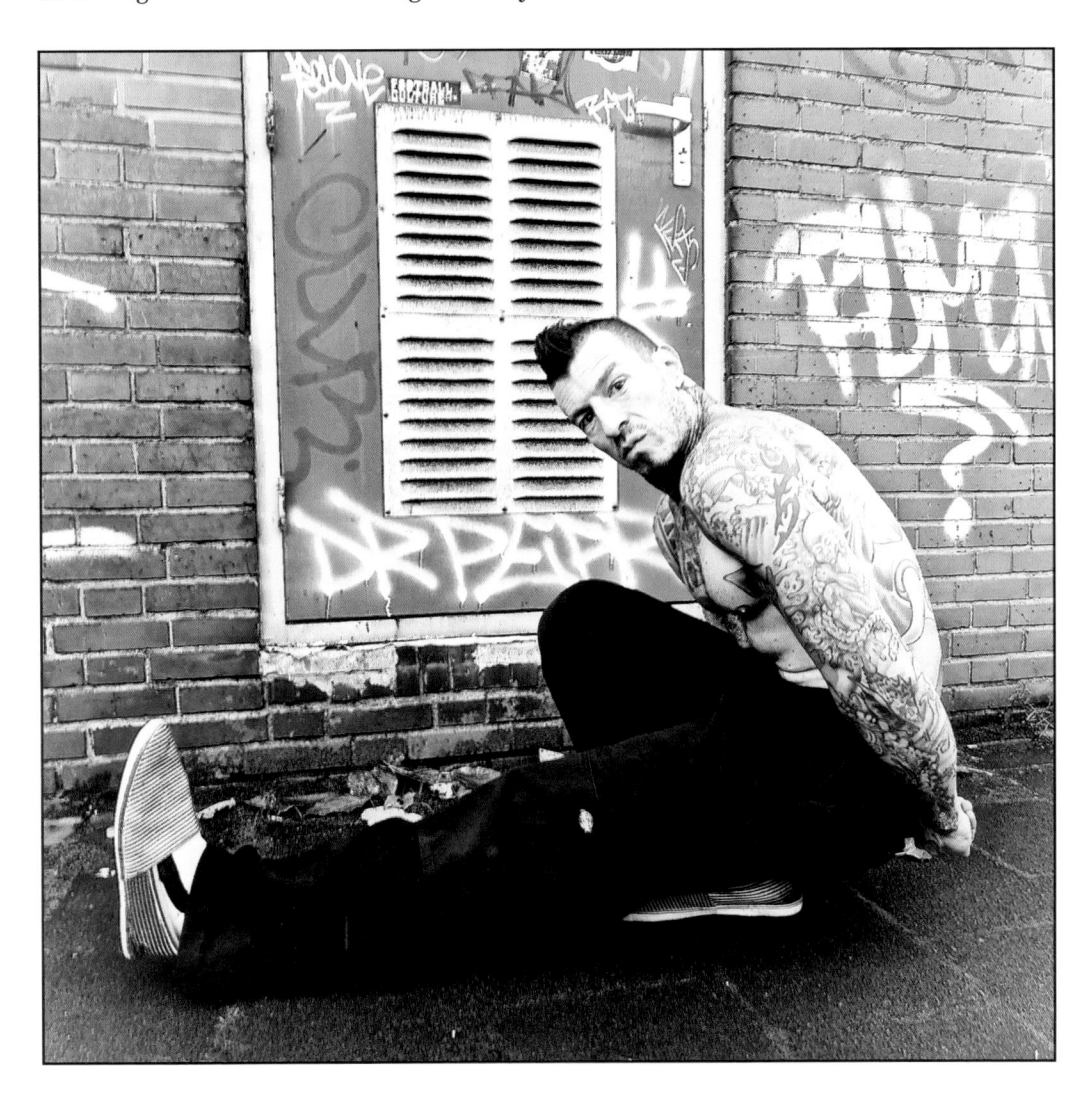

RAIL PISTOL

Performing a pistol squat while standing on a rail or bar takes the balance component to a whole other level. The narrower the rail, the more difficult this becomes, so start out with something relatively wide and take it from there.

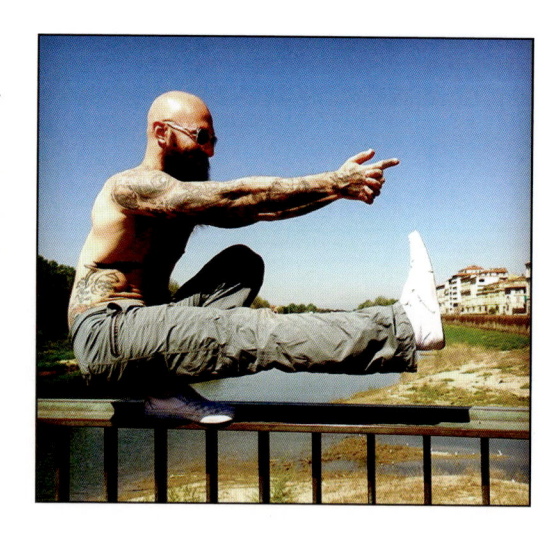

DRAGON PISTOL

The dragon pistol resembles a standard pistol squat, only with the extended leg threaded behind the squatting leg.

Like the traditional pistol squat, the dragon pistol requires serious strength, balance and mobility—but in a very unique way. This advanced variant can be surprisingly taxing on your inner thighs as well as your deep glute and hip muscles. And of course, all the other muscles that you work in a standard pistol will get hit as well.

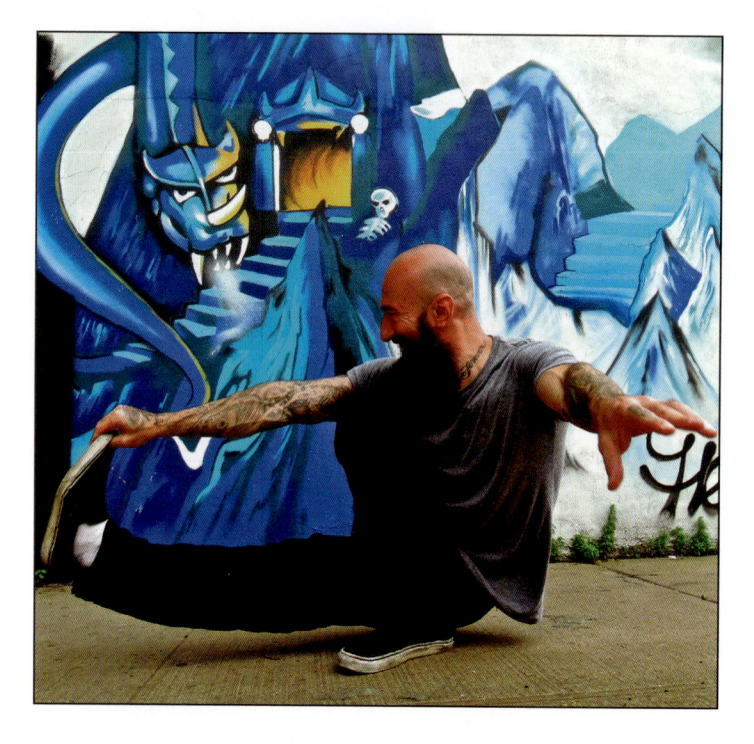

Like the standard pistol, beginning on an elevated surface and/or holding onto the foot of your non-squatting leg are both great ways of easing into the full dragon pistol.

HOVER LUNGE

The hover lunge is a one-legged squat that finds the non-squatting leg positioned behind the body, rather than in front, as it is with the pistol. It looks almost like a split squat or lunge, except the back foot never touches the floor (hence the name hover lunge). Unlike a lunge, however, you will need to reach your arms in front of your body and lean your torso forward to stay balanced, due to the fact that your rear foot never reaches the ground. As with many of the other squat variations, you may hold onto a pole or other sturdy object for assistance when starting out.

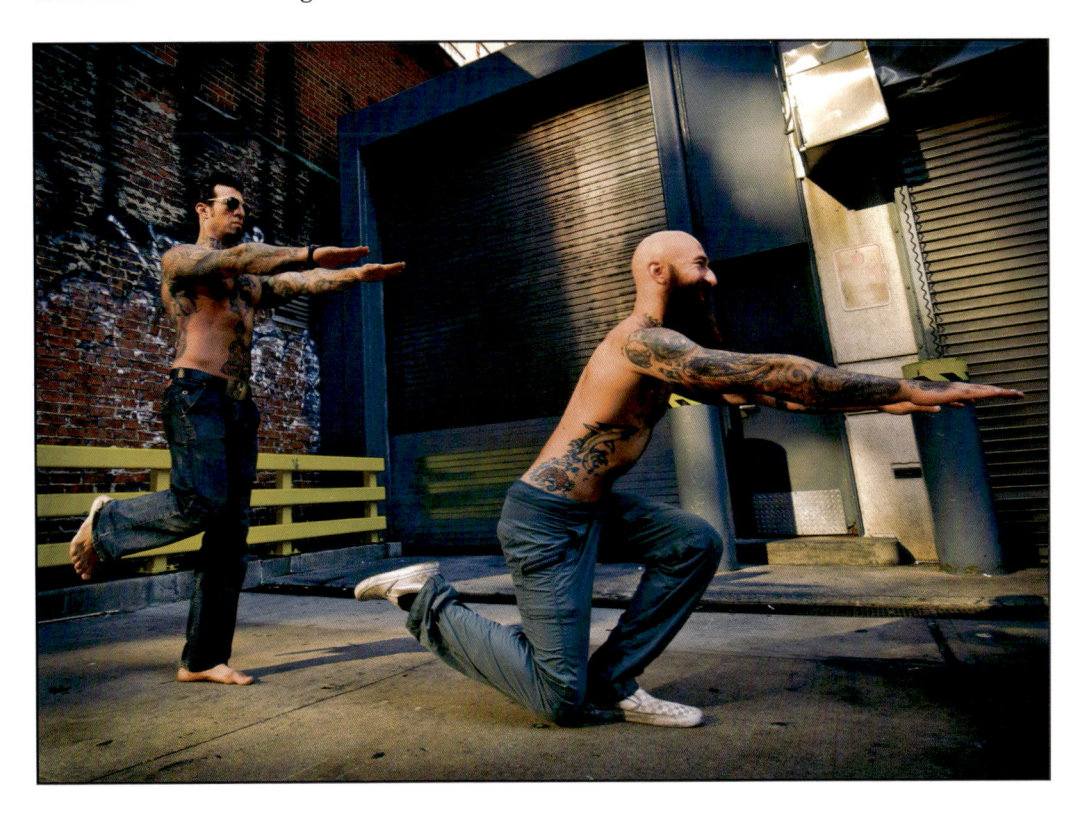

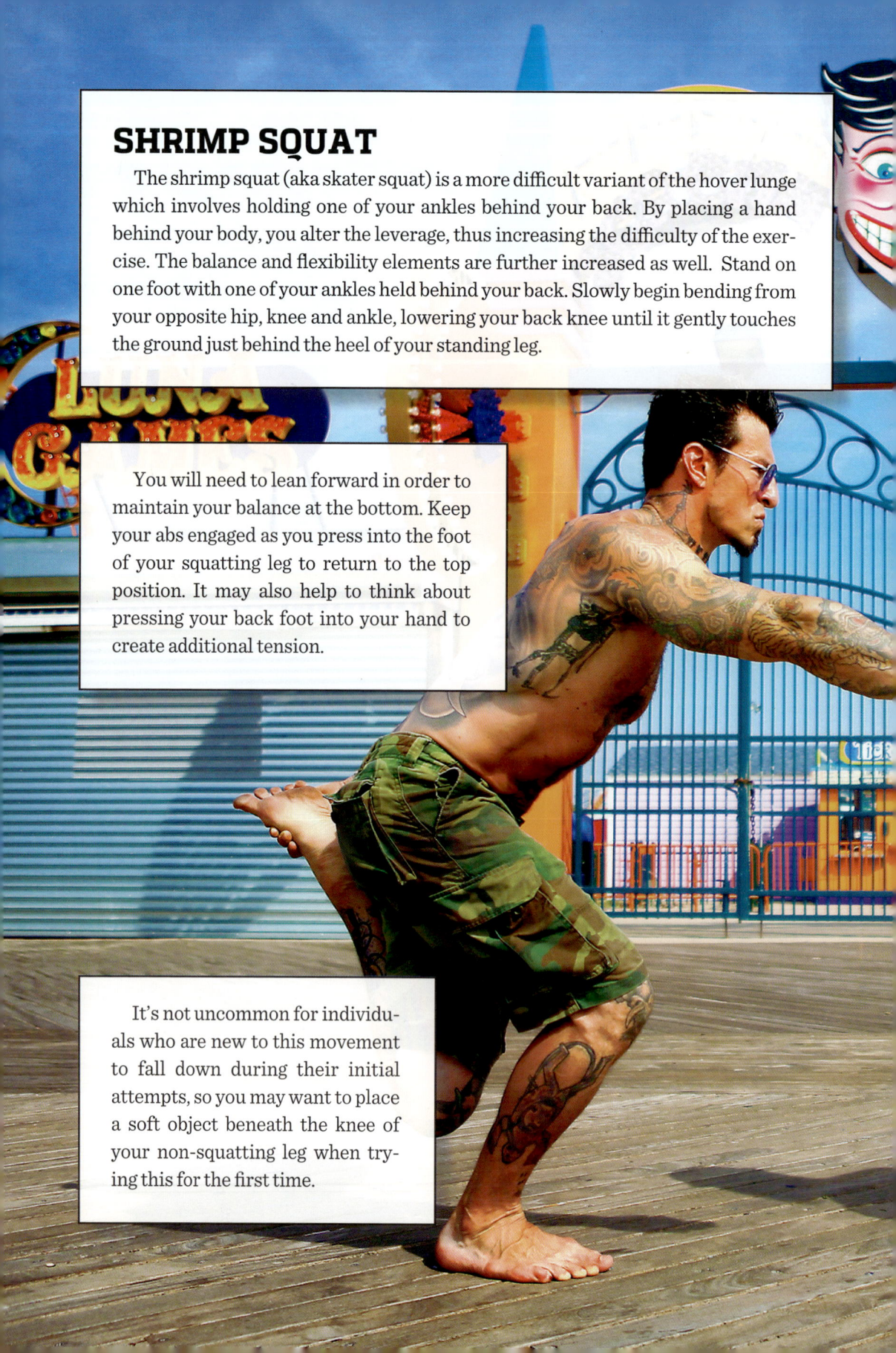

SHRIMP SQUAT

The shrimp squat (aka skater squat) is a more difficult variant of the hover lunge which involves holding one of your ankles behind your back. By placing a hand behind your body, you alter the leverage, thus increasing the difficulty of the exercise. The balance and flexibility elements are further increased as well. Stand on one foot with one of your ankles held behind your back. Slowly begin bending from your opposite hip, knee and ankle, lowering your back knee until it gently touches the ground just behind the heel of your standing leg.

You will need to lean forward in order to maintain your balance at the bottom. Keep your abs engaged as you press into the foot of your squatting leg to return to the top position. It may also help to think about pressing your back foot into your hand to create additional tension.

It's not uncommon for individuals who are new to this movement to fall down during their initial attempts, so you may want to place a soft object beneath the knee of your non-squatting leg when trying this for the first time.

ADVANCED SHRIMP

Just like pistols, you can make shrimp squats significantly harder by placing both hands behind your back. This simple change in positioning may not look like much, but it can make the move significantly more difficult. Make sure to lower yourself down slowly in order to avoid banging your back knee into the ground on the way down. Having both hands behind your back may also require you to lean farther forward to account for the change in balance.

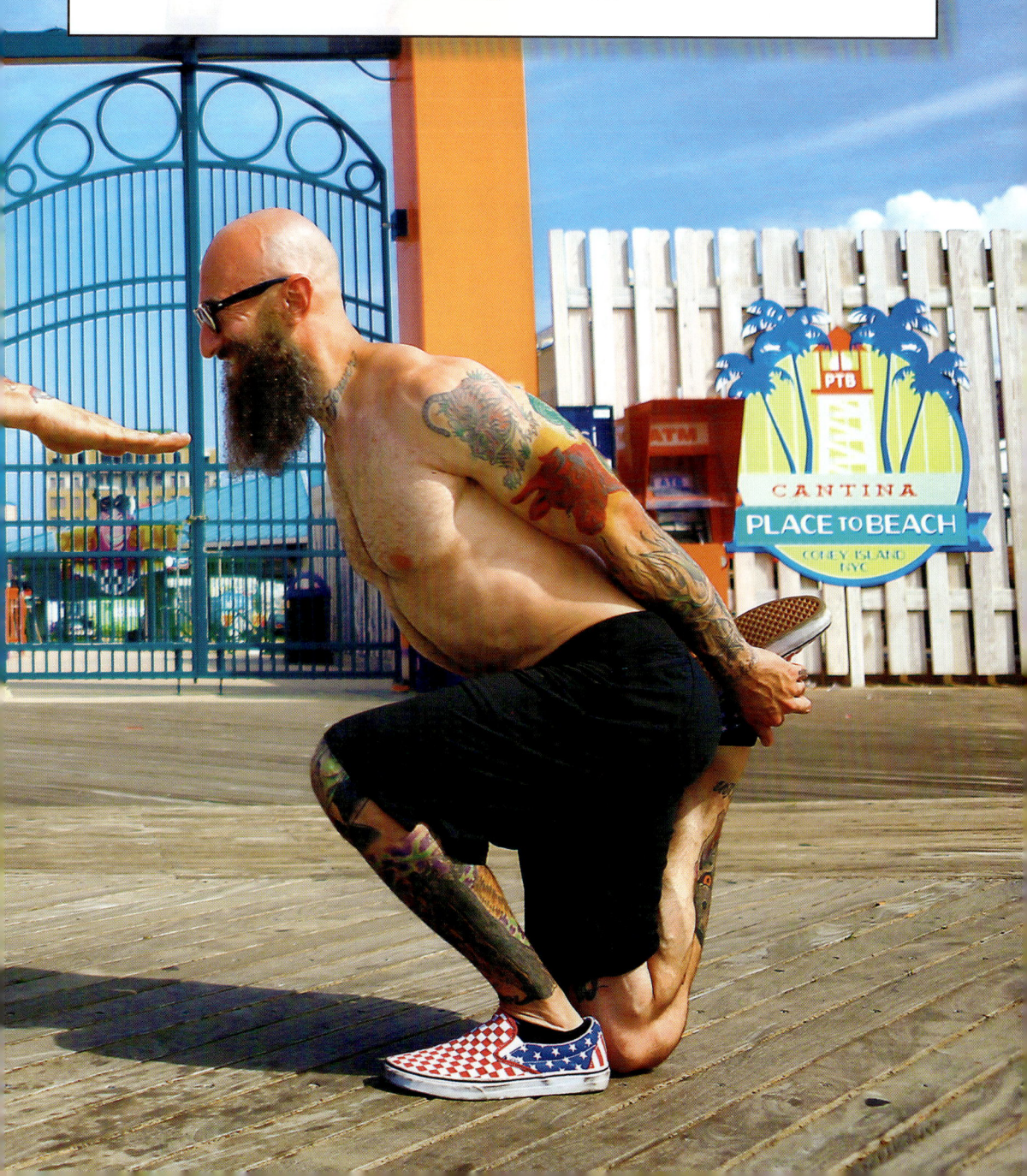

HAWAIIAN SQUAT

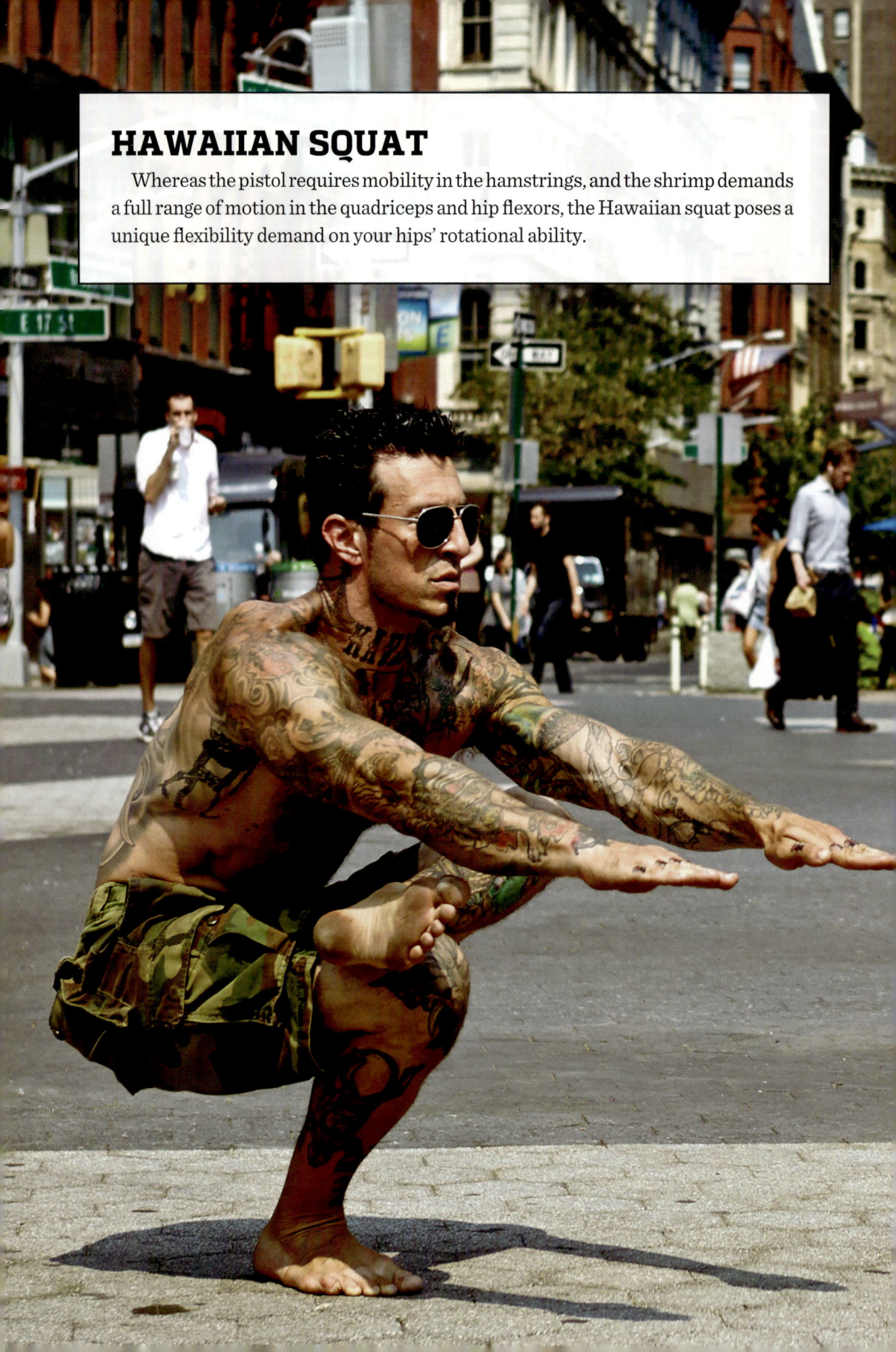

Whereas the pistol requires mobility in the hamstrings, and the shrimp demands a full range of motion in the quadriceps and hip flexors, the Hawaiian squat poses a unique flexibility demand on your hips' rotational ability.

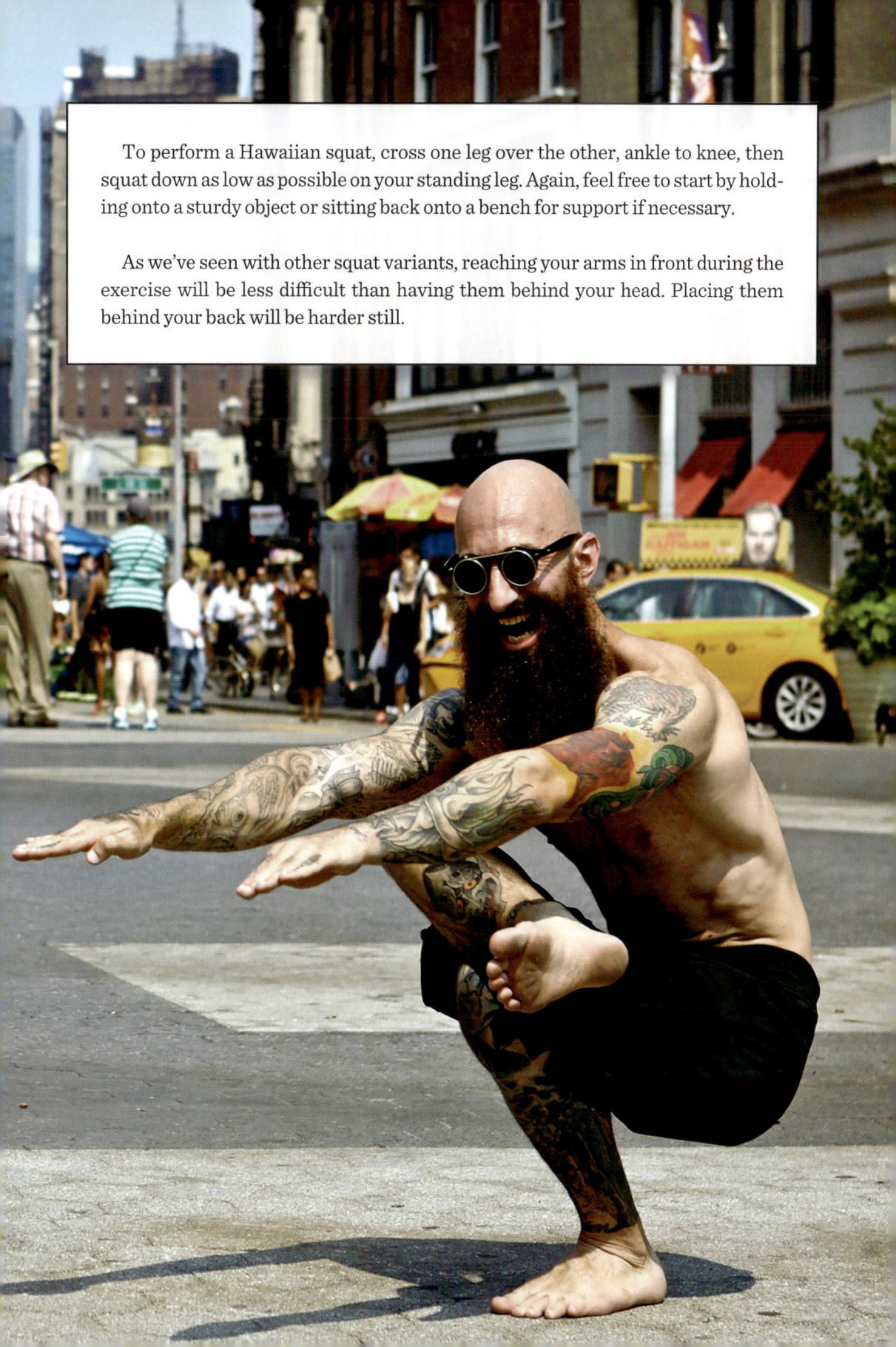

To perform a Hawaiian squat, cross one leg over the other, ankle to knee, then squat down as low as possible on your standing leg. Again, feel free to start by holding onto a sturdy object or sitting back onto a bench for support if necessary.

As we've seen with other squat variants, reaching your arms in front during the exercise will be less difficult than having them behind your head. Placing them behind your back will be harder still.

JUMBO SHRIMP

Unlike the pistol, which becomes easier when elevated, performing a shrimp on an elevated surface increases the range of motion, as your knee can now drop down deeper than the level of your foot. The increased range of motion can make an already challenging exercise considerably more difficult.

The flexibility demands of the jumbo shrimp are also greater due to this additional range of motion. You'll likely need to allow your bottom knee to come forward as you pass below the depth of the elevated object on which you're positioned.

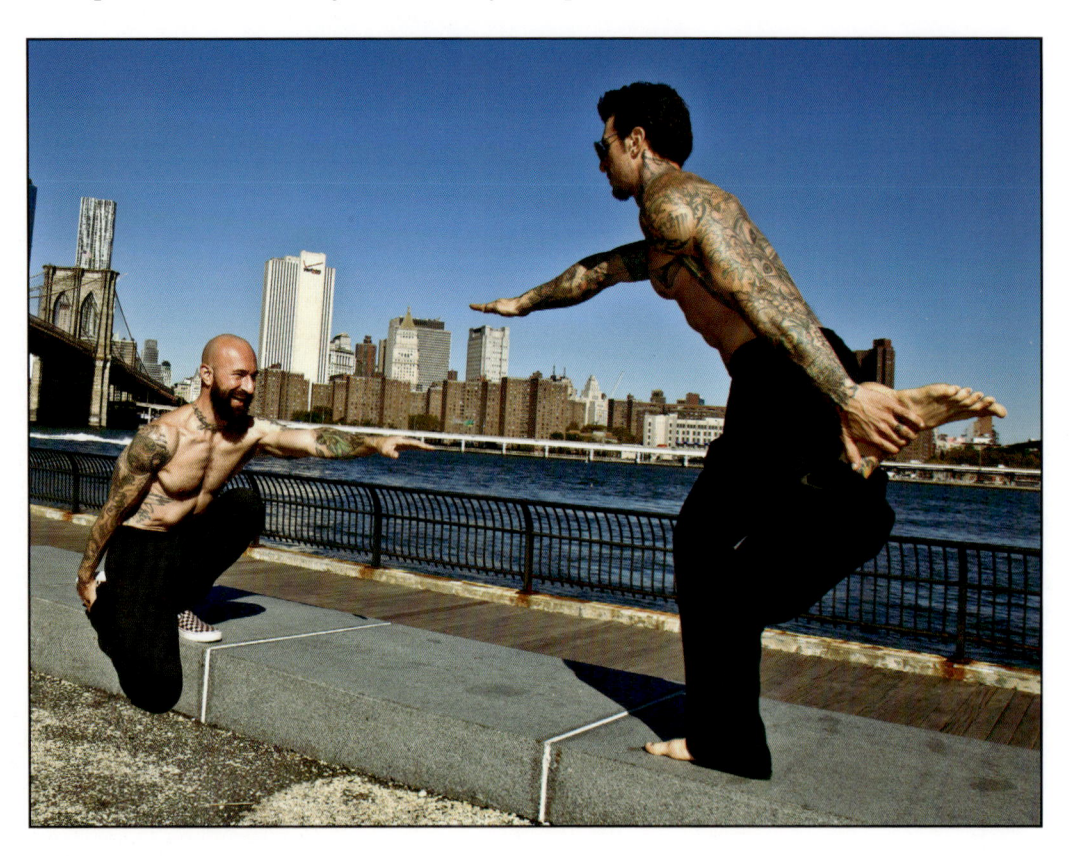

The Plyo-Matrix Jump Around

Any type of jump is a form of plyometrics. When you perform jump squats, it is helpful to think of pushing off with your feet with so much force that you explode off the floor.

Plyometrics are not limited to squats and can be applied to just about every variant, including split squats, lunges, step-ups, pistols and just about anything you can imagine.

It is important to bend into your hips, knees and ankles when you land, so as to absorb the impact. Training your legs in this capacity fires up numerous muscle fibers and is an amazing conditioning workout for the heart, as you will be demanding a lot of blood flow to the largest muscles in your body.

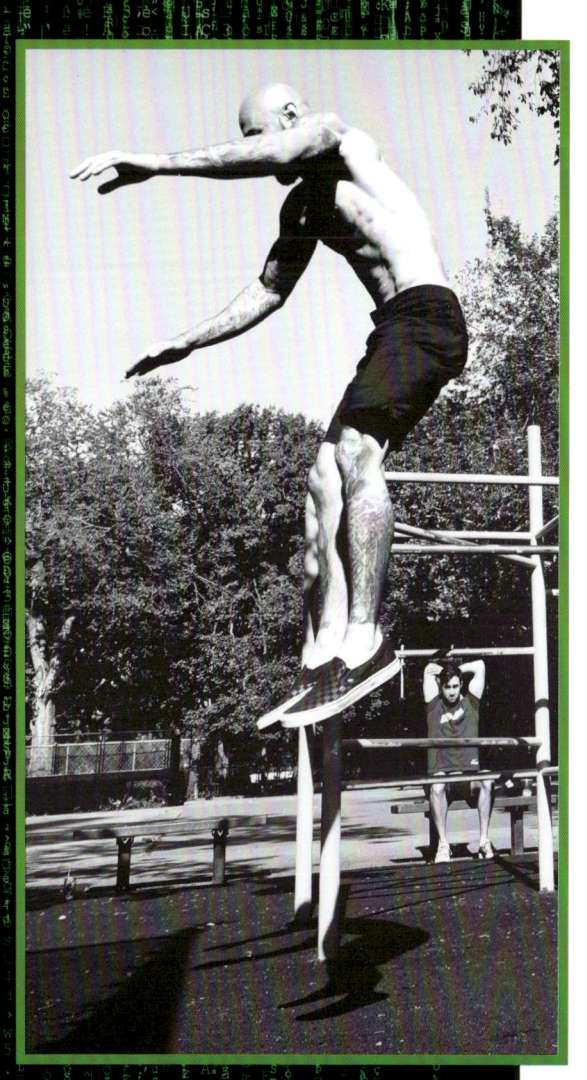

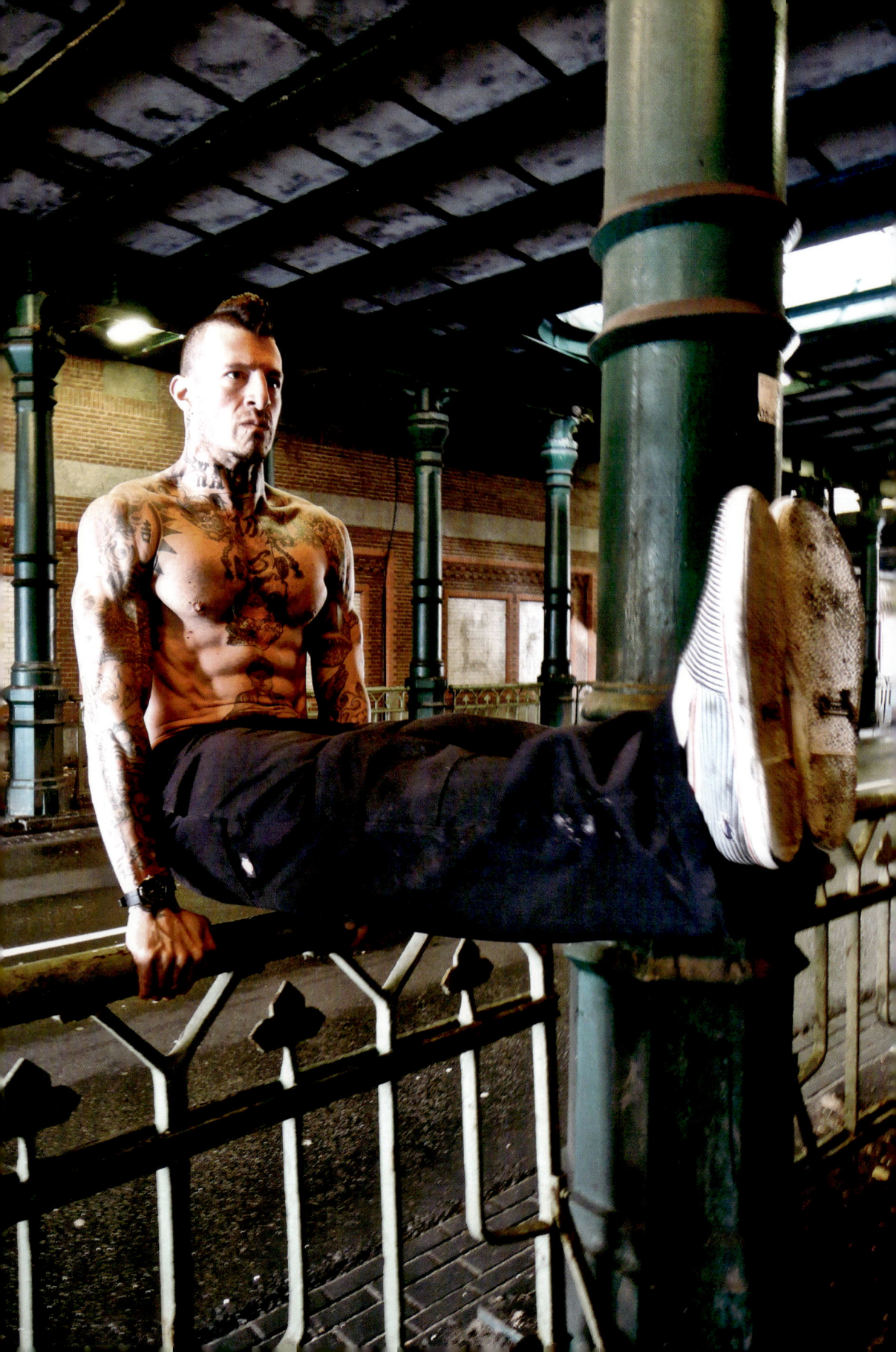

CHAPTER 7

Flex

Full body forward flexion is sometimes inappropriately simplified to mean "abs exercise." And while it's true that the abdominal chain is the primary mover in these activities, to dismiss these exercises as exclusively abs workouts would irresponsibly misrepresent the situation. Yes, these exercises emphasize the core, but many of them will also challenge your arms, legs, chest, shoulders and more.

This is not to discount the importance of your abs; they play a large role in stabilizing the trunk every time you do a squat, a push-up or even get out of bed in the morning, so it's critical to train all abs muscles including the sides (obliques) and the deep abs stabilizers (transverse abdominals) to get a powerful, unbreakable center.

This section is separated into two categories: Grounded Flex and Hanging Flex, as dictated by the body's placement in its environment. Changing the spatial plane in which we train alters the difficulty of the exercises by affecting leverage, a key component of bodyweight training in all its glorious forms.

GROUNDED FLEX PROGRESSIONS

These exercises are performed lying or seated. If you are a beginner, it is recommended that you start out with the first few exercises in this category before moving onto Overhead Flexion, but make no mistake: the advanced grounded exercises are absolutely a force to be reckoned with in their own right.

LYING KNEE TUCK

Lie on your back with your hands by your sides, then lift your heels a few inches off the ground. Keeping your feet close to the floor, tuck your knees all the way to your chest, allowing your lower back to come off the ground slightly at the top. Stay in control as you extend your legs back to the start position, pressing your lower back into the ground to engage your deep abdominal stabilizers. This start position is essentially the same as the hollow body hold discussed on page 30.

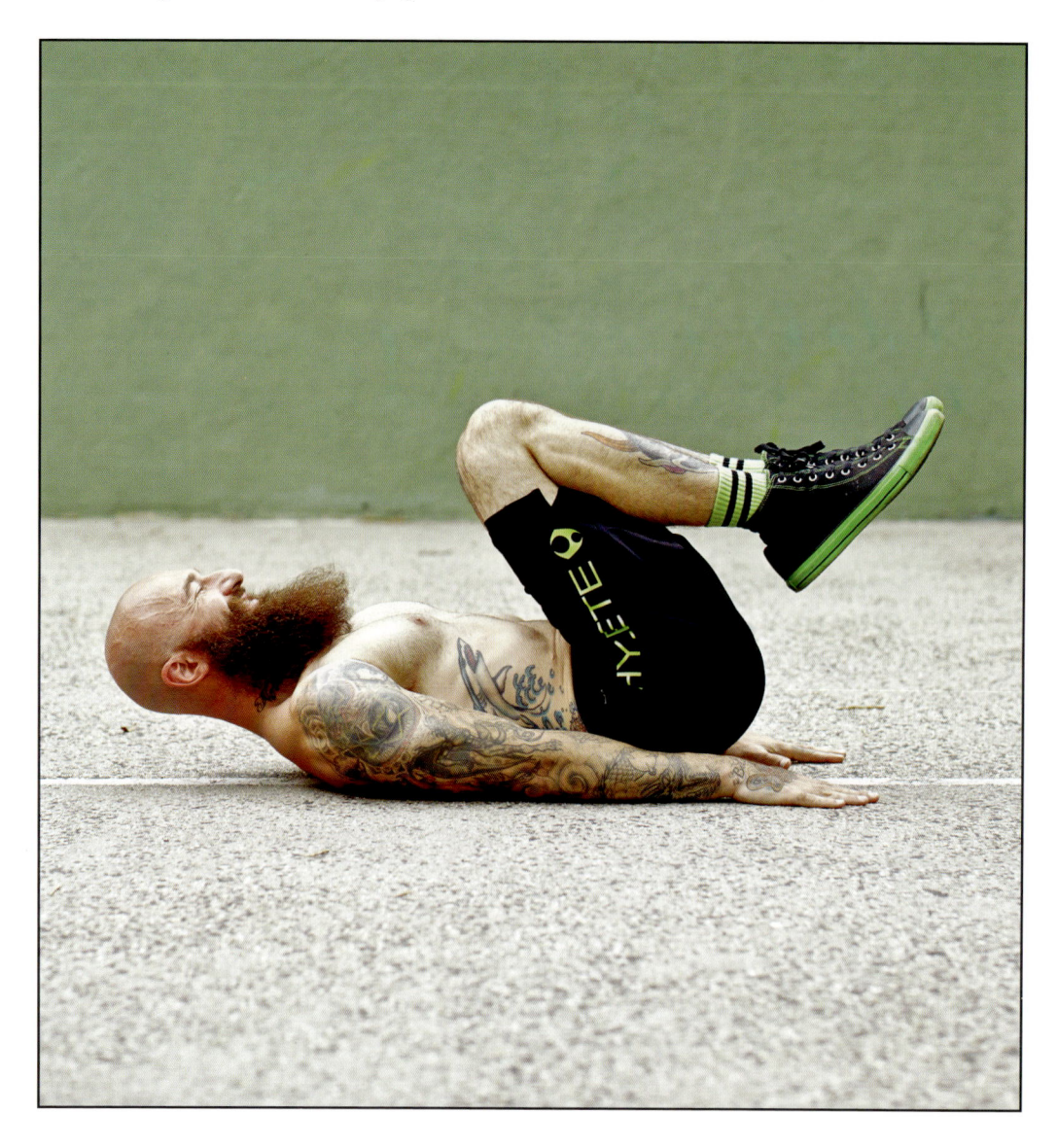

LYING BENT KNEE RAISE

Lie on your back with your feet flat on the floor, knees bent and hands at your sides. Draw your navel inward and roll your hips away from the ground, bringing your knees toward your chest. Carefully lower your legs back down and repeat. The angle at your knees should remain consistent throughout the range of motion, with the movement primarily taking place at the hips.

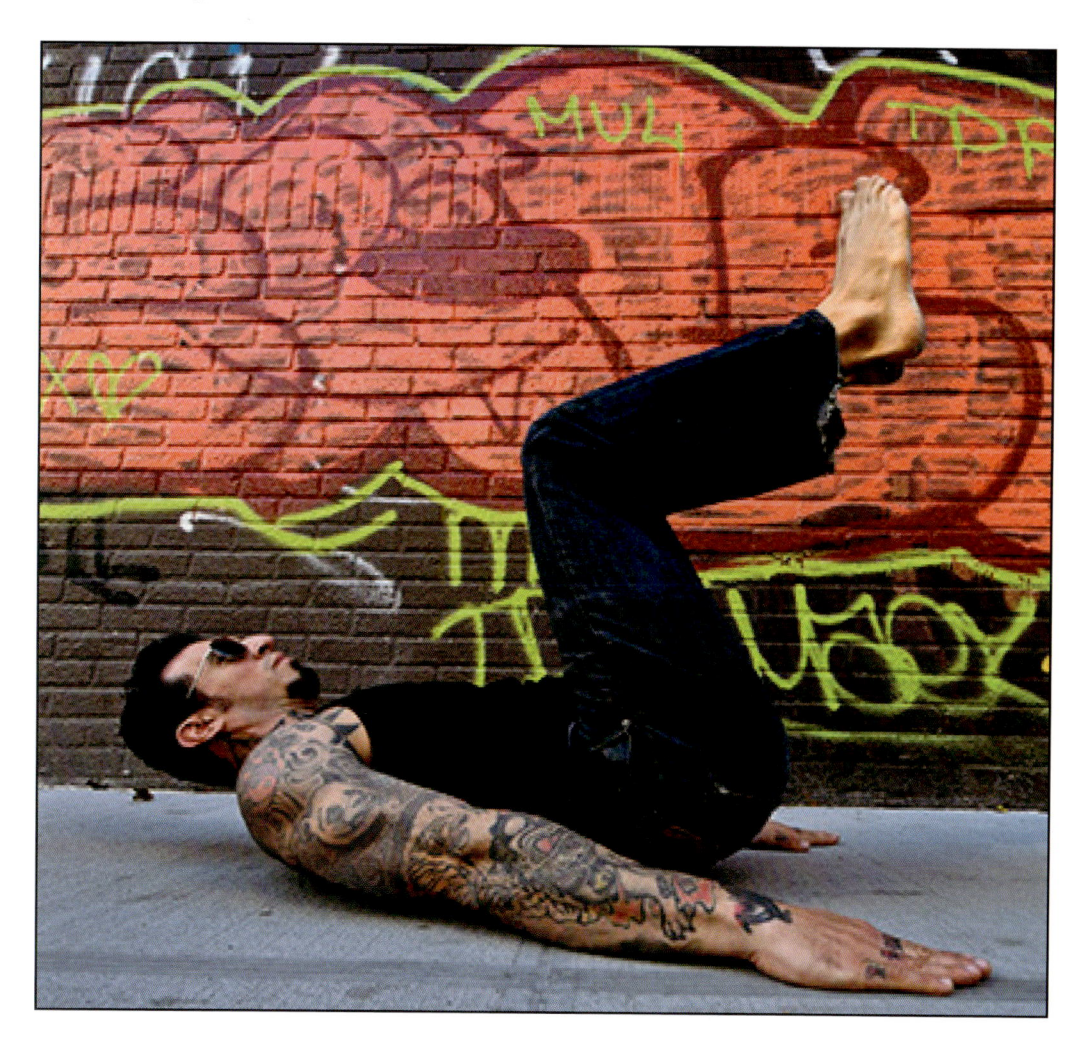

STRAIGHT LEG RAISE

Lie on your back with your legs straight and hands at your sides. Draw your navel inward and roll your hips away from the ground, raising your legs straight into the air until they are perpendicular to the ground, then carefully lower them back down and repeat. To add difficulty, raise your hips at the top of the range of motion.

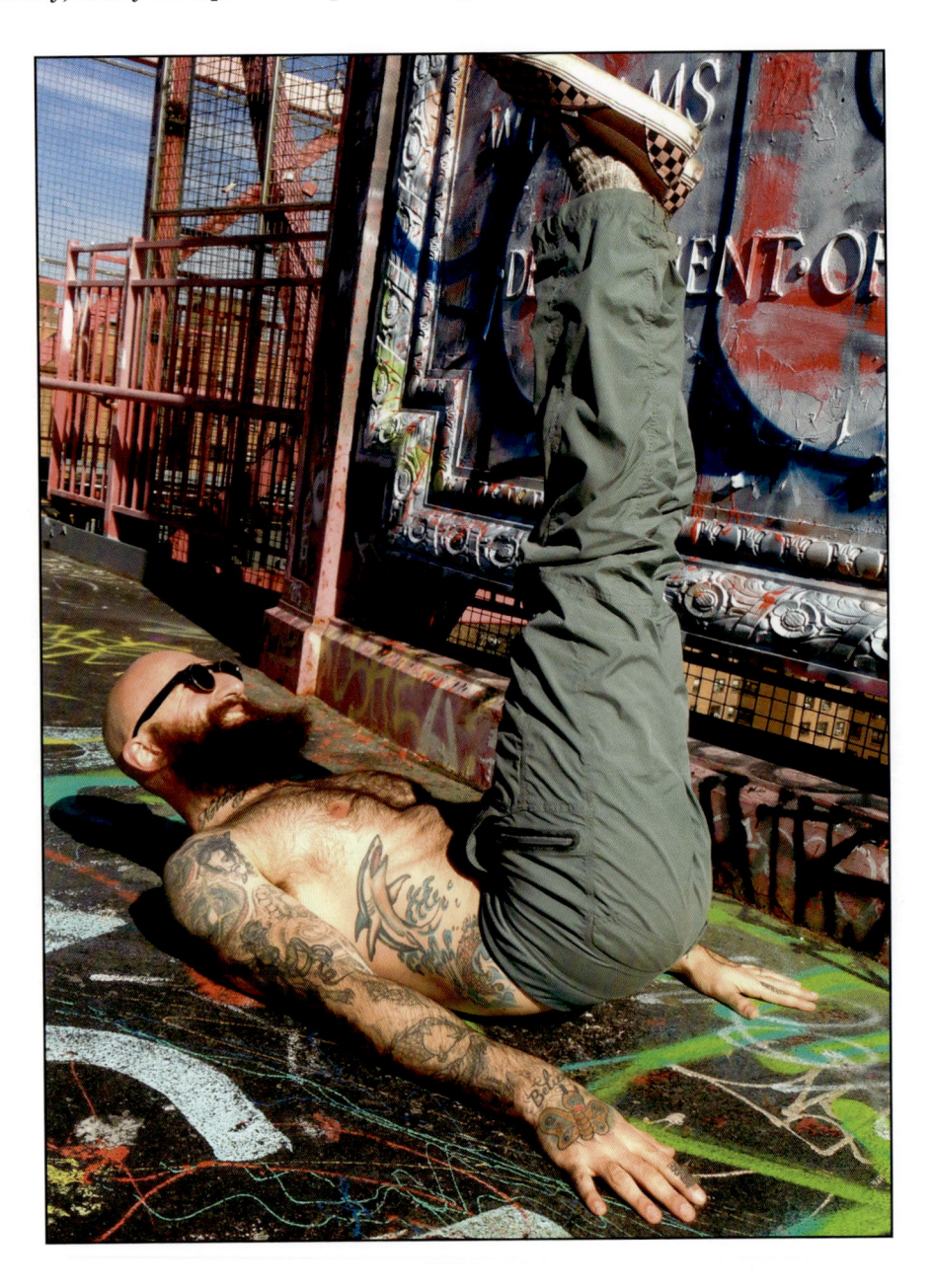

GROUNDED WINDSHIELD WIPER

Lie on the floor with both legs straight in the air above your hips. Reach your arms out to the sides for stability and begin rotating your hips and legs toward the left until they form a 45 degree angle to the ground. Pause briefly, then reverse direction and lower your hips and legs to the opposite side, alternating left and right on each rep. The twisting movement at the trunk emphasizes your obliques in addition to working the "six pack" muscles on the front of the body.

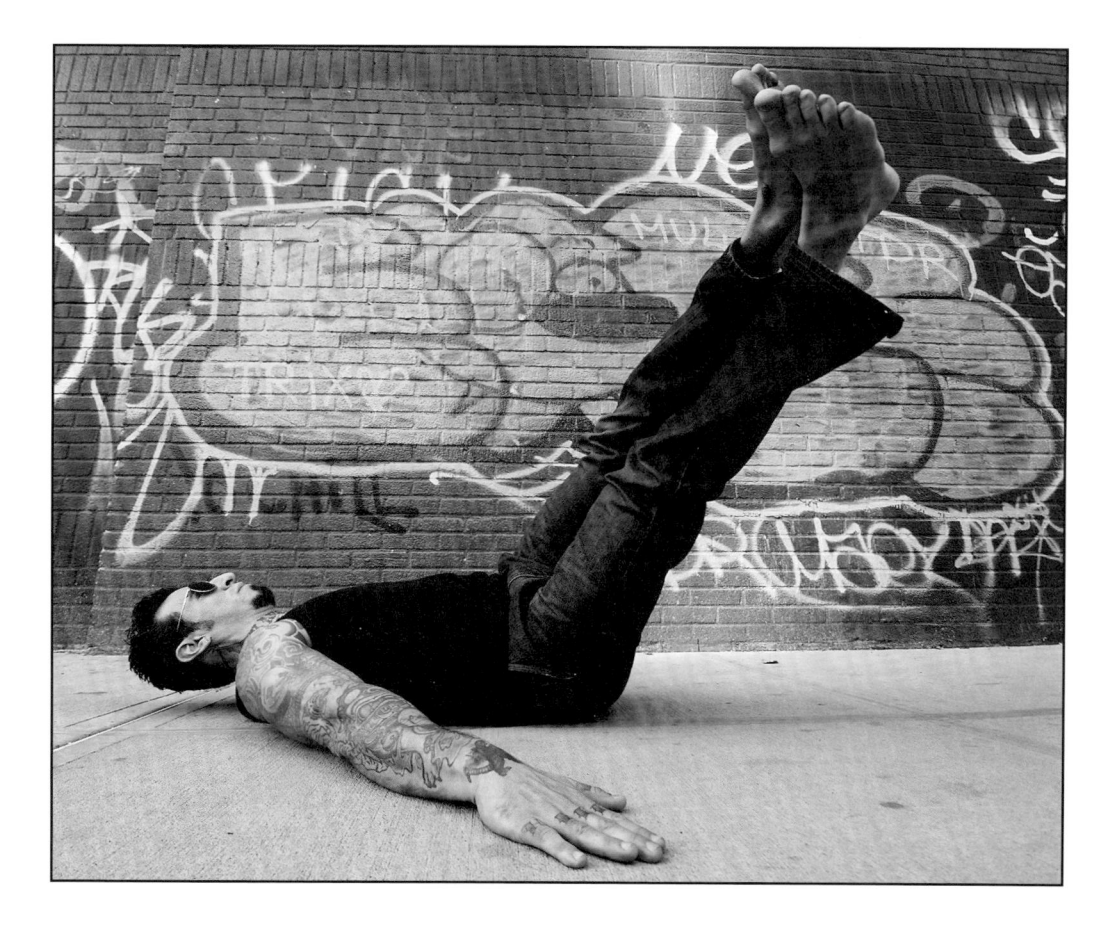

SEATED KNEE RAISE

Sit on a bench, chair or other object with your arms by your sides, gripping the bench for stability. Lean back and tuck your knees to your chest, then extend them out in front of your body, maintaining tension in your trunk throughout the range of motion. You may need to lean back a bit farther as your extend your legs away from your torso to maintain balance.

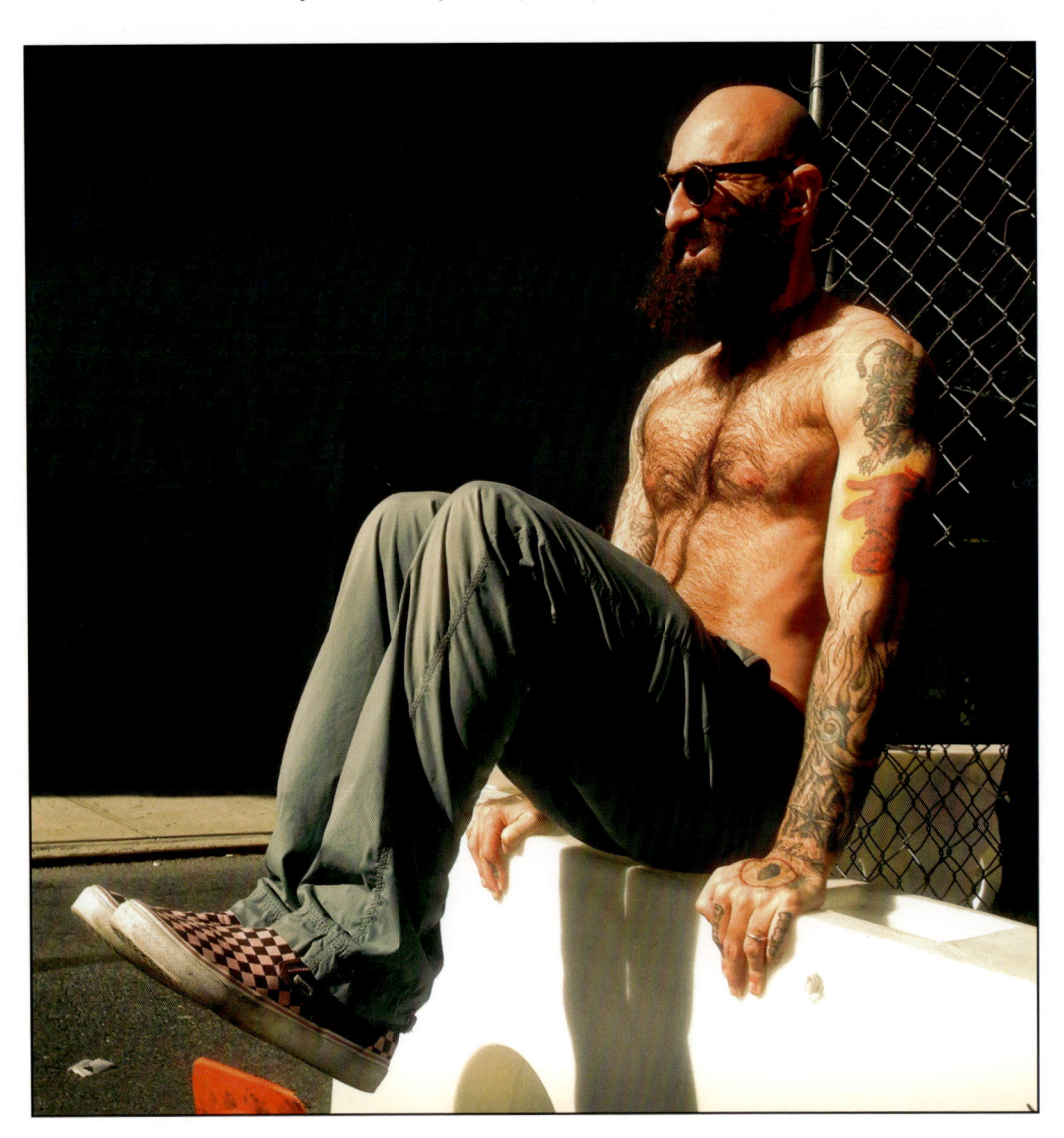

BENT KNEE HOLD

Sit on the floor with your hands flat on the ground just outside of your hips. Extend your arms and push your hands into the ground, lifting your legs and upper-body into the air with your knees tucked toward your chest.

If you are having a hard time getting into position from the floor, practice on a raised object instead, as elevating your hands provides more leeway to lift into position.

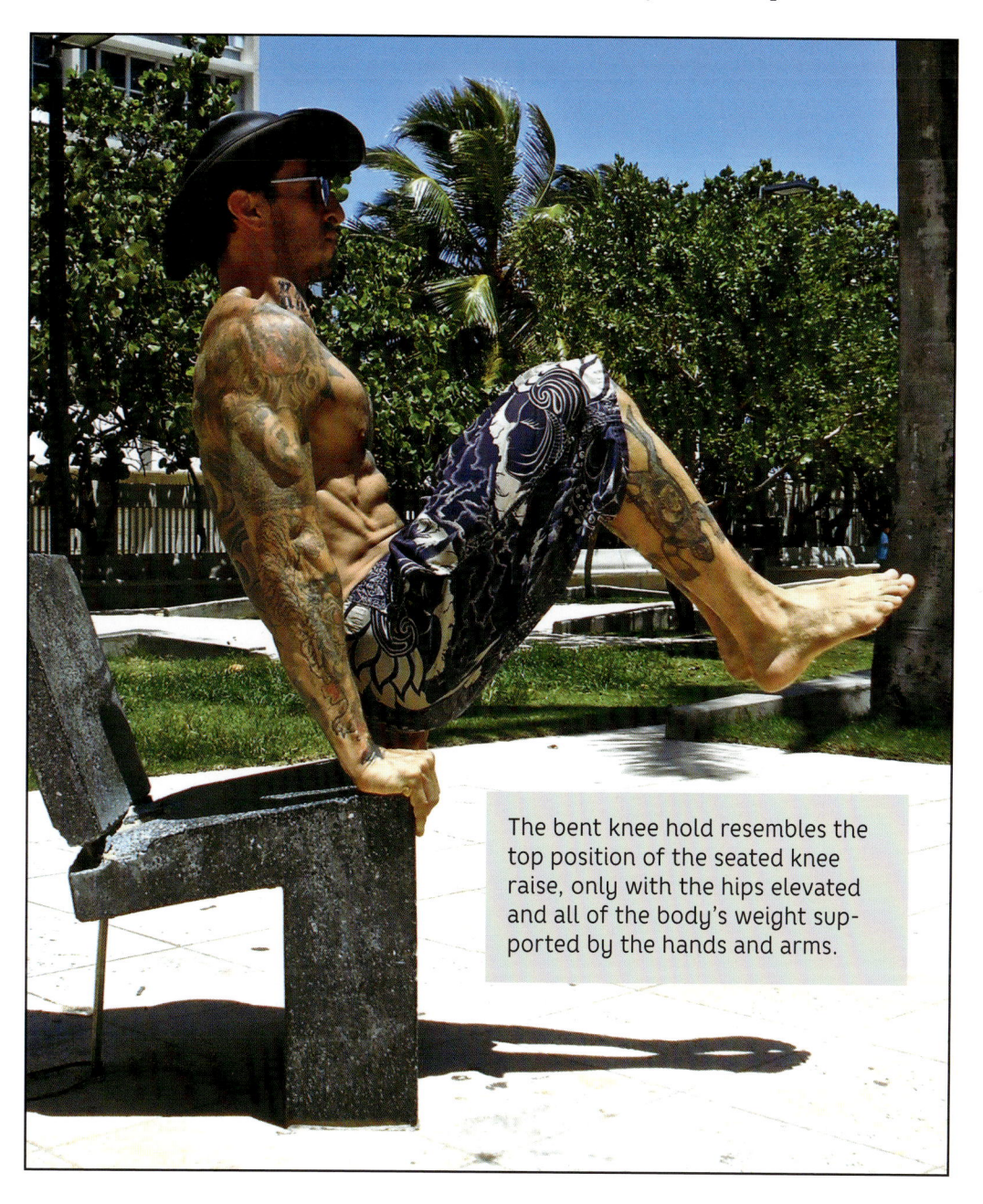

The bent knee hold resembles the top position of the seated knee raise, only with the hips elevated and all of the body's weight supported by the hands and arms.

L-SIT

Sit on the floor with your hands flat on the ground just outside of your hips. Extend your elbows and push your hands into the ground, lifting your legs and upper body into the air with your legs straight so your body resembles a capital letter L, hence the name L-sit.

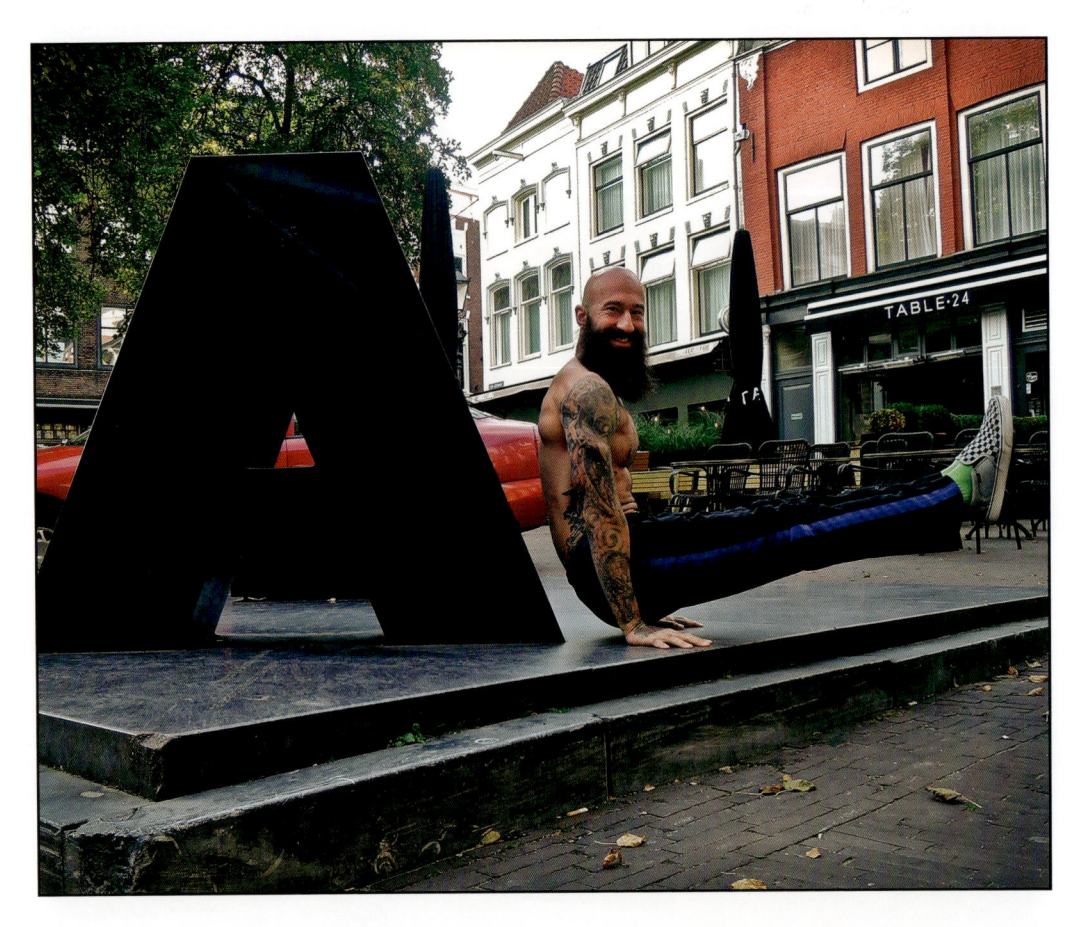

If you are having a hard time getting into position from the floor, practice on a raised object instead, as elevating your hands provides more leeway to lift into position. Additionally, performing the L-sit on parallel bars allows you to use your grip strength, which can make the exercise more achievable for some. You may also bend one knee to reduce the difficulty as you progress toward the full L-sit.

Whichever method you employ, think about keeping your arms close to your body, with your elbows locked and pointed back behind you as much as possible. Focus on creating tension with every muscle in your entire body. Though the L-sit is often classified as an "abs" exercise, you may be surprised by how much you'll need to use your arms and legs.

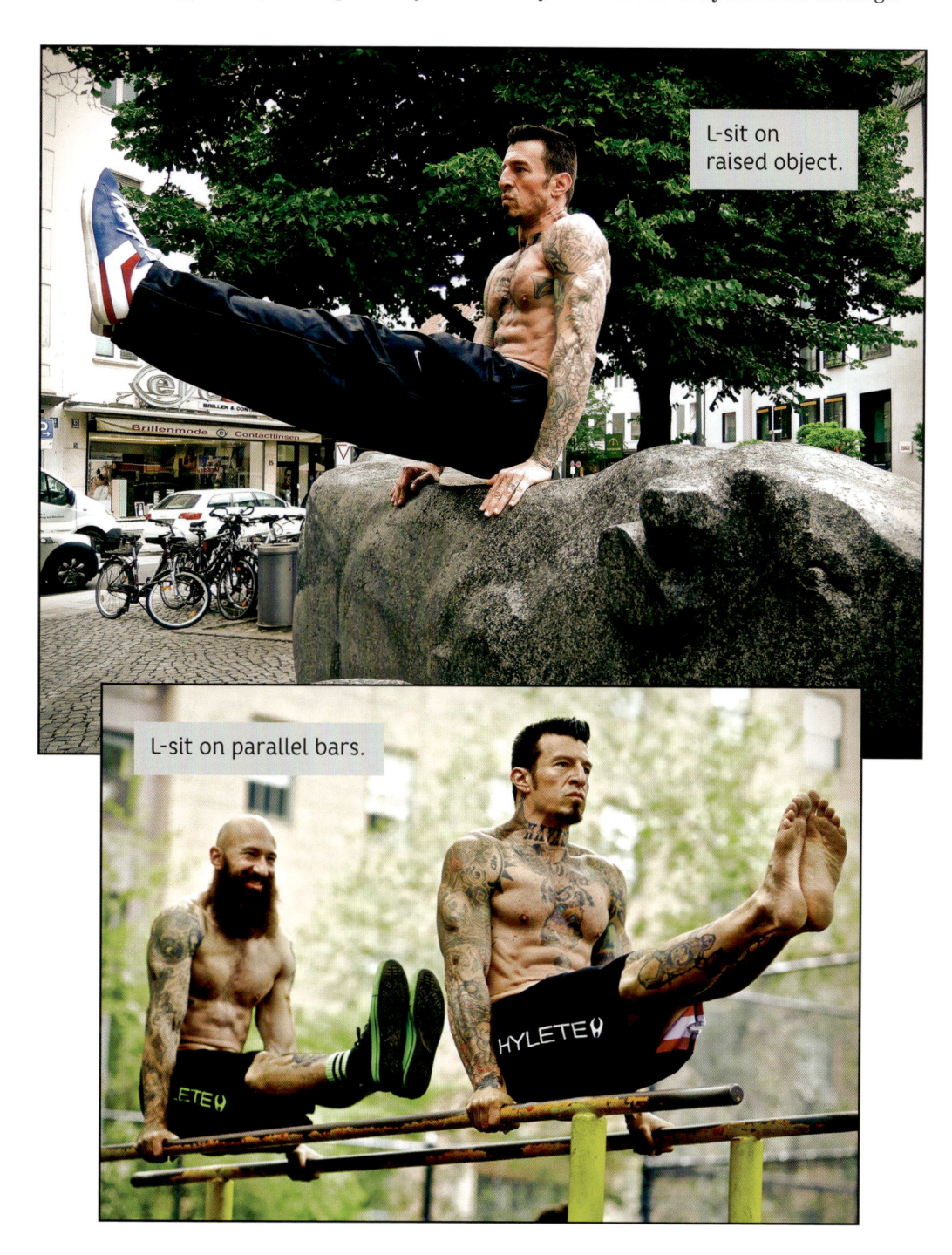

L-sit on raised object.

L-sit on parallel bars.

STREET WORKOUT

V-SIT

Sit on the floor with your hands flat on the ground just outside of your hips. Extend your elbows and push your hands into the ground, lifting your legs and upperbody into the air with your legs as vertical as possible. You will need to lean your torso back and move your hips forward in order to get your legs close to perpendicular with the ground. As such, your body will resemble a capital letter V, hence the name V-sit.

Like the previous two exercises, practicing on an elevated surface will allow for better leeway to lift into position. Additionally, holding onto parallel bars can give you better leverage to lean back farther, thus achieving a more vertical leg position.

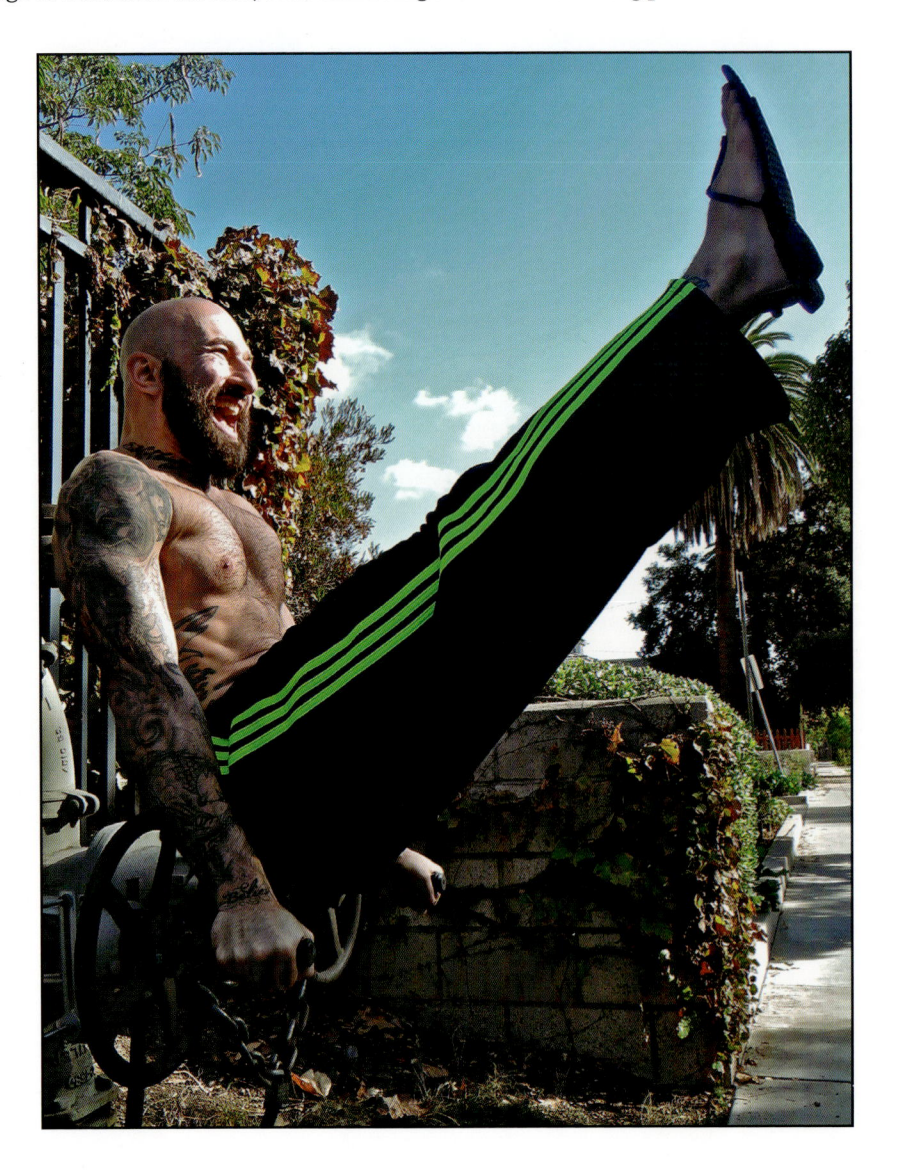

"WRISTY" BUSINESS

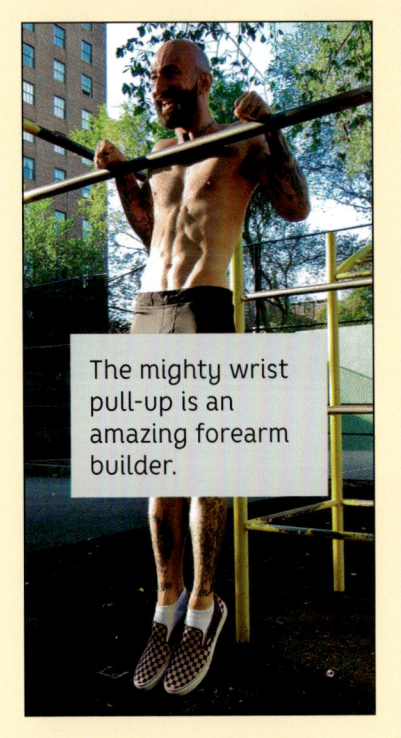

Training with an unconventional grip is fantastic for building monstrous strength in your forearms. But training with no grip at all is a way to take it to the next level! While not for beginners, the following examples are great for anyone whose lifestyle demands wrists that can accept massive impact without buckling under pressure, or anyone up for a new and unique challenge. You don't need to be a boxer, martial artist or Street Workout competitor to give these a try.

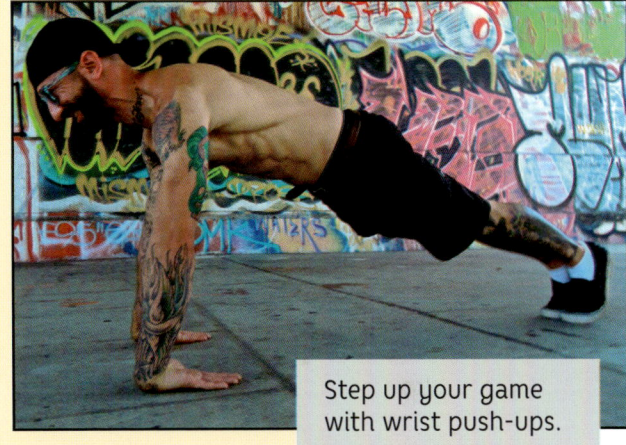

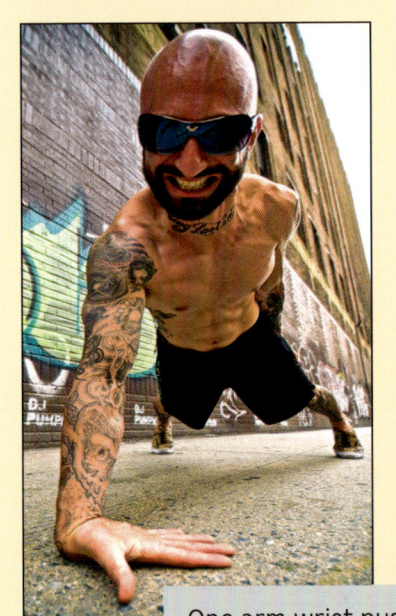

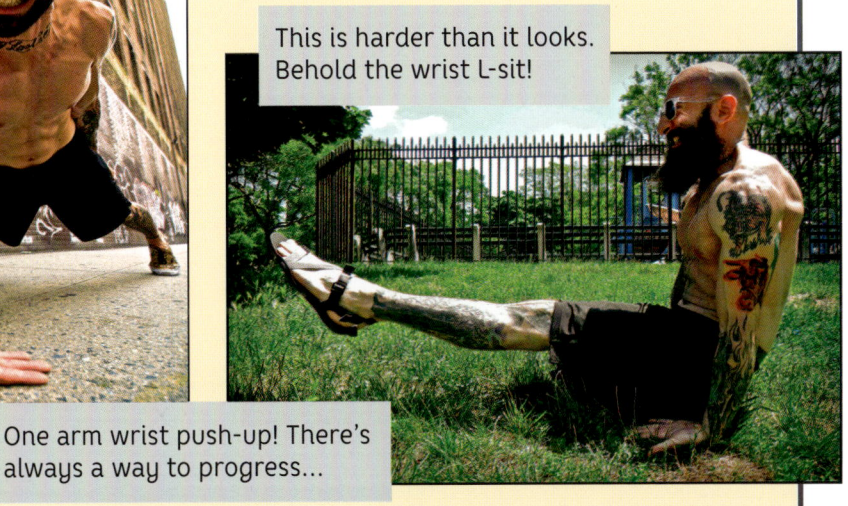

The mighty wrist pull-up is an amazing forearm builder.

Step up your game with wrist push-ups.

This is harder than it looks. Behold the wrist L-sit!

One arm wrist push-up! There's always a way to progress...

STREET WORKOUT

DRAGON FLAG

Lie on the ground or a bench, gripping a sturdy object behind your head. Tense your entire body as you lift your hips and legs into the air, stacking your body vertically above your shoulders. In addition to engaging your core, use your arms to lift yourself into position. Be careful not to pull too hard against the back of your neck.

From the top position, carefully lower yourself down until you are hovering just above the ground, maintaining a straight line from your shoulders to your toes, then raise back up to the top position. Be mindful to avoid folding at the hips. In fact, it may even be useful to imagine overextending your hips in order to compensate for the body's tendency to do the opposite.

While the full dragon flag requires both legs to be fully extended, it can be helpful to use a modified version with one or both knees tucked as a progression.

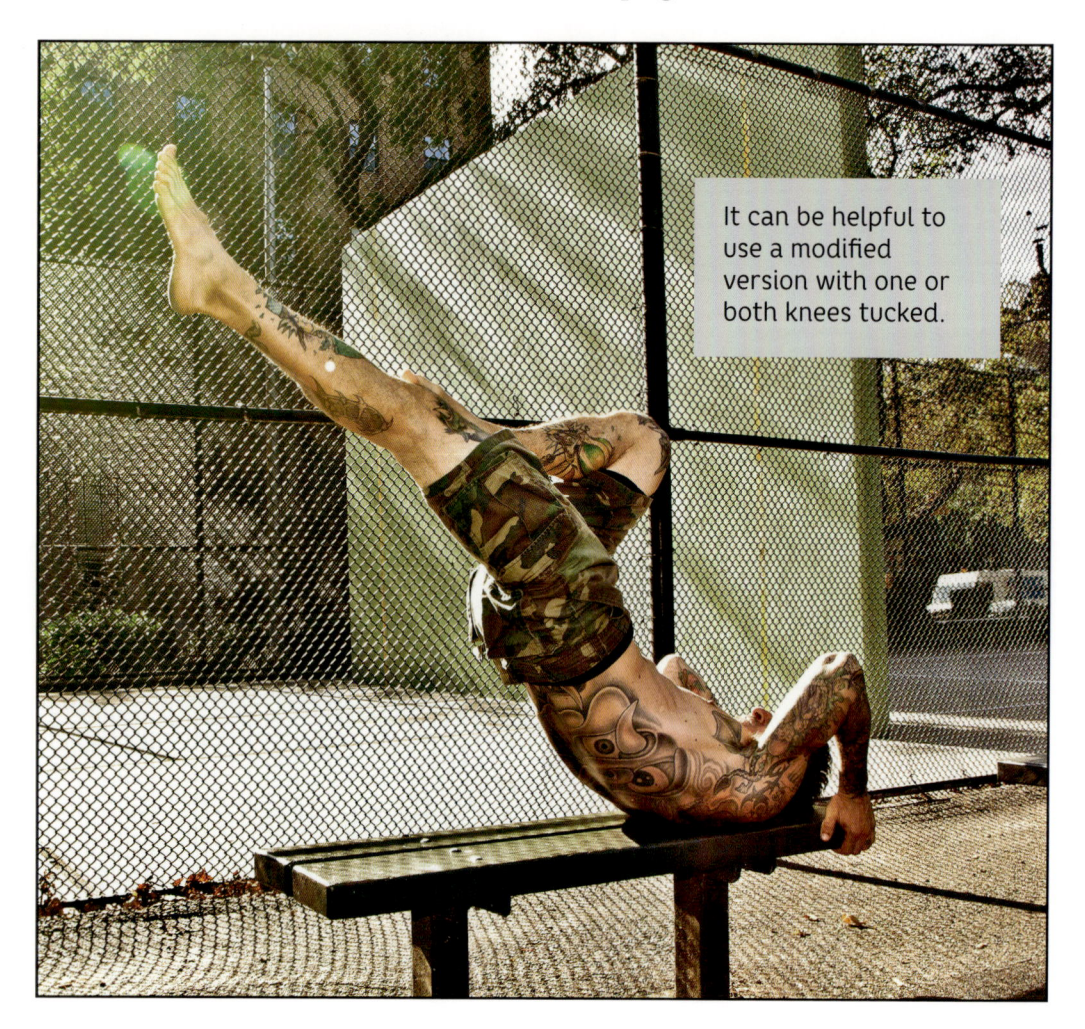

It can be helpful to use a modified version with one or both knees tucked.

It can also help to start by practicing the negative phase. The idea behind this method is to gradually increase the load so that you can prime your neurological system for the full dragon flag. Once you get confident with negatives, you can start working on doing a static hold with your body hovering a few inches over the ground. After you can hold this position for a few seconds, you should be ready to start working on full dragon flags for reps.

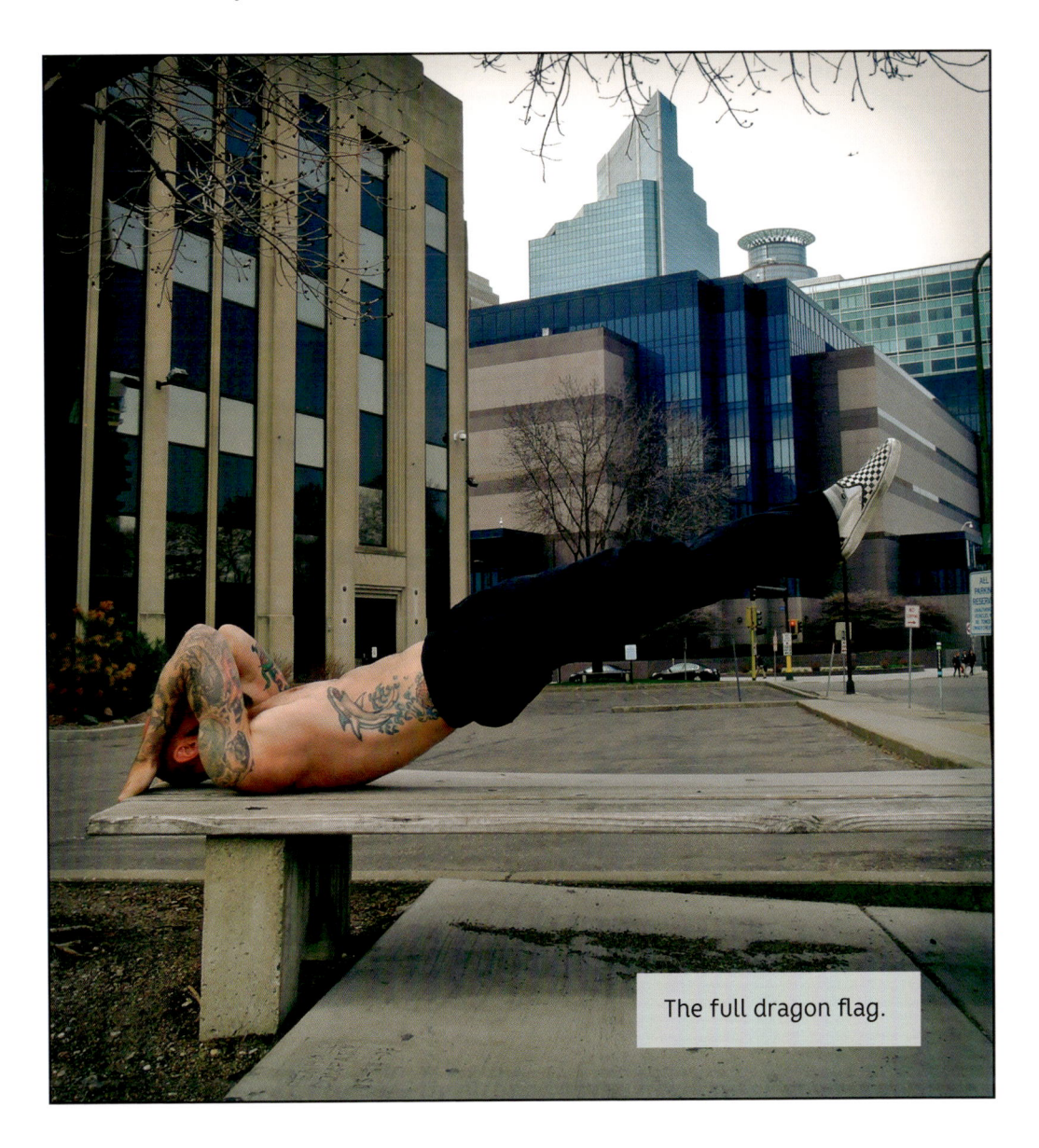

The full dragon flag.

HANGING FLEX PROGRESSIONS

These exercises are performed hanging from a bar (or tree, scaffold or lamppost, for those who truly embody the essence of Street Workout). The hanging position places your body in the vertical plane, thus increasing the mechanical disadvantage against gravity, as well as limiting your points of contact to only your hands. That's why the following movements recruit your arms, legs, chest, shoulders, back and grip to a greater degree than the grounded exercises.

HANGING KNEE RAISE

Hang with an overhand grip, then carefully lift your knees toward your chest. Focus on tilting your pelvis forward at the top in order to fully engage your abdominals. Lower your legs back to the bottom, being mindful not to swing or pick up momentum on the way down. Keep your elbows locked, squeeze the bar tightly and brace your trunk to maintain control.

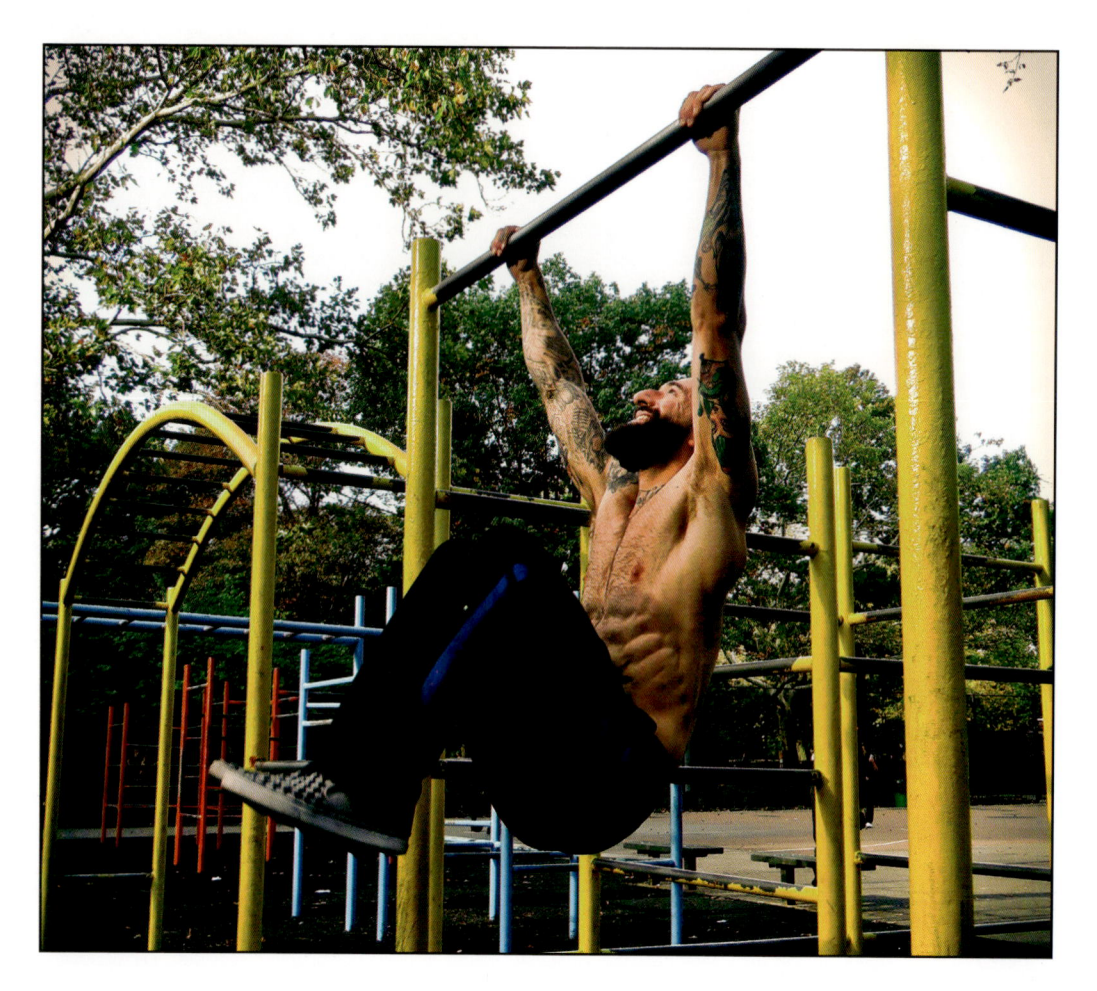

TWISTING HANGING KNEE RAISE

Hang with an overhand grip, then twist your trunk and pull your knees toward the opposite armpit. Focus on tilting your pelvis forward at the top in order to fully engage your abdominals. Lower your legs back to the bottom, being mindful not to swing or pick up momentum on the way down, then repeat the movement on the opposite side. Keep your elbows locked, squeeze the bar tightly and brace your trunk to maintain control. Twisting at the trunk involves additional recruitment of the obliques and serratus muscles.

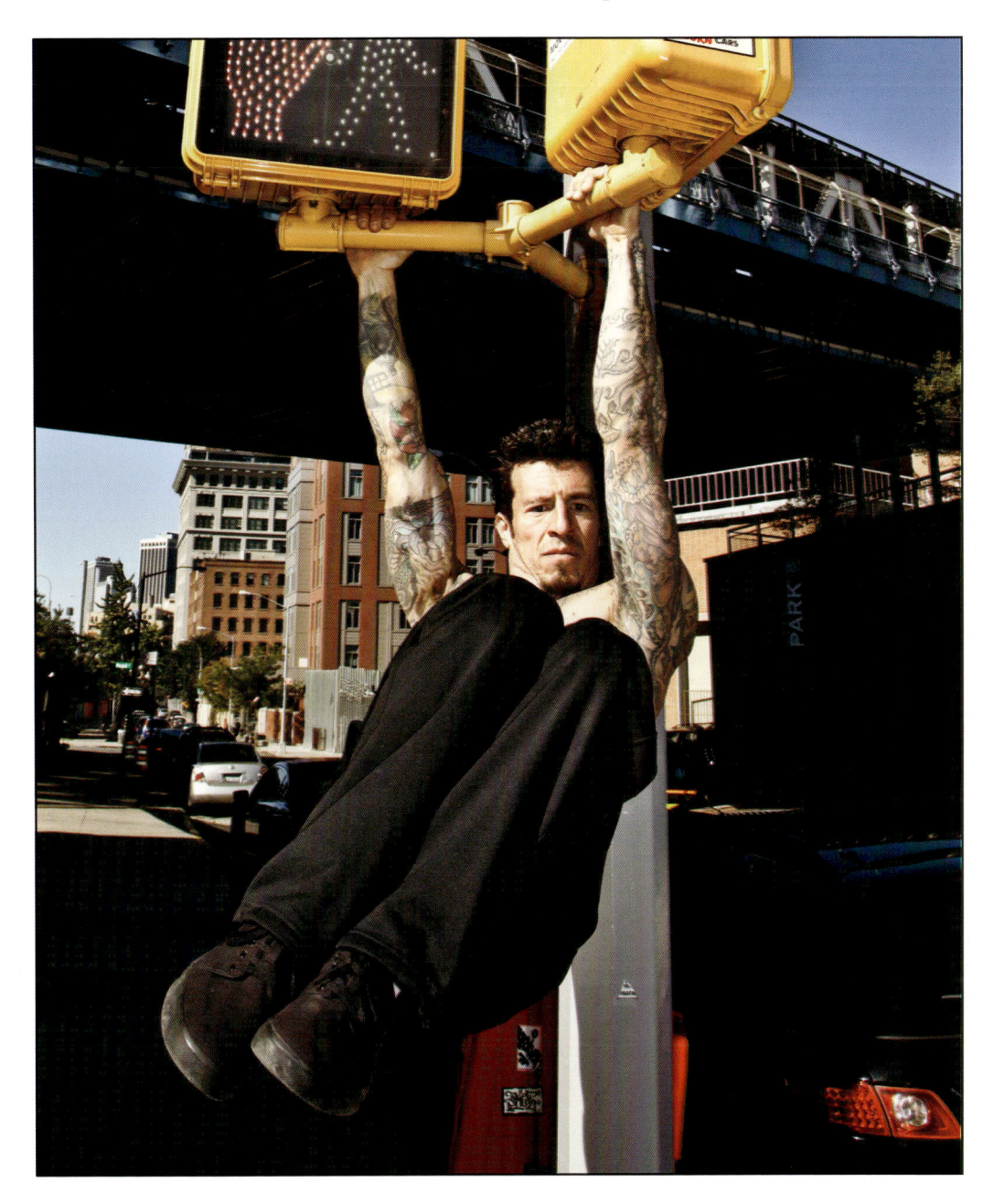

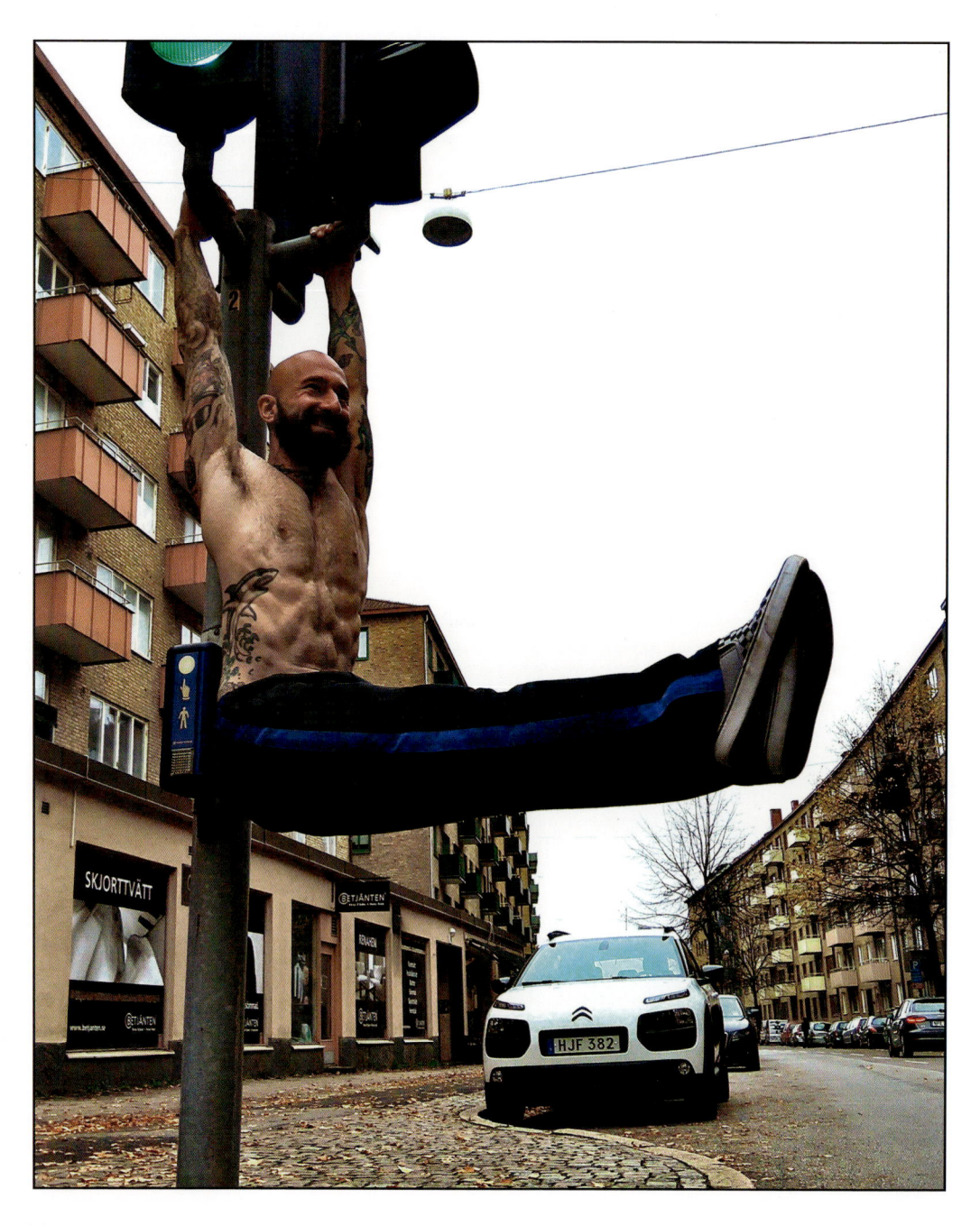

HANGING LEG RAISE

Hang with an overhand grip, then carefully raise your legs to hip height. Focus on tilting your hips and pelvis forward at the top in order to fully engage your abdominals. Lower your legs back to the bottom, being mindful not to swing or pick up momentum on the way down. Keep your elbows locked, squeeze the bar tightly and brace your trunk to maintain control.

TOES-TO-BAR HANGING LEG RAISE

Hang with an overhand grip, then raise your legs all the way up until your toes gently touch the bar. Focus on tilting your hips and pelvis forward in order to fully engage your abdominals, but do your best to maintain an upright torso. Lower your legs back to the bottom, being mindful not to swing or pick up momentum on the way down. Keep your elbows locked, squeeze the bar tightly and brace your trunk to maintain control.

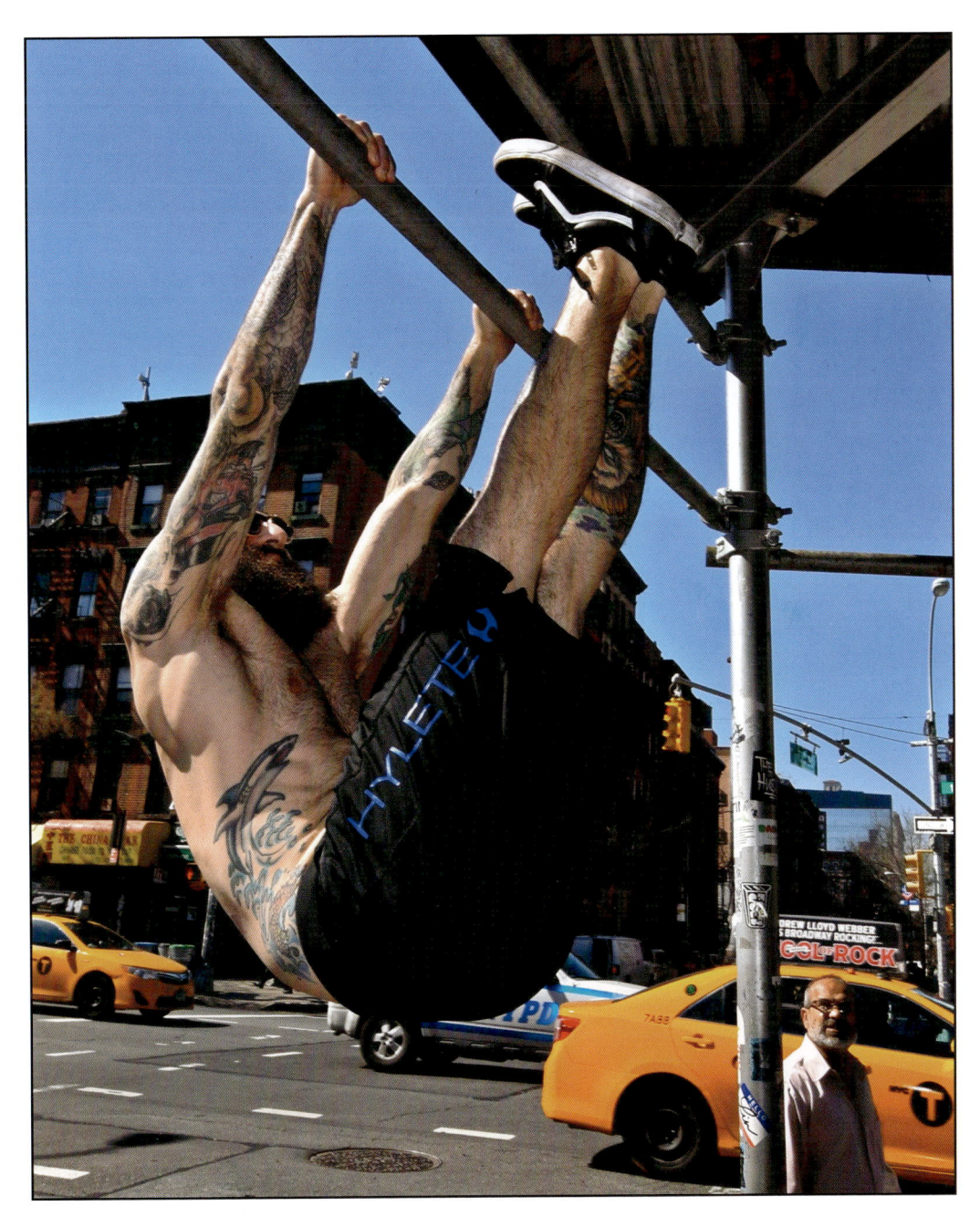

PARALLEL UNIVERSE

Hanging abs exercises such as knee raises and leg raises can also be performed while holding yourself upright between a pair of parallel bars. This is a more forgiving alternative for practitioners who are having an issue with grip strength or stability. Although generally less difficult than the hanging version, parallel bar knee and leg raises remain viable exercises in their own right.

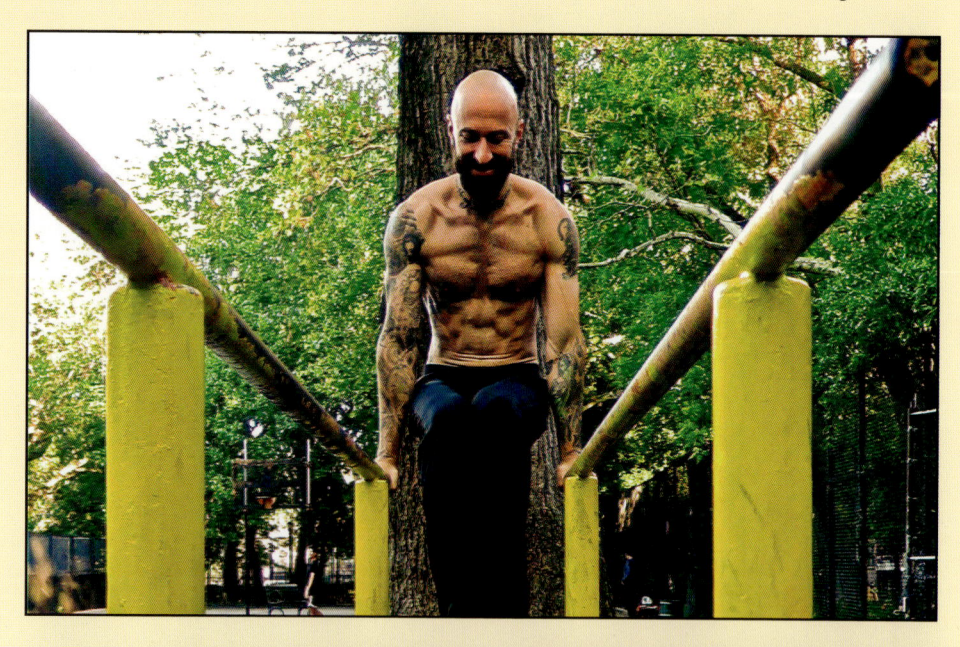

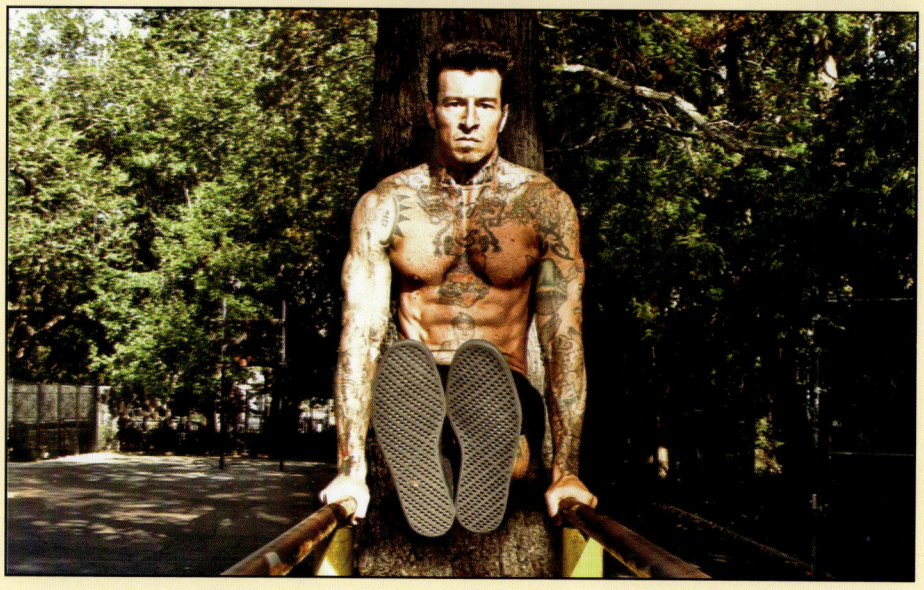

ROLLOVER

Perform a toes-to-bar hanging leg raise, then continue lifting your legs and hips until they are above your shoulders with your body fully inverted. Simultaneously give a pull with your arms, bending your elbows as you throw your hips over the bar until you roll around to the other side. You will end up with your torso above the bar in an upright position.

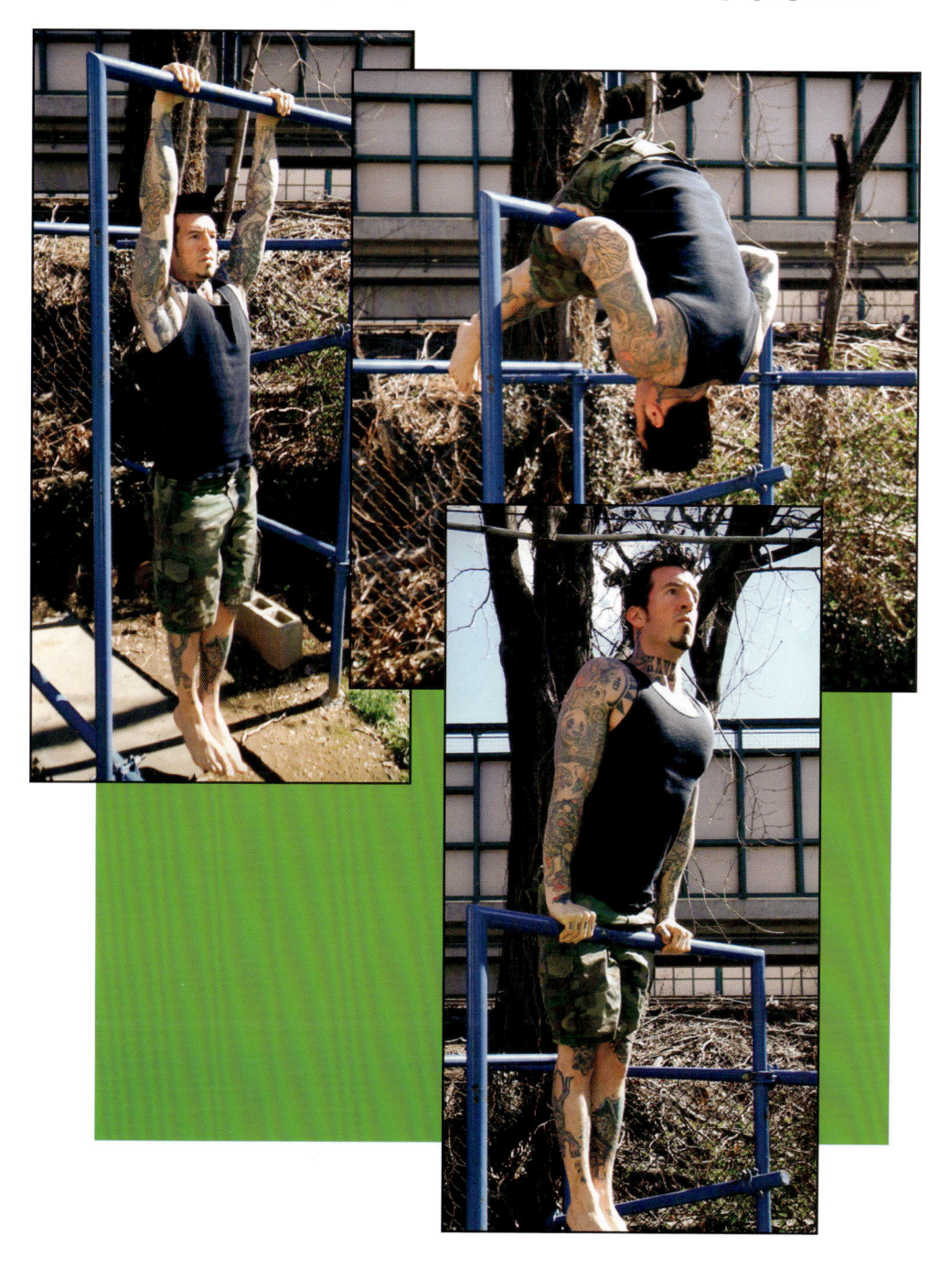

HANGING WINDSHIELD WIPER

Hang with your hands in an overhand grip, then lift your toes all the way to the bar as you would in a toes-to-bar leg raise. When you get to the top, begin rotating your legs toward one side. Aim to get your legs parallel to the ground before reversing direction and lowering them to the opposite side. The twisting movement at the trunk emphasizes your obliques and serratus muscles. Do your best to avoid bending your elbows when performing windshield wipers, though a slight kink may be unavoidable at first.

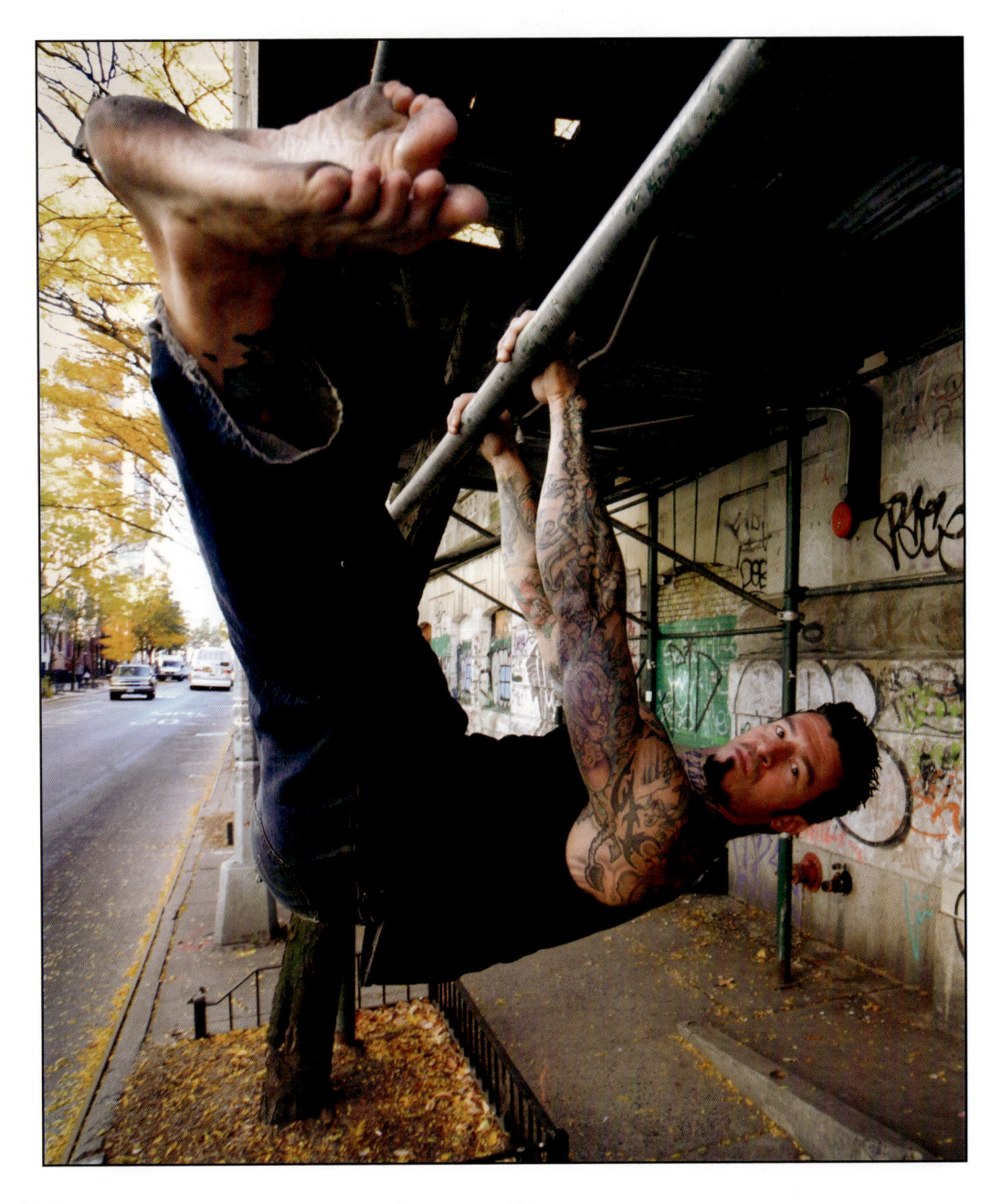

ONE ARM HANGING LEG RAISE

Grab an overhead bar with two hands, then carefully take one away. Squeeze the bar tightly with your remaining hand, making sure to keep your shoulder, back and entire arm engaged as you raise your legs until they are parallel to the ground. For an added challenge, you can try lifting your legs all the way up until your toes touch the bar.

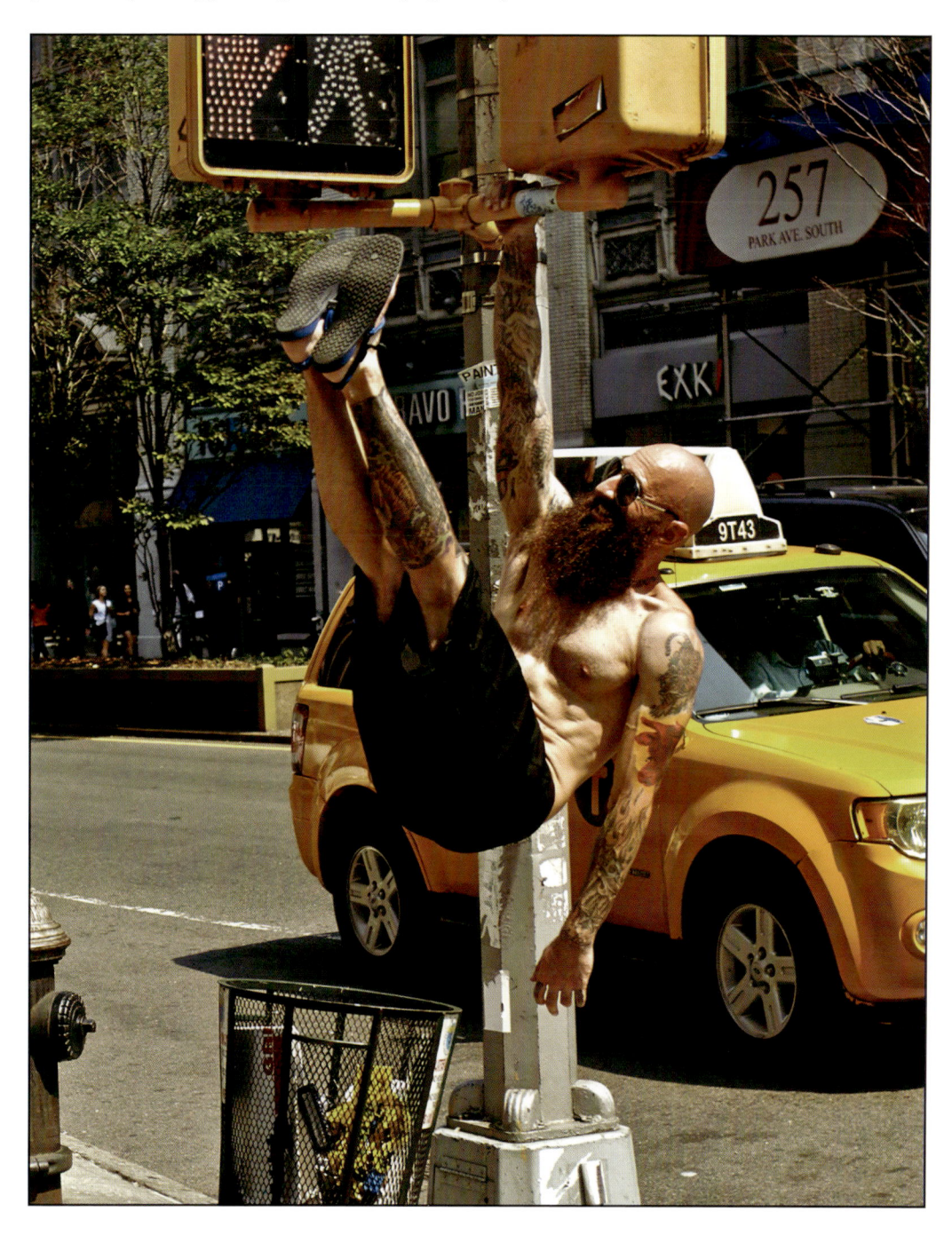

MEATHOOK

Begin by performing a windshield wiper toward your dominant arm. When your legs are all the way over to the side, lift your hips toward your elbow, folding your body around your arm. The elbow pit of your primary arm should wind up by your hip. It may take some trial and error to get a feel for finding the "sweet spot" but at a certain point, you will feel your balance shift.

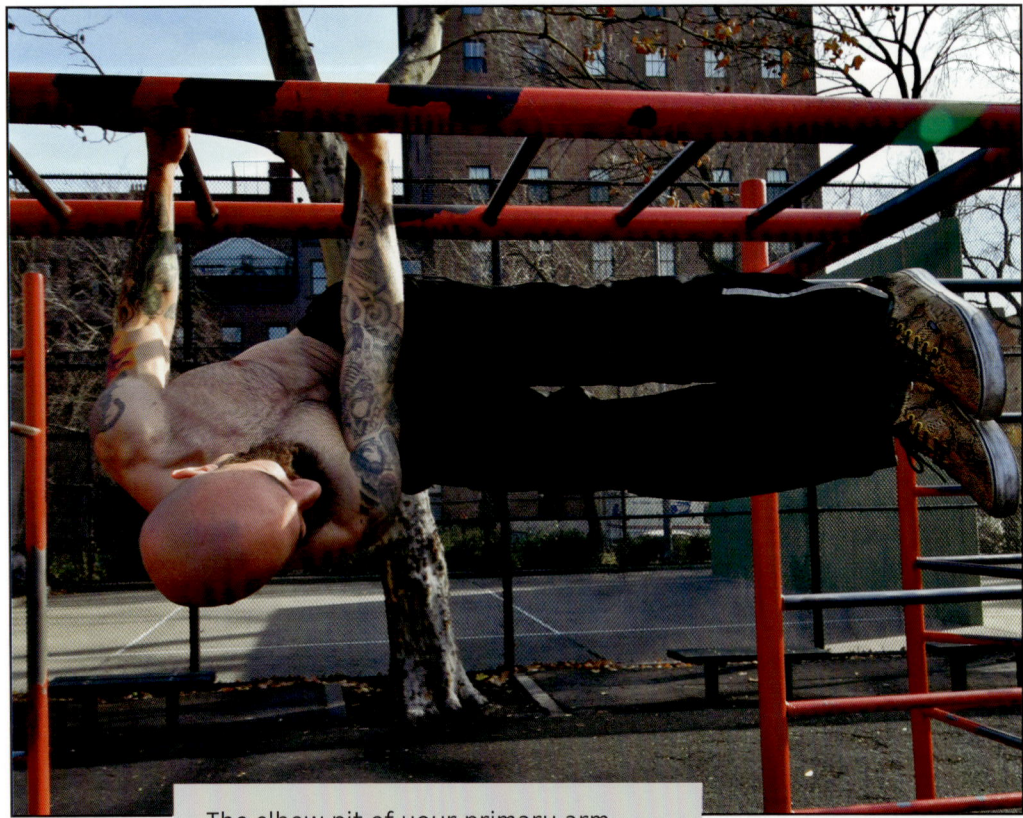

The elbow pit of your primary arm should wind up by your hip before you remove the other arm.

Once your hips are in position, begin to loosen the grip on your secondary arm, gradually transferring all of your weight to the other side. When you feel confident enough to completely release your secondary hand from the bar, do so carefully. You're now holding a meathook—congratulations! Stay here for a few seconds, then slowly reverse the movement and try it on the other side.

If you are unable to take your other hand away, try removing a finger or two instead. Over time you can work toward relying on your secondary arm less as you progressively build the strength to perform the full meathook.

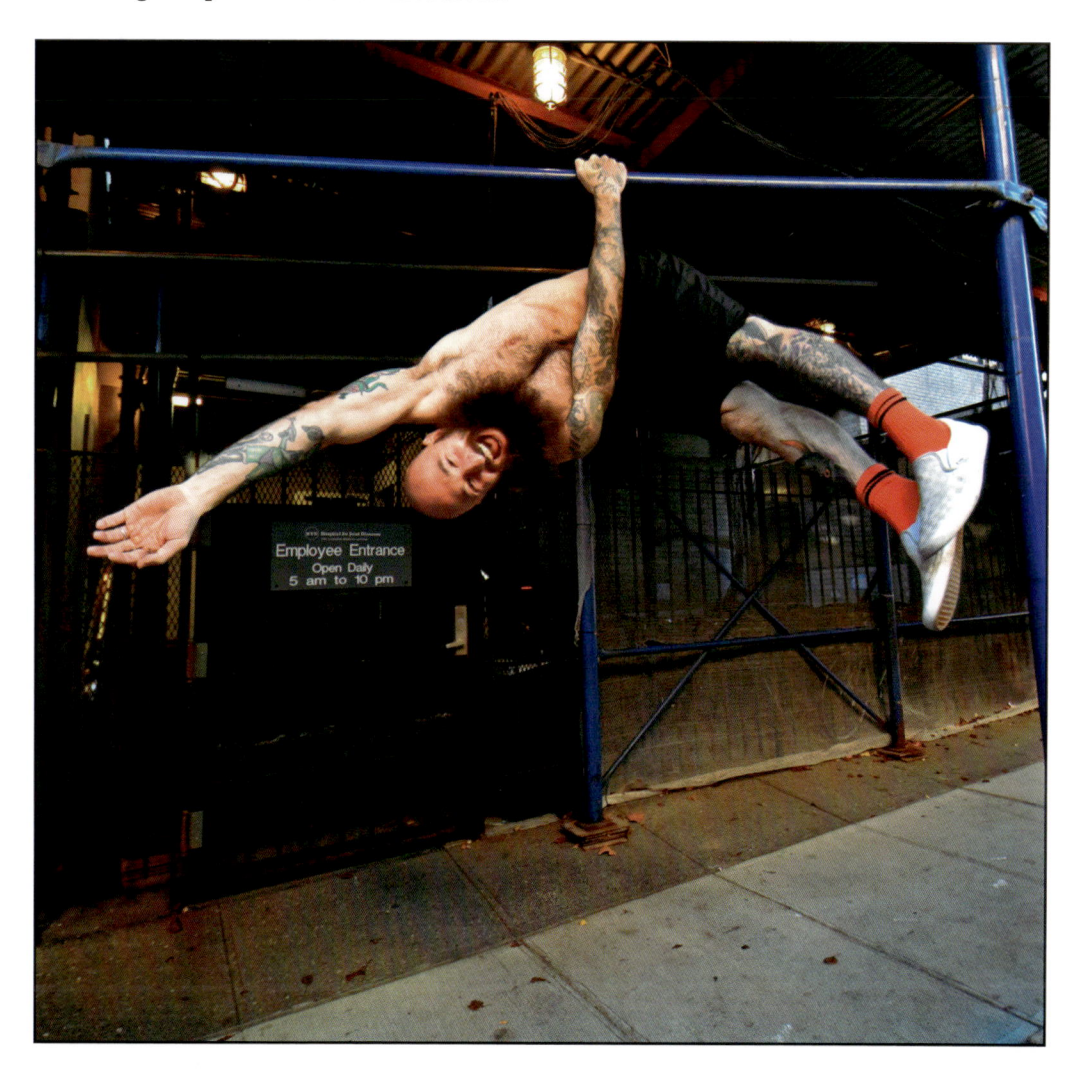

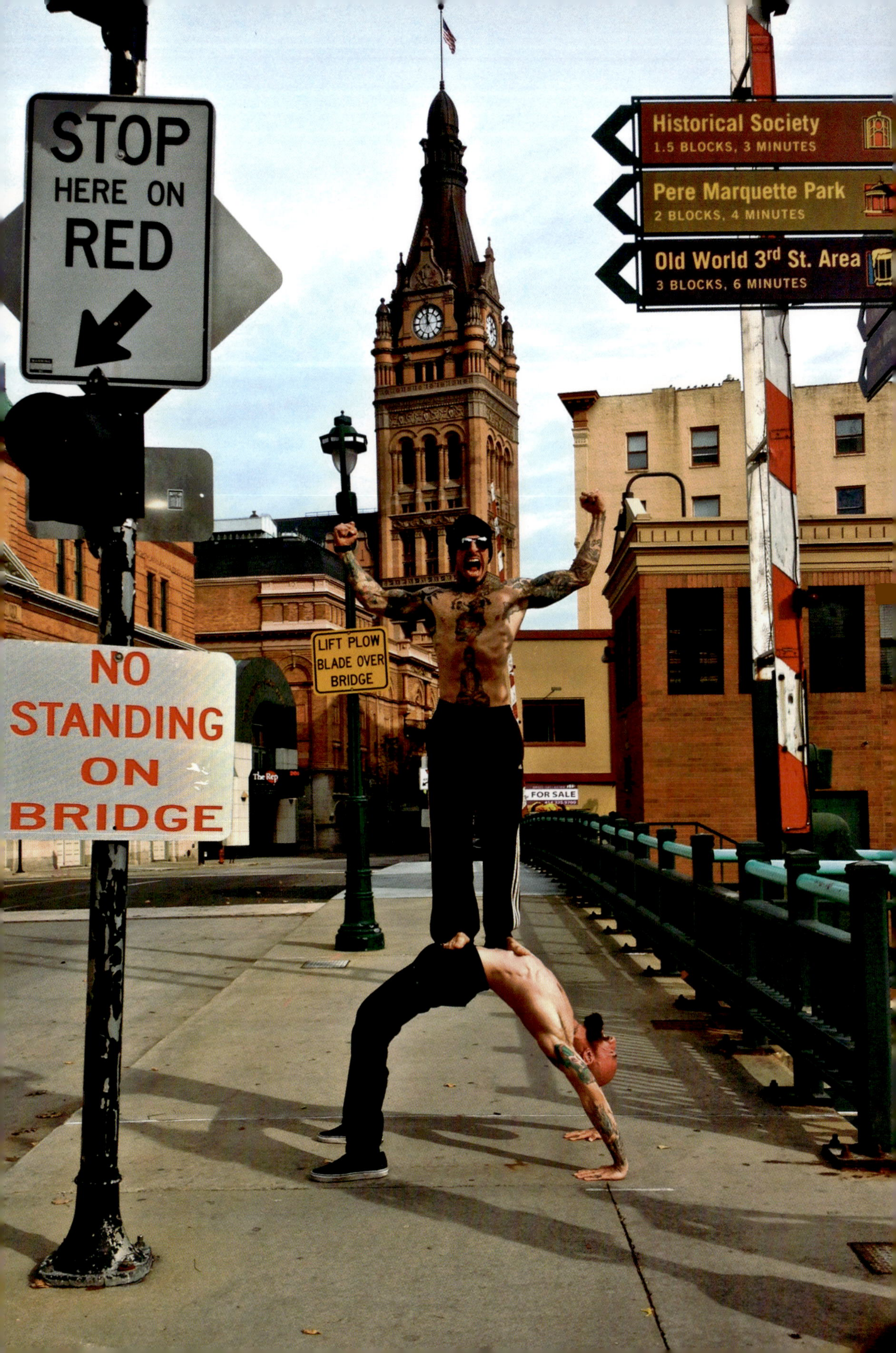
STOP
HERE ON
RED
Historical Society
1.5 BLOCKS, 3 MINUTES
Pere Marquette Park
2 BLOCKS, 4 MINUTES
Old World 3rd St. Area
3 BLOCKS, 6 MINUTES
LIFT PLOW
BLADE OVER
BRIDGE
NO
STANDING
ON
BRIDGE
The Rep
FOR SALE

Chapter 8

Bridge

Sir Isaac Newton's third law states that for every action there is an equal and opposite reaction. Well sadly, this is not always true in the fitness world... but it should be! Consider bridging to be the sober yang to trunk flexion's raging yin. Or something like that.

Americans tend to spend so much time slouching over (at the computer, for example), that we often get stuck walking around all day with our backs rounded and heads drooped forward. Couple this with the fact that everyone seems so focused on wanting to look good in the mirror that they forget to work the muscles they can't see. Like the pulling exercises previously discussed, bridging is an invaluable and often overlooked component of full body fitness. Bridge work will have a dramatic impact on your power, balance and flexibility.

The following bridge variants recruit the muscles along the back side of your body (glutes, legs, shoulders, upper and lower back), while at the same time stretching the ones in the front (chest, abs, hip flexors). This poses a unique set of circumstances depending on the body type of the practitioner. In the case of a highly muscular body, flexibility may be a great obstacle. Conversely, more mobile individuals will find the strength element to be the biggest challenge.

This leads to the often-asked question: what's "better," performing a bridge for reps or as an isometric hold? The truth is that they are both beneficial. Sets and reps cause the muscle to contract repeatedly and are more likely to lead to muscle gains. Meanwhile static holds allow the body to take its time and slowly stretch out, which may make it preferable for mobility. You really can't go wrong if you work on both.

Additionally, there are many types of bridges, requiring different points of contact with the earth beneath you. When training any unilateral or asymmetrical bridge, make sure you train both sides evenly. But enough talk. Like James Brown used to say, "Take 'em to the bridge!"

HIP BRIDGE

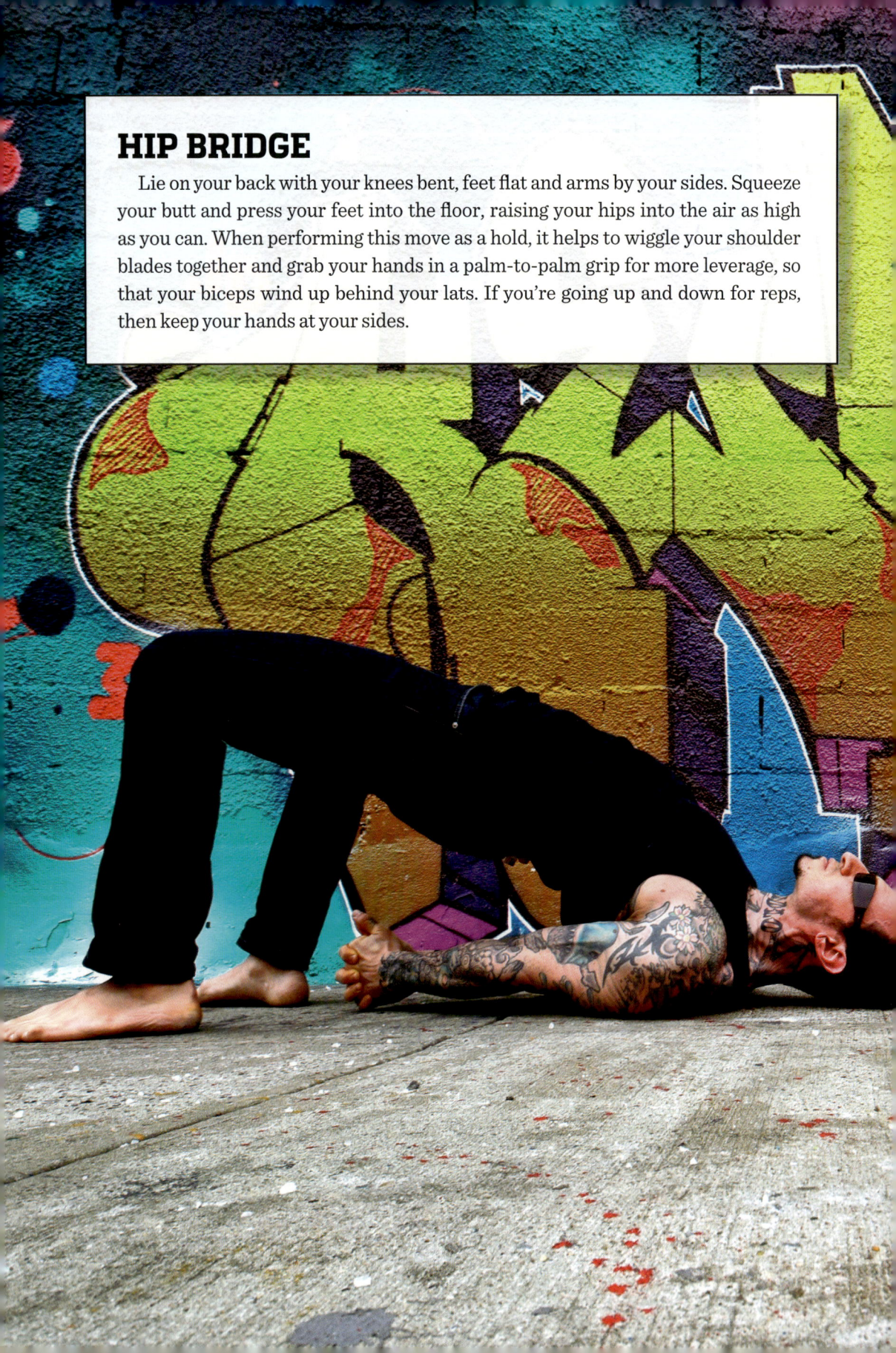

Lie on your back with your knees bent, feet flat and arms by your sides. Squeeze your butt and press your feet into the floor, raising your hips into the air as high as you can. When performing this move as a hold, it helps to wiggle your shoulder blades together and grab your hands in a palm-to-palm grip for more leverage, so that your biceps wind up behind your lats. If you're going up and down for reps, then keep your hands at your sides.

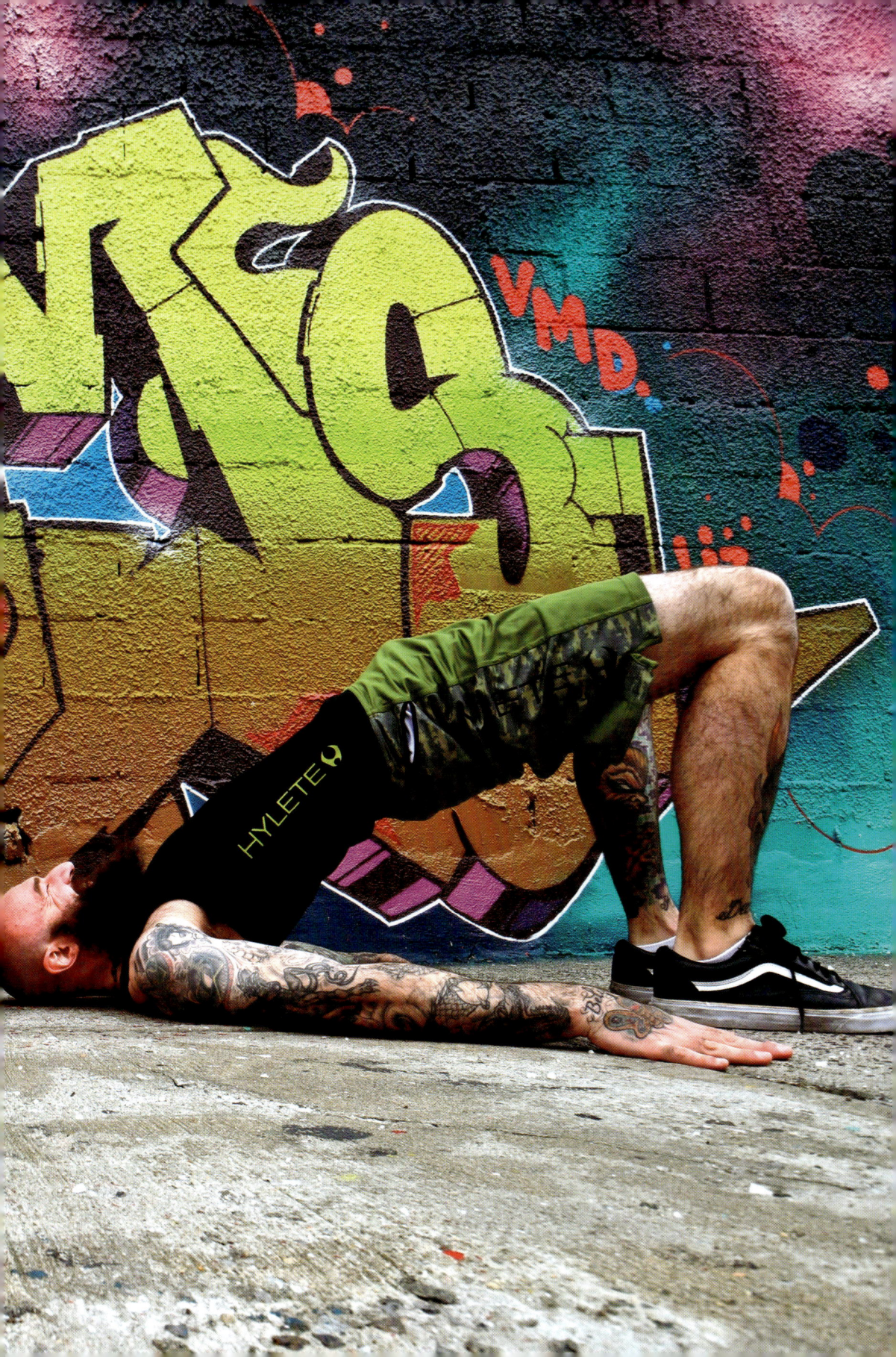

TABLE BRIDGE

Sit on the floor with your legs bent and feet flat on the ground in front of you, then place your hands palms-down outside of your hips. From here, squeeze your butt and press your heels into the ground, lifting your hips to shoulder height. Drop your head back and press your chest out to help open your shoulders and neck. Point your fingers away from your feet to further help open up your chest and shoulders. Feel free to experiment with different hand positions as well.

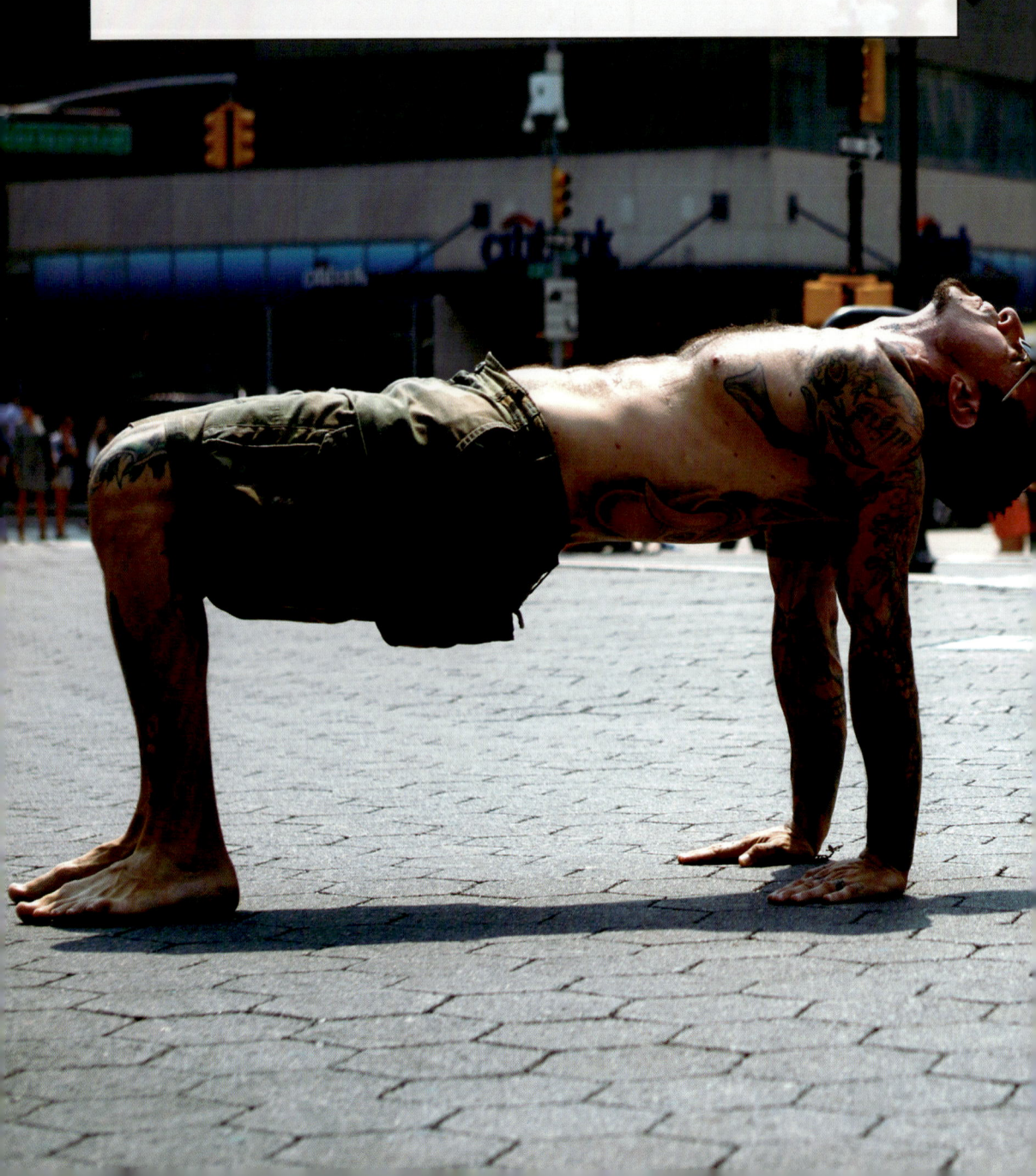

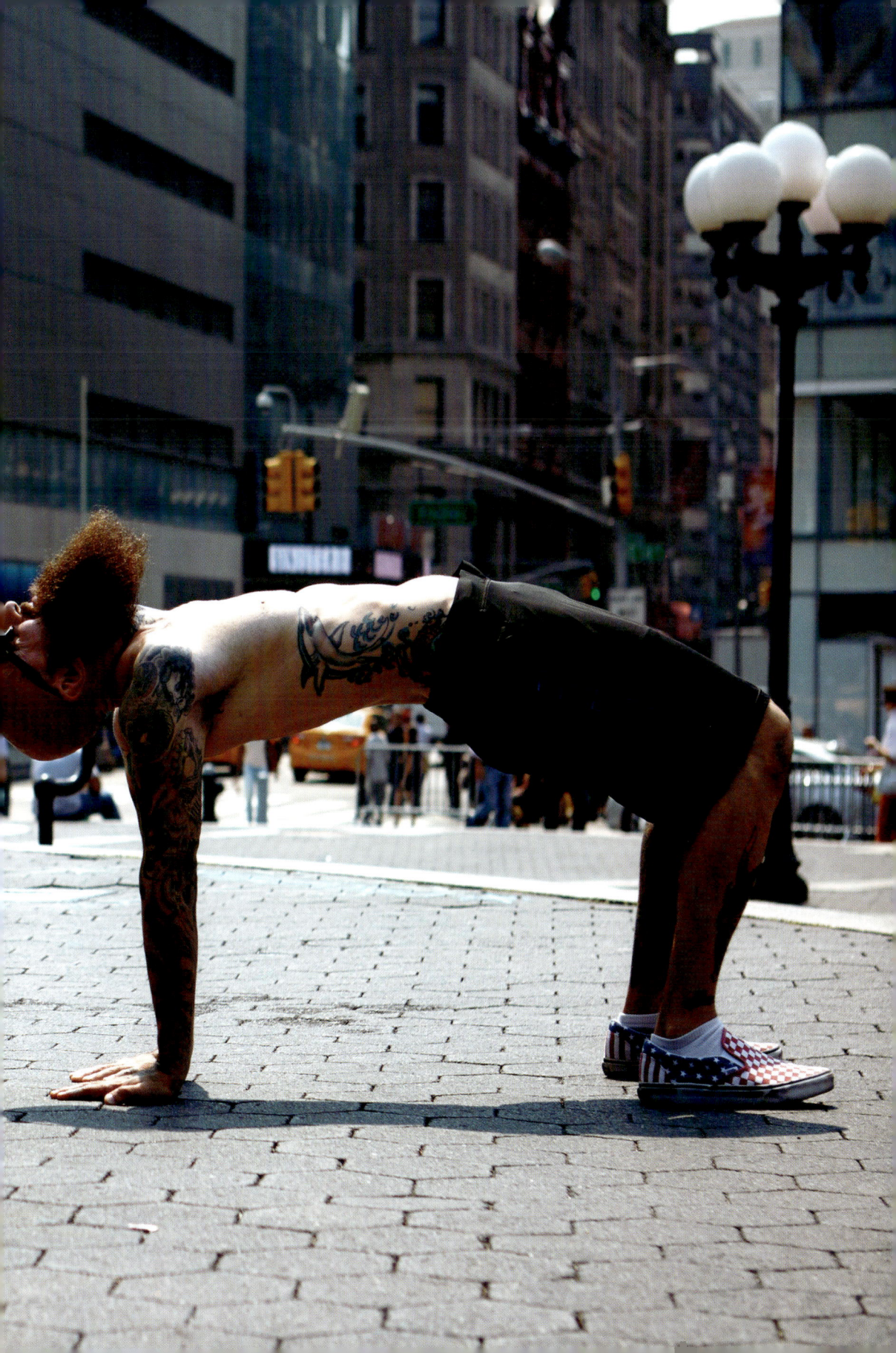

STRAIGHT BRIDGE

Sit with your legs directly in front of you and your hands on the ground just behind your hips. From here, lift yourself up and straighten out your body by contracting your hamstrings, glutes, lower back and other posterior musculature. Drop your head back, press your chest out and try to look behind you. You'll wind up looking like an upside-down plank. Feel free to experiment with various hand positions.

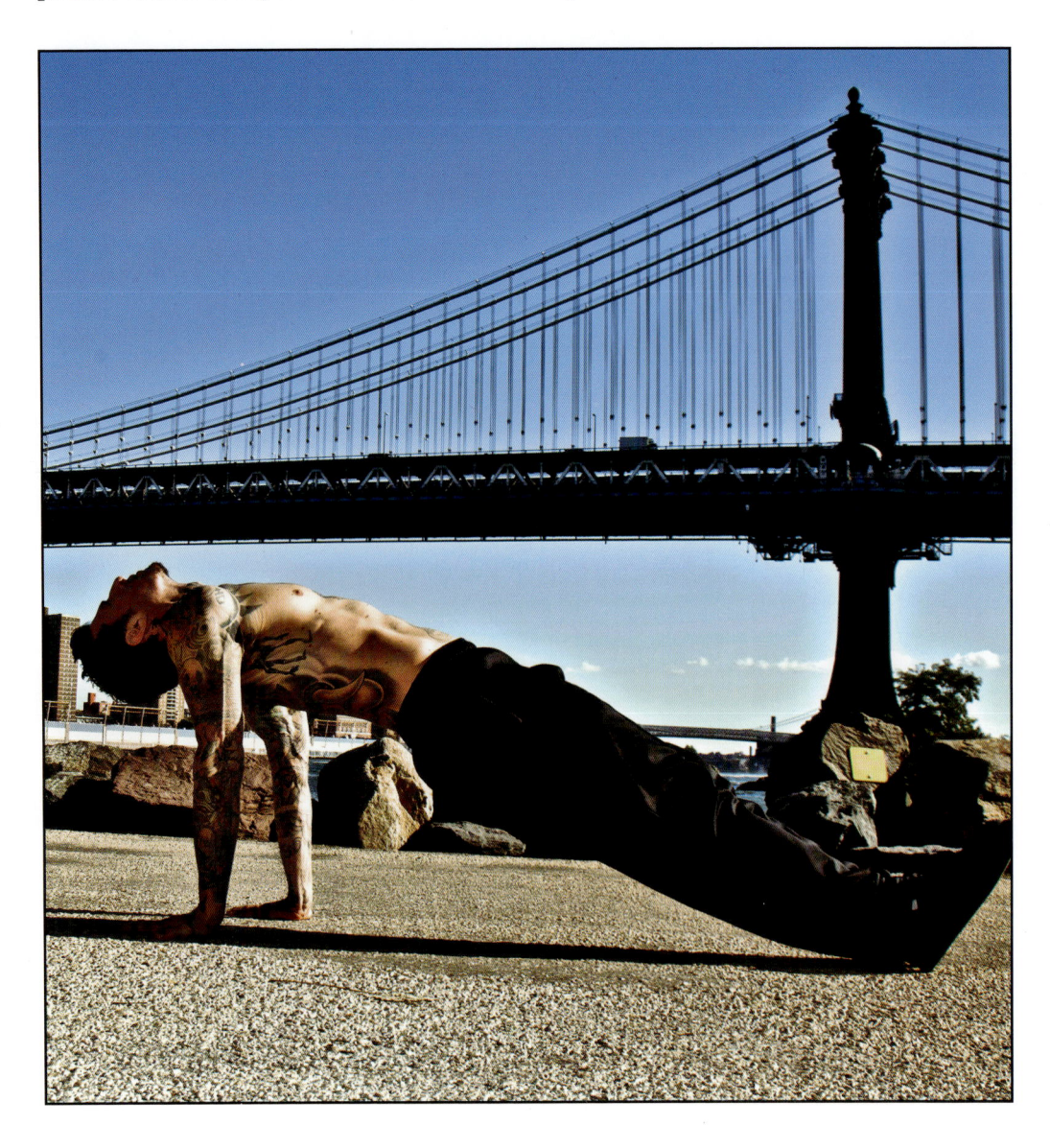

SHOULDER BRIDGE

Lie on your back with your hands at your sides and legs straight. Without bending your knees, dig your heels into the ground and roll onto your shoulders. Use your arms if needed to create an arch from your feet to your shoulders. Eventually you can try it with your arms off the ground, but don't be in a rush. This bridge variant is more difficult than it may appear.

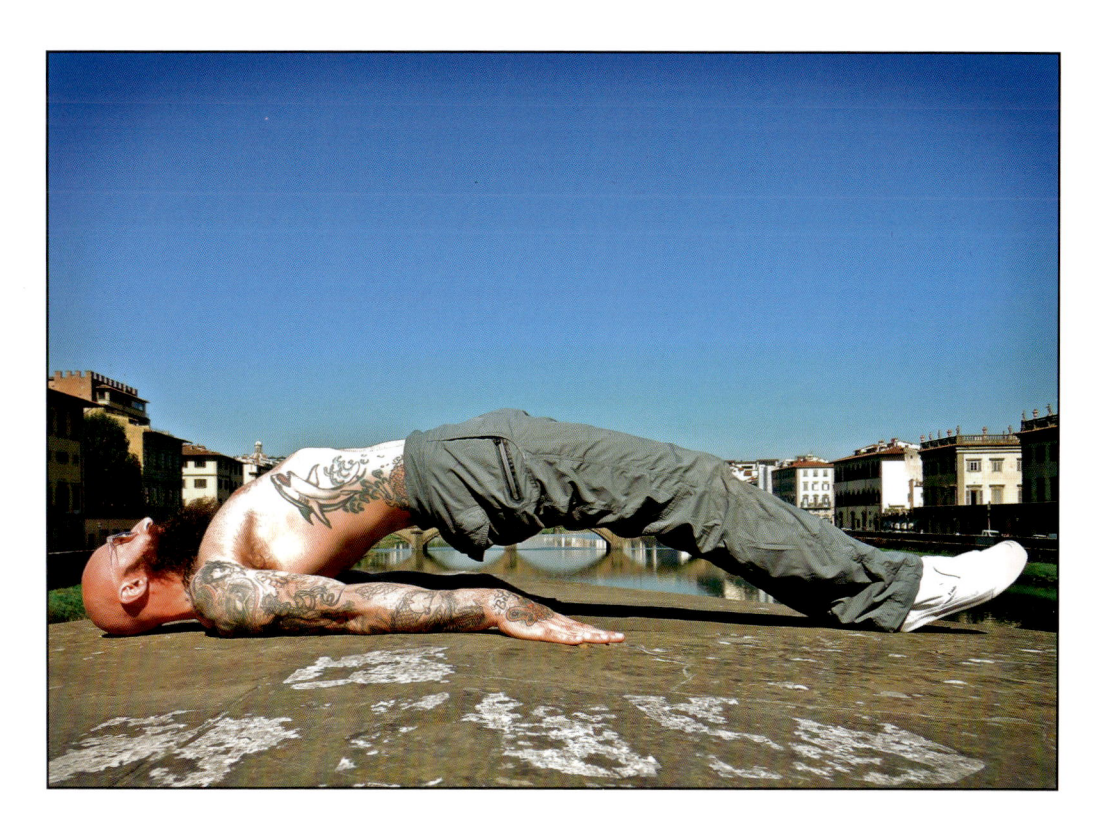

CANDLESTICK BRIDGE

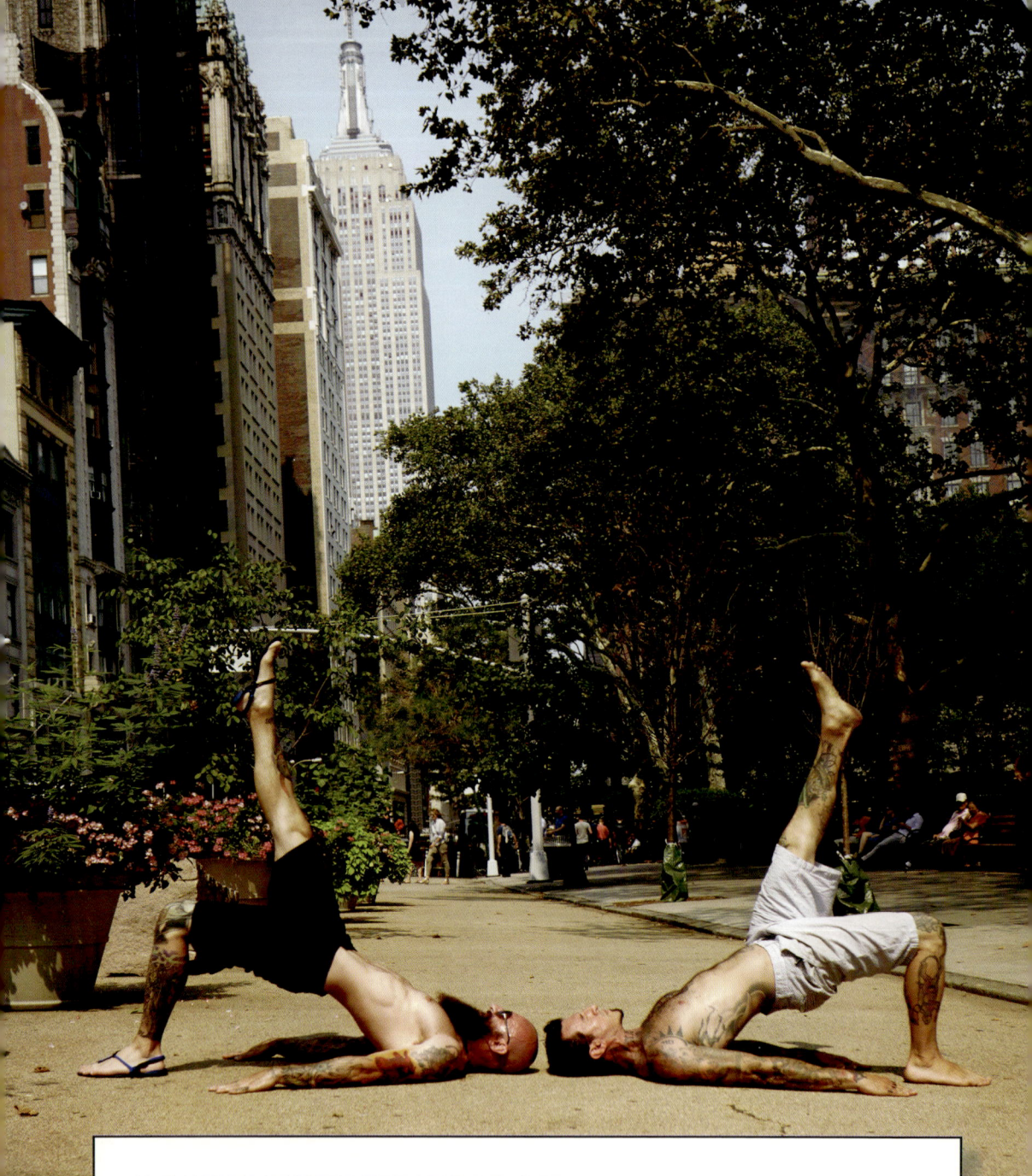

The candlestick bridge is basically a one-legged version of the hip bridge. As such, the strength requirement is doubled and a balance element is introduced. Lie on your back with your knees bent, feet flat and arms by your sides. Lift one leg straight above your hips and press into the ground with your opposite foot to raise your body up into the air. Beginners can start out in a hip bridge and then remove one leg once they are stable.

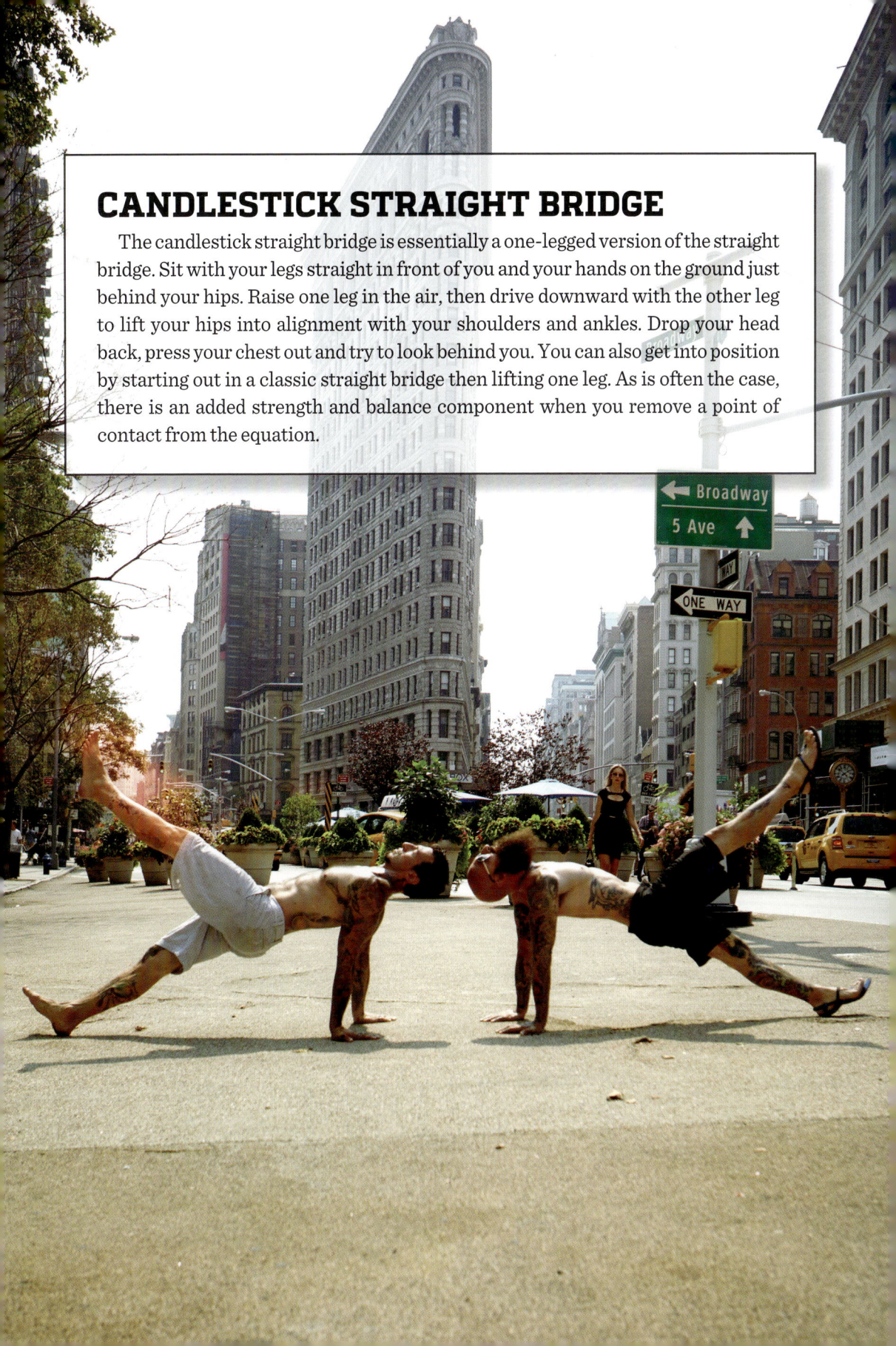

CANDLESTICK STRAIGHT BRIDGE

The candlestick straight bridge is essentially a one-legged version of the straight bridge. Sit with your legs straight in front of you and your hands on the ground just behind your hips. Raise one leg in the air, then drive downward with the other leg to lift your hips into alignment with your shoulders and ankles. Drop your head back, press your chest out and try to look behind you. You can also get into position by starting out in a classic straight bridge then lifting one leg. As is often the case, there is an added strength and balance component when you remove a point of contact from the equation.

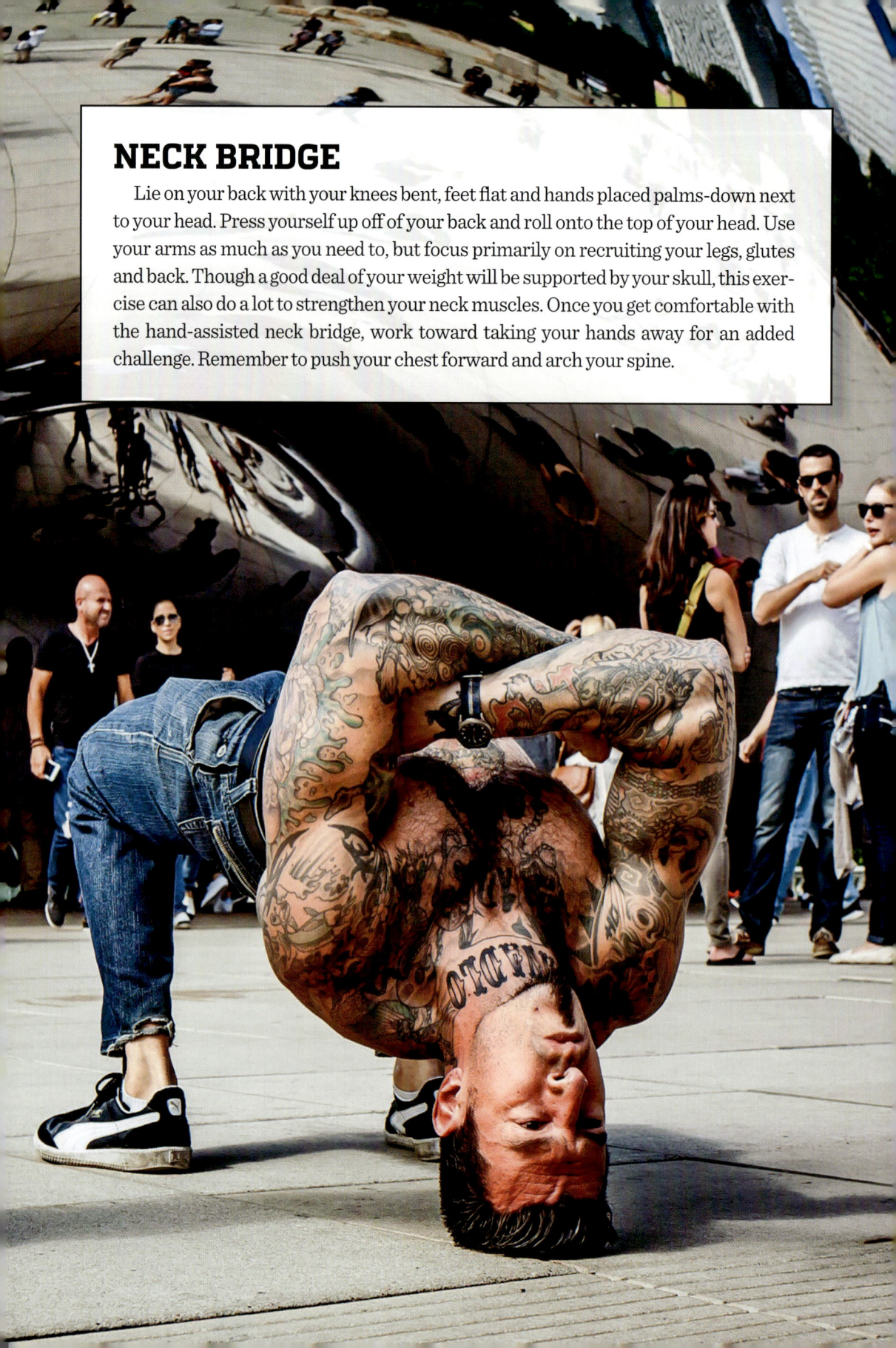

NECK BRIDGE

Lie on your back with your knees bent, feet flat and hands placed palms-down next to your head. Press yourself up off of your back and roll onto the top of your head. Use your arms as much as you need to, but focus primarily on recruiting your legs, glutes and back. Though a good deal of your weight will be supported by your skull, this exercise can also do a lot to strengthen your neck muscles. Once you get comfortable with the hand-assisted neck bridge, work toward taking your hands away for an added challenge. Remember to push your chest forward and arch your spine.

FOREARM BRIDGE

From the neck bridge position, lower your forearms and elbows toward the ground and bring your hands behind your head. You can interlace your fingers or place them flat on the floor, whichever feels better. Once your forearms are on the ground, press your chest outward, bringing your shoulders directly above your elbows. From here, lift your head off the floor (if you are able to) and continue pressing your chest outward to intensify the stretch in your upper-back and shoulders.

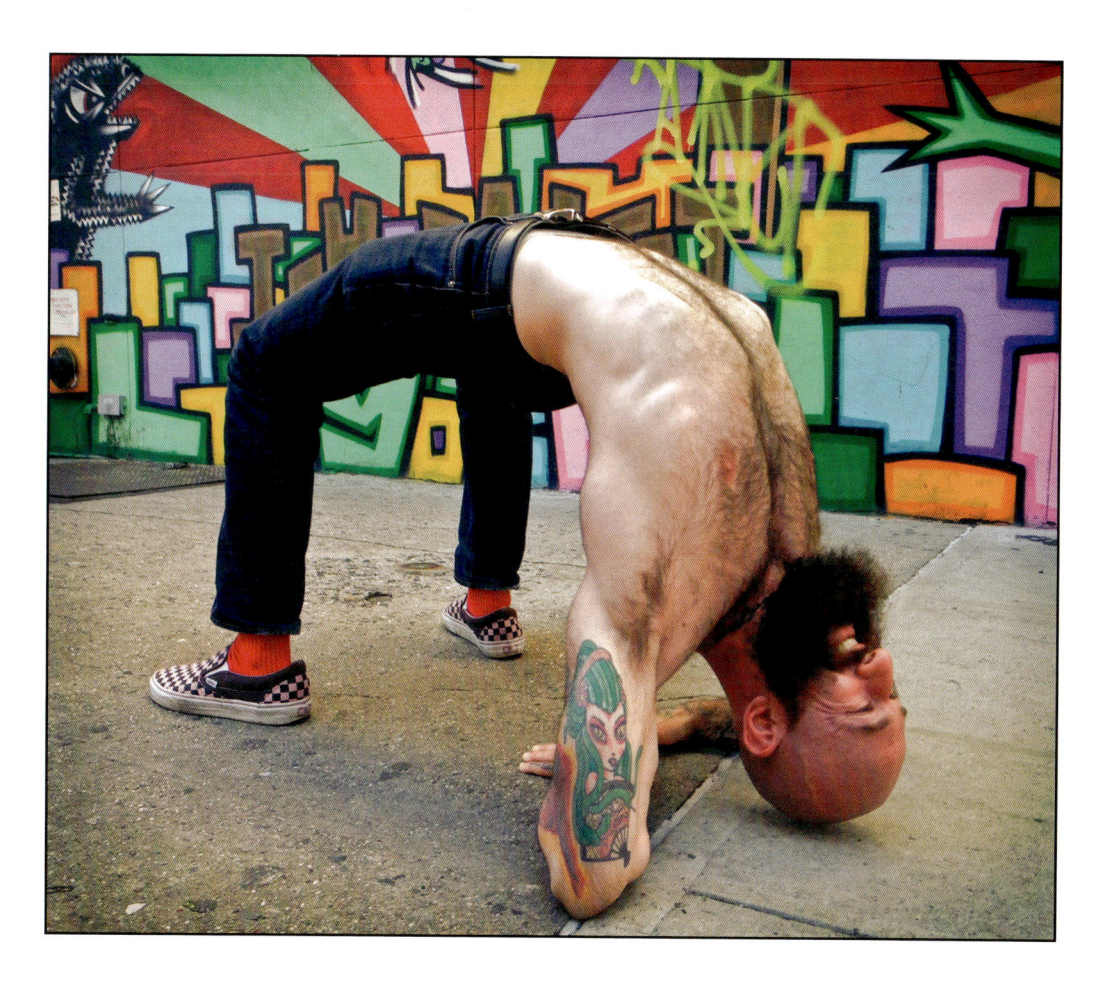

BACK BRIDGE

Lie on your back with your knees bent, feet flat and hands placed palms-down next to your head. Press into the floor with your hands and feet, arching your back to extend your chest forward and raise your hips into the air. Aim to get your elbows fully locked in the top position (though a partial bend is acceptable when starting out).

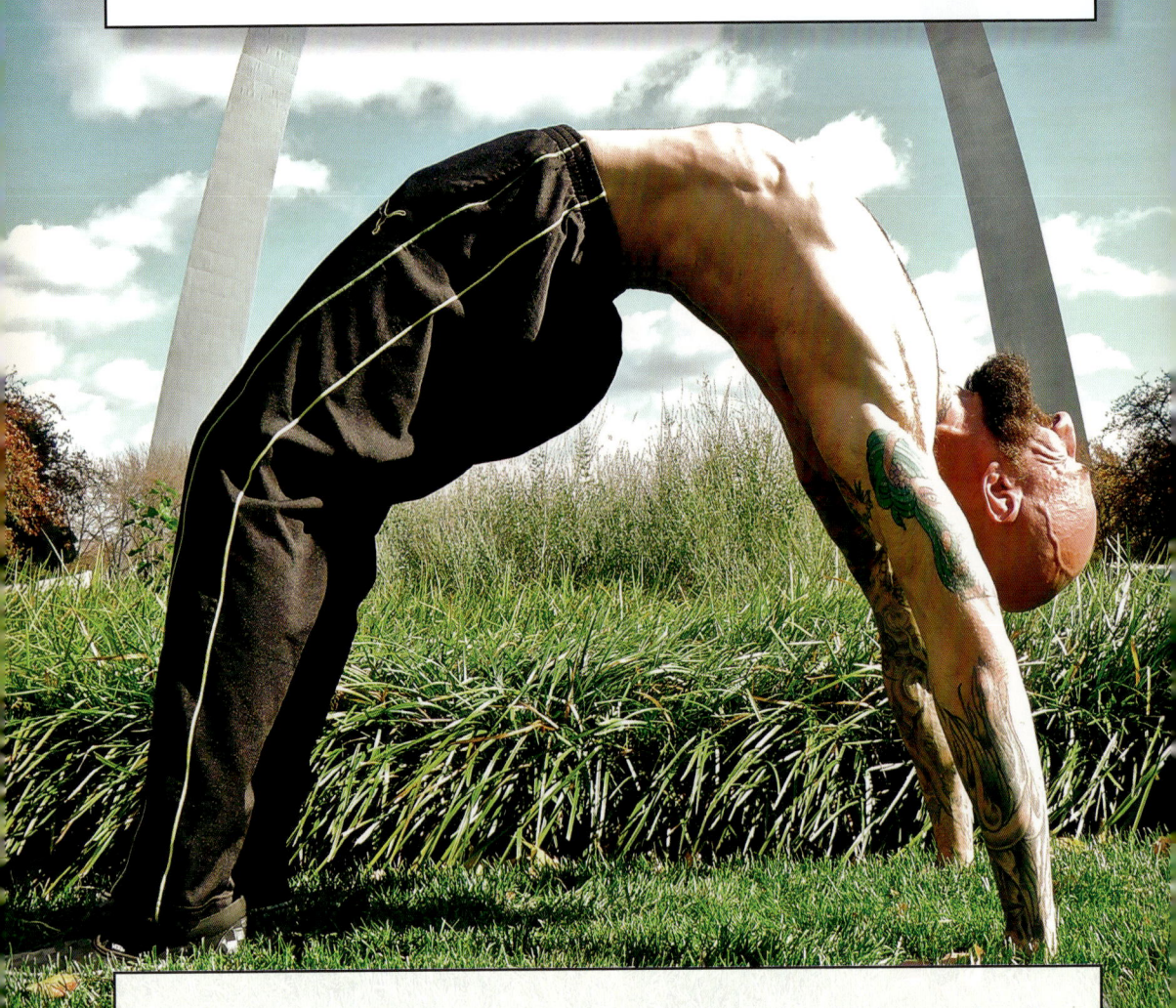

Do your best to keep the arc of your spine even throughout, and not too heavily pronounced in the lumbar region. If your upper back is stiff, which is quite common, you'll need to be especially mindful of this. The better your flexibility, the closer together you'll be able to get your hands and feet.

ONE LEG BACK BRIDGE

Removing a point of contact increases the strength demands and adds a balance component to the back bridge. There are two ways you can approach the one leg bridge. The less difficult method is to first get into a back bridge, then carefully lift one leg, placing that foot back down before switching sides. The more advanced method is to first lift one leg, then press up into your bridge with just the other leg.

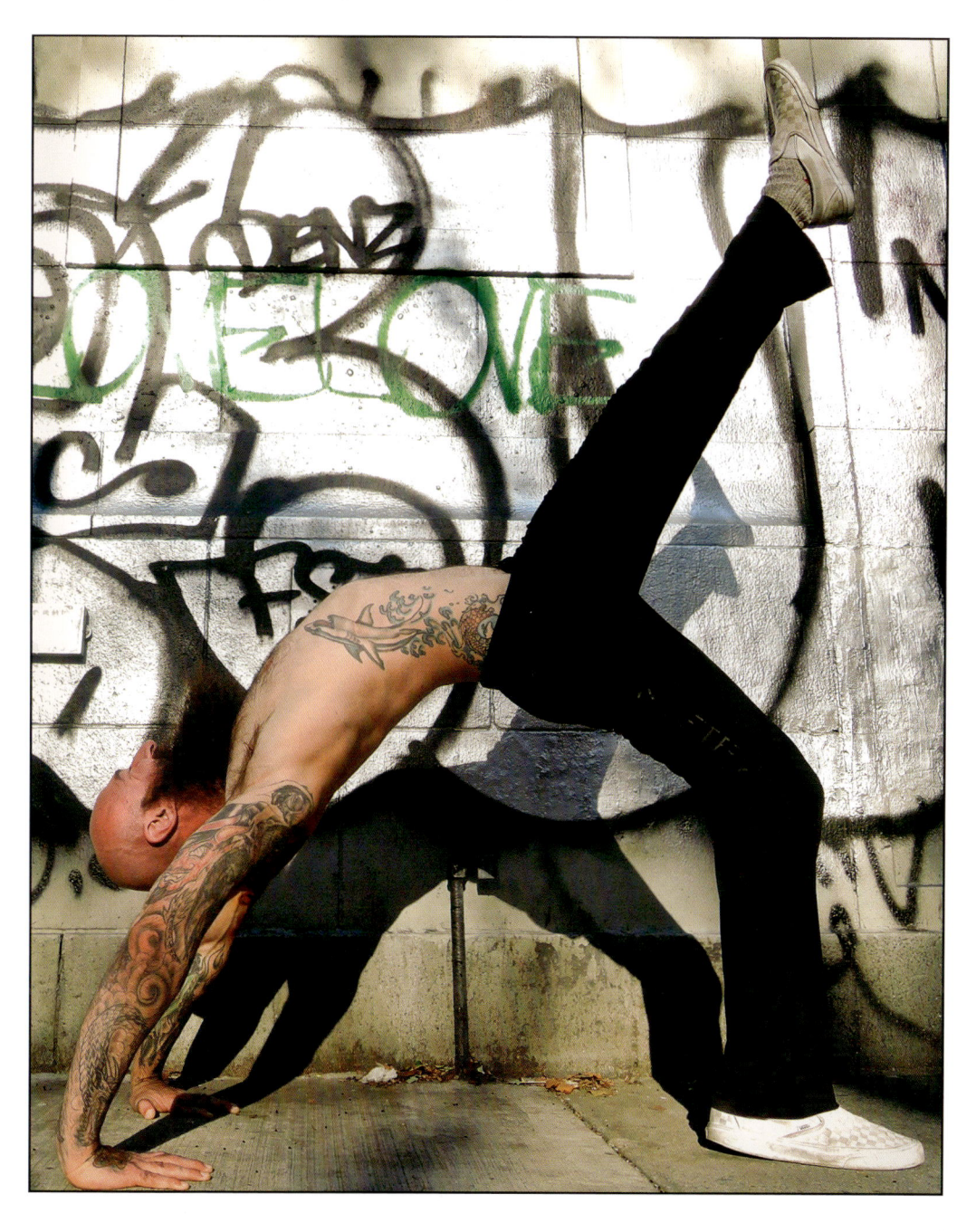

ONE ARM BACK BRIDGE

Like the one leg version, there are two ways you can approach the one arm bridge. Again, the less difficult method is to first get into a back bridge, then carefully lift one arm and hold, placing that hand back down before switching sides. The more advanced method is to press up into your bridge with just one arm, which is considerably more difficult. To improve your leverage slightly, you can go with a wide foot stance when first attempting this exercise. By spreading your contact points further apart, you will be more stable.

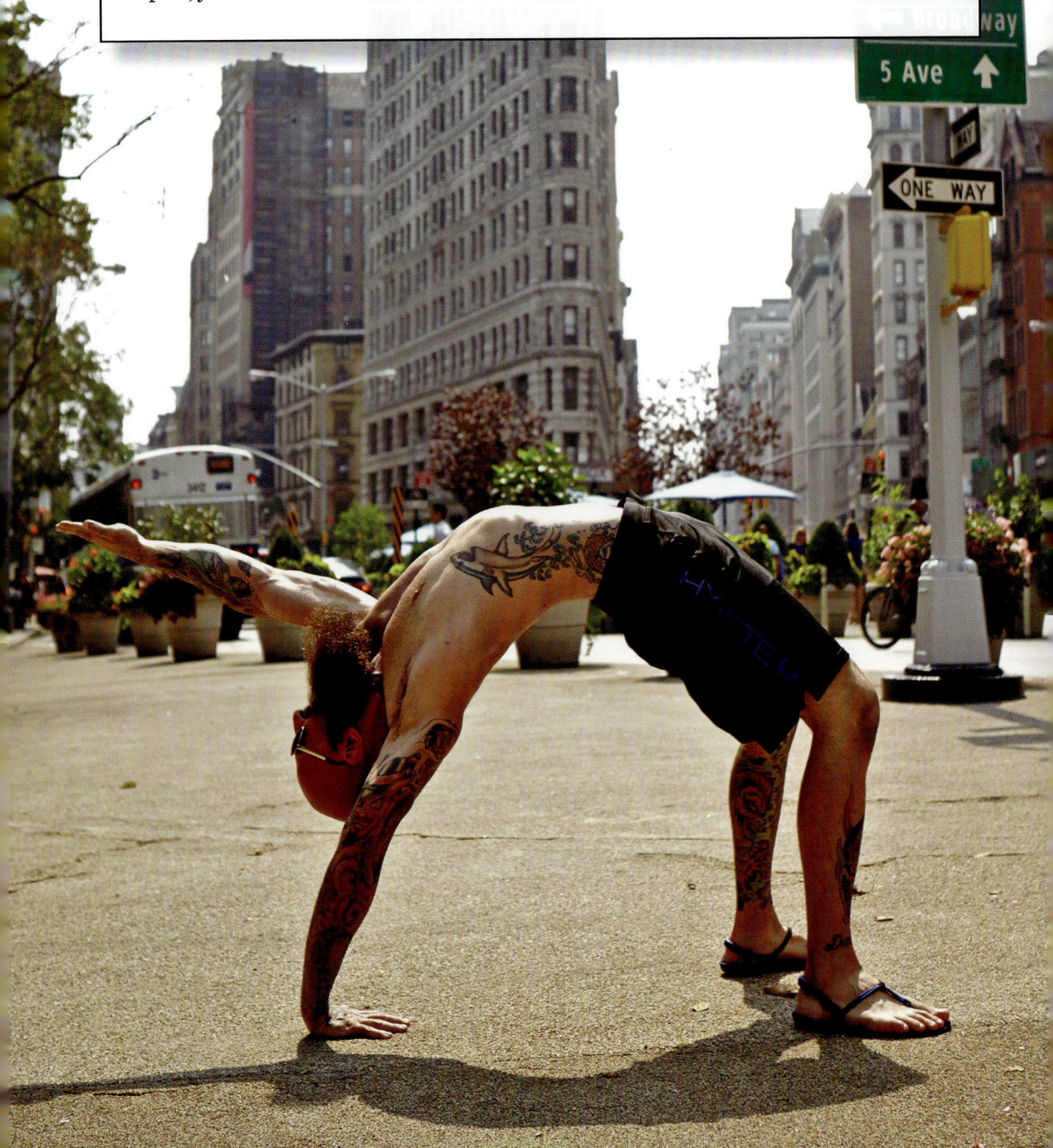

GECKO BRIDGE

A bridge held on just one arm and one leg is called a gecko bridge. The balance and stability it requires is tremendous, and it also demands major posterior chain strength. We recommend easing into this bridge gradually. Some will find that picking up one hand first, then lifting the opposite foot feels best. For others lifting the foot first feels better.

Though the gecko bridge is typically performed right leg/left arm or left leg/right arm, you can also experiment with lifting the arm and the leg on the same side. In time, you can work towards lifting the hand and foot simultaneously and holding it for longer periods of time. Eventually you may be able to press into a gecko bridge with one arm and one leg elevated from the start. Experiment with different hand and foot positions to see what works best for you.

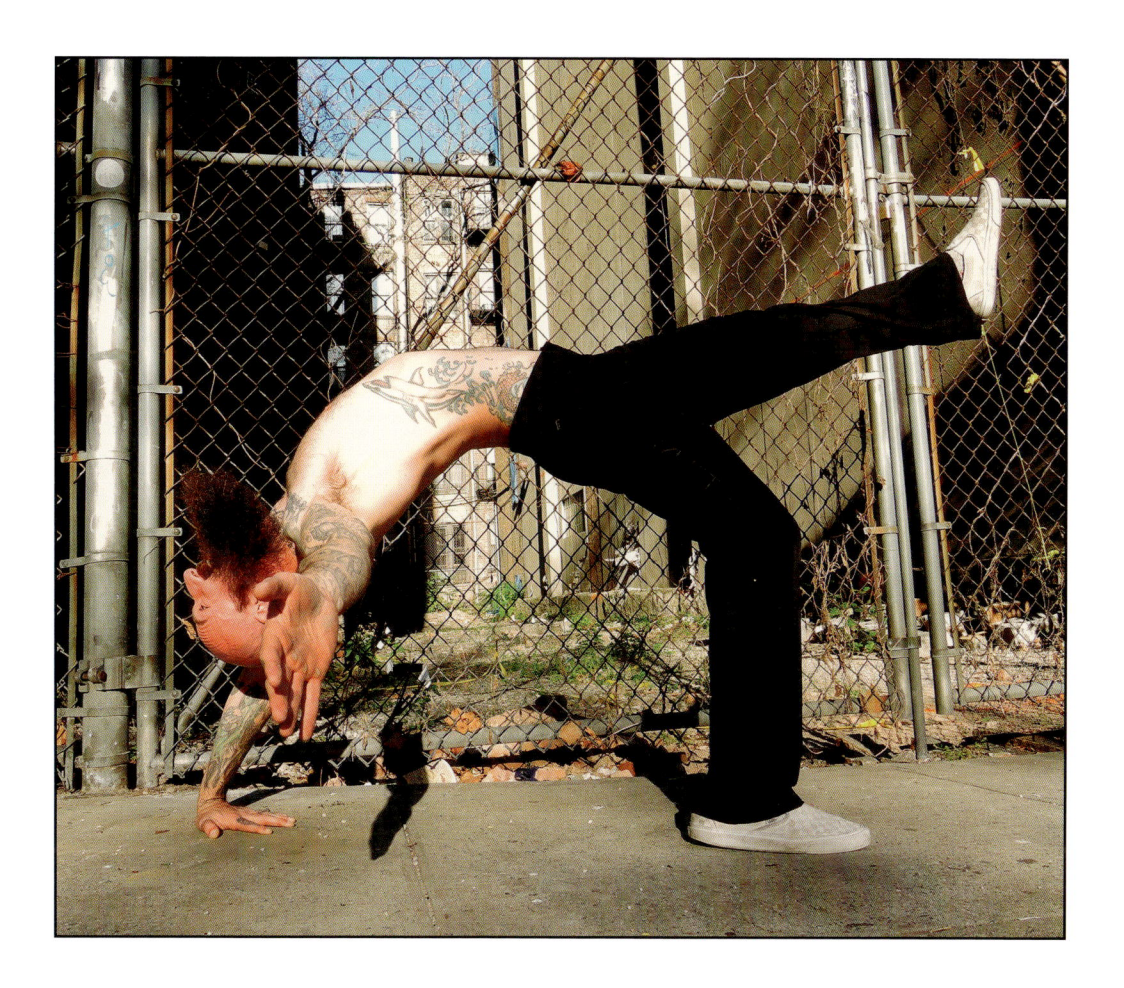

BRIDGE ROTATION

Begin on the ground in a seated position with your hands by your sides, knees bent and feet flat on the floor in front of your body. Turn your wrists out away from your body, press your weight off of your butt and reach one arm into the air. Slowly begin to spin your body around on your opposite palm, eventually bringing the other hand to the floor, so you wind up in a back bridge position. Though you will likely need to bend your elbows in order to rotate all the way around, aim to minimize any arm flexion. Once you are in a bridge, you can return to the start position, or lift the opposite hand and rotate to the other side.

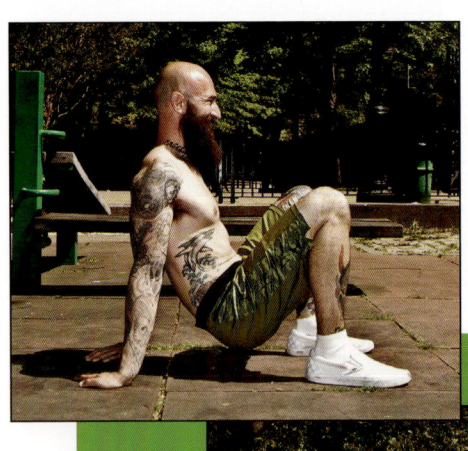

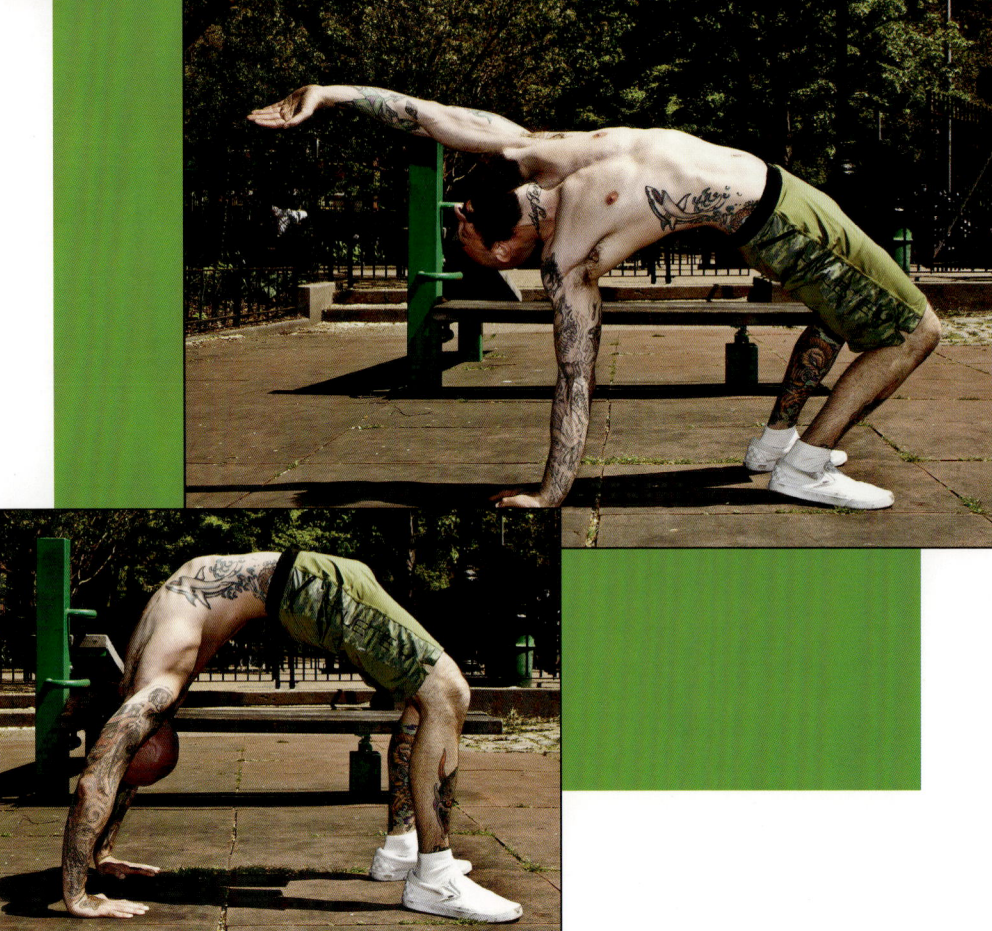

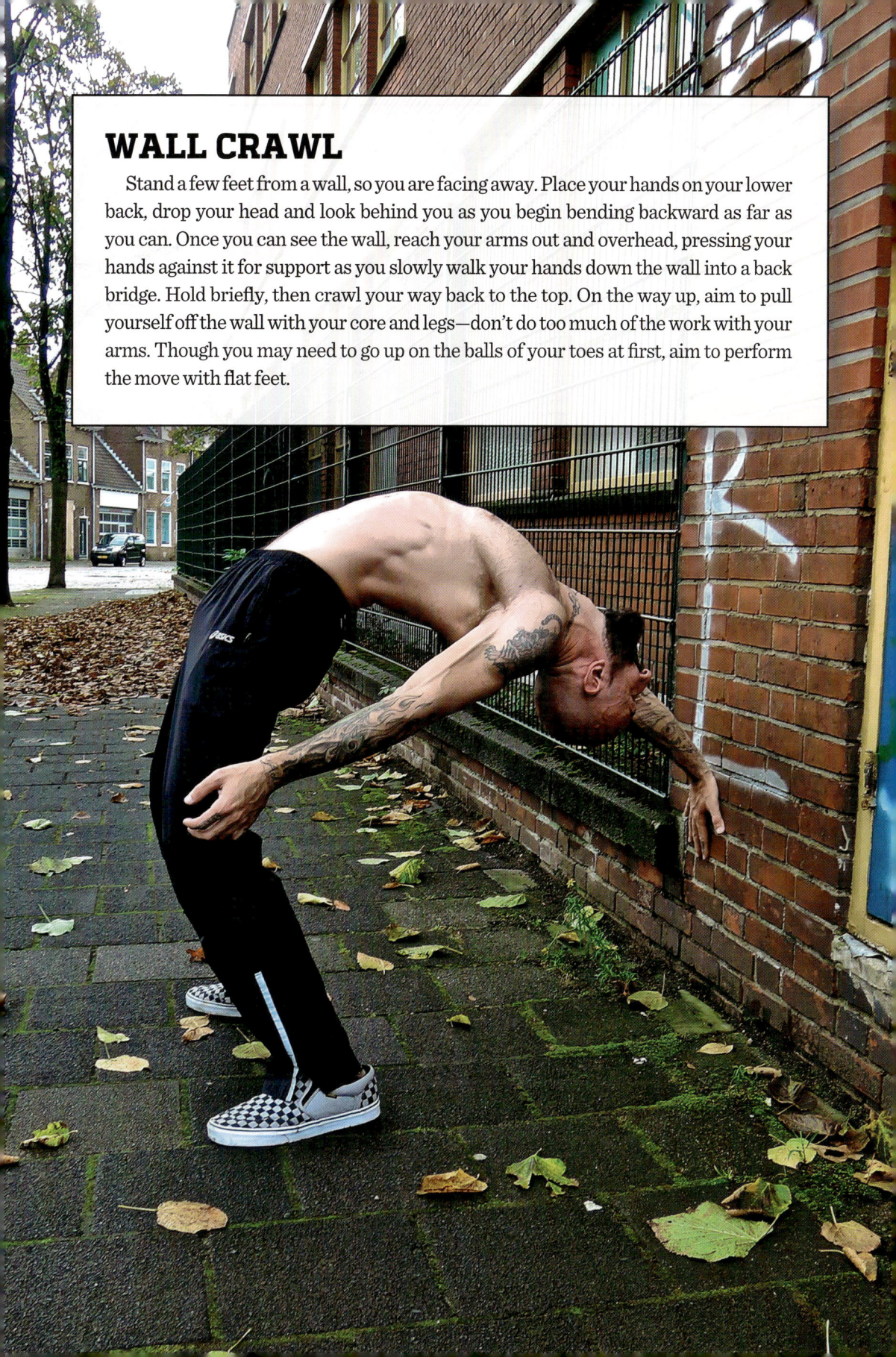

WALL CRAWL

Stand a few feet from a wall, so you are facing away. Place your hands on your lower back, drop your head and look behind you as you begin bending backward as far as you can. Once you can see the wall, reach your arms out and overhead, pressing your hands against it for support as you slowly walk your hands down the wall into a back bridge. Hold briefly, then crawl your way back to the top. On the way up, aim to pull yourself off the wall with your core and legs—don't do too much of the work with your arms. Though you may need to go up on the balls of your toes at first, aim to perform the move with flat feet.

STAND-TO-STAND BRIDGE

The stand-to-stand bridge is essentially a wall crawl without the wall. Stand tall, push your hips forward and bend backward as far as you can. Once you can see the ground behind you, reach your arms away from your body and reach for the floor. Be prepared to actively press the ground away the moment your hands make contact. Failure to do so can result in crashing down on your head.

From the back bridge position, press into the ground with your arms and aim your hips up and out over your toes to shift your weight back completely onto your feet. It may be helpful to reach one arm in the air before the other and/or go on the balls of your feet for better leverage, though the ultimate aim should be to perform the movement with the heels down.

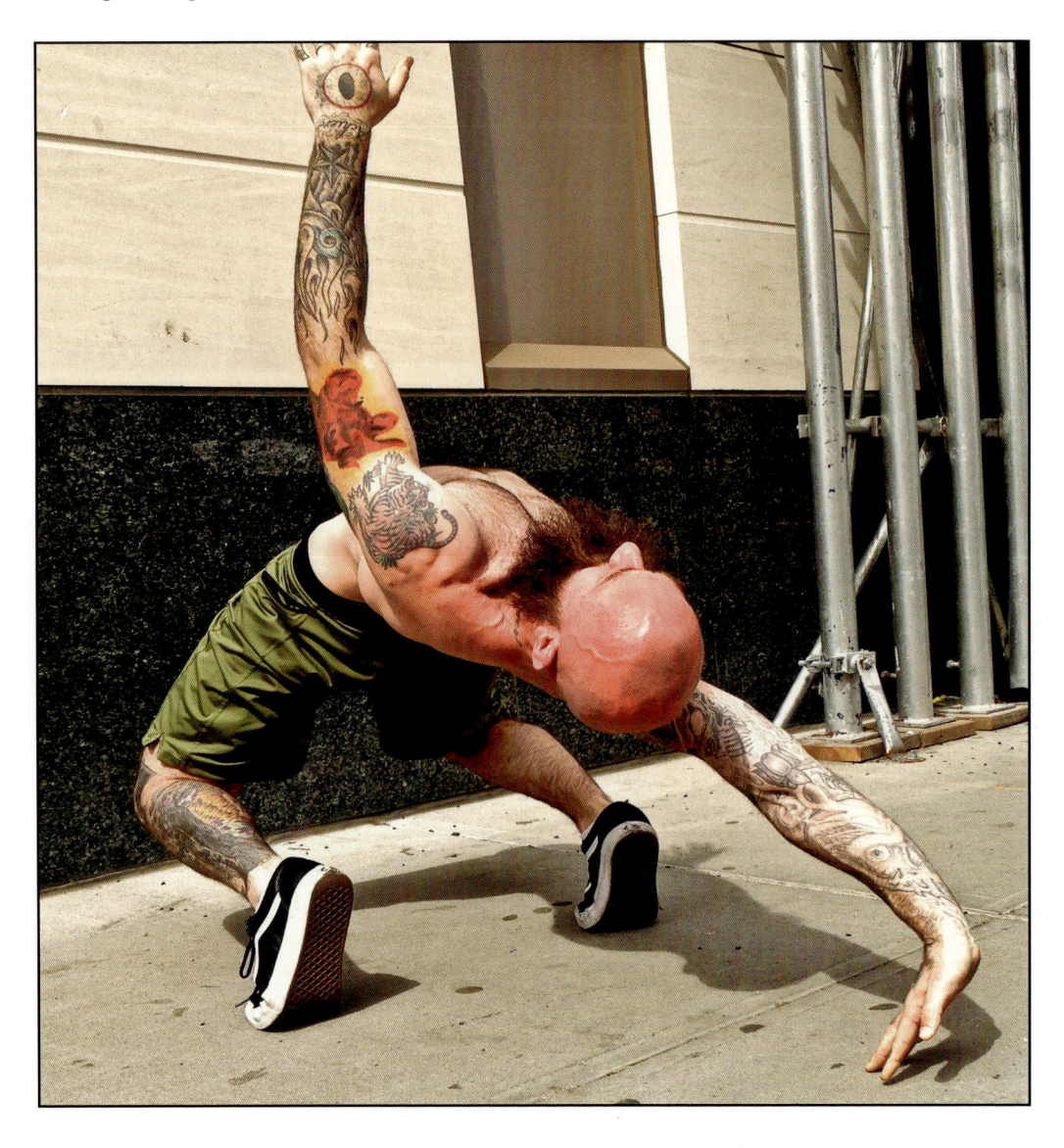

The Plyo-Matrix
Kipping Up

The realm of plyometric movements is not limited to your classic strength training exercises. Although not a strict arch per se, the kip-up is still considered an explosive variant of the bridge nonetheless. It is a fantastic drill in full body coordination and plyometric power, as well as a breathtaking visual.

To perform it, start by lying on your back with your palms flat on the floor and on either side of your head. Roll your thighs up toward your shoulders, then kick your legs up as you push off with your hands and arms. Explode from the hips and land your feet on the ground, in a full standing position. Timing is of the essence.

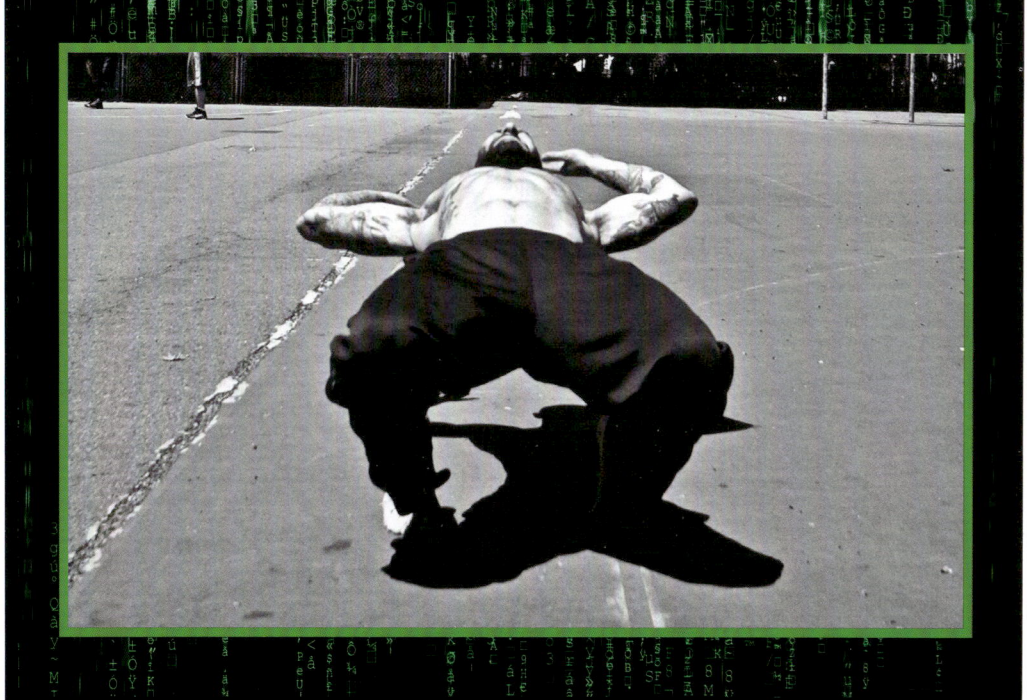

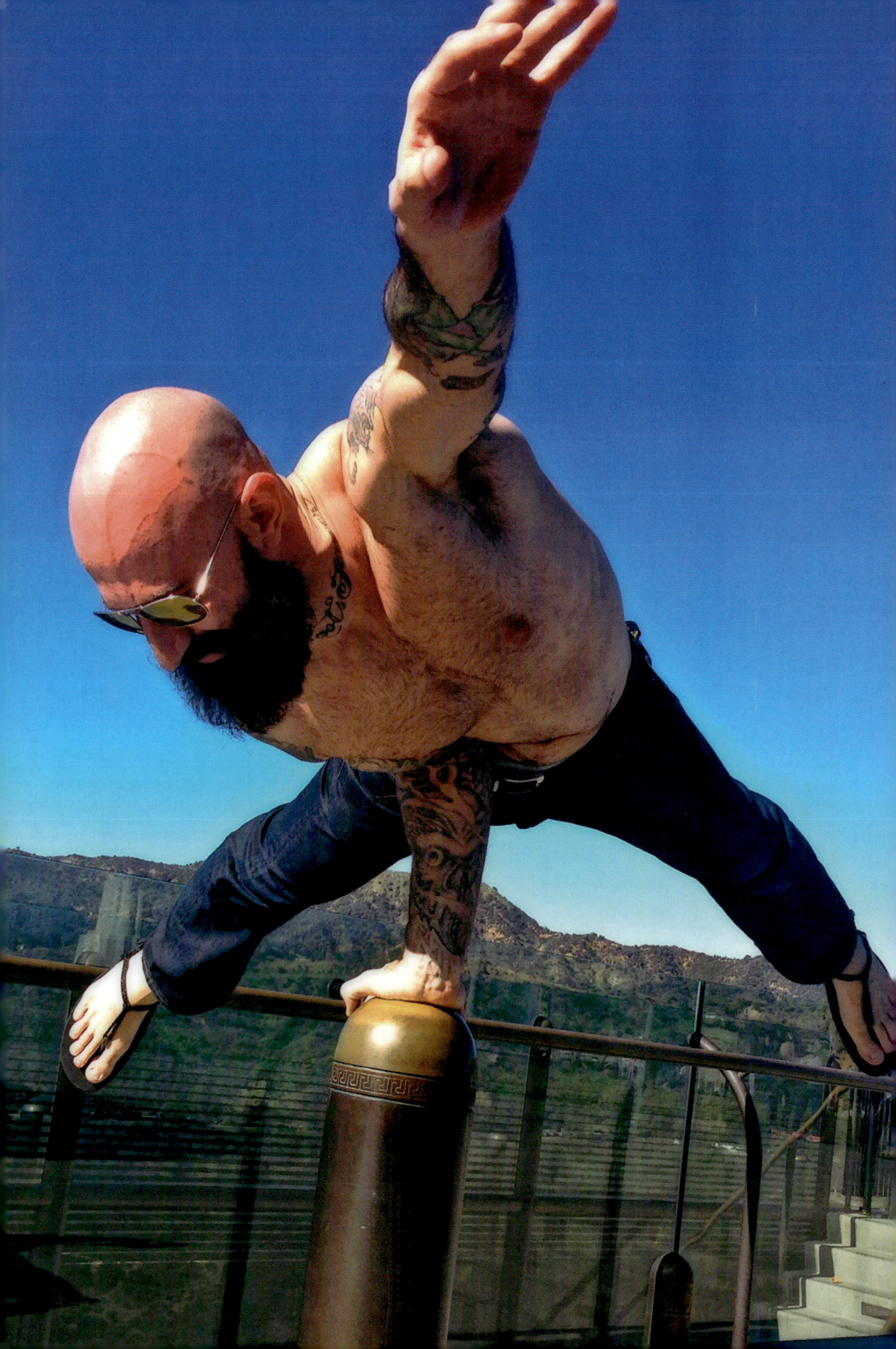

Skills & "Tricks"

First things first. There are no tricks. The following exercises embody strength and proficiency in all their magnificent splendor. They reflect patience, practice and perseverance in the face of adversity.

Detractors often claim that many of these moves do not represent functional strength or absolute power, even implying that there is some sort of "hack" to performing them, but that is far from the truth. These moves are only learned—or rather, earned—through countless hours of technical and muscular training. Whether it's muscle-ups, handstands or human flags, you must put in the time and train hard. That's right. There are no tricks. As for skill, well, that's another story...

Skill training is very much a practice. Just like learning a foreign language or a musical instrument, consistency and effort are key. For many of these exercises, you are better off training with frequency, but not necessarily to failure, so your body can "rehearse" the movement pattern on a regular basis. You might want to take a video of yourself or have a spotter to let you know when you're in the correct position, as it can be difficult to feel where you are in space.

The beautiful thing about making your priority learning a skill is that you will very likely, along the way, increase your strength and improve your overall fitness. Often it's more enjoyable to immerse yourself in skill training rather than chasing numeric goals. If we had to tell you what the "trick" is, the answer would be days, months and years in the humble pursuit of the seemingly unachievable.

The following section is broken down into three categories, Floor Holds, Bar Moves and Human Flag. Within each, the moves are shown in approximate order of difficulty, though different individuals will discover their own strengths and weaknesses.

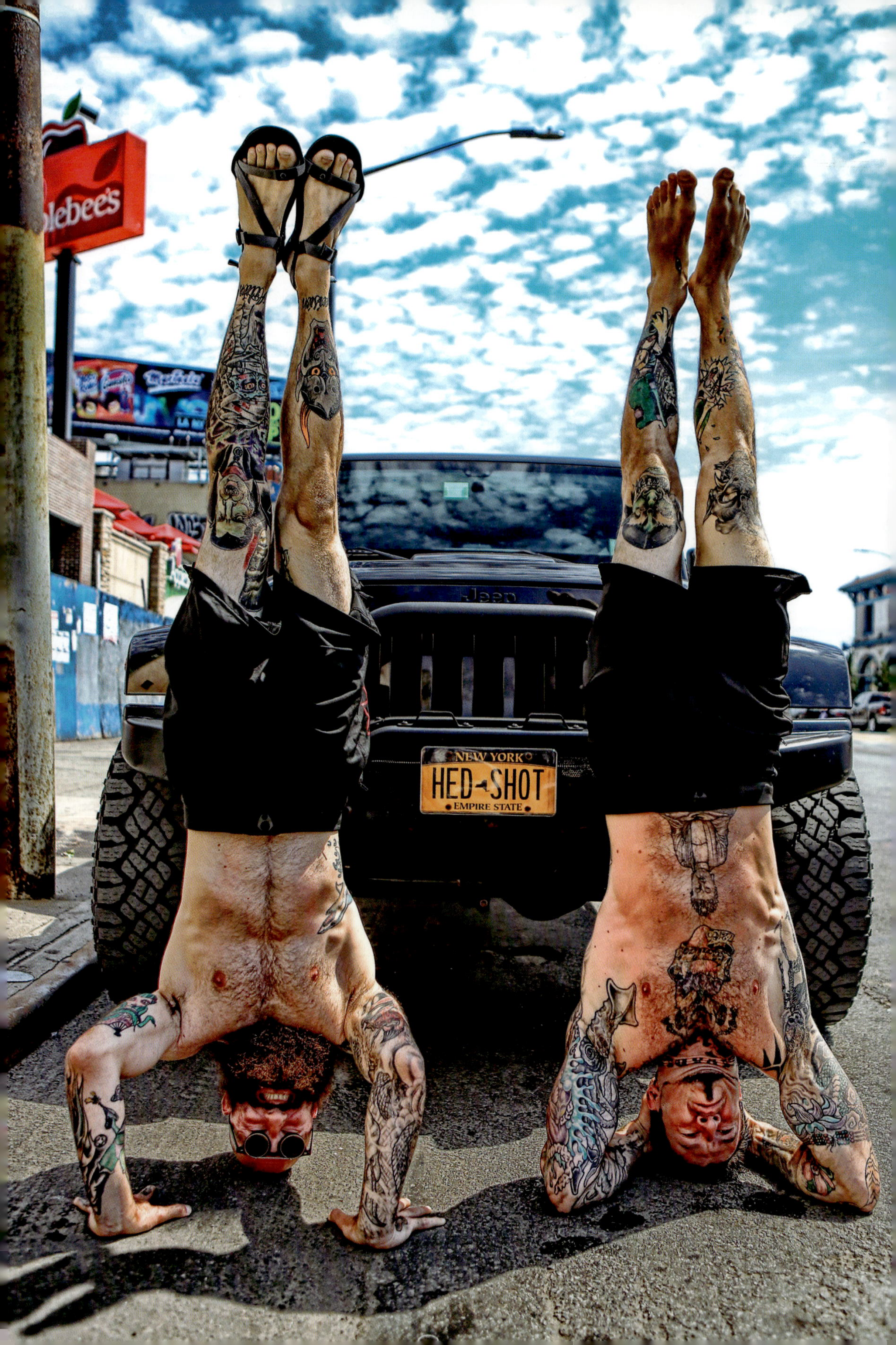
NEW YORK
HED-SHOT
EMPIRE STATE

CHAPTER 9

Floor Holds

The pure minimalism of training with nothing but your own physical body and the raw earth beneath you is the ultimate expression of primal simplicity and animal splendor. This section represents directness, clarity and integrity in training.

The exercises contained herein are divided into four categories: Frog, Crow & Crane serves as an introduction to hand balancing. The Headstand & Handstand section is a comprehensive guide to inversions from the most basic to the most advanced, as well as a history lesson on how the current standards came to be. The Elbow Lever grouping takes us to a realm where we exploit our skeletal anatomy and physical awareness in order to literally find a balance. The final category, Planche, represents calisthenics strength, precision, skill and fortitude in its most advanced forms.

Are you ready to work hard?

FROG, CROW AND CRANE PROGRESSIONS

Because the body is kept closer to the ground in these exercises than it would be with full inversions (handstands, headstands, etc.), it is shorter in length, giving a mechanical advantage when starting out. However, although more favorable leverage is provided, you will see that these exercises can be progressed from very basic to extremely advanced.

The frog, crow and crane have their origins in yoga. One of the most profound aspects of Street Workout is that it fuses elements from many different styles and disciplines of movement. Calisthenics, break dancing, martial arts and, yes... yoga! It's all bodyweight training. The body moves the way the body moves, in spite of any classification. There is no need to over categorize things. These exercises demand a certain skill level, but make no mistake: in addition to rehearsing the skill, a baseline of strength in the hands, arms, shoulders and core is required.

FROG STAND

Get into the bottom of a deep squat, then place your palms flat on the floor, just wider than shoulder width. Bend your elbows back and rest the insides of your thighs and calves against your triceps, almost like you're using your arms as a shelf to support your lower body. The more contact you have between your arms and legs, the easier it will be to balance. From here, continue to bend your elbows until they are around 90 degrees and tip all of your weight forward, lifting your feet off the ground. Think about looking in front of your hands rather than in between them in order to stay balanced.

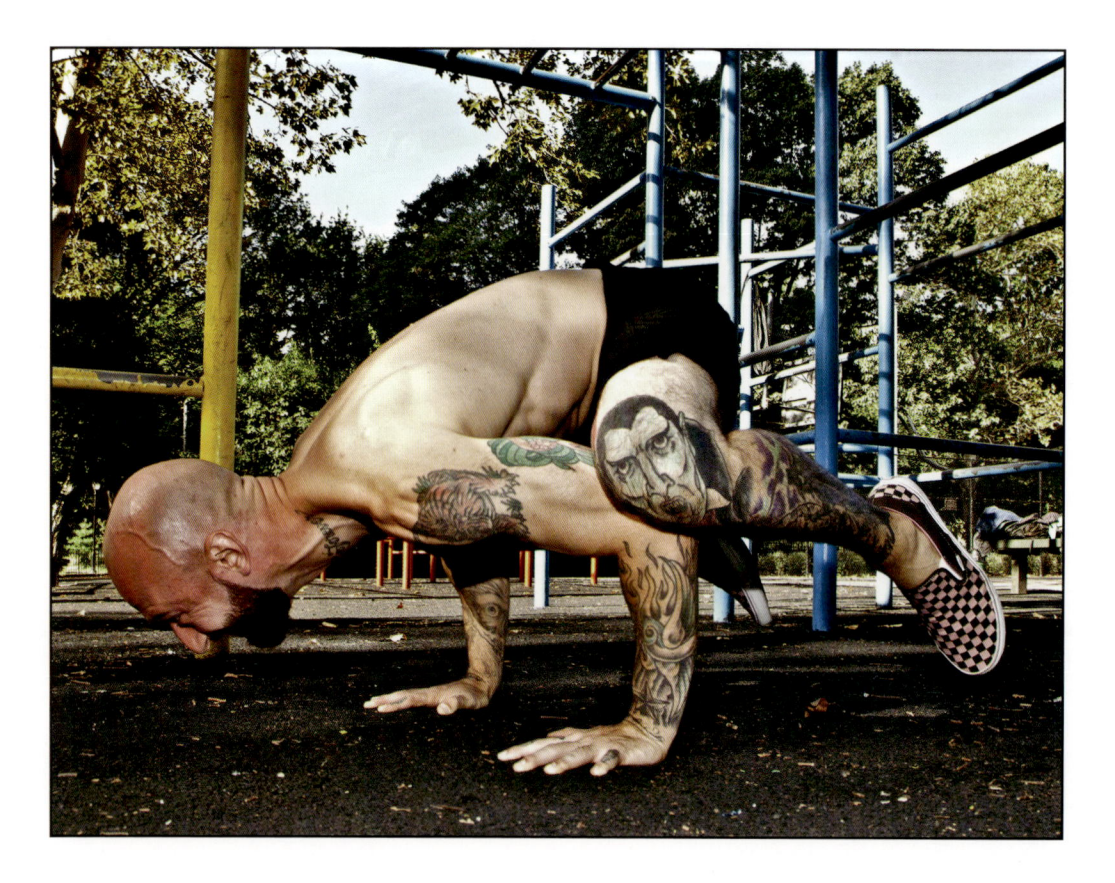

CROW HOLD

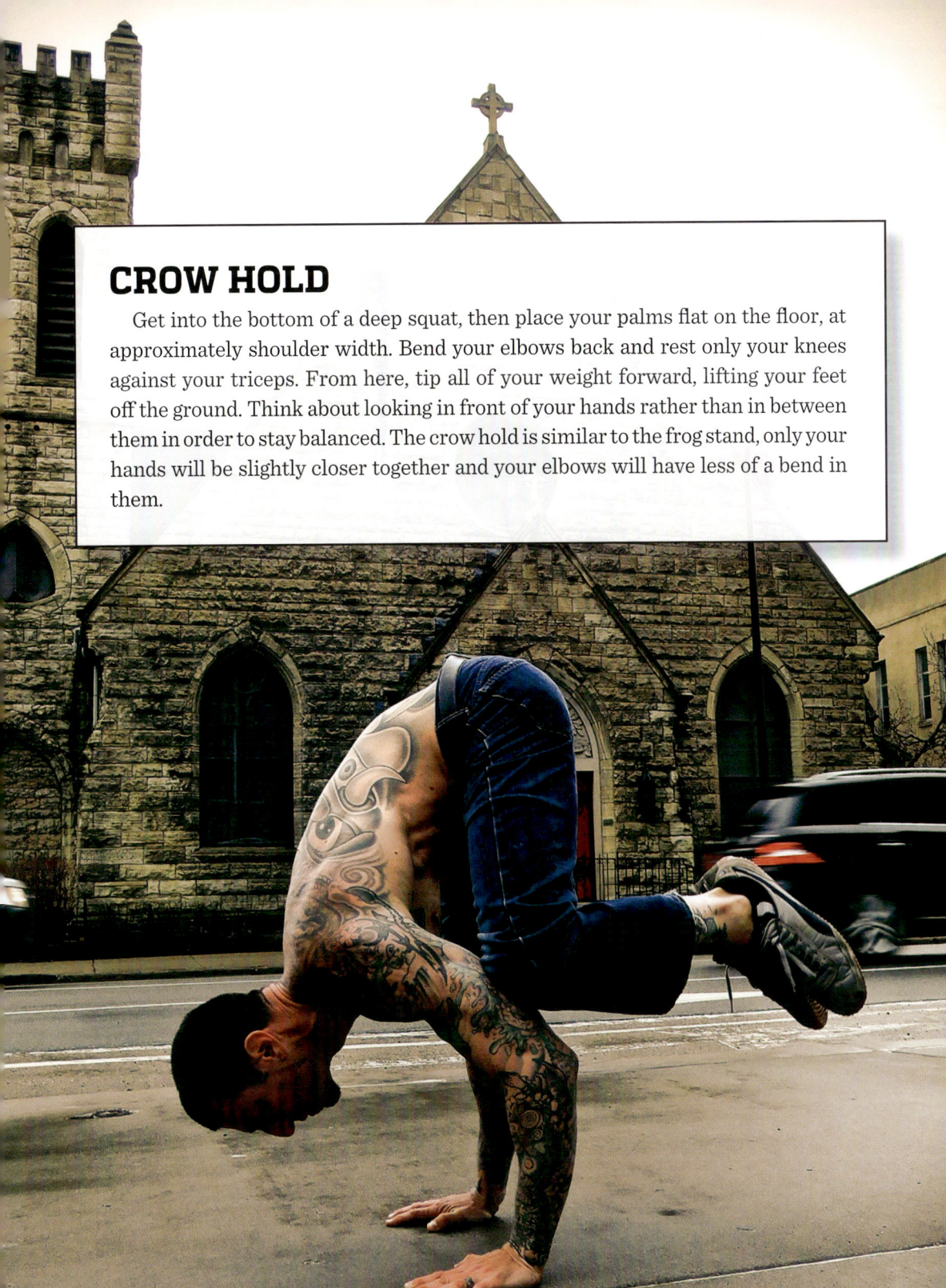

Get into the bottom of a deep squat, then place your palms flat on the floor, at approximately shoulder width. Bend your elbows back and rest only your knees against your triceps. From here, tip all of your weight forward, lifting your feet off the ground. Think about looking in front of your hands rather than in between them in order to stay balanced. The crow hold is similar to the frog stand, only your hands will be slightly closer together and your elbows will have less of a bend in them.

CRANE POSE

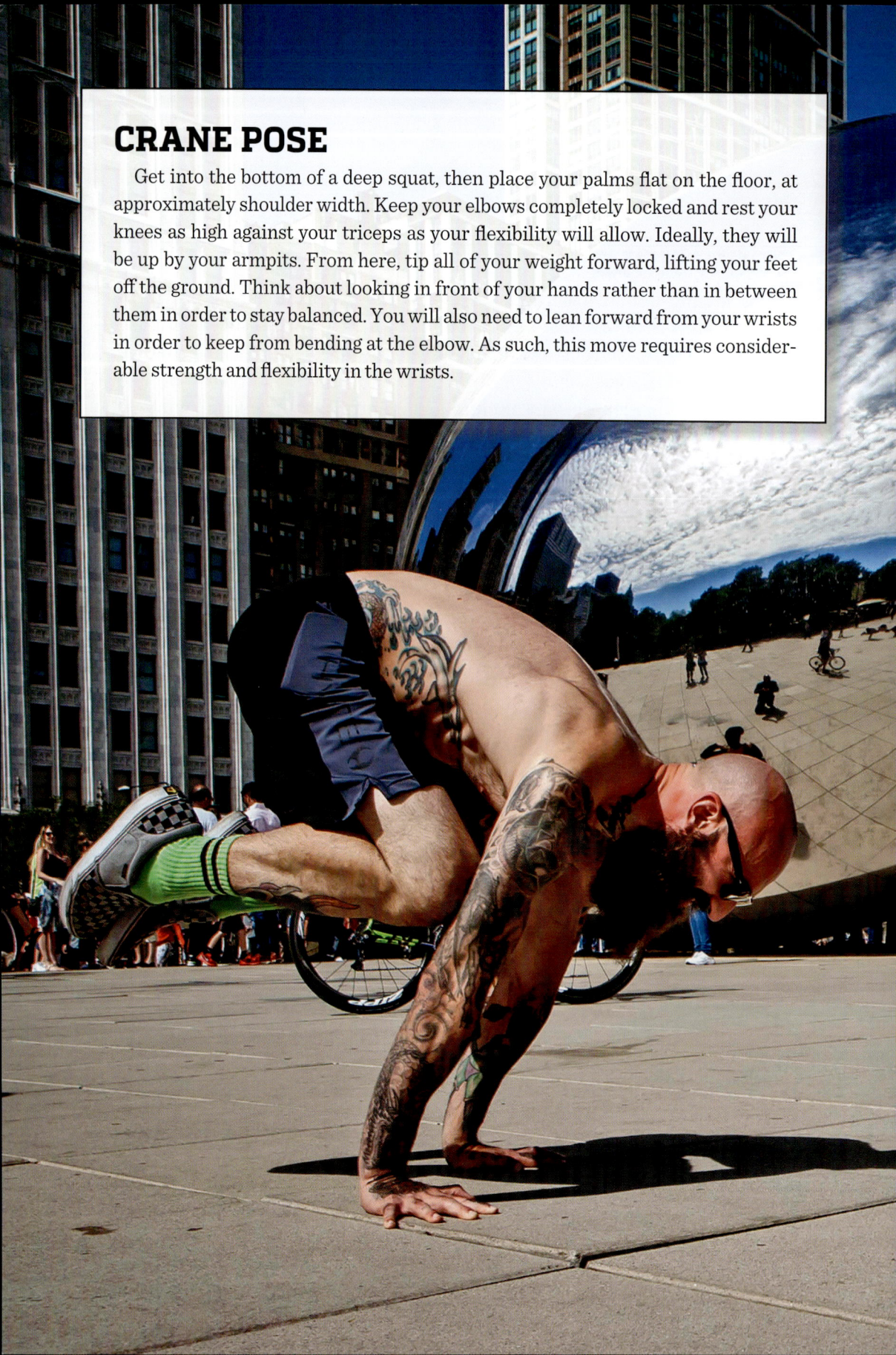

Get into the bottom of a deep squat, then place your palms flat on the floor, at approximately shoulder width. Keep your elbows completely locked and rest your knees as high against your triceps as your flexibility will allow. Ideally, they will be up by your armpits. From here, tip all of your weight forward, lifting your feet off the ground. Think about looking in front of your hands rather than in between them in order to stay balanced. You will also need to lean forward from your wrists in order to keep from bending at the elbow. As such, this move requires considerable strength and flexibility in the wrists.

SIDE CROW

Get into the bottom of a deep squat, then twist to one side and place both arms on the outside of one leg with your hands on the ground. Similar to the standard crow hold, your elbows should bend back toward your legs, except this time making contact with only one leg and at two points: near your knee and the other by your hip. Lift your hips and shift all your weight onto your hands, with your knees stacked together.

If you do not have the flexibility to do the above variation, you can start by placing your hands further apart and only use one elbow as a contact point. Try to line up your elbow mid-thigh, before lifting your hips and shifting your weight onto your hands. Make sure to practice the balance on both sides.

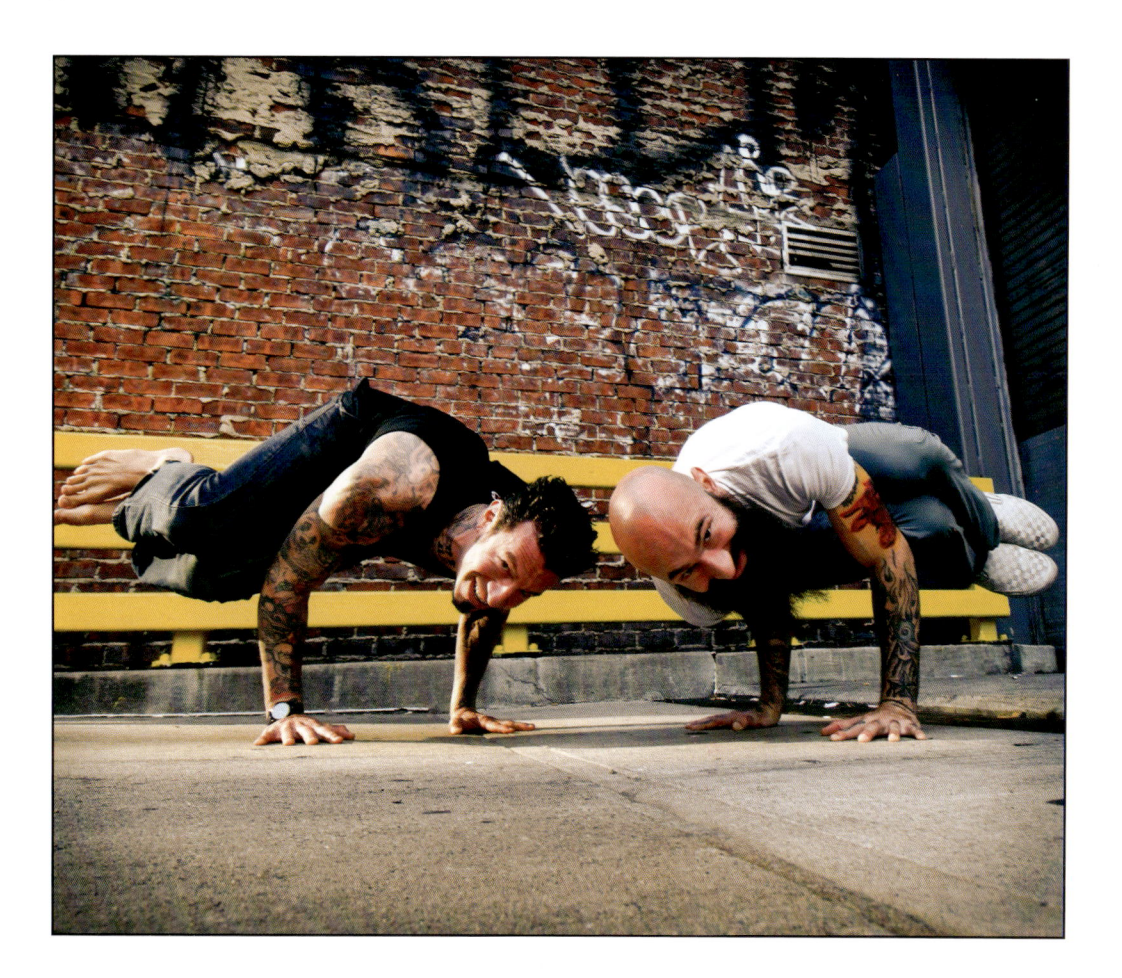

ONE LEG CROW

By removing a leg from the equation, you can quickly and easily increase the difficulty of the standard crow pose in both the balance and strength departments. Start in a basic crow, then carefully shift one leg off of your arm and bring it toward the center. Once you have a feel for this, you can begin extending that leg to add further difficulty.

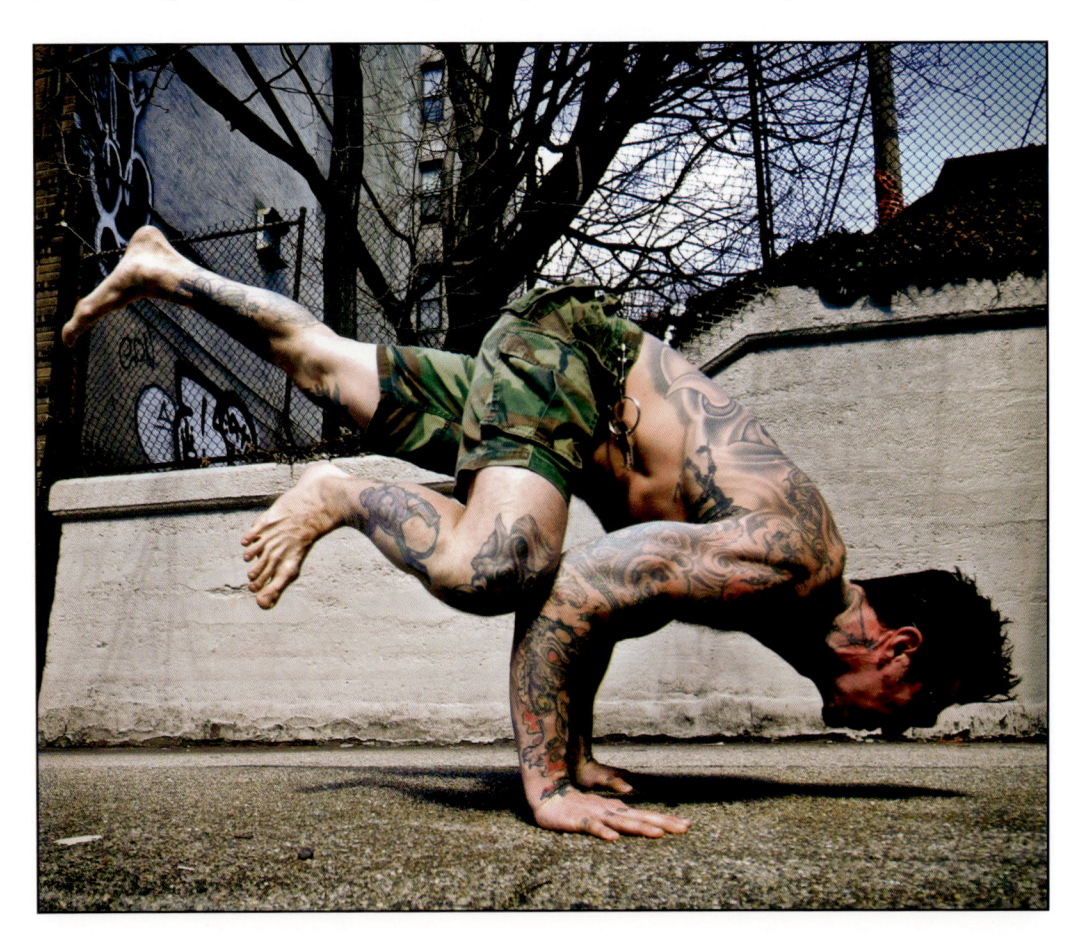

ONE ARM/ONE LEG CROW

The one arm/one leg crow, or "air baby" as it's known in the breakdancing world, is one of the most challenging and visually impressive moves in all of calisthenics.

Begin in a one leg crow, then start to stack your hips vertically as you gently begin taking some of the weight off of the hand that is not supporting your leg. Try to gradually shift weight away from that side, removing contact points one finger at a time, until only one remains on the ground. Eventually you will learn to float that finger up and off the ground as well, leaving all your weight supported on just one hand.

Bear in mind that this move requires a lot of strength as well as very precise balance. Think about actively pressing the ground away with your primary arm as you shift your weight off of the other side.

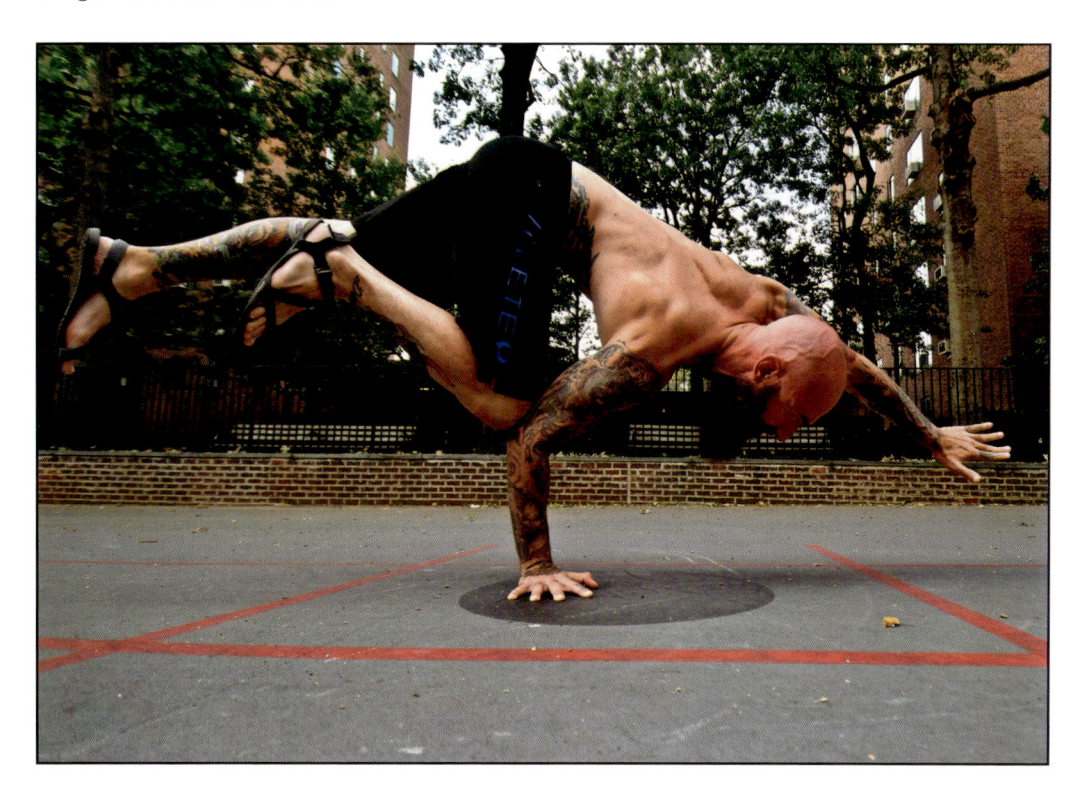

HEADSTAND & HANDSTAND PROGRESSIONS

When it comes to calisthenics training, the handstand is often overlooked (even dismissed) as a "skills-only" practice, rather than a strength move. But we assure you: one cannot attain a solid handstand without a foundation of physical power in the arms, core, chest, back and, particularly, the shoulders and traps. In fact, many well-meaning members of the fitness community have wondered how they can emphasize those sensational shoulder muscles when performing bodyweight exercises. Well, the answer is the handstand and its many forms. Because a handstand involves supporting your entire body in an inverted position, with arms extended and hands flat on the floor, a great degree of overhead pressing capability, along with hand and finger strength, is involved. Of course, there is also a huge skill component. Hand balancing is an entire discipline unto itself, even beyond the realm of Street Workout. We encourage you to pursue all forms of training.

The headstand allows you to use your head as an additional point of contact and is often seen as a progressive step leading up to the handstand, but it is a legitimate pursuit in its own right. Both these exercises require a tremendous degree of balance, as well as a necessary capacity for spatial adaptation, as everything appears literally upside-down and backward to the practitioner. These inversions require both strength and skill.

Beyond the aforementioned elements, handstands and headstands place your heart over your head, reversing your blood flow. This invigorates the circulatory and immune systems. Many believe it rejuvenates the spirit as well.

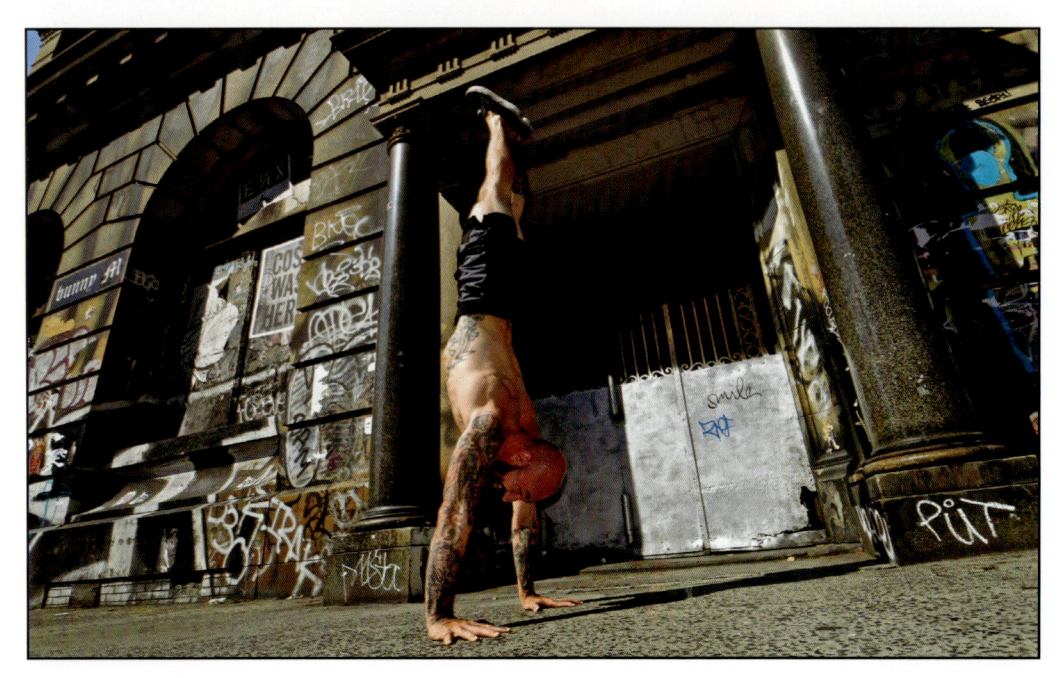

TRIPOD

Get into the bottom of a deep squat, then place your palms flat on the floor in front of you at approximately shoulder width. Bend your elbows back and place the top of your head on the floor, higher than your hands, not in between them, so that the three points of contact form a triangle, hence the name tripod. Raise your hips over your shoulders and bring your knees to rest on the backs of your arms. Engage your abdominal and lower back muscles and begin lifting your knees off of your arms. You can think of this move like a headstand with your knees tucked. Shortening the length of the body makes the balance easier while letting you get a feel for being completely inverted.

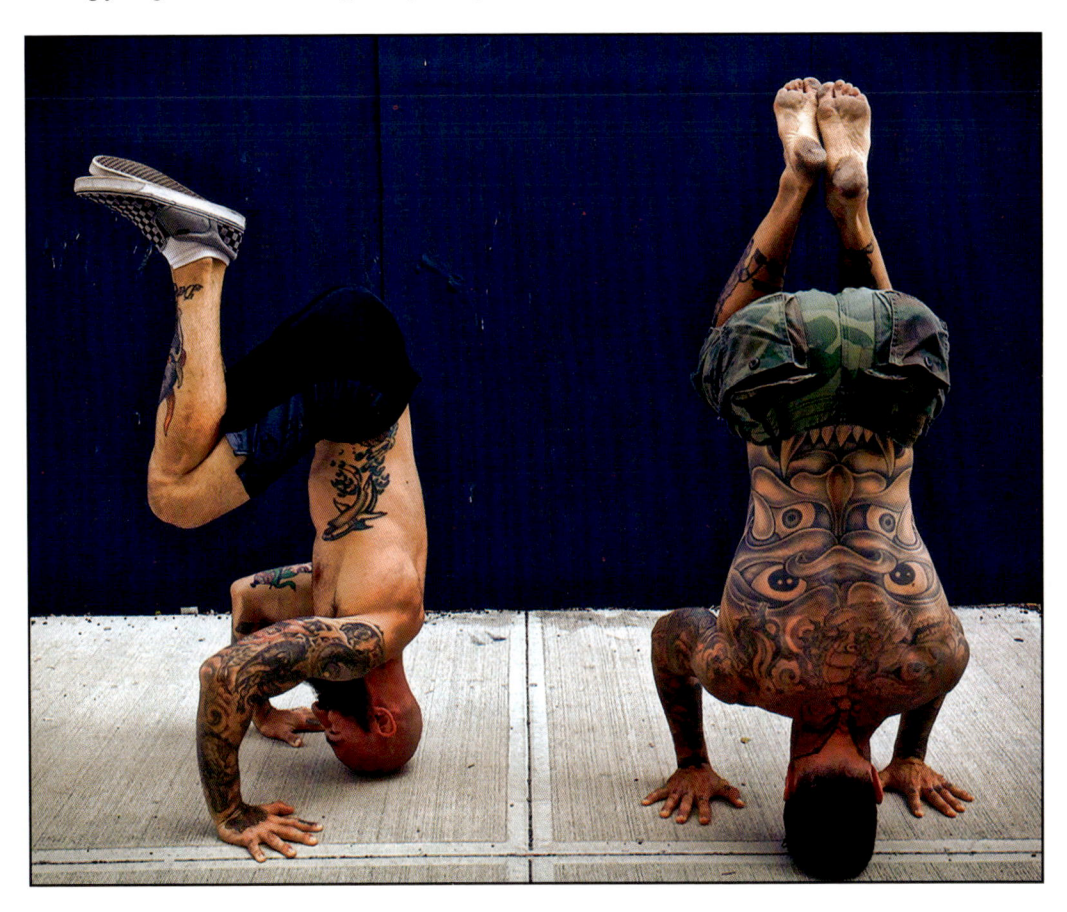

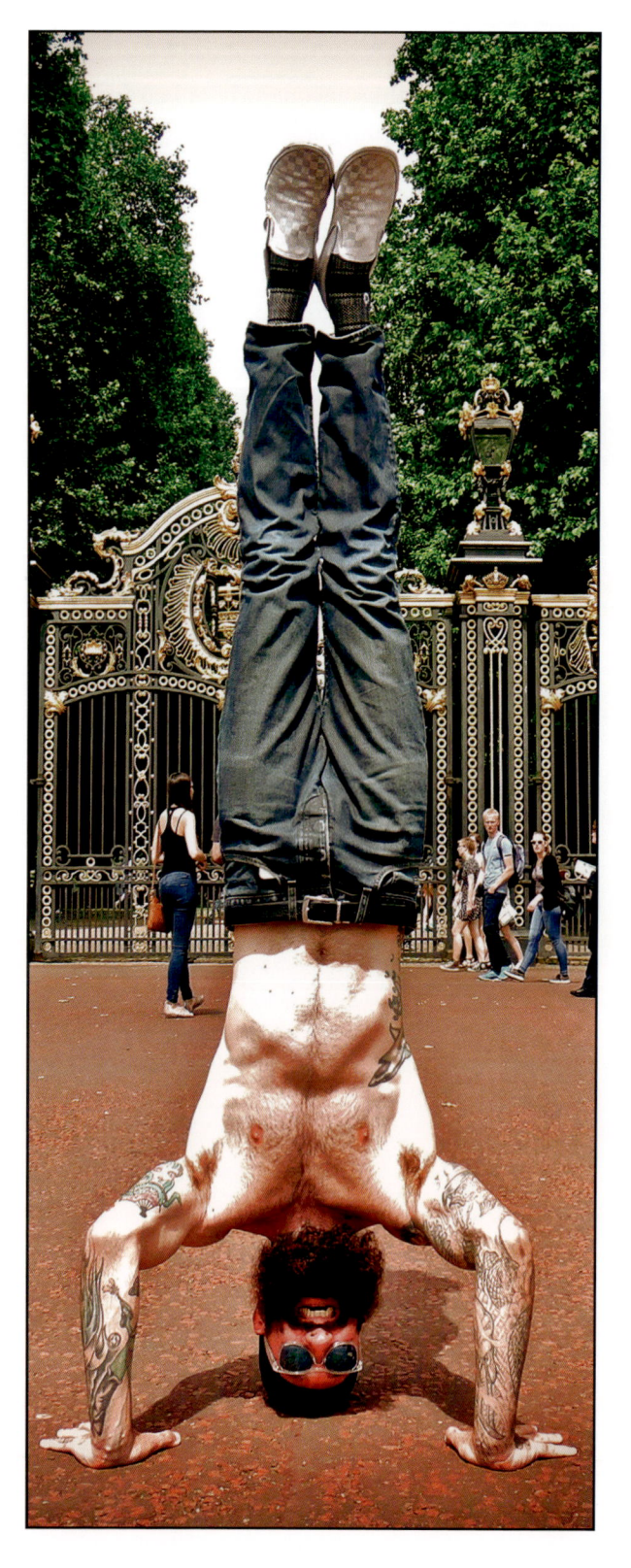

TRIPOD HEADSTAND

From the tripod position, begin lifting your legs off your arms and carefully extend them over your head. Squeeze your glutes and engage your legs in order to get your body fully extended. You can also use your shoulders, arms and hands to stay balanced by pressing into the ground. You can start out with your back to a wall if you are worried about tipping over.

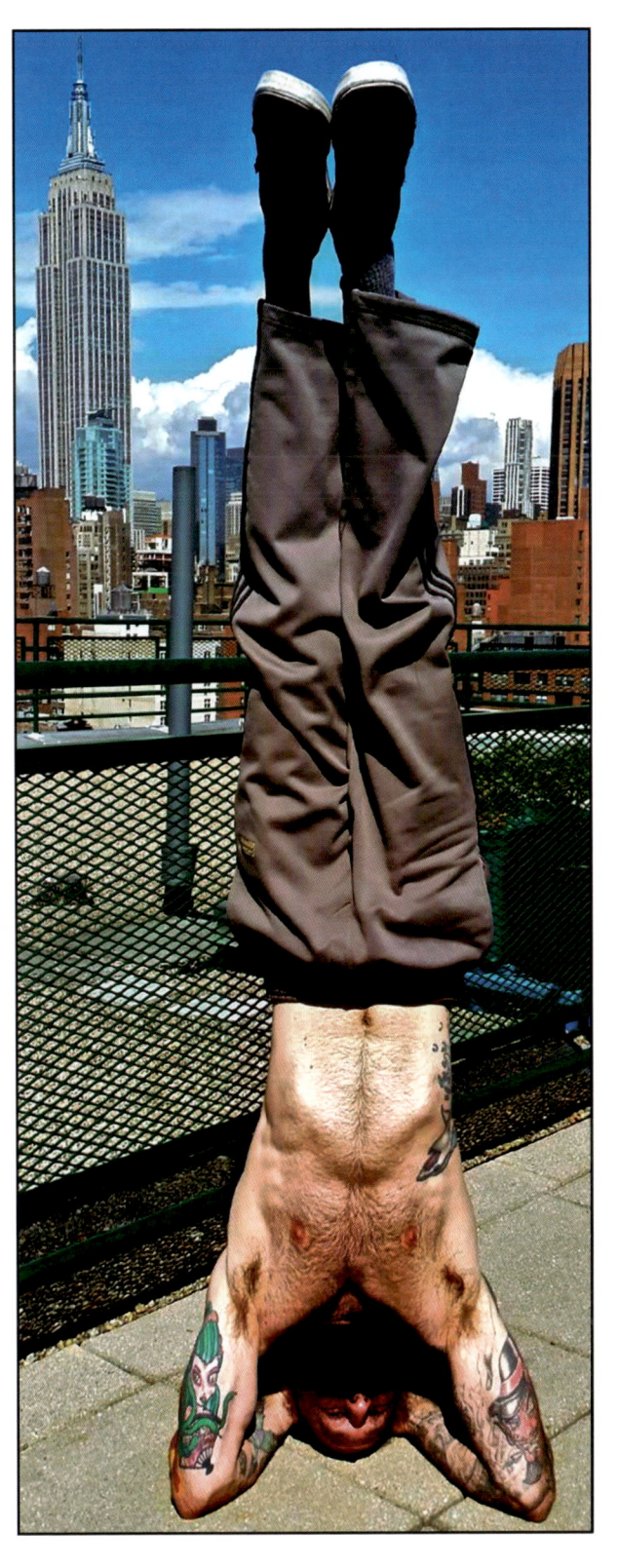

ELBOW HEADSTAND

Place the top of your head on the ground with your fingers interlaced behind the back of your head. Your forearms will rest on the ground with your elbows on the floor in front of your shoulders, rather than off to the sides. Walk your feet in toward your head and raise your hips above your shoulders. When your hips get high enough, lift or kick your legs up, stacking your body in a straight line. Start out with your back to a wall if you are worried about tipping over.

STRADDLE HEADSTAND

From either the tripod or elbow headstand, spreading your legs into a straddle can make extended holds less difficult. When you reach your legs out to the sides, you're essentially shortening the length of your body while simultaneously lowering your center of gravity, both of which make it easier to balance. Straddling your legs also takes some weight off your head and relieves pressure from your lower back.

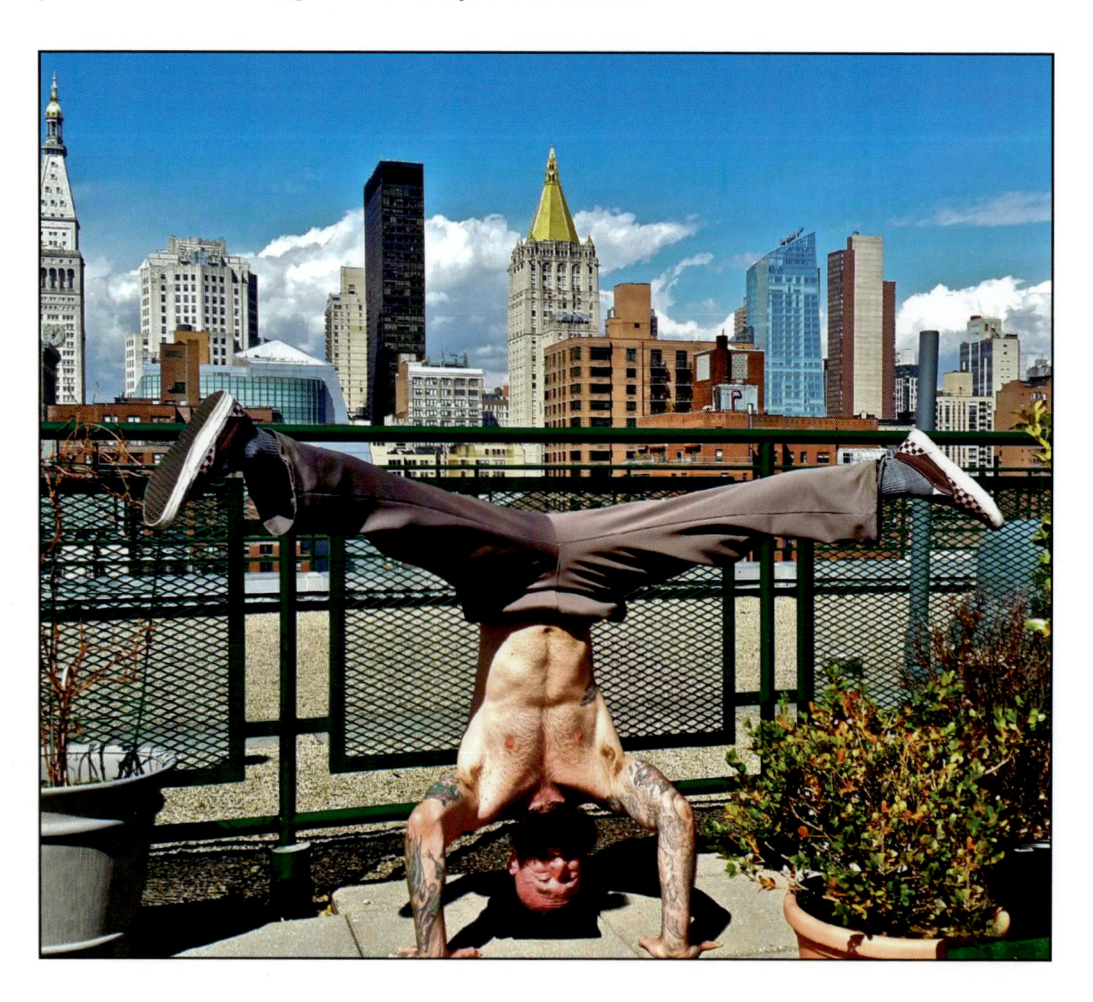

ULTIMATE HEADSTAND

Performing a headstand with no point of contact other than your skull is the ultimate progression. Begin in a tripod headstand and gradually shift your weight off of your hands until you are supported only by your head and fingertips. At this point, experiment with taking fingers away. As discussed previously, straddling your legs can help. Though it will take much trial and error, you may eventually be able to shift all of your weight to your head and remove your hands from the ground completely. The ultimate headstand requires tremendous neck strength and even greater balance. Holding it for even one full second takes lots of practice.

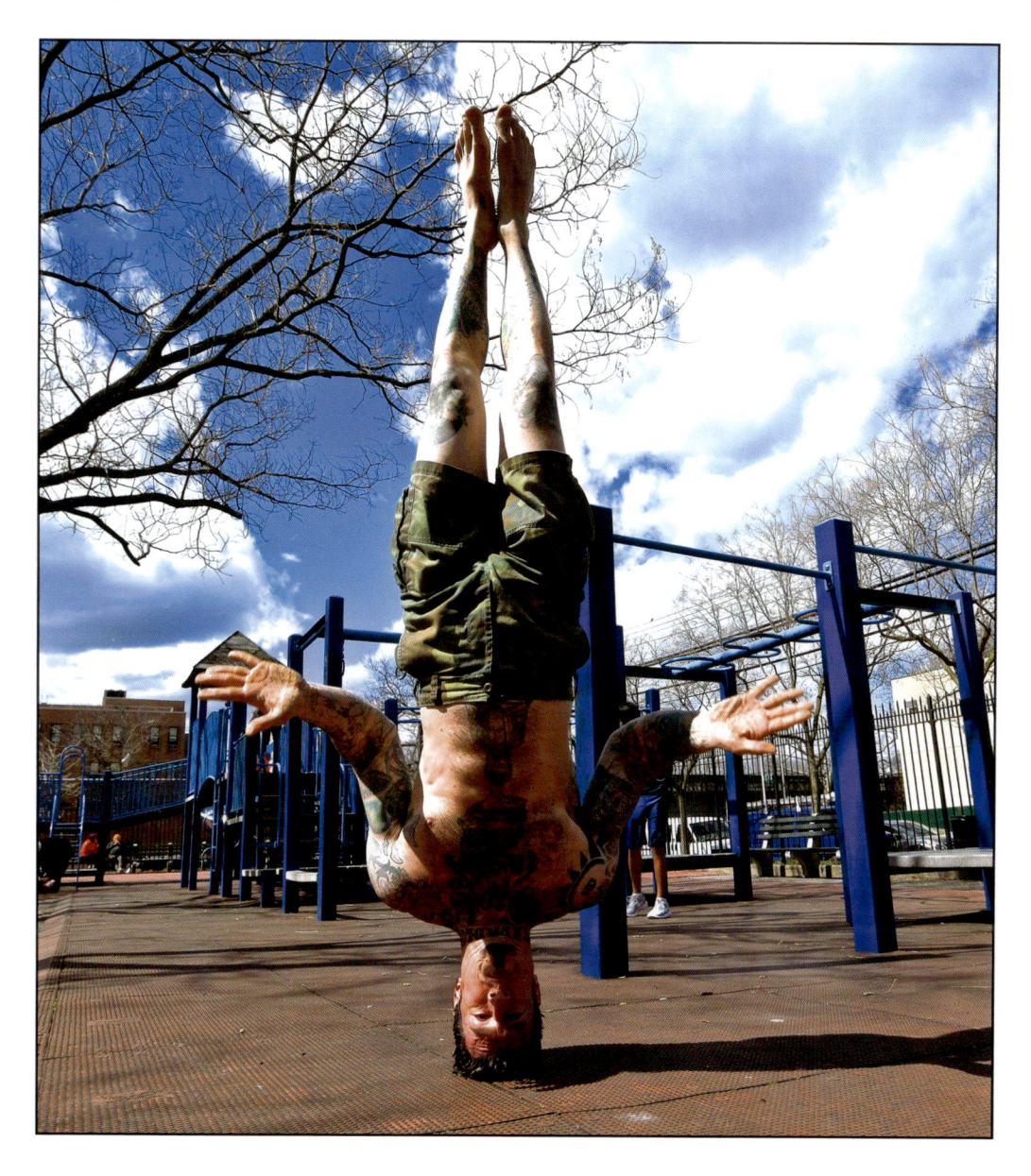

WALL HANDSTAND

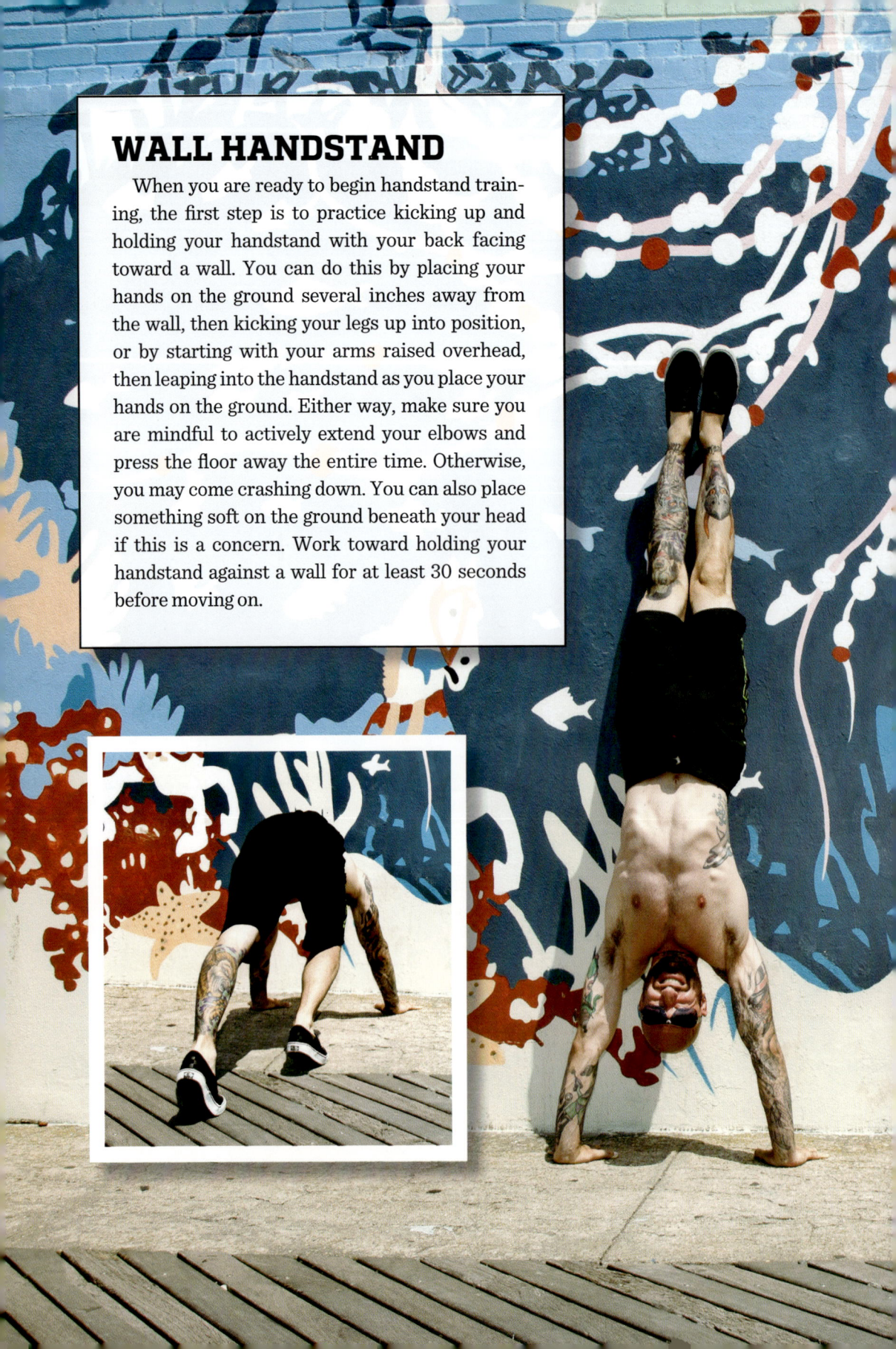

When you are ready to begin handstand training, the first step is to practice kicking up and holding your handstand with your back facing toward a wall. You can do this by placing your hands on the ground several inches away from the wall, then kicking your legs up into position, or by starting with your arms raised overhead, then leaping into the handstand as you place your hands on the ground. Either way, make sure you are mindful to actively extend your elbows and press the floor away the entire time. Otherwise, you may come crashing down. You can also place something soft on the ground beneath your head if this is a concern. Work toward holding your handstand against a wall for at least 30 seconds before moving on.

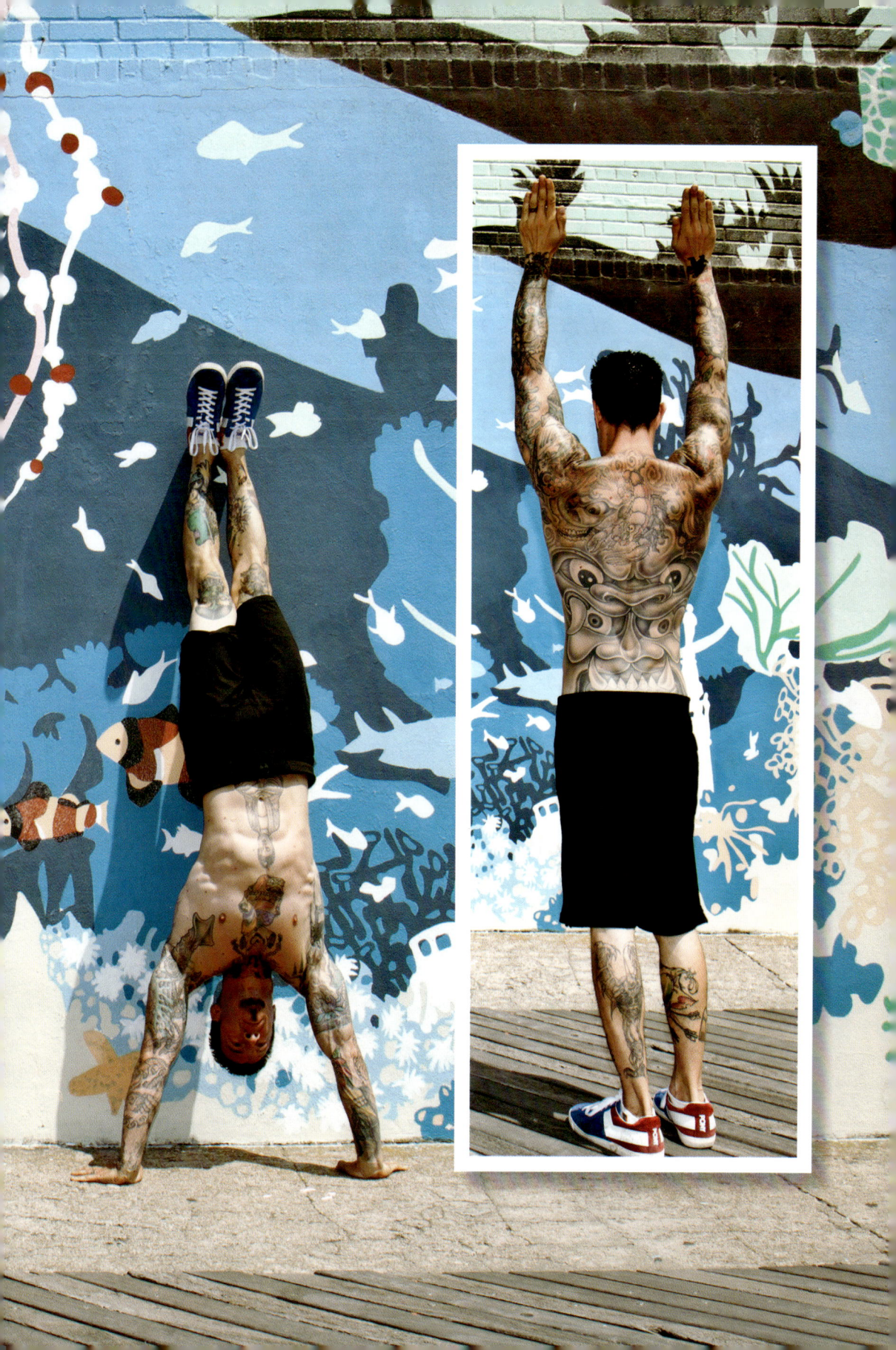

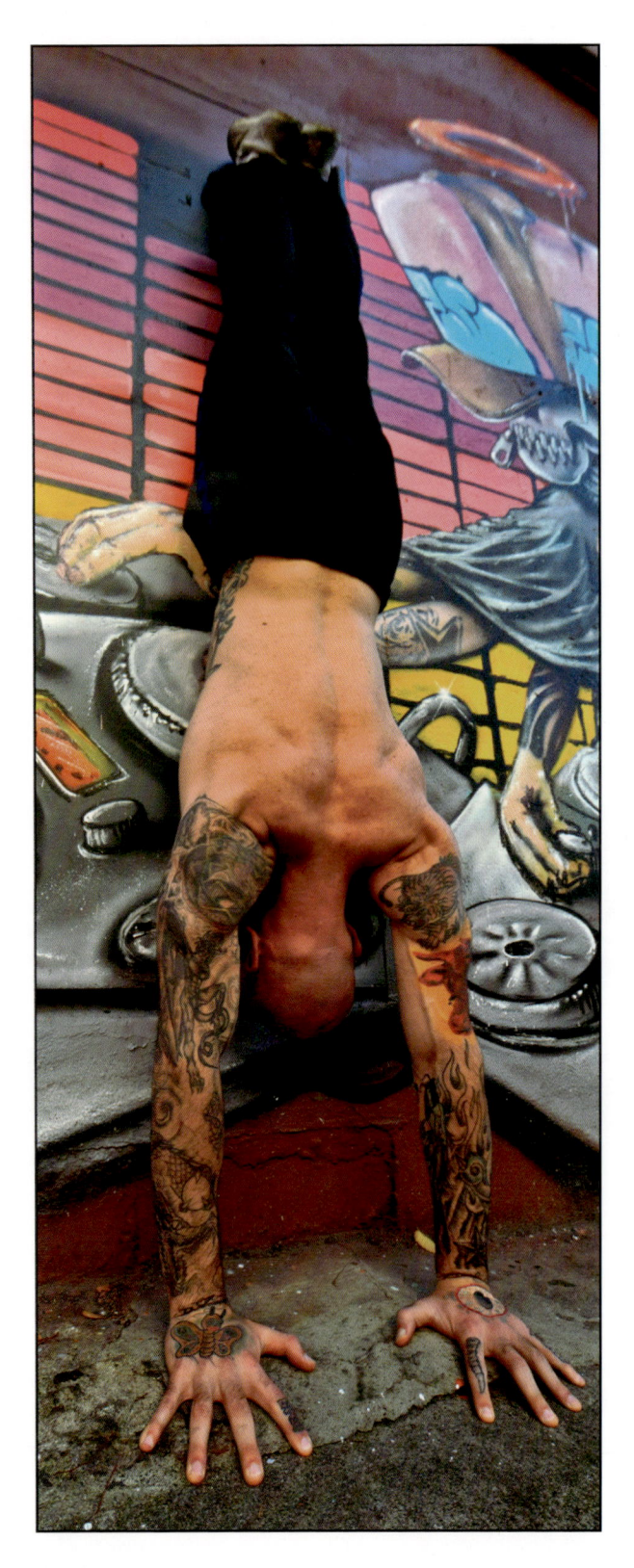

HANDSTAND FACING THE WALL

Begin in a plank position with your feet against the wall, then start walking your feet up as you gradually crawl your hands back toward it. Get your palms as close to the wall as possible while lengthening your entire body and pressing the ground away. When you've gotten as close as you can, actively shrug your shoulders, press your chest toward the wall and point your toes. Practicing your handstand while facing a wall is a great way to start to get the feel for the gymnastic style straight-back handstand.

When you need to come down, you can reverse the movement that you used to get up, or cartwheel your legs to the side.

FOREARM STAND

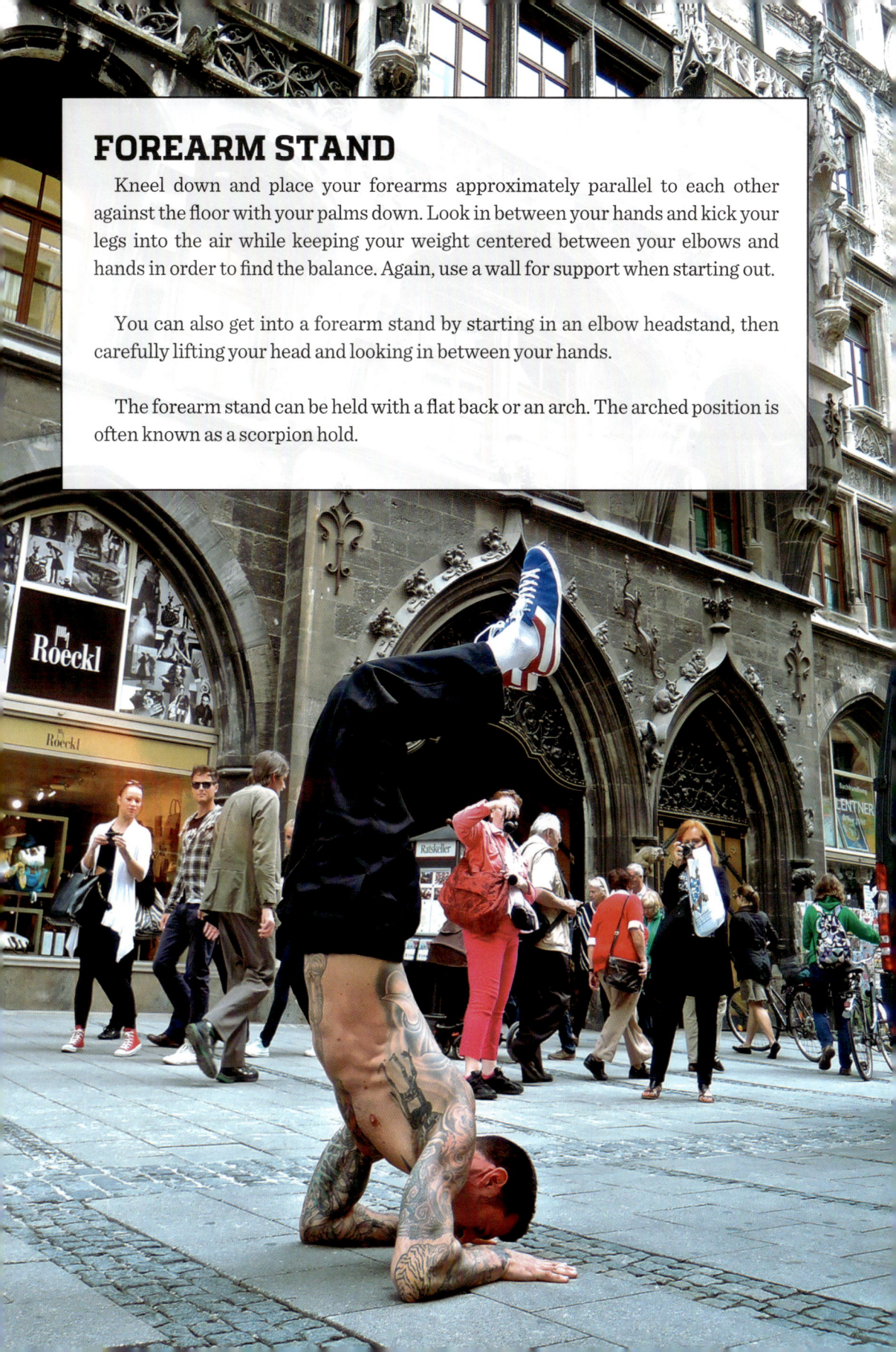

Kneel down and place your forearms approximately parallel to each other against the floor with your palms down. Look in between your hands and kick your legs into the air while keeping your weight centered between your elbows and hands in order to find the balance. Again, use a wall for support when starting out.

You can also get into a forearm stand by starting in an elbow headstand, then carefully lifting your head and looking in between your hands.

The forearm stand can be held with a flat back or an arch. The arched position is often known as a scorpion hold.

STRADDLE HANDSTAND

Spreading your legs into a straddle position during a handstand can make holding the position less difficult. When you reach your legs out to the sides, you're essentially shortening the length of your body while simultaneously lowering your center of gravity, both of which make it easier to balance. Straddling your legs also distributes mass away from your balance point, which further decreases your chances of toppling over.

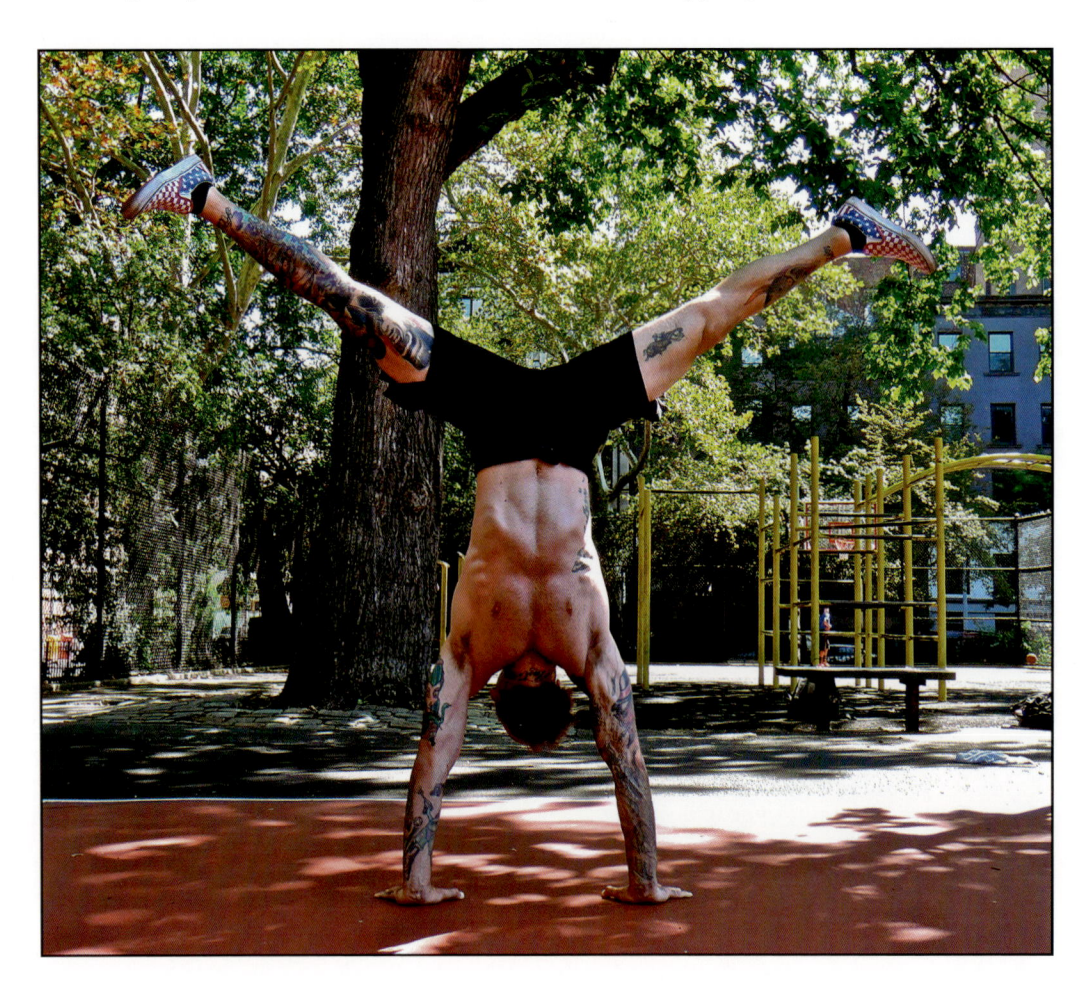

ARCH RIVALS

The old school strongmen of yesteryear were often seen performing handstand holds with an arched back. In modern gymnastics, however, it was decided that the flat back (hollow body) handstand would be the standard within that sport. Arched handstands are considered incorrect in the world of gymnastics. As a result, some people are under the unfortunate misconception that the strongman style or arched back handstand is universally wrong and/or dangerous. The truth is, both styles of handstand are valuable and worth pursuing, though most people will find the arched handstand comes more naturally when starting out. The straight handstand is typically more difficult as it requires significantly more shoulder flexibility and stricter body alignment. (For those who have that range of motion, however, the straight handstand may prove less difficult.)

We ultimately recommend training both versions, though you are encouraged to work toward balancing on your hands in any way that suits your interests. No matter which style you choose to practice, there is going to be a lot of trial and error in the beginning. Nobody learns to hold a freestanding handstand without lots of practice, patience and falling.

Why were so many of the old school strongmen practicing arched handstands? Here's one theory: When holding a freestanding handstand, it can be helpful to look in between your hands, as having a visual connection to the ground directly beneath you provides a lot of proprioceptive feedback. When you look in between your hands, however, it automatically encourages arching the spine. This is one of the reasons why the straight back handstand can be more difficult to learn; it's tough to look between your hands while keeping your back totally straight. Instead, you need to tuck your chin and look toward the horizon. The other reason is that having your arms completely vertical over your head requires more mobility than many adults naturally have. As such, a lot of flexibility work tends to be required in order to achieve a straight body handstand.

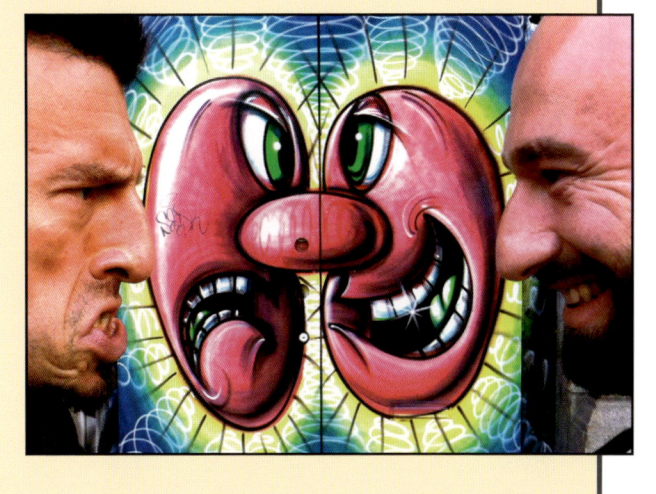

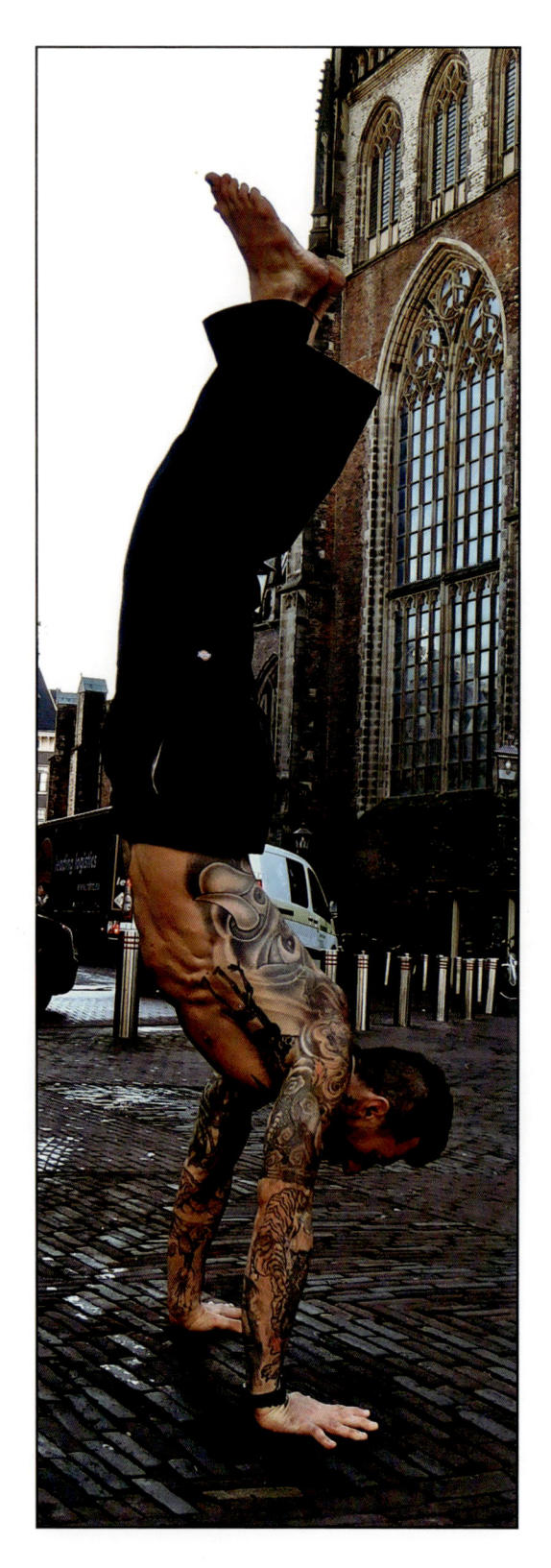

STRONGMAN STYLE HANDSTAND

To begin practicing the strongman style handstand, start by kicking up into a wall handstand, as described earlier, then gradually begin to take your heels away from the wall. You can experiment with removing them one at a time or together.

It can help to think about initiating this movement from your hands by pressing into the floor with your fingers and flexing your wrists against the ground, rather than initiating it from your legs or feet. This technique of "grabbing the ground" can also be useful to correct your balance should you find yourself about to tip over onto your back while practicing away from the wall.

Do your best to avoid flaring your elbows out to the sides when practicing your handstand. Remember to keep your elbows in a fully locked position during the kick up. You want your arms to be as straight as possible so that your bones can do some of the work to hold you up.

Focus on keeping your hips stacked above your hands. Your hips are your center of gravity and if they go forward or backward, the rest of you probably will as well.

Eventually you will get comfortable enough to begin practicing the strongman handstand in an open space by kicking up or pressing your body into position without relying on a wall for support.

GYMNASTIC STYLE HANDSTAND

Get into a handstand while facing a wall with your chin tucked toward your chest as described earlier. Pull your hips away from the wall slightly and stack them directly above your shoulders so that only your toes and the tops of your feet are against the wall. Shrug your shoulders, suck in your stomach and squeeze your glutes as you carefully pull your feet away from the wall while maintaining a hollow body position and tensing your fingers against the ground for support.

Eventually you will get comfortable enough to begin practicing the gymnastic style handstand away from the wall by kicking up or pressing your body into position.

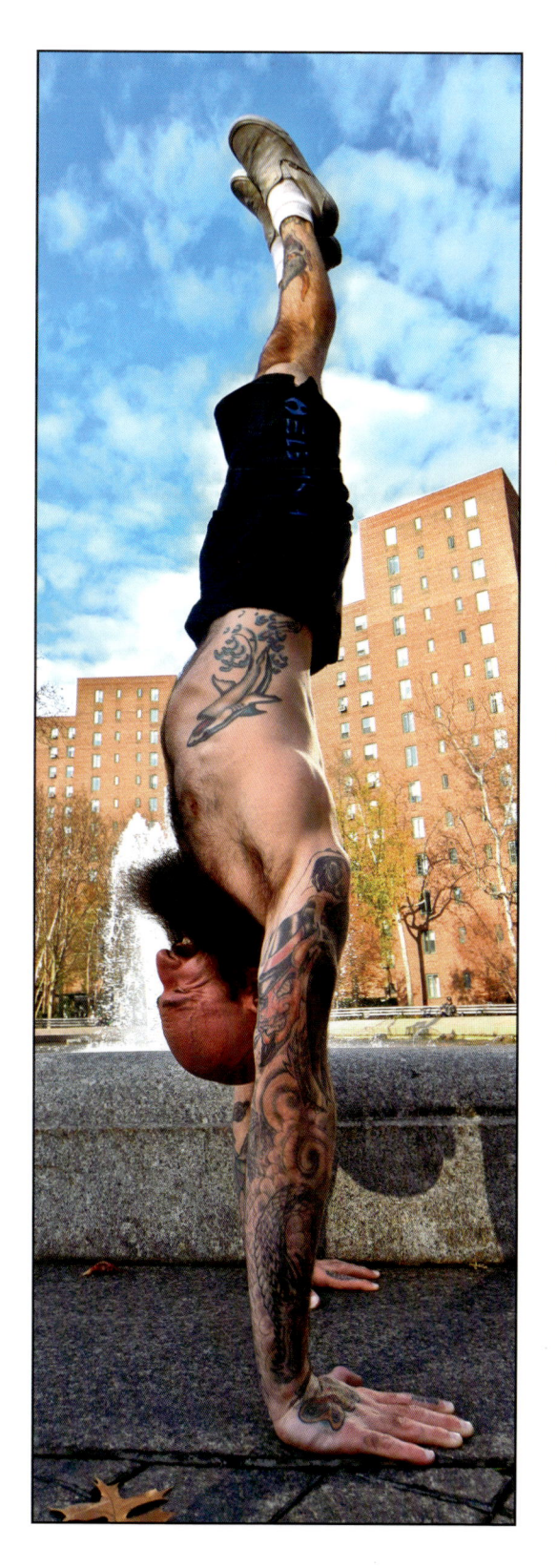

HOLLOWBACK HANDSTAND

For this variant, also known as a Mexican handstand, you'll not only be arching your back, you will intentionally aim to make that arch as significant as possible. It's almost like combining a handstand with a back bridge. As such, make sure you are comfortable with both handstands and back bridges individually before attempting the hollowback handstand. Like the other handstand variants, it's helpful to practice with a wall for support in the beginning, although for this variant, you'll need to kick up a bit farther from the wall to allow room to arch your back and reach your legs behind you. Focus on pressing your chest away from your legs to counterbalance their weight. Eventually you can work toward performing a freestanding hollowback handstand.

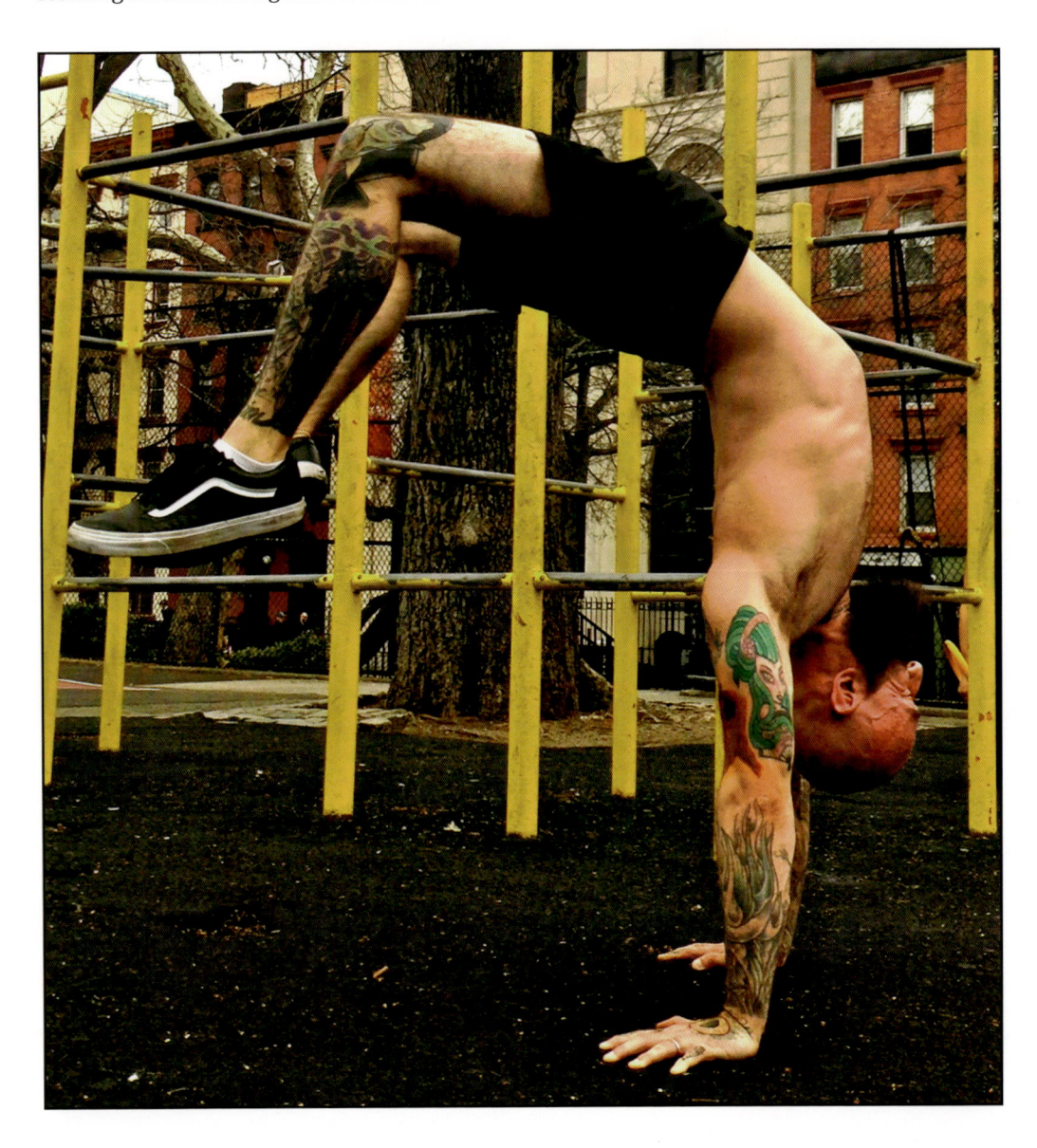

PIROUETTE

If you feel like you are about to tip over while attempting to hold a freestanding handstand, the pirouette is a great way to bail out safely. This involves lifting one hand and placing it in front of your body, then immediately turning your hips and letting your legs come down one at a time, almost like they would if you were performing a gymnastic cartwheel. It may seem intimidating, but performing a pirouette is not particularly difficult. In fact, it will happen pretty naturally for most people.

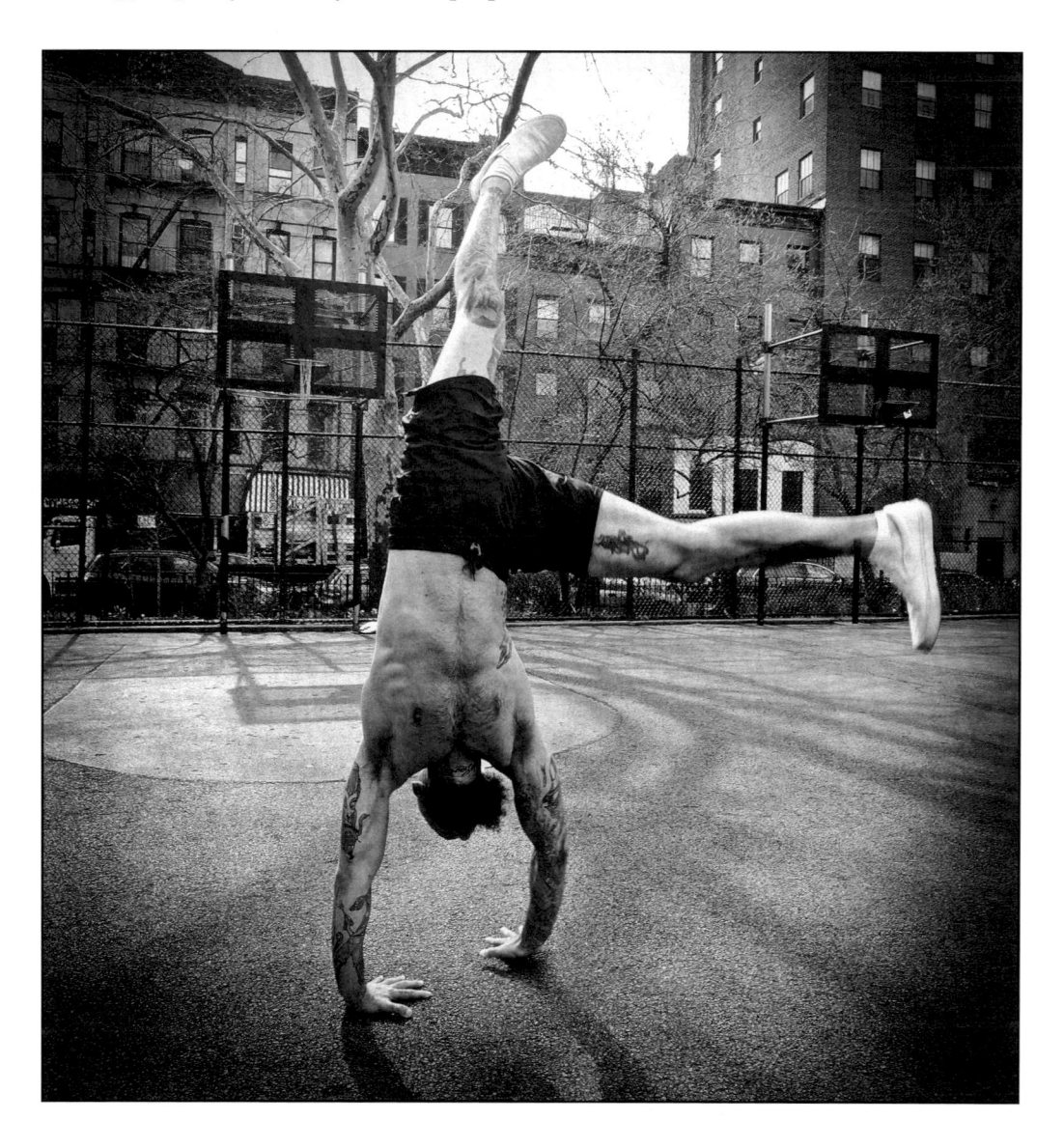

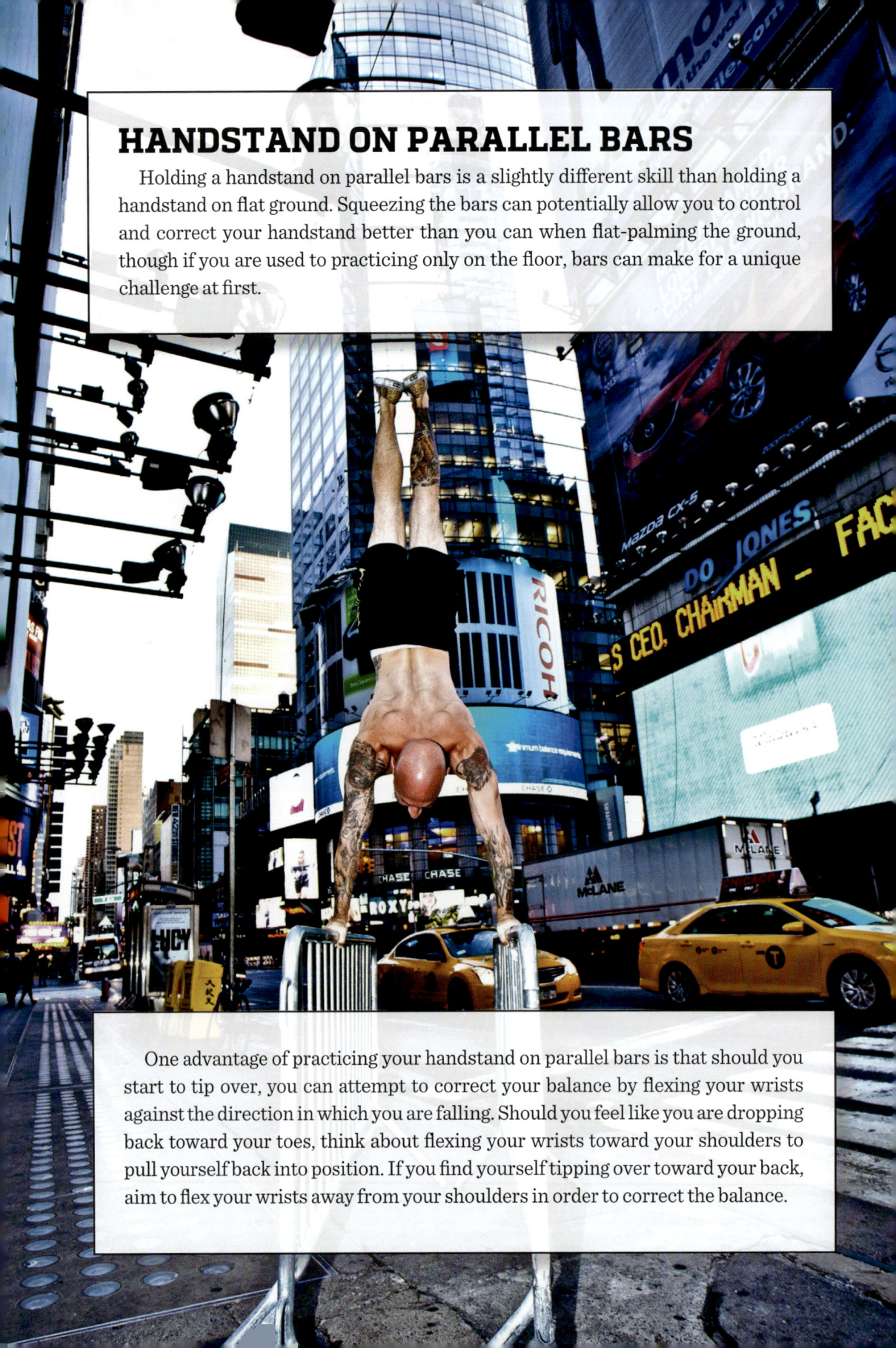

HANDSTAND ON PARALLEL BARS

Holding a handstand on parallel bars is a slightly different skill than holding a handstand on flat ground. Squeezing the bars can potentially allow you to control and correct your handstand better than you can when flat-palming the ground, though if you are used to practicing only on the floor, bars can make for a unique challenge at first.

One advantage of practicing your handstand on parallel bars is that should you start to tip over, you can attempt to correct your balance by flexing your wrists against the direction in which you are falling. Should you feel like you are dropping back toward your toes, think about flexing your wrists toward your shoulders to pull yourself back into position. If you find yourself tipping over toward your back, aim to flex your wrists away from your shoulders in order to correct the balance.

FREESTANDING HANDSTAND PRESS-UP

A merger of balance, control and strength, the freestanding handstand press-up (aka freestanding handstand push-up) is a fantastic display of overall calisthenics prowess. Before you attempt this move, make sure you are comfortable holding a freestanding handstand as well as performing handstand press-ups against a wall.

When working toward a freestanding handstand press-up, it's helpful to practice holding a bent arm freestanding handstand, which is essentially the bottom position of the exercise. In this position, it's important to look in front of your hands rather than right in between them (or behind them) as you might when holding a handstand with your arms straight. In order to stay balanced with your arms bent, you will need to have your head in front of your hands. It's almost like a tripod headstand except that your body will be at a slight angle and your head will be off the floor.

To press yourself up from this bottom position, maintain tension in your trunk and legs as you extend your arms overhead. Shift your gaze back between your hands as you straighten your elbows.

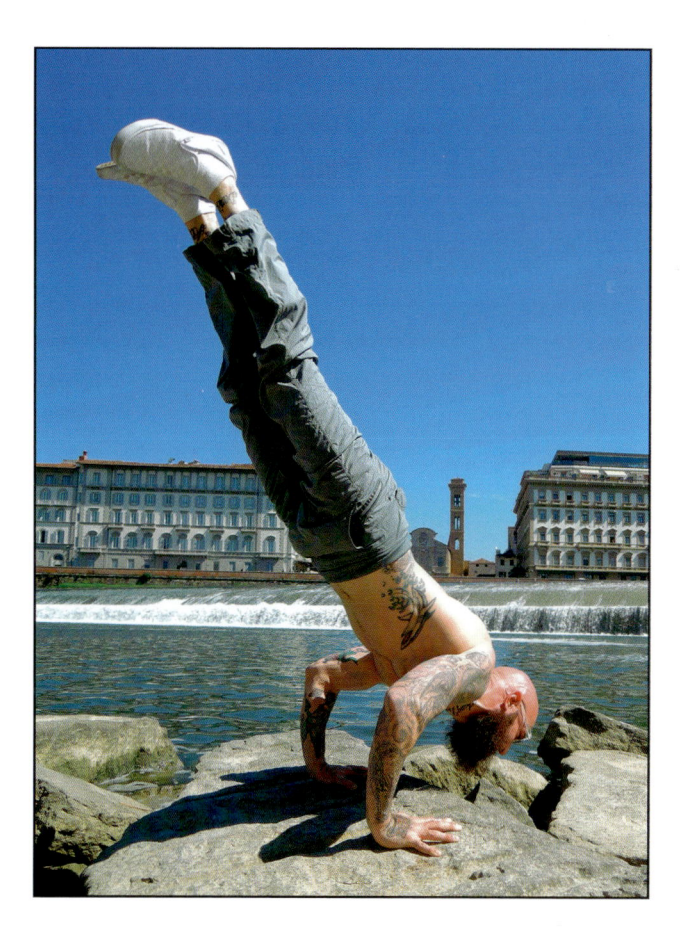

ONE ARM HANDSTAND

Once you've gotten comfortable with handstands, you can up the ante significantly by practicing on just one arm. When starting out, use a wall for support the same way you would when learning the two-arm version; practice both with your back to the wall as well as facing it.

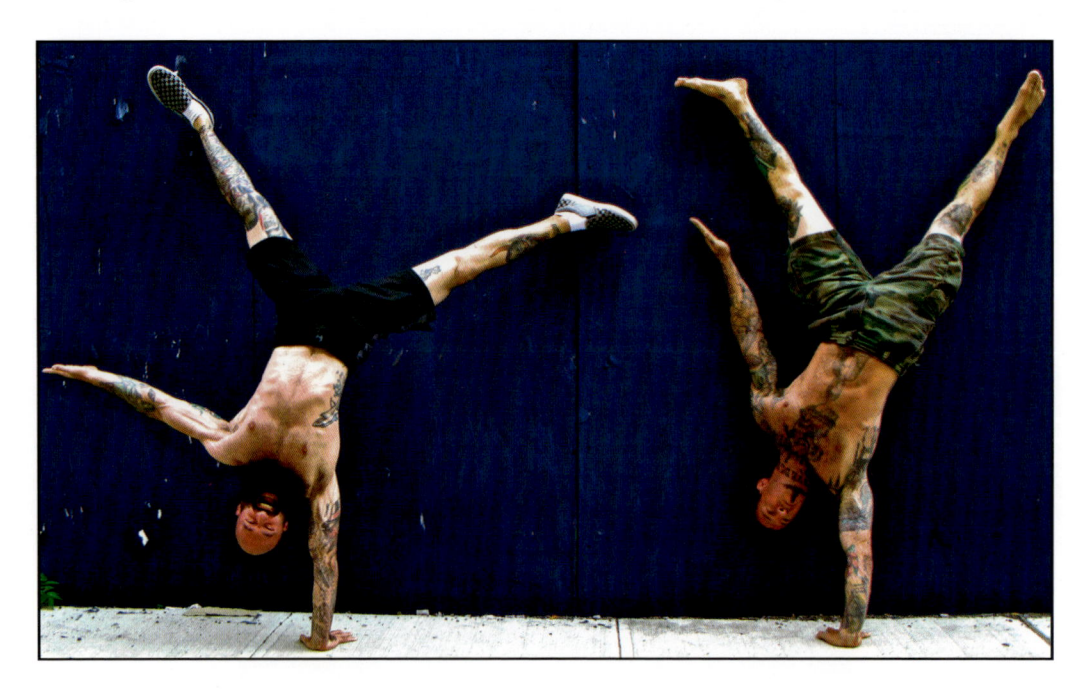

Once you're able to hold a one arm handstand against a wall and can hold a freestanding handstand for a minute or longer, you can begin working toward a free standing one arm handstand. Even more than with the two-arm version, holding your legs in a straddle will make the balance much more favorable in a one arm handstand.

Start in a straddle handstand, then slowly begin shifting your weight towards one hand. If and when you feel ready, attempt to lift the other hand onto the fingertips. Spread your legs as wide as you can and stack your hips over your primary hand. Then you can gradually remove one finger at a time from the assisting hand. With enough patience and practice, you may eventually be able to completely remove your opposite hand from the ground.

The freestanding one arm handstand is one of the most difficult and elusive skills in the world. Do not expect to get it without putting in a tremendous amount of work.

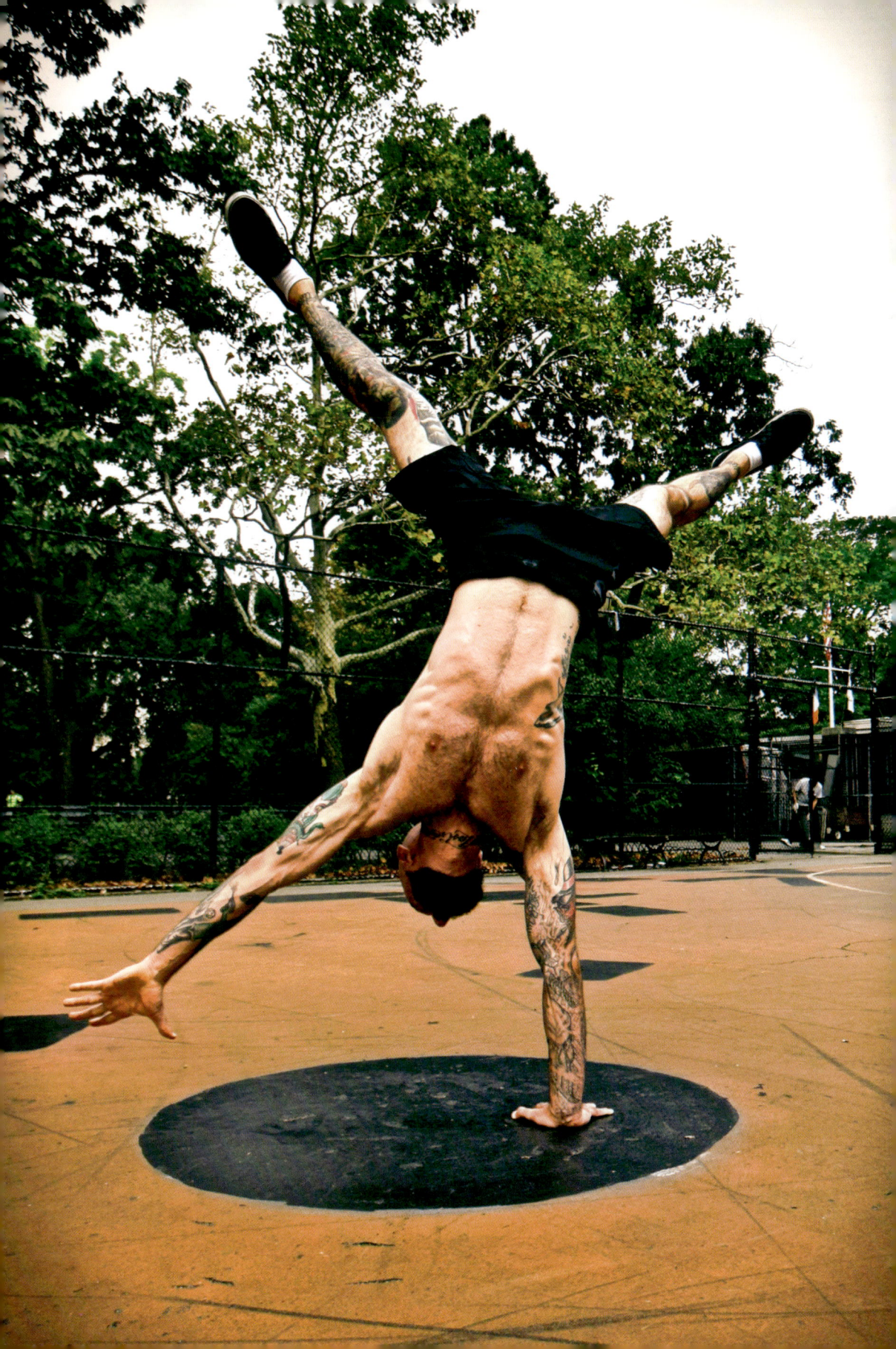

ELBOW LEVER PROGRESSIONS

The classic elbow lever is a calisthenics staple and a breathtaking visual demonstration. The move involves holding your body extended horizontally over the ground, supported only by your two hands, with your elbows leveraged against your sides. It fuses precise balance, physical prowess and an iron will.

When learning the early elbow lever progressions, it's generally helpful to start on a bench, step or any other flat, raised object. This will allow more room to lift your legs into position, as opposed to the limited amount of space available when your hands are placed on the floor. But once you get a feel for it, you can perform this move just about anywhere!

Like many bodyweight exercises, the elbow lever has roots in several styles of physical culture, and while some may know this move by other names, such as peacock pose, it remains a fantastic exercise no mater what you call it.

To the untrained eye, the elbow lever can be mistaken for a planche. And although they do look similar, the elbow lever is a less difficult skill, due to the fact that your upper body rests on your arms (or just one arm, in more advanced versions). But make no mistake: the elbow lever stands on its own as a remarkable exercise in its own right.

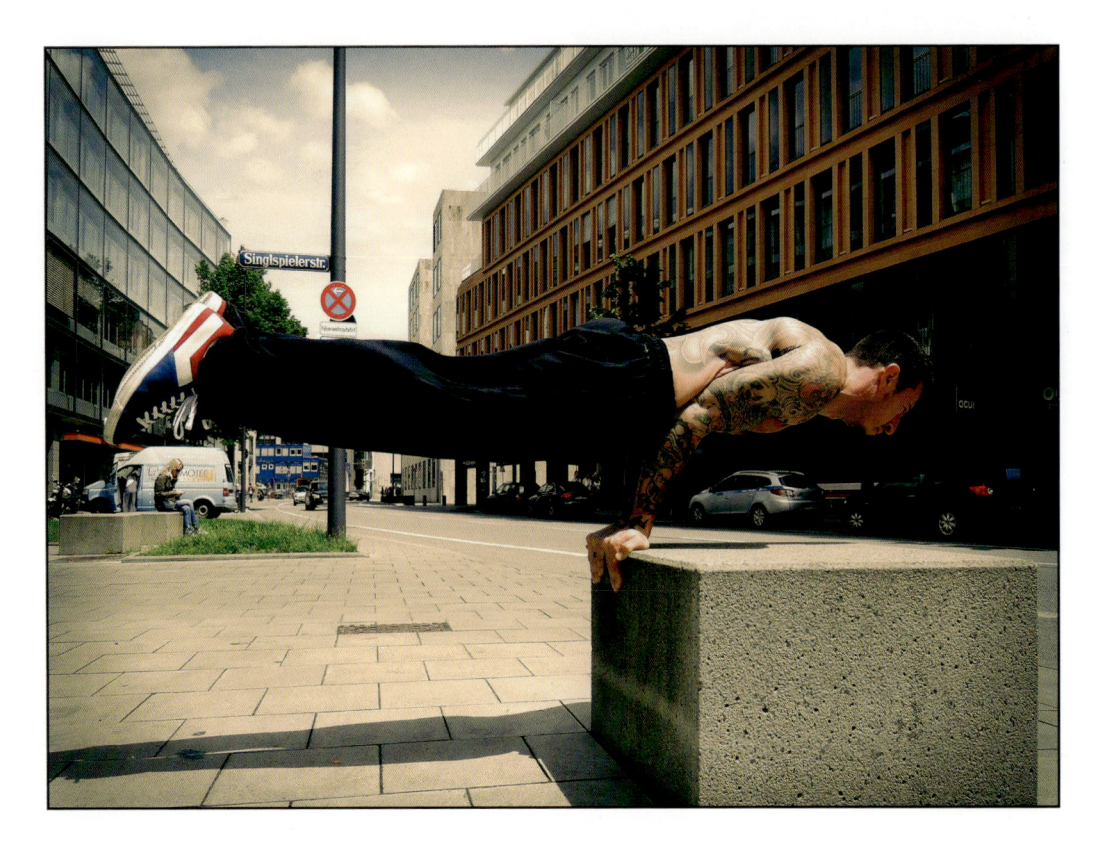

CLOSED UMBRELLA

Begin by placing your hands flat on an elevated object with your fingers facing toward your feet and your palms a few inches apart. You can also wrap your fingers around the edge if you prefer. Bend your elbows and think about making a shelf with the backs of your arms upon which you will rest your hip bones and torso. Lean forward and bend your knees as you place your elbows against your abdomen. Next, tense your midsection and shift your weight forward until your feet start to lift up off the floor. Let your legs hang for now and just get a feel for this position before moving on.

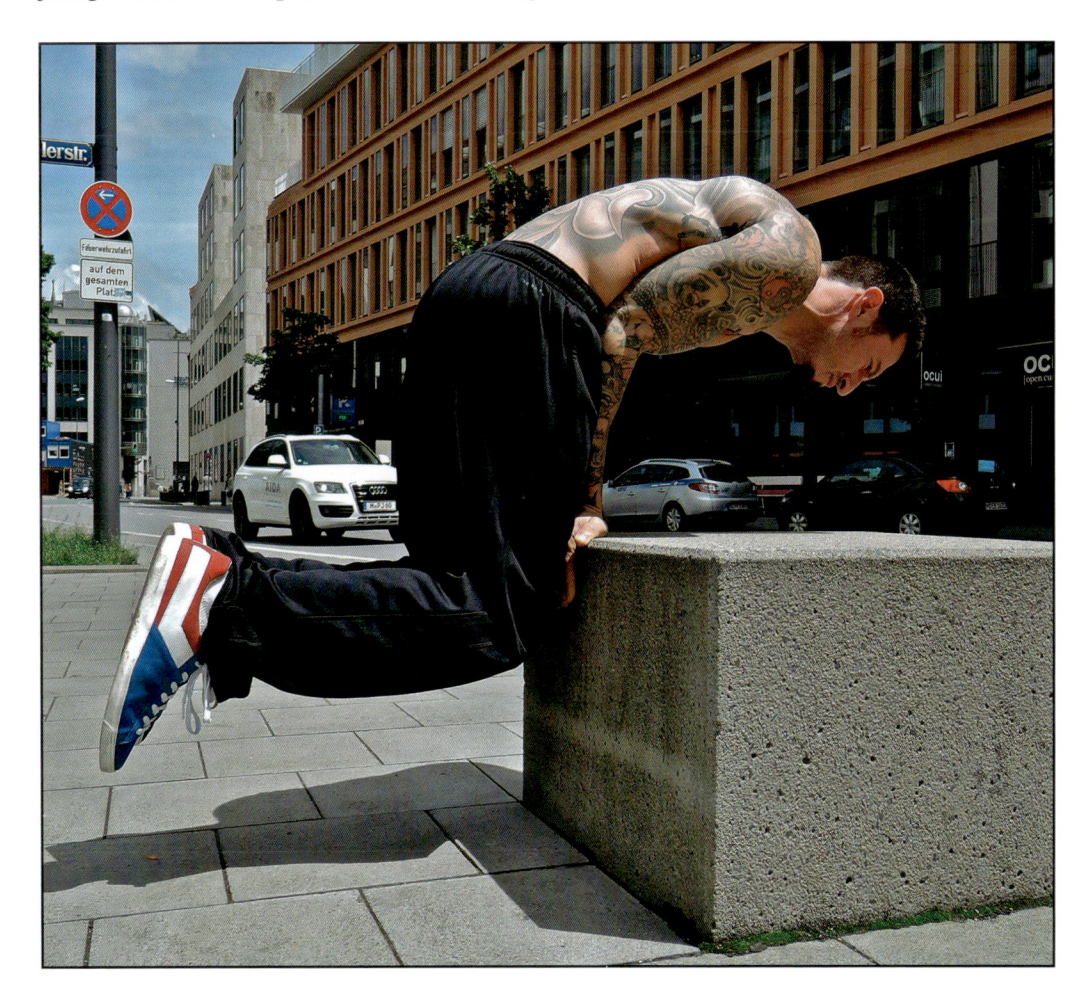

STRADDLE ELBOW LEVER

Once you get a feel for supporting yourself on your elbows, you can start to work toward straightening your back and extending your legs out to the sides. A straddle-leg position is the perfect intermediate step after you can hold the closed umbrella but before you are ready for a full elbow lever.

As you lengthen your legs and extend your chest forward, you'll need to alter the angle at your elbows. Many people will bend the elbows too much, while others will not bend them enough. The ideal angle for your elbows is somewhere around 130 degrees.

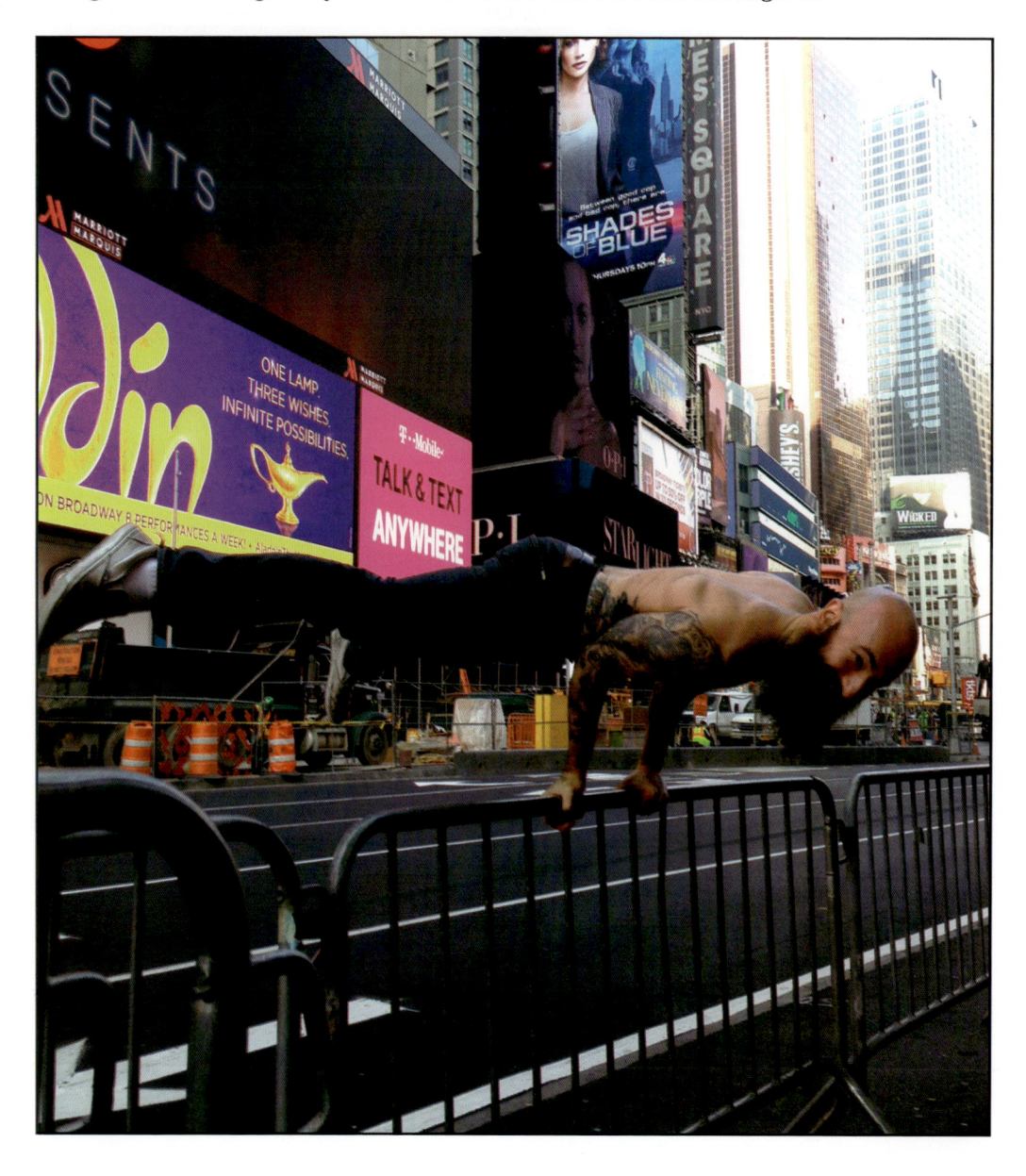

ELBOW LEVER

One way to learn the full elbow lever is to transition from the straddle elbow lever. Carefully close your legs together while pitching your torso slightly farther forward. Go slowly in order to avoid losing your balance.

When you get more confident holding the elbow lever, you can lift your legs directly into position, bypassing the straddle. When performing it this way, be mindful to keep your abs contracted and extend your lower back as you lift your feet off the floor. Your legs tend to feel heavier when they're straight.

For either method, it is important to pitch your upper body forward in order to counterbalance the weight of your bottom half. Open your elbows while doing so; make sure the fulcrum point remains just below waist level. Remember, the ideal angle for your elbows is around 130 degrees. You may also experiment with different hand positions.

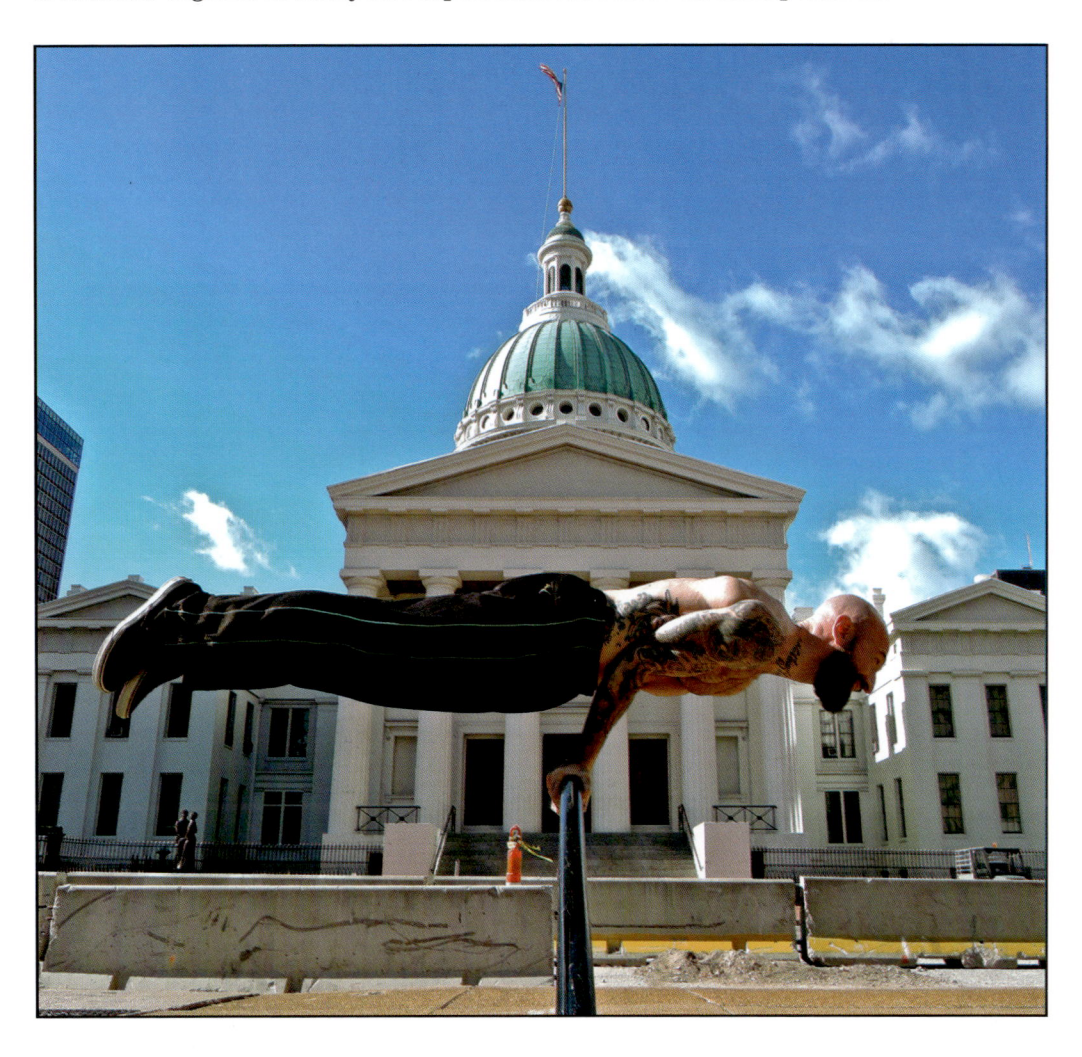

ELBOW LEVER SETUP

To set up for the elbow lever, your elbows must be inside of your hips. As such, a certain amount of rotational ability is required at the shoulders. If you are experiencing difficulty getting or keeping both arms into position simultaneously, or if you feel your elbows slipping out, you can try practicing the bound eagle stretch to increase your mobility.

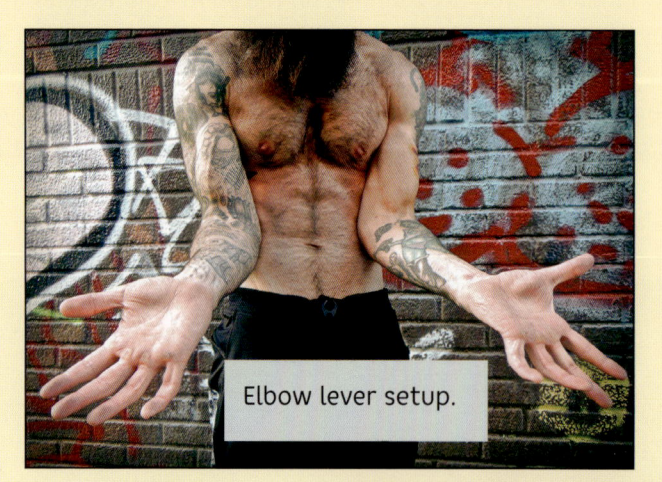

Until it improves, you may be better off trying a variant where one arm is inside of the hip while the other arm remains off to the side until you achieve a better range of motion in your shoulders. This one arm in/one arm out variant is a more viable option for folks with mobility issues.

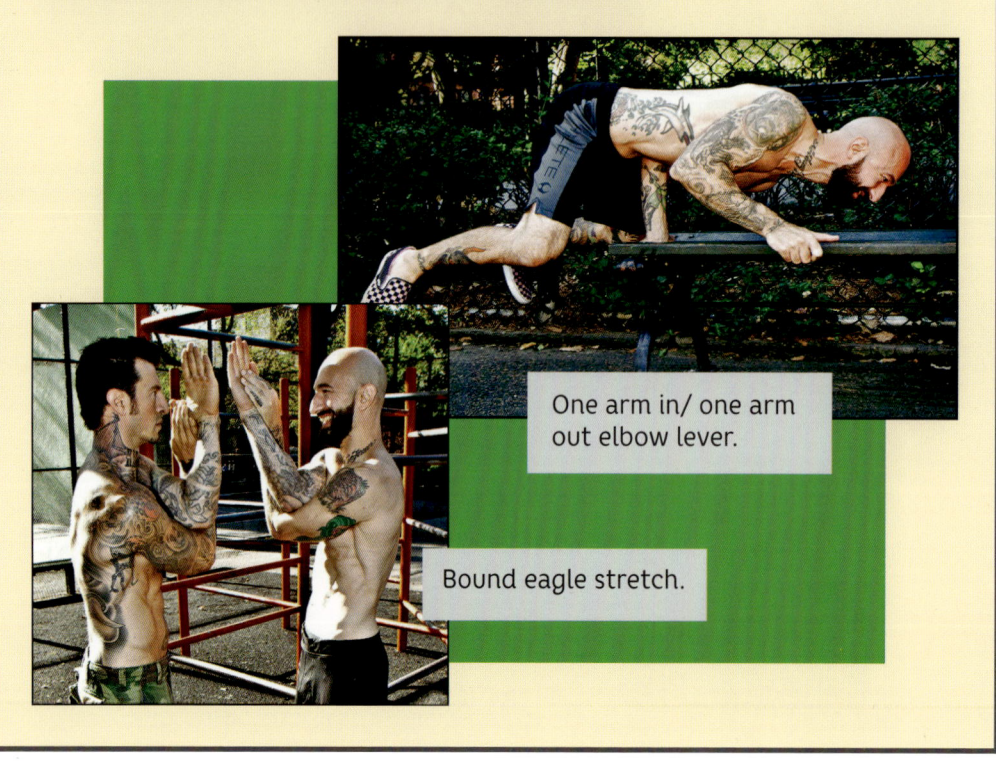

Elbow lever setup.

One arm in/ one arm out elbow lever.

Bound eagle stretch.

ONE ARM ELBOW LEVER

When you need a new challenge beyond the classic elbow lever, you can begin working toward a one arm elbow lever. Start on an elevated surface with one arm in and one arm out—the same position we advised on the two arm elbow lever for those experiencing shoulder mobility issues. From there, you can spot yourself with your outside hand and gradually shift your weight off your fingers and onto your main hand.

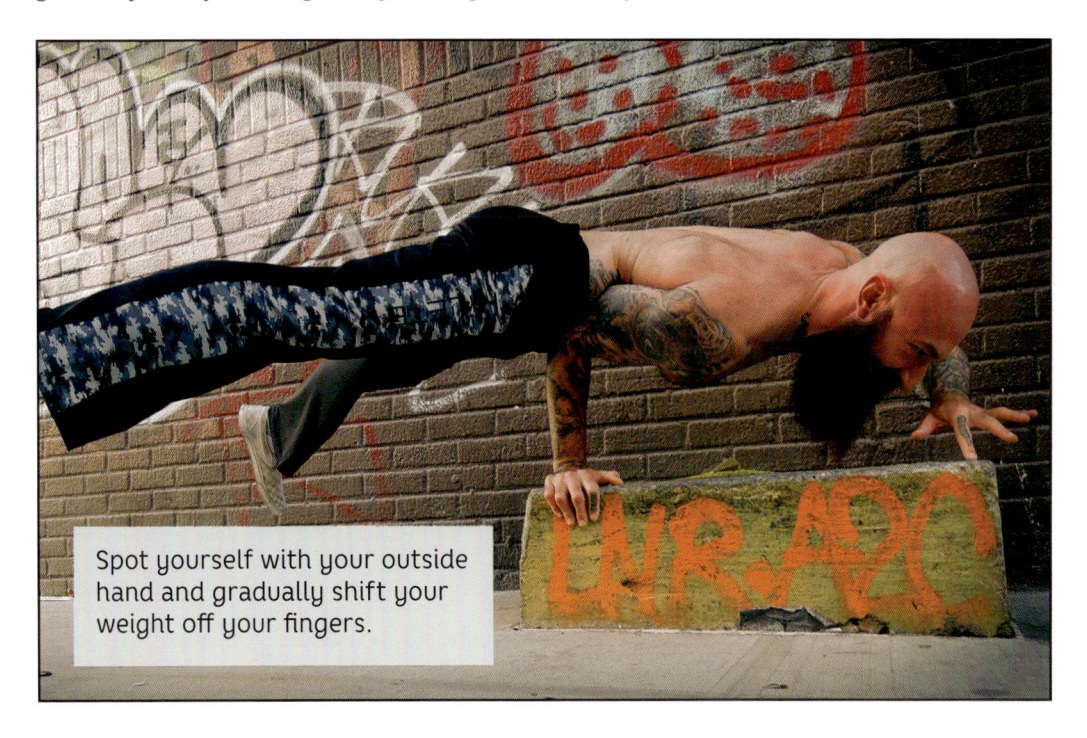

Spot yourself with your outside hand and gradually shift your weight off your fingers.

It takes a lot of trial and error to find the sweet spot for the one arm elbow lever, so be patient. With enough practice, however, you will eventually get the feel for completely removing your assisting arm and holding all of your weight on just one side. Then you can start to work toward longer holds.

It takes a lot of trial and error to find the sweet spot for the one arm elbow lever.

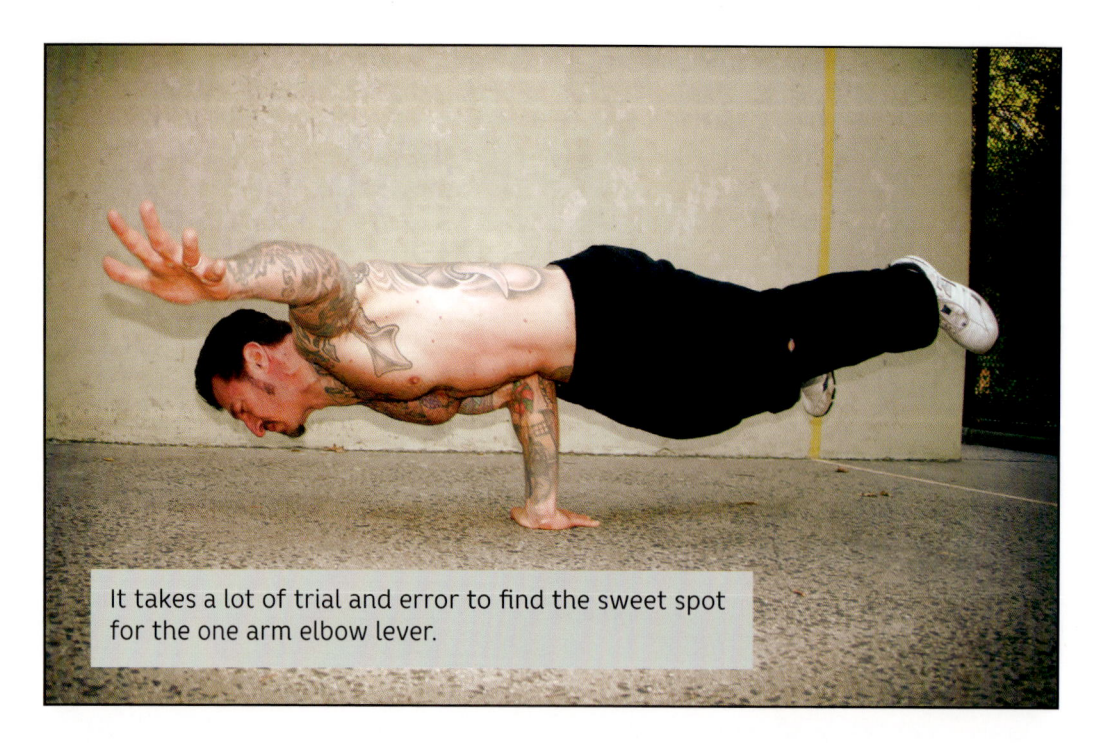

Begin with your legs in a straddle, reaching your free arm out and away from your body to help counterbalance your legs. Holding the position with your feet together requires significantly more balance and stability.

Though sometimes people mistakenly put their elbow too close to their navel, the point of contact between your elbow and your body should be pretty much the same as in the two arm version. The ideal elbow placement can vary a bit from person to person, but it is generally best to keep your elbow close to your hip. As such, you will need to rotate your body ever so slightly toward your primary arm in order to stay balanced.

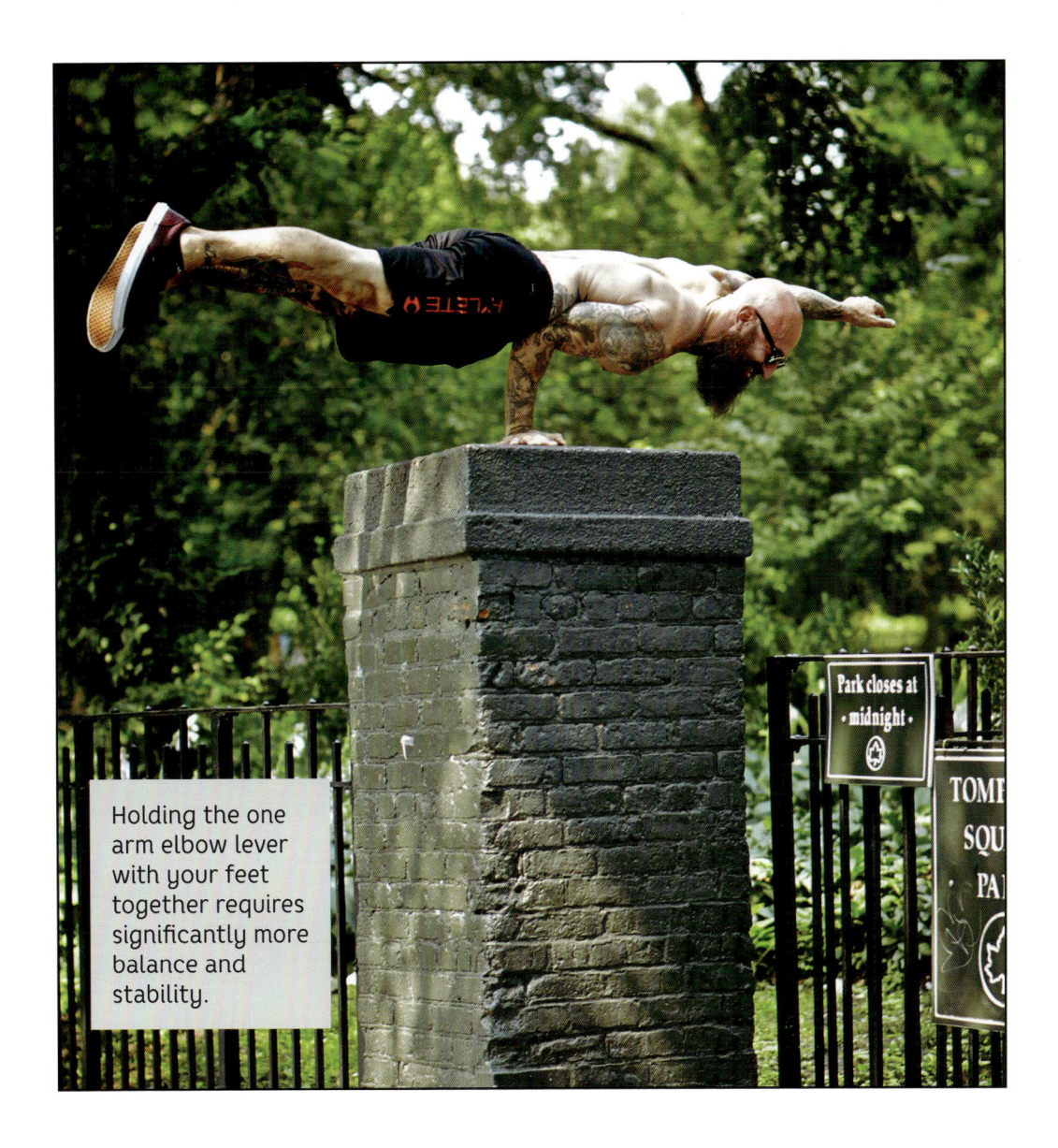

Holding the one arm elbow lever with your feet together requires significantly more balance and stability.

STREET WORKOUT

ADVANCED ONE ARM ELBOW LEVER

When you hold a one arm elbow lever, having your opposite arm outstretched is helpful for balance. Therefore, removing that assistance from the equation by placing the free arm along your side makes the balance considerably more difficult. Like the conventional one arm elbow lever, start with your legs in a straddle, then gradually work toward closing them as you gain strength and confidence in the position. Try gripping onto your side to create more tension.

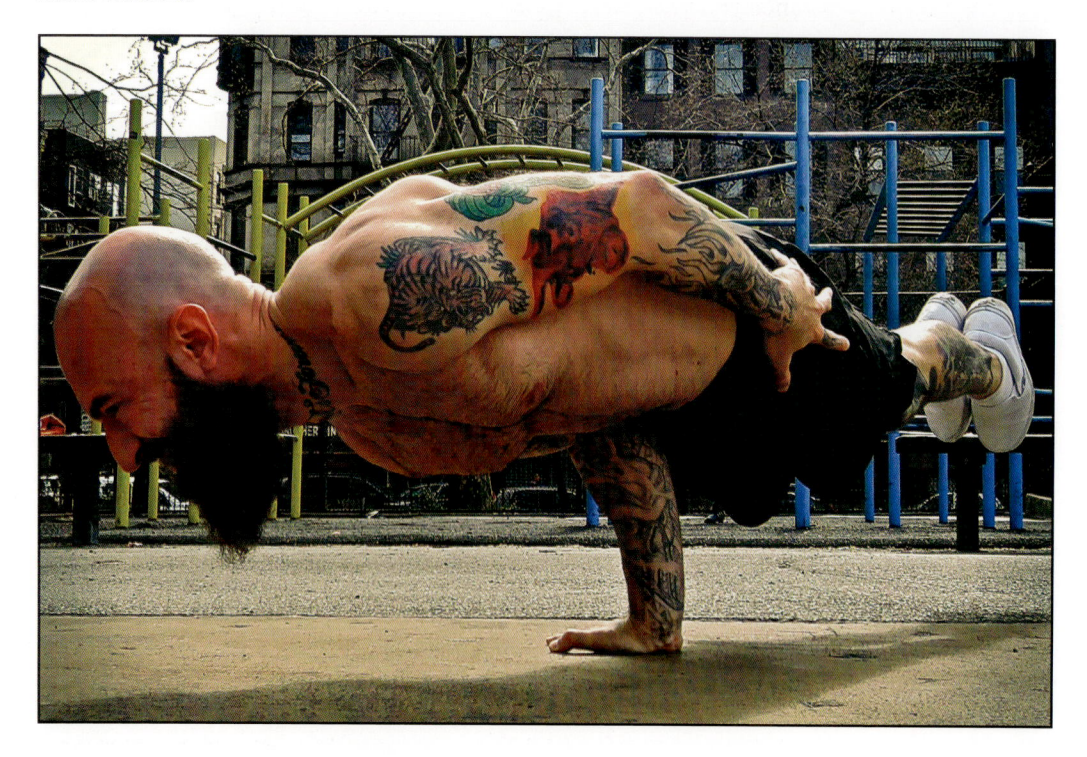

SIDE ONE ARM ELBOW LEVER

For this variation, your torso will be turned to the side instead of facing down toward the ground as it is in the standard one arm elbow lever. As such, you will need to rotate your elbow farther outside of your hip, requiring a great degree of mobility at the shoulder.

It's common to find this side-on position more difficult as compared to the standard one arm elbow lever. Since you can't really straddle your legs here, try bending your bottom knee to shorten the lever and make the balance a bit easier. Eventually you can work toward holding the position with both legs straight.

Like the standard one arm elbow lever, using your non-balancing arm to spot yourself can be very helpful. As you get more comfortable with the move, you can gradually start to shift your weight off that arm until you can take the hand away from the ground altogether.

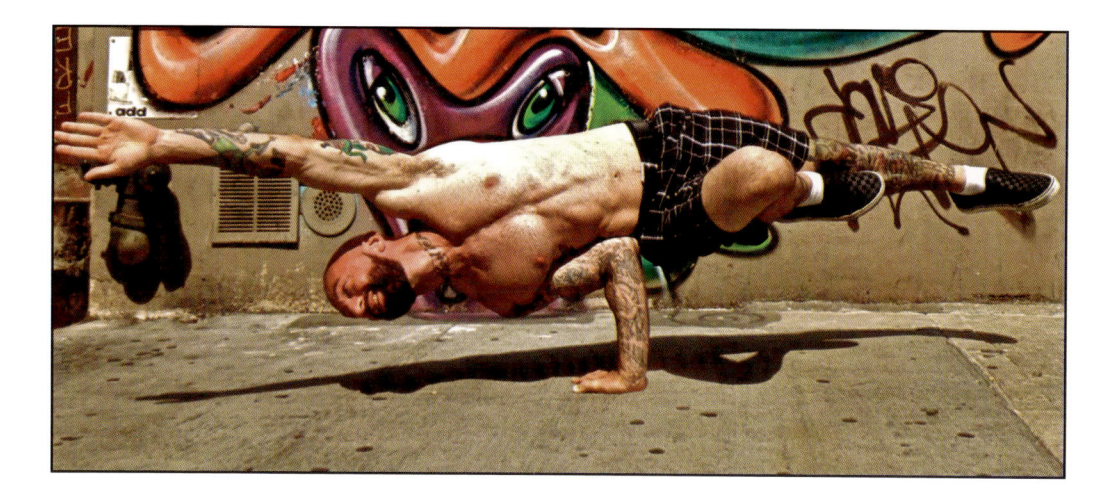

PLANCHE PROGRESSIONS

The planche is the "Big Kahuna" of all floor holds. It is one of the beastliest displays of brute strength, sound technique and implausible balance in the entire domain of calisthenics training.

With its roots in gymnastics, the planche has been widely adapted and celebrated in the Street Workout world. It really is a sight to behold: the human body parallel to the ground, with a straight line from the shoulders to the hips to the feet. The only point of contact with the ground is the hands. We discussed how the planche is sometimes confused with the elbow lever, but they are clearly birds of a different feather. The planche requires the practitioner's arms to be totally straight, without supporting the rest of the body. It looks almost like a plank with the feet floating in the air. Astonishing!

Without a doubt, the planche is a hard-won move, unbelievably difficult and extraordinarily advanced. Be prepared to spend a long time with this one. Take it slow and stay the course.

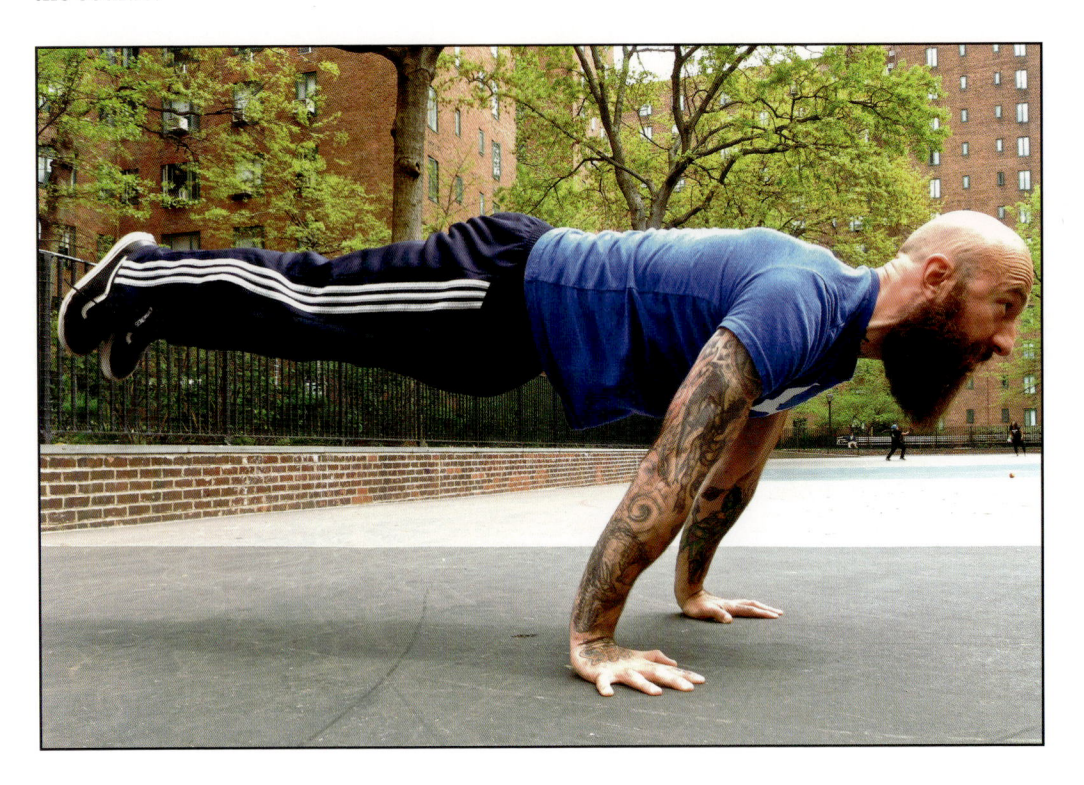

PLANCHE LEAN

Start at the top of a push-up with your hands and fingers turned out partially toward the sides. Begin to gradually shift your weight forward as you flex into your wrists and walk your toes forward, actively pushing the ground away in order to maintain straight arms. Spread your shoulder-blades apart and continue slowly taking weight off your feet until your hands are supporting as much of the load as they can handle. In a full planche, all of your weight will be in your hands; this position can start to give you a feel for what that entails.

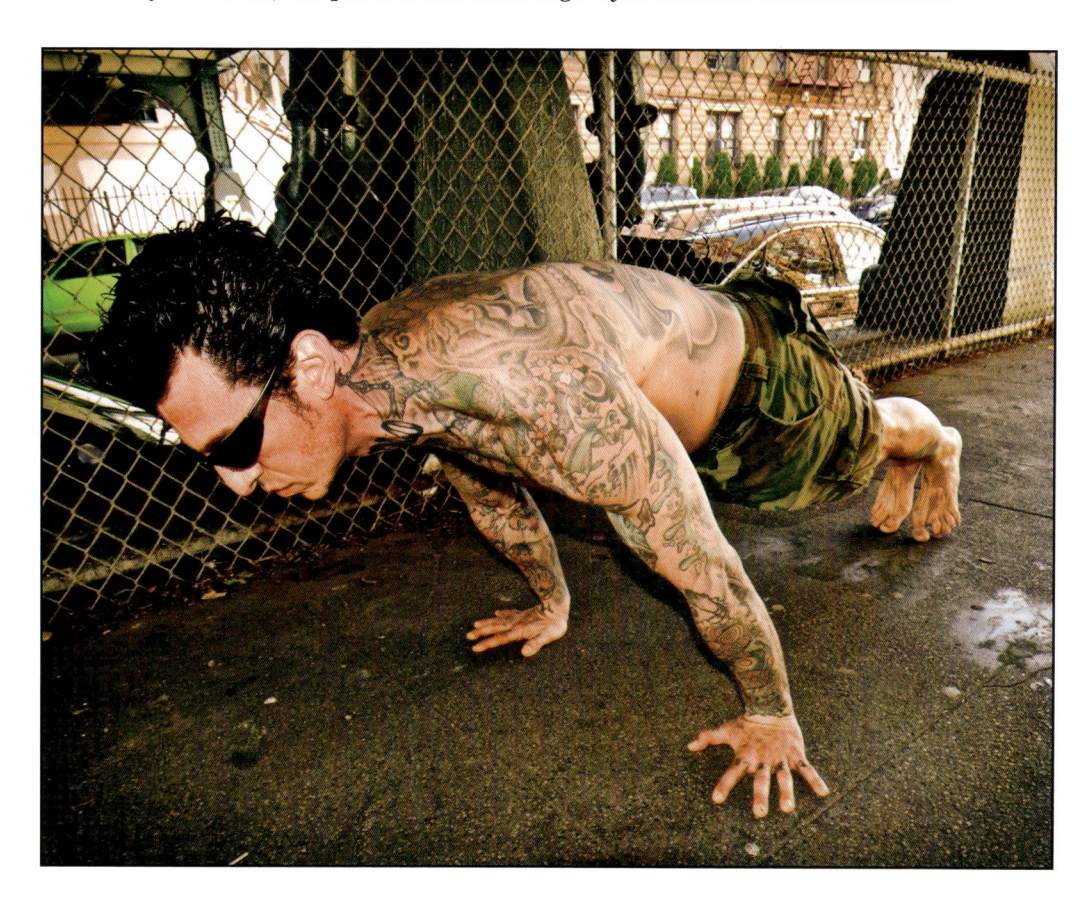

TUCK PLANCHE

Once again, we will be shortening the length of the body in order to scale a difficult exercise down to a more approachable level. Make no mistake, however, the tuck planche is a fairly early progression toward a full planche, but it is still an intense move in its own right. Think of it like the crane pose discussed earlier, only without any contact between your arms and legs.

Get into a narrow squat position with your heels off the ground and knees tucked by your chest. Place your hands on the floor partially turned out and begin gradually shifting your weight into your fingers and palms. Flex into your wrists, spread your shoulder-blades apart and press into the ground with your hands, arms and the rest of your upper body. Finally, raise your hips into the air and pick your feet up off the floor, transferring all of your weight into your hands.

At first, you can allow your lower back to round in order to shorten your body length as much as possible. Once you've gotten a feel for this, you can begin to extend through your lower back and slide your knees and feet farther from your trunk.

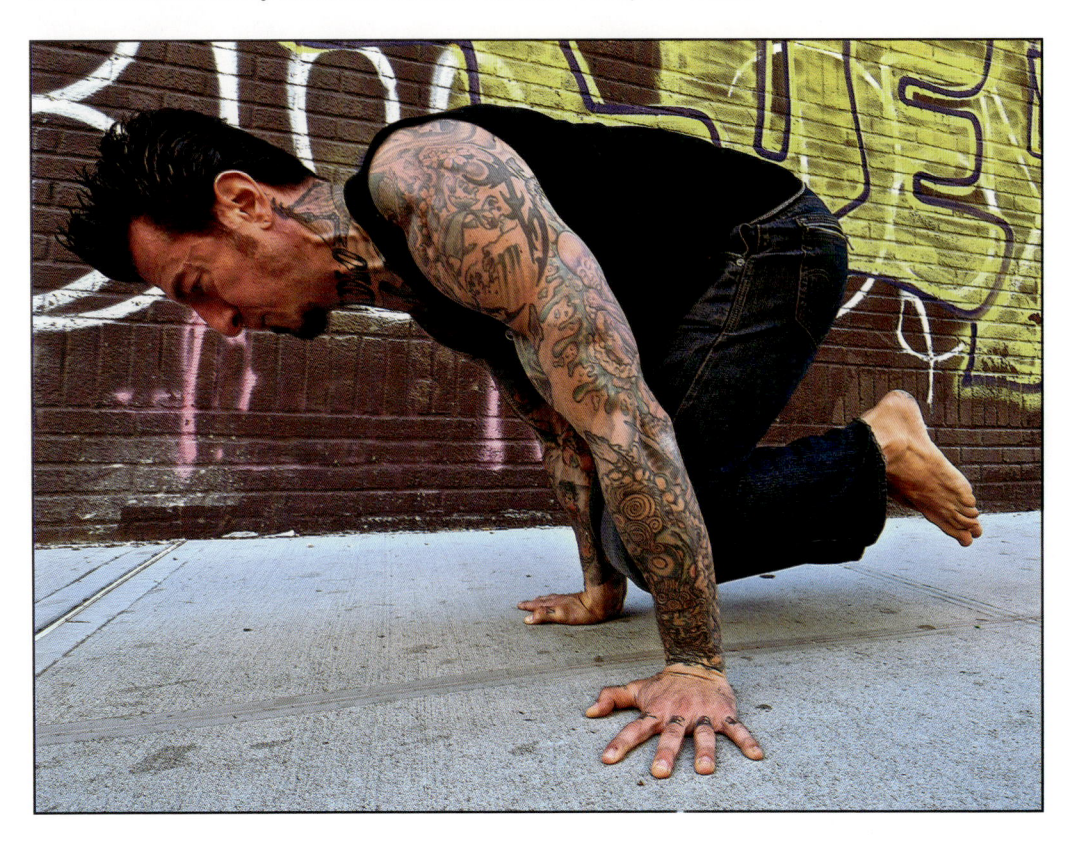

STRADDLE PLANCHE

From the tuck planche position, continue leaning farther forward into your wrists and reach your legs out to the sides. The leap from the tuck planche to the straddle planche is fairly significant, so be prepared to put in a lot of time with the tuck position before moving on to the straddle. As is often the case, the farther you can spread your legs, the more favorable your leverage will become.

You can also experiment with lowering into the straddle planche from a straddle handstand. If you choose this method, be mindful to pitch your chest forward and flex deep into your wrists as you descend, actively pressing into the ground and flaring your lats on the way down.

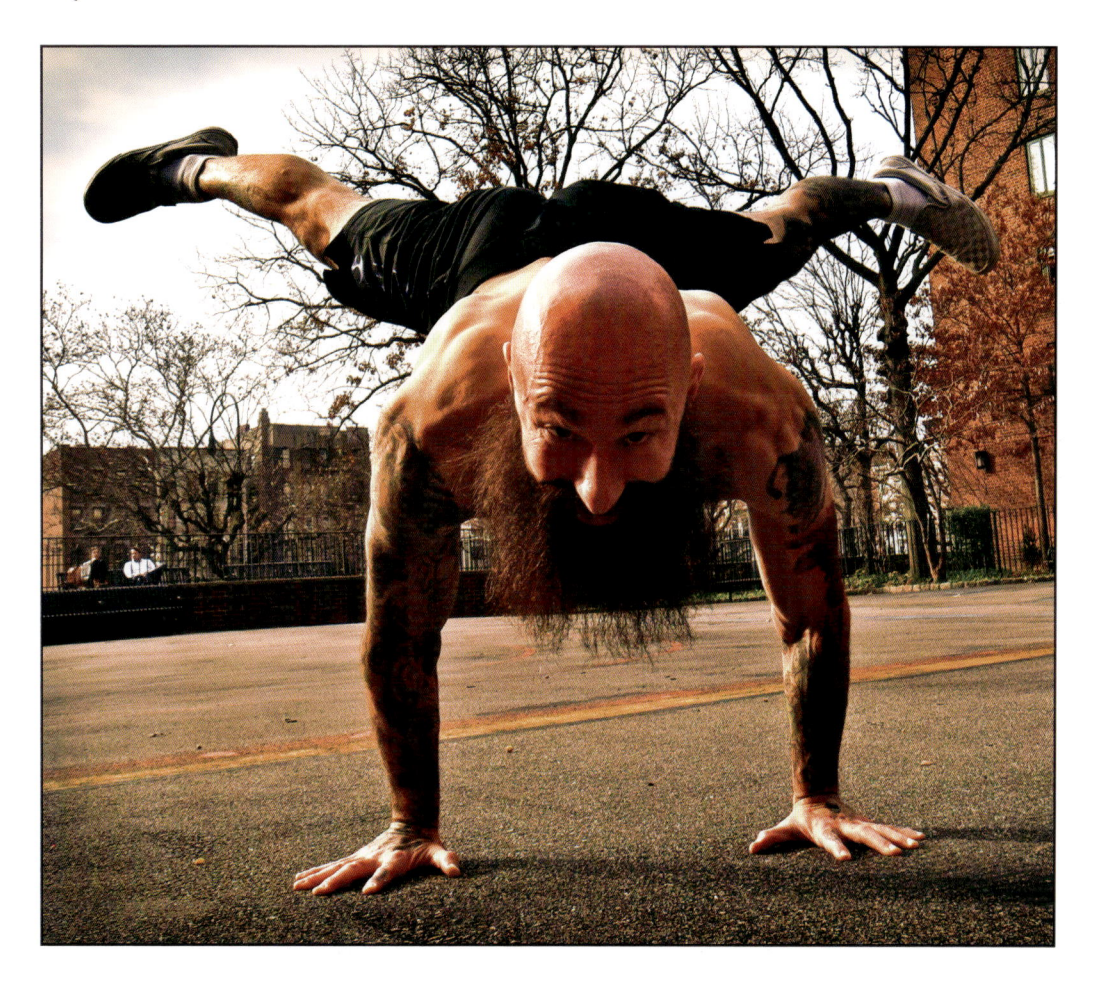

SCORPION PLANCHE

This planche variation again shortens the length of the body for increased leverage, this time by keeping the knees bent above and behind the body, rather than beneath. Begin in a handstand with your hands turned out slightly, then bend your knees, arch your back and gradually begin to lower your hips down while pitching your torso forward and bending into your wrists. As with the other planche variants, make sure to actively spread your shoulder blades apart and press into the ground with your hands and arms.

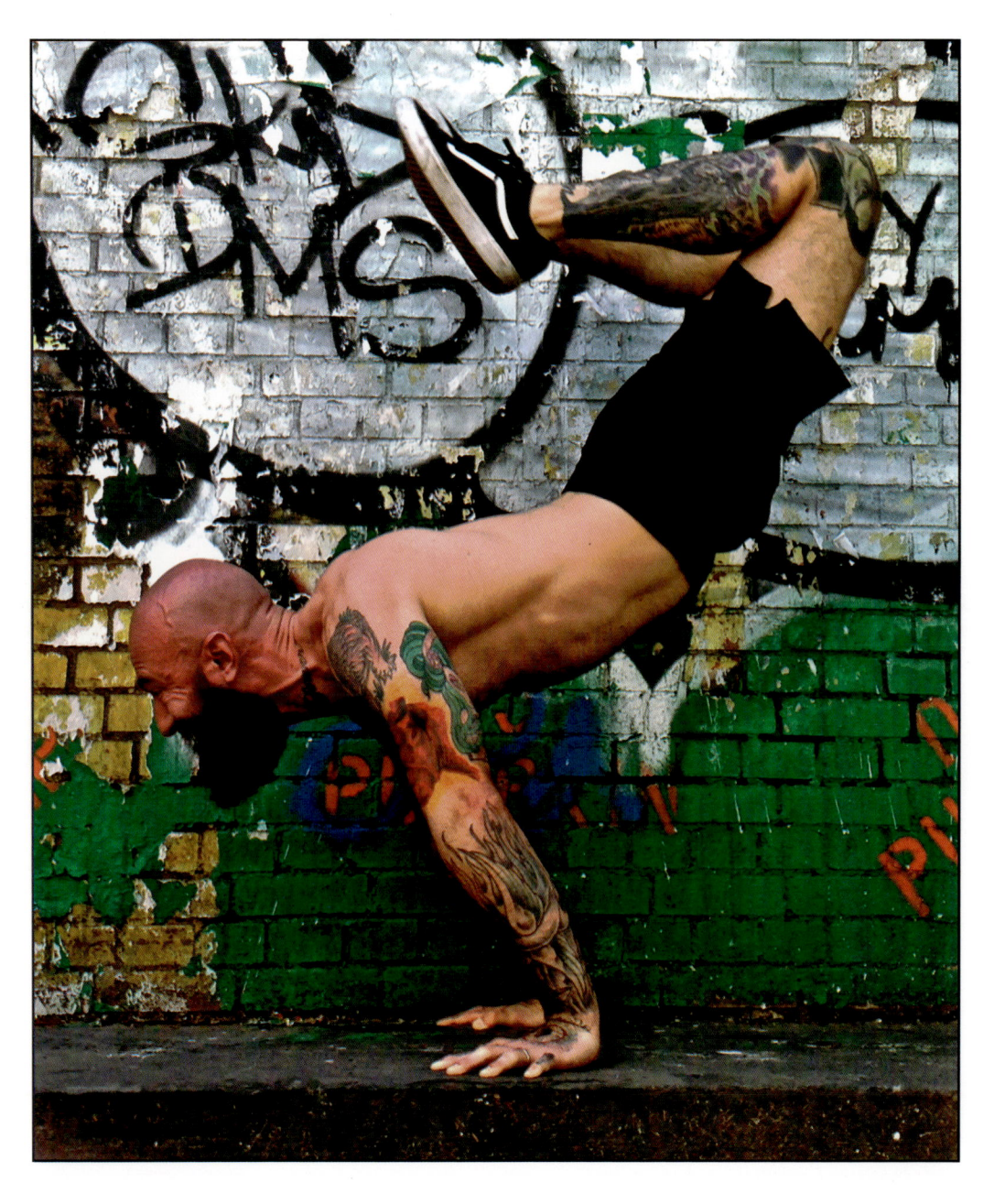

PLANCHE

After you've spent adequate time on the previous progressions, you can start to explore the full planche, which can be approached in a few different ways.

The first method is to begin in a tuck planche, then slowly extend your body out into the full planche position, transitioning through the advanced tuck and straddle planche positions along the way. Gradually increasing the load on your muscles by starting in a tuck position allows you to prime your nervous system for the incredibly unfavorable leverage involved with holding your body completely horizontal to the ground with your feet in the air.

You can also lower into the planche from a freestanding handstand, which again gives you the opportunity to "charge up" neurologically as you increase the load on your arms. Remember to pitch your chest forward and bend into your wrists as you descend into position. Again, it can be helpful to turn your hands outward to allow for deeper wrist flexion.

Like the freestanding handstand, you may find that practicing the planche while holding parallel bars can be slightly less difficult than performing the hold with your hands flat on the ground. Using parallel bars allows you to fully engage your grip strength and does not require as much mobility in the wrists. Additionally, being elevated can provide more room to lift into position.

Regardless of which method you employ, be mindful to avoid bending at your elbows or sagging at the hips when executing the planche.

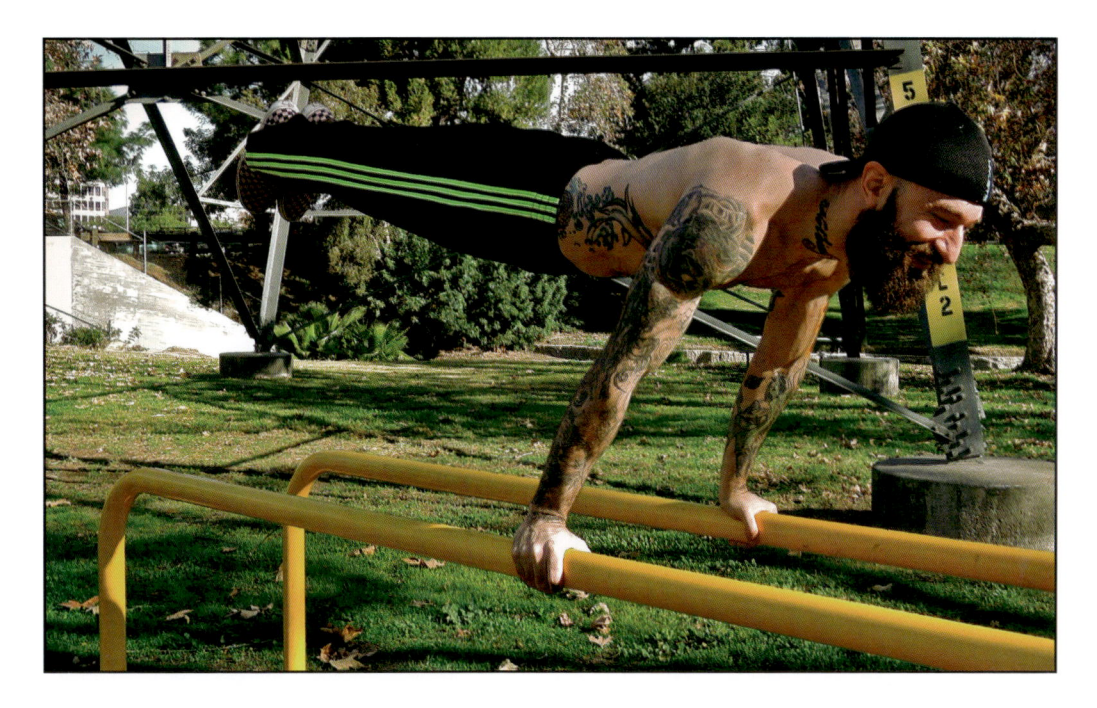

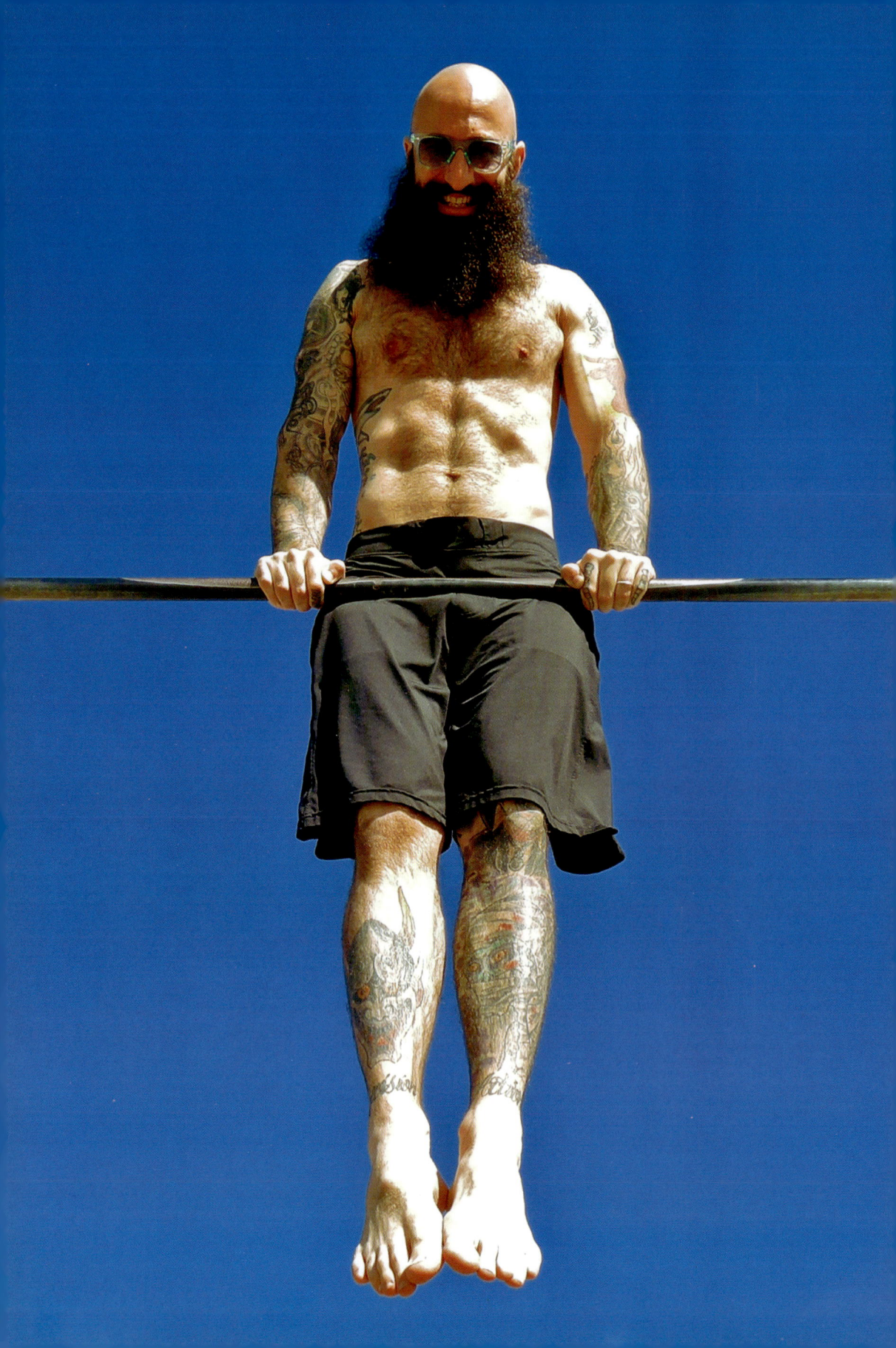

Chapter 10

Bar Moves

Nothing screams "Street Workout" like bar moves. Many practitioners of advanced calisthenics were roped in the first time they saw these advanced exercises because they are such a spectacular visual to behold. We sure were!

But there's more to these moves than just looking cool. They require strength, technique and perseverance. The muscle-up, back lever and front lever are all full body exercises even if they emphasize different muscle groups as primary movers; none of them isolate the upper body completely.

The following gravity-defying feats will suspended you in mid-air, as if you're flying over the earth beneath you, and will make you feel like the king or queen of the world!

MUSCLE-UP PROGRESSIONS

The muscle-up is a gatekeeper of sorts between intermediate and advanced bar-work. Muscle-ups beckon us to take our game to the next level, as they work the entire upper body in a way that no other single exercise can. They're also a lot of fun!

To the untrained eye, the muscle-up appears to simply be a combination of a pull-up and a dip, but be assured, it's a unique animal unto itself. It's the only upper-body exercise that combines both a pull and a push. Beyond that, muscle-ups also require an explosive generation of power, along with a notoriously difficult transition around the bar. In the calisthenics county, the muscle-up is tops!

EXTENDED RANGE-OF-MOTION PULL-UP

Once you can do several clean pull-ups with your chin going over the bar, extending the range of motion can be the next step toward a muscle-up. Yank down hard on the bar as fast and powerfully as you can, using your entire body to generate force.

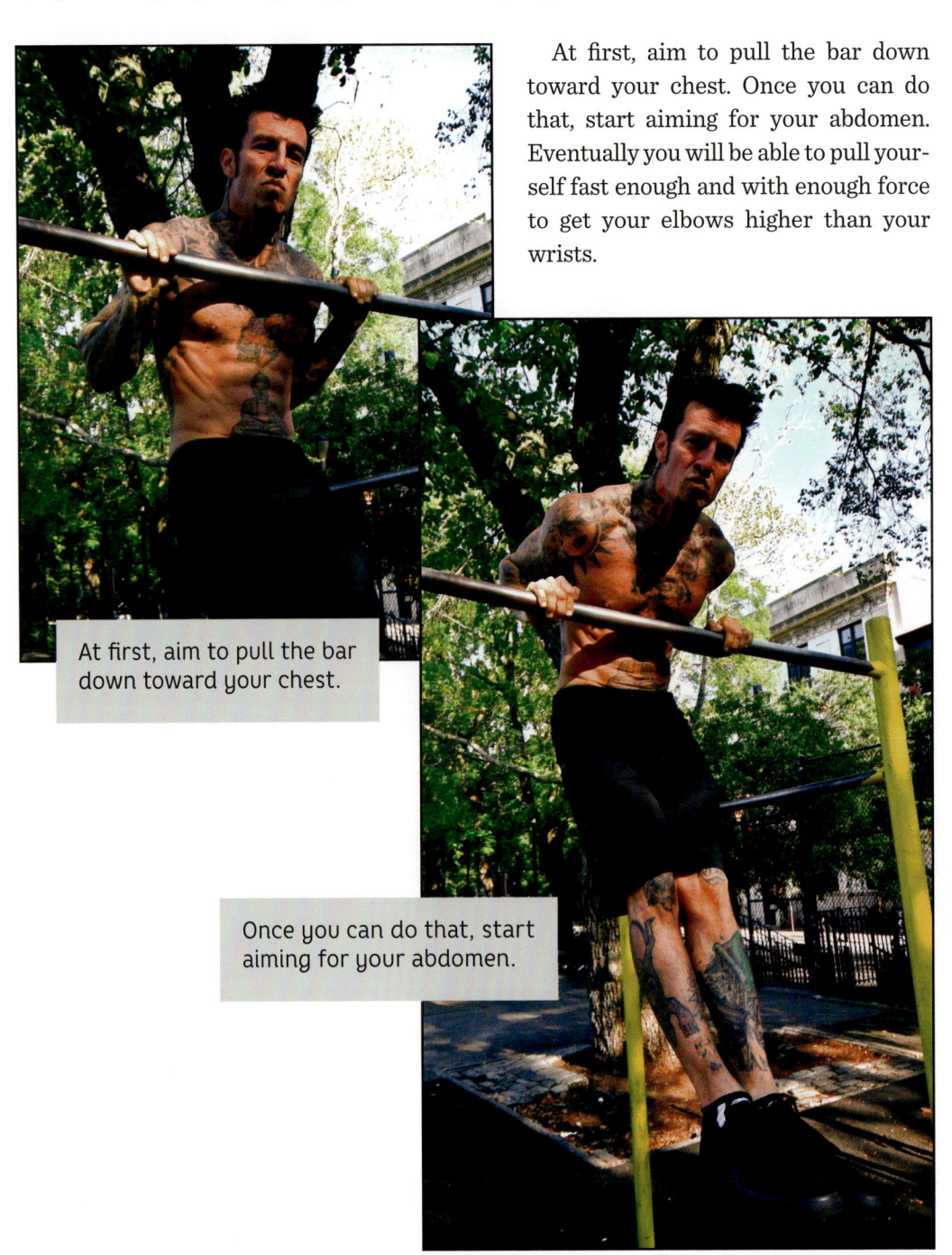

At first, aim to pull the bar down toward your chest. Once you can do that, start aiming for your abdomen. Eventually you will be able to pull yourself fast enough and with enough force to get your elbows higher than your wrists.

At first, aim to pull the bar down toward your chest.

Once you can do that, start aiming for your abdomen.

216 STREET WORKOUT

NEGATIVE MUSCLE-UP

Training the negative (or eccentric) phase of a movement pattern is a useful technique for learning many Street Workout exercises, though it can be especially helpful for the muscle-up. Practicing the negative phase helps you get a feel for the movement pattern from the top down.

Get above the bar just like you would for a straight bar dip, then carefully lower yourself to the bottom of your dip position. From here, continue lowering yourself as slowly as you can while you extend your legs forward, bracing your entire body and squeezing the bar as hard as possible as your hand rolls from the dip position into the pull-up position. At first, you may drop very quickly, but you'll gain control of the descent with practice. Eventually, that control will transfer into reversing the movement.

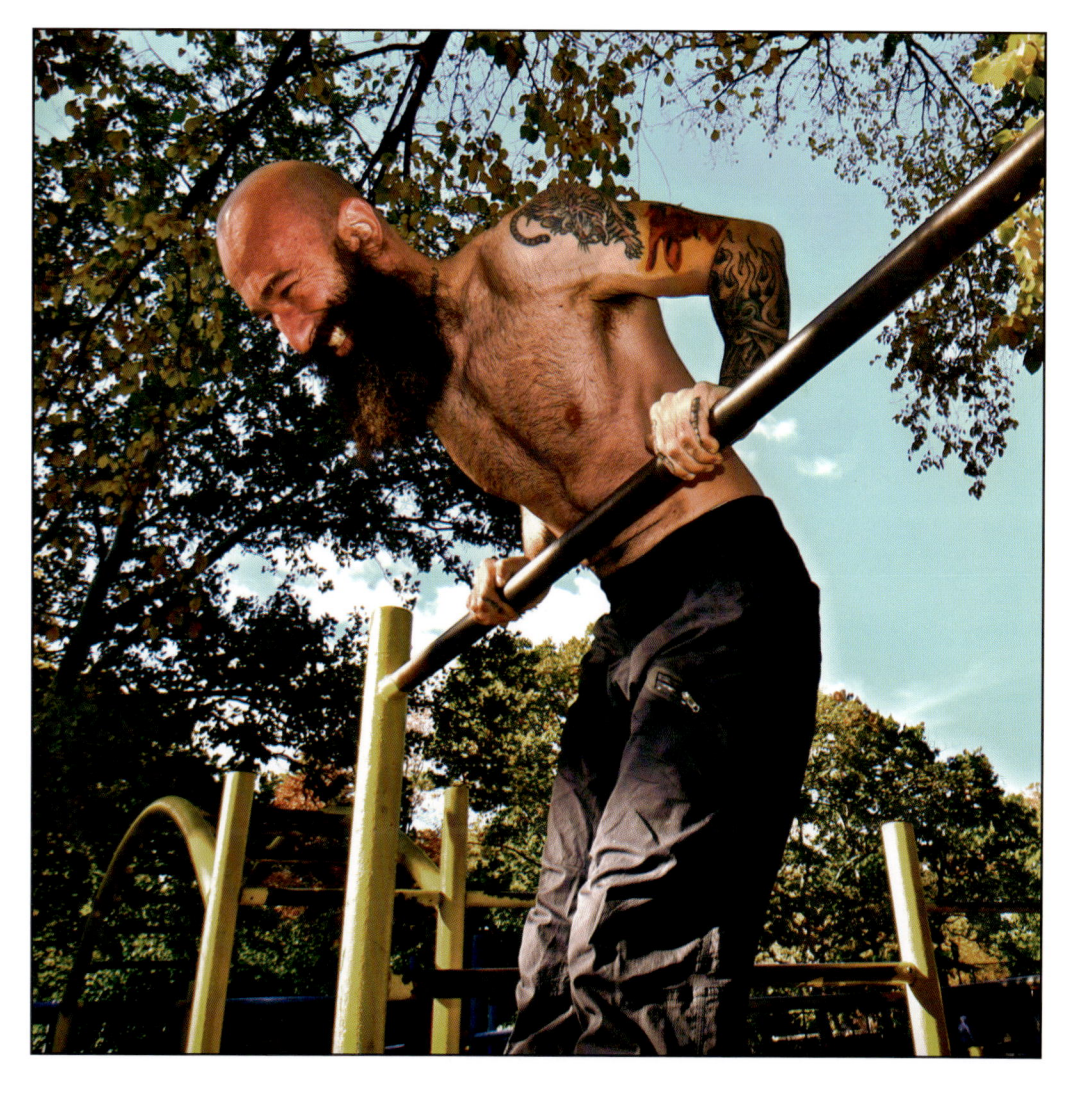

FALSE GRIP

Part of the challenge of the muscle-up is timing the transition so your hands roll from the pull-up grip into the dip position at just the right time. Using a "false grip" can sometimes fix this issue.

The false grip involves cocking your wrists over the bar before you start your pull so they won't need to roll around it during the transition. By starting with your palms facing toward the ground rather than away from your body, you will automatically be in the right position to begin the pushing phase once you get to the top of your pull. The false grip can be especially helpful when working on performing a strict muscle-up.

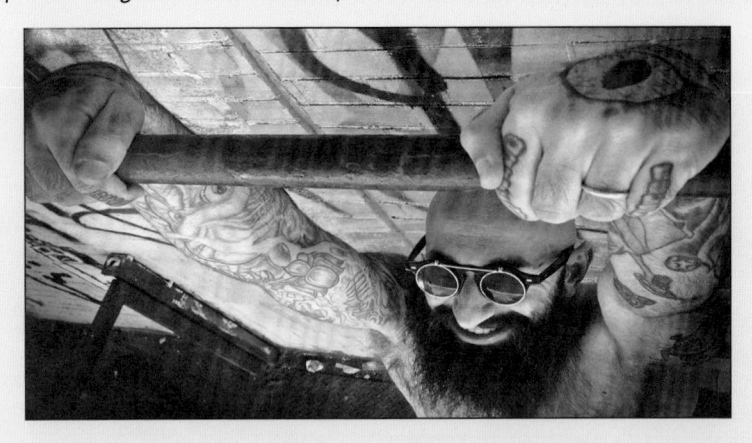

Some people find an exaggerated false grip with their closed fists resting on the bar to be ideal. In this variant, the bar will wind up in the crook of your wrists, allowing for more of your hand to be on top of the bar. This can create better leverage, particularly if you lack the wrist mobility for a standard false grip muscle-up.

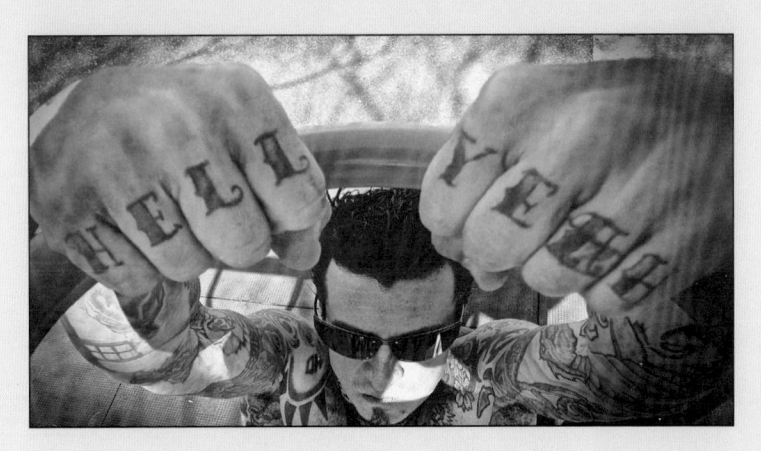

MUSCLE-UP

The mighty muscle-up begins like a pull-up, but continues until your entire torso goes up and over the bar. Grip the bar slightly narrower than you would for a pull-up, then lean back and pull the bar down your body as low as possible. At the top of your pull, reach your chest over the bar and extend your arms.

Though the first phase of the muscle-up shares a lot in common with the pull-up, the two movement patterns are subtly different. When you do a muscle-up, you'll be driving your elbows behind your body, rather than toward your sides as you would in a standard pull-up. This is why a narrower grip tends to work better for the muscle-up.

It's also helpful to think about leaning away from the bar during the pulling phase before pitching forward at the top. This creates a movement pattern that's more of an "S" shape than a straight line, allowing you to better maneuver your body around the bar.

When starting out, we encourage you to use momentum and be explosive. It may take a lot of practice to get a feel for the timing, though if you are solid on your pull-ups and diligent in practicing the previous steps, the muscle-up will eventually be yours.

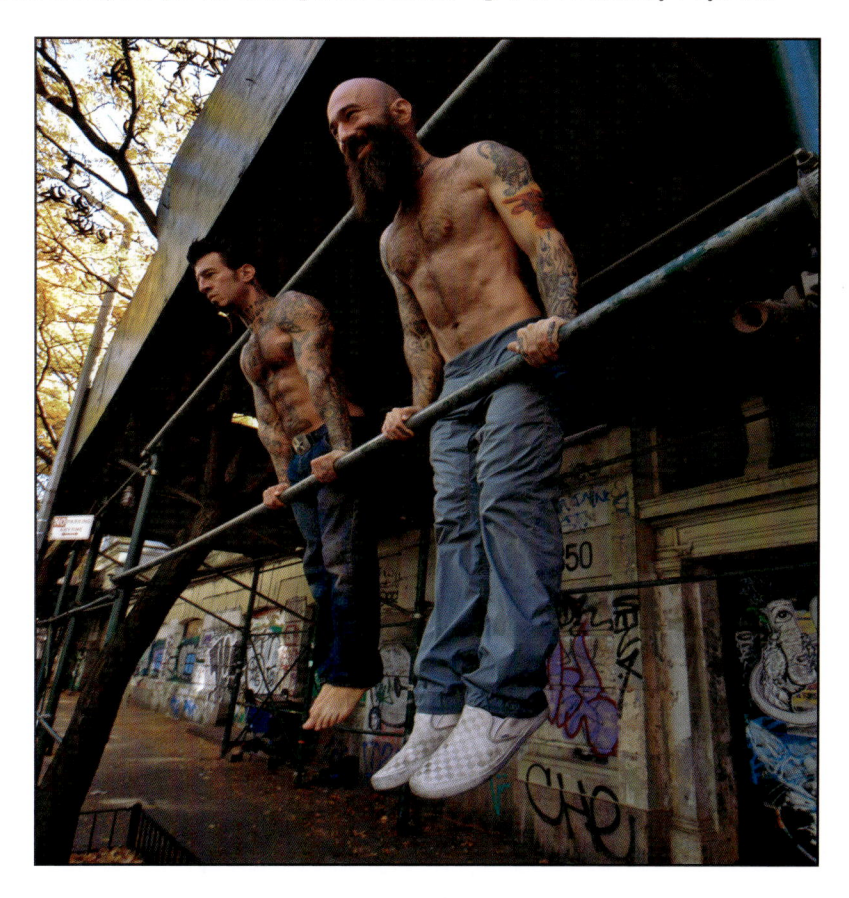

CHICKEN WINGING

It is common for people new to muscle-ups to find that one arm will get over the bar before the other. Though "chicken-winging" can be a helpful way to first get a feel for the crucial transition from pull to push, it's best to try to shake this habit as soon as possible, as doing so can be stressful on the shoulders and elbows.

If you have to chicken wing in the beginning, it's not necessarily a problem, but make it your mission to learn to get both arms over the bar at the same time.

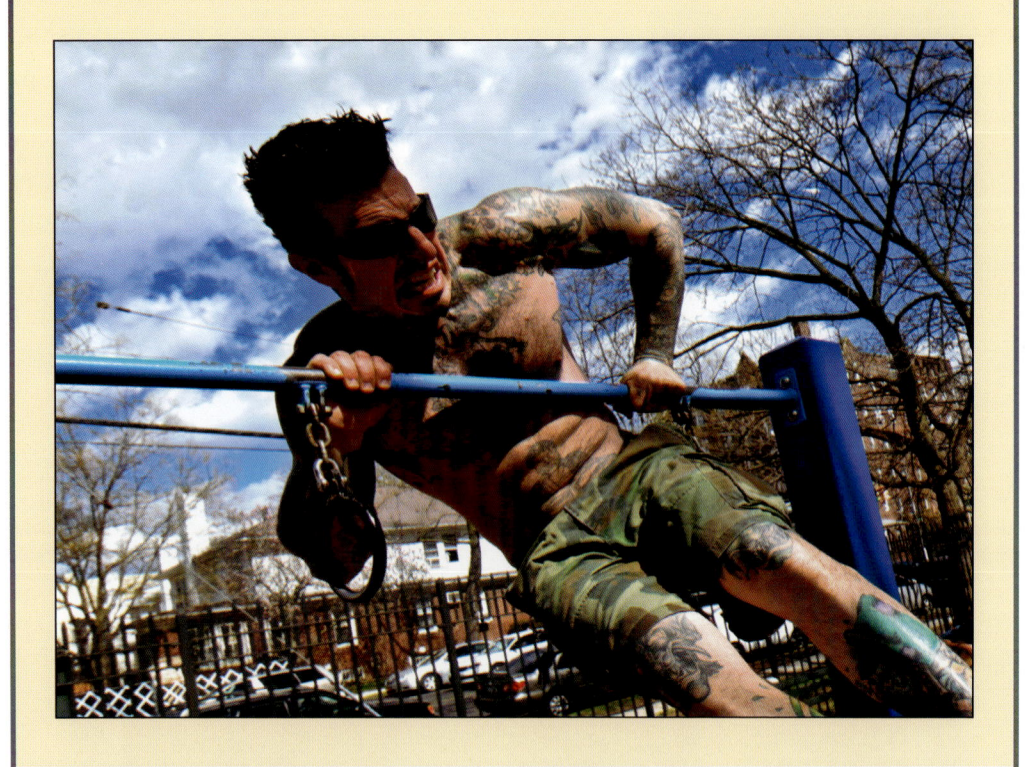

STRICT MUSCLE-UP

Once you can do a few muscle-ups in a row, it's time to begin eliminating the use of any momentum, instead performing the move with nothing more than solid technique and raw strength.

A strict muscle-up involves maintaining straight legs while avoiding any swinging or hip movement as you pull and push your entire torso over the bar from a dead hang. You will need to brace your abs and tense your legs to in order to perform a strict muscle-up. You may also find it helpful to reach your legs forward as you transition from the pulling phase into the pushing phase.

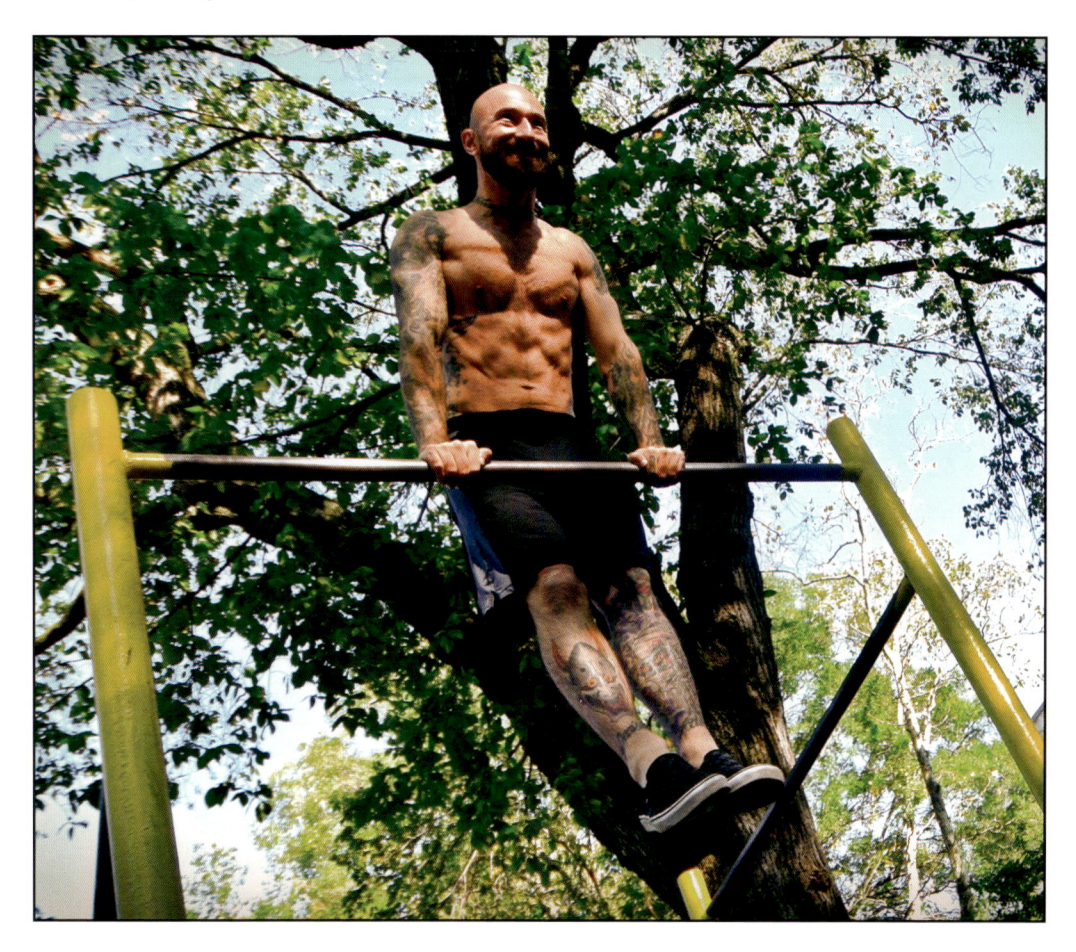

REVERSE GRIP MUSCLE-UP

Unlike pull-ups, which are typically harder with an overhand grip, the muscle-up is significantly more difficult to perform using an underhand grip. Due to the change in hand position, the transition from pulling to pushing becomes even more challenging. As such, you will need to generate even more explosive force during the pull in order to roll your hands around. It's also important to be careful to avoid placing too much pressure on your thumbs during the transition. A mixed grip muscle-up (one arm in an overhand position and the other one underhand) can serve as a helpful step toward learning a reverse grip muscle-up.

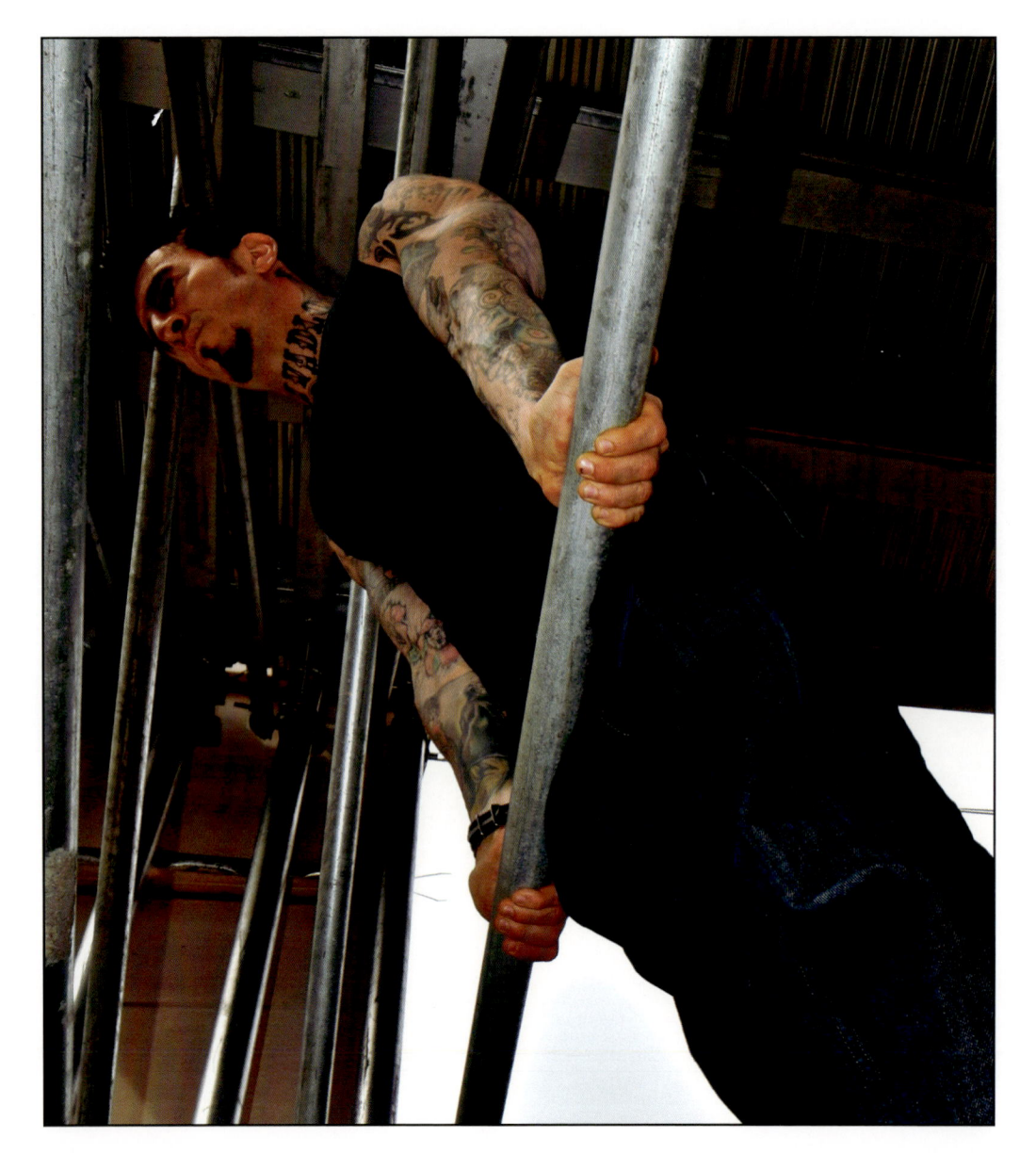

The Plyo-Matrix Muscle-Mania

Performing a plyometric muscle-up is the ultimate expression of explosive power. In order to execute this exercise, you must go for as much height as possible. In other words, keep practicing those explosive pull-ups and dips.

Once you can generate enough height on the bar, try removing your hands at the top of the muscle-up for just a moment. This is how the plyometric muscle-up begins. In time, you can try keeping your hands off the bar for longer, adding a clap, putting your hands behind your back or even crossing your hands over one another.

The most advanced plyometric muscle-ups entail jumping over the bar (sometimes referred to as a "muscle-over") or doing a complete 360, if you can believe it. Indeed, this exercise embodies the true essence of street workout in all its splendor!

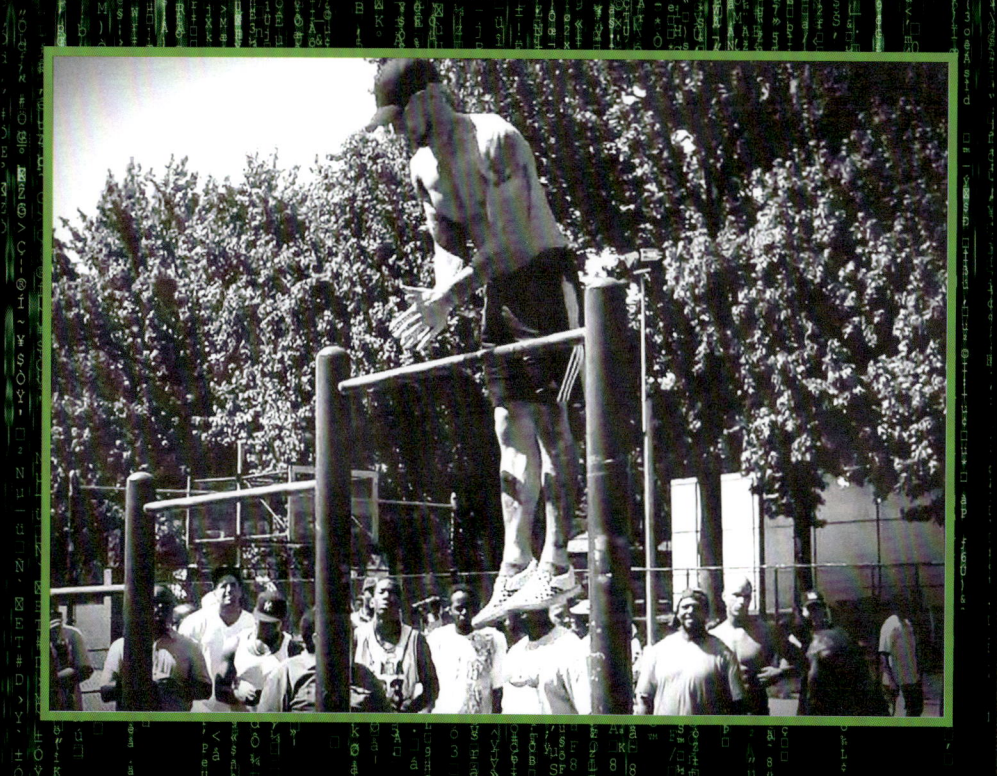

BACK LEVER PROGRESSIONS

It's a bird. It's a plane. It's... a back lever!

While a back lever will not actually give you the power of flight, executing this incredible feat is sure to make you feel like Superman.

The full back lever involves gripping the bar with your body in a prone position, parallel to the ground. A superhuman amount of strength is required, as you'll be recruiting your many muscle groups, including your arms, abs, shoulders, back, glutes and even your legs. Because this incredible spectacle trains your sensory awareness in addition to rocking your muscles, back lever practice provides a fantastic workout for your mind, body and spirit.

SKINNING THE CAT

Before you embark on learning the back lever, you need to familiarize yourself with a calisthenics skill commonly referred to as skinning the cat.

Hang from a pull-up bar in an overhand grip, then pull your knees all the way toward your chest. When you can't get them any higher, begin rotating your body beneath the bar so your legs and feet pass behind it on the other side. Continue lowering yourself until your legs are fully extended with your arms positioned behind your back. This is known as a German hang. It's a great stretch for your shoulders. Pause here briefly, then tuck your knees toward your chest, raise your hips up toward the bar and thread your legs back around, returning to the start position.

When starting out, you may have to cross your ankles in order to get your legs under the bar. Folks with limited mobility tend to have a particularly hard time with this. There is also a great deal of shoulder flexibility required. Do your best to avoid bending your elbows during this exercise.

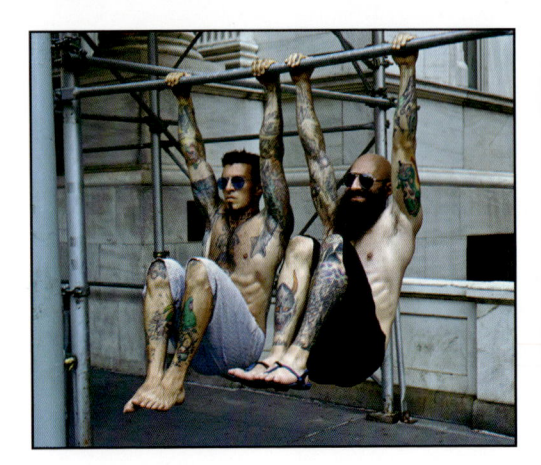

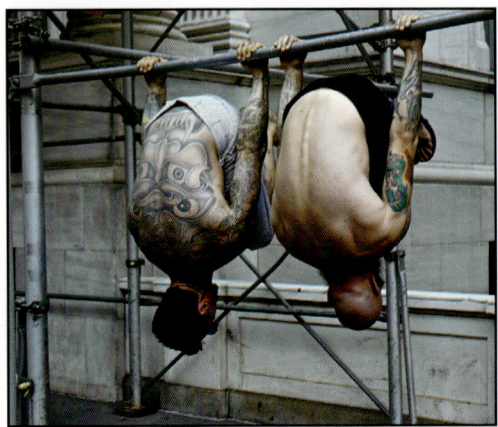

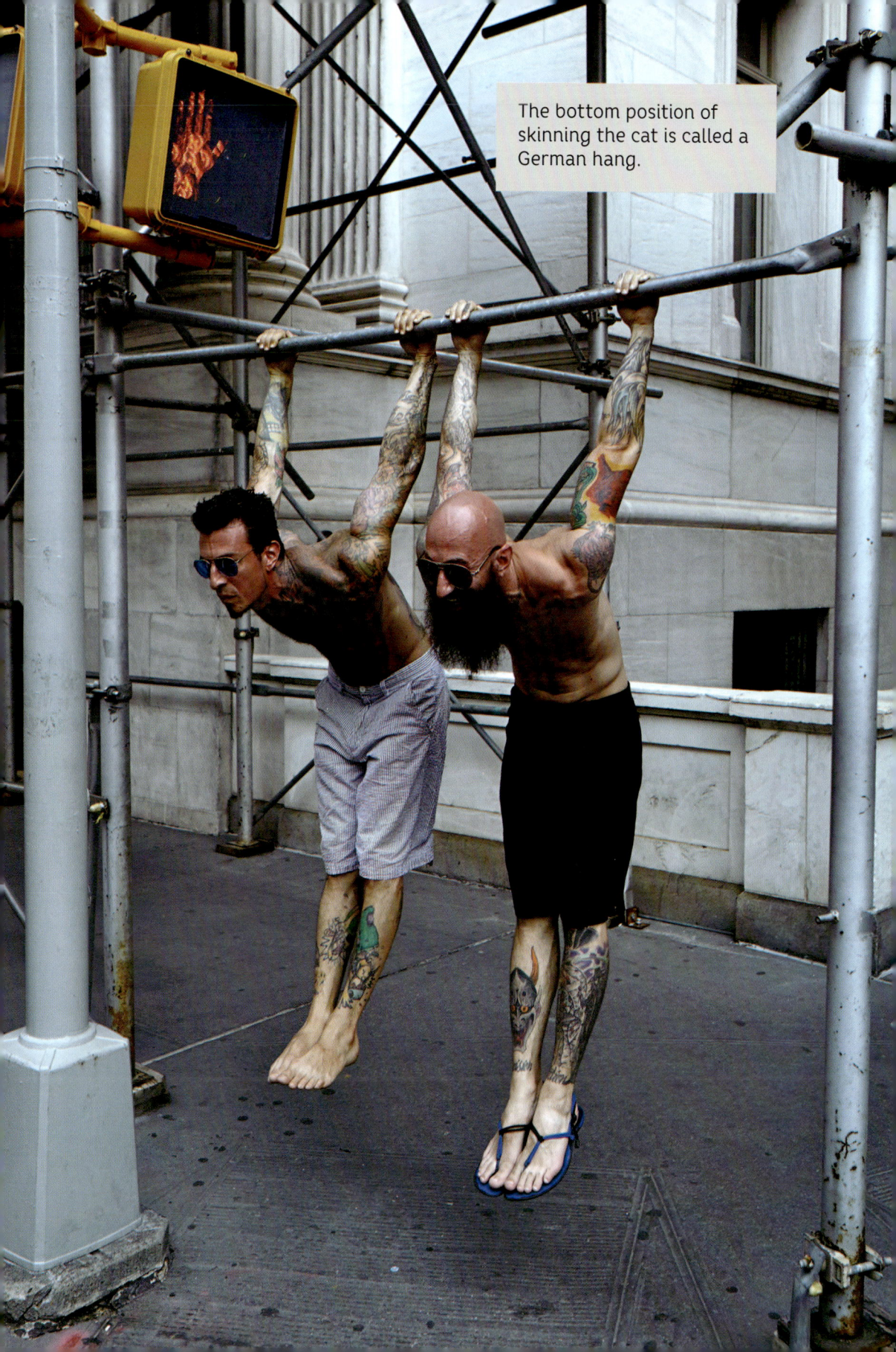

The bottom position of skinning the cat is called a German hang.

TUCK BACK LEVER

From a German hang, begin lifting your hips, pulling your knees toward your chest and flattening out your back. Aim to get your torso parallel to the ground with your heels up by your butt. Focus on extending through your lower back to avoid excessive rounding.

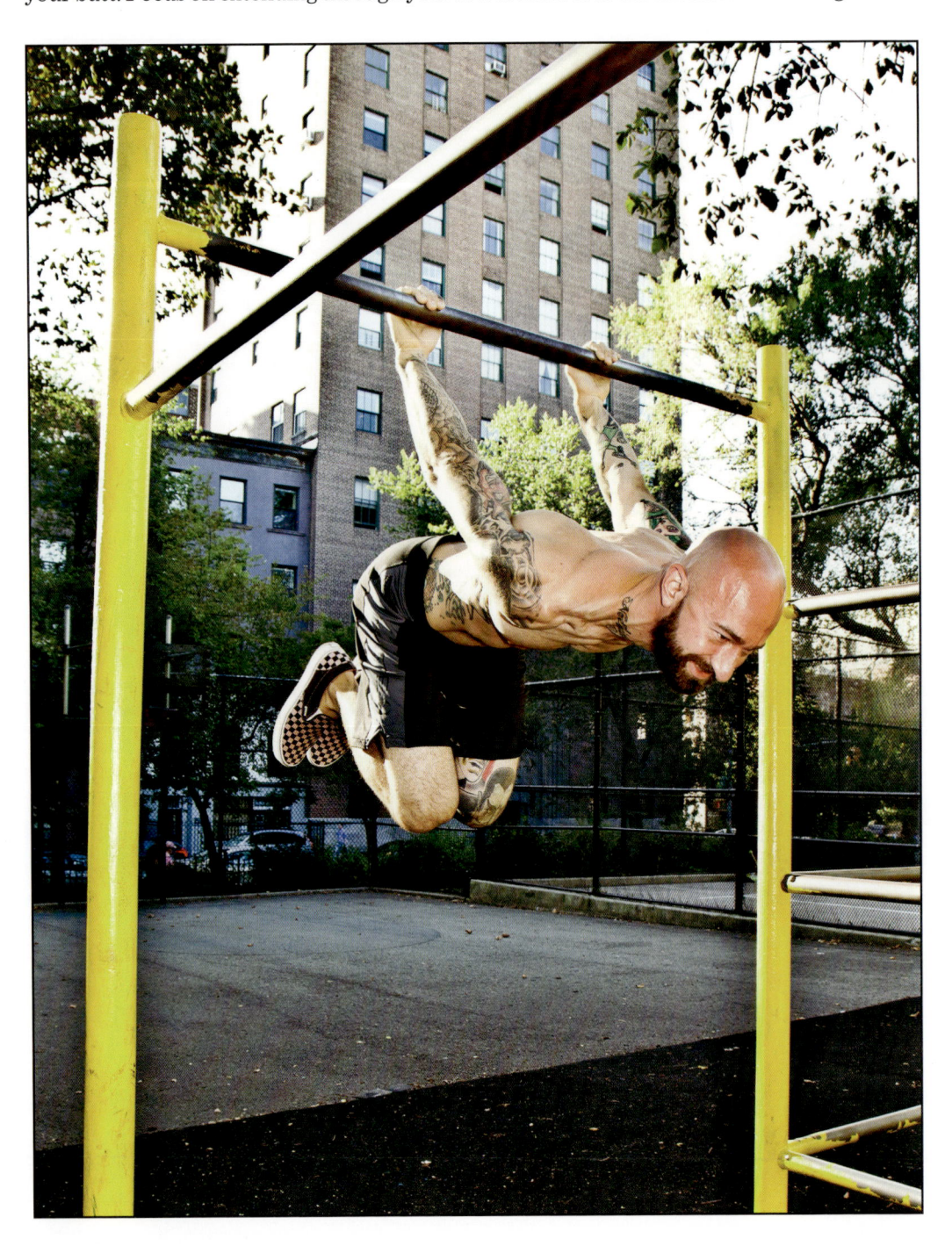

ONE LEG BACK LEVER

Extending one leg while keeping the other tucked is a helpful intermediate step between a tuck back lever and the full version. From the tuck back lever position, carefully reach one leg behind while pitching your chest forward and increasing the tension in the rest of your body.

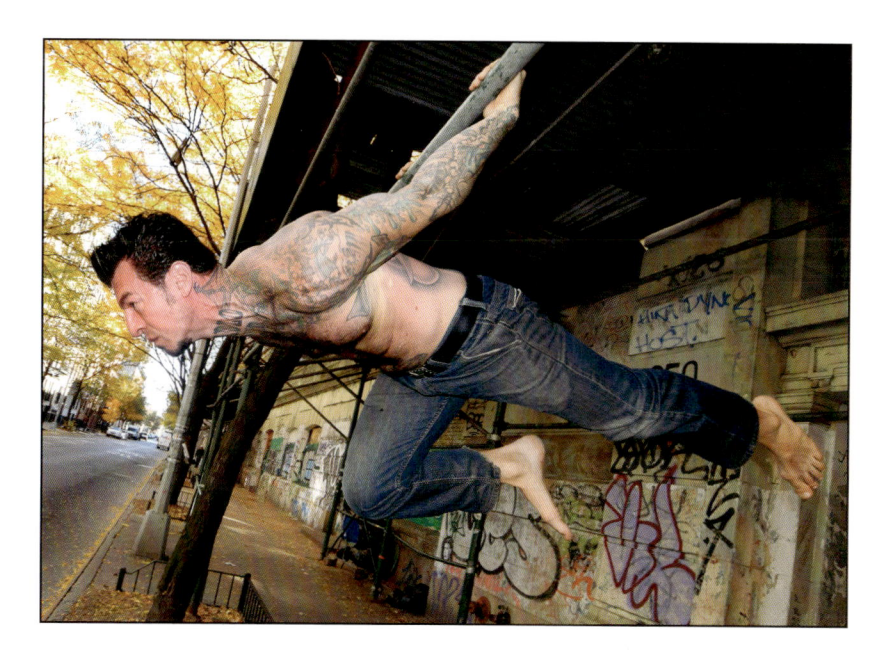

STRADDLE BACK LEVER

Holding your legs outstretched to the sides is a bit less difficult than holding the full back lever, as the straddle leg position shortens your body length slightly. Give it a shot once the single leg version is no longer as challenging, yet the full back lever still remains out of reach.

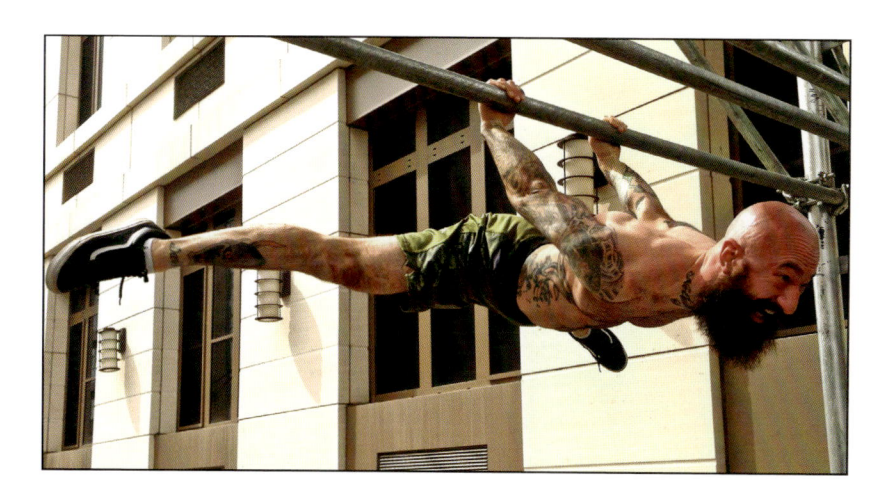

BACK LEVER

The Street Workout style back lever is typically performed with an overhand pull-up grip, holding the entire body horizontally above the ground with your hands grasping the bar behind your lower back. Full body tension is very much necessary, as you must squeeze not only with your hands against the bar, but with your arms against your body.

Once you've gotten comfortable with the previous steps, there are a few different ways you can experiment with getting into position for a full back lever. You are encouraged to experiment with all three.

The first method is to lift your body in the air vertically so you wind up facing downward with your feet above the bar and the bar behind your waist. Once you establish tension in your entire body, you can slowly begin lowering yourself until you are parallel to the ground. This gradually increases the muscular load and primes your neurology for the feeling of supporting your full body weight in a back lever. Pitch your torso forward as you come down in order to control the descent and avoid being pulled down too forcefully by the weight of your legs.

Slowly lowering yourself into position is one method of getting into a back lever.

The second method is to start in a tuck back lever, then carefully unfurl your legs (one at a time or simultaneously). As you extend your legs, remember to pitch your chest forward to keep the length of your body even on both sides of the bar. Your hands should wind up behind your hips rather than behind your shoulders.

The last method (and typically the most difficult) is to lift your body into position from a German hang without ever bending at the hips or knees. You'll need to think about pulling the bar toward your back as you extend through your back and legs in order to lift into position.

One of the most common issues with the back lever is excessive curvature of the back. Actively engage your abs, legs and glutes to avoid falling into this trap. It might even help to think about folding forward slightly as a means of overcompensating, almost like an upside down version of the hollow body position. Furthermore, maintaining a narrow grip can help facilitate greater tension between your torso and your upper arms, which can aid in holding the back lever, whereas a wider grip will make the move more difficult.

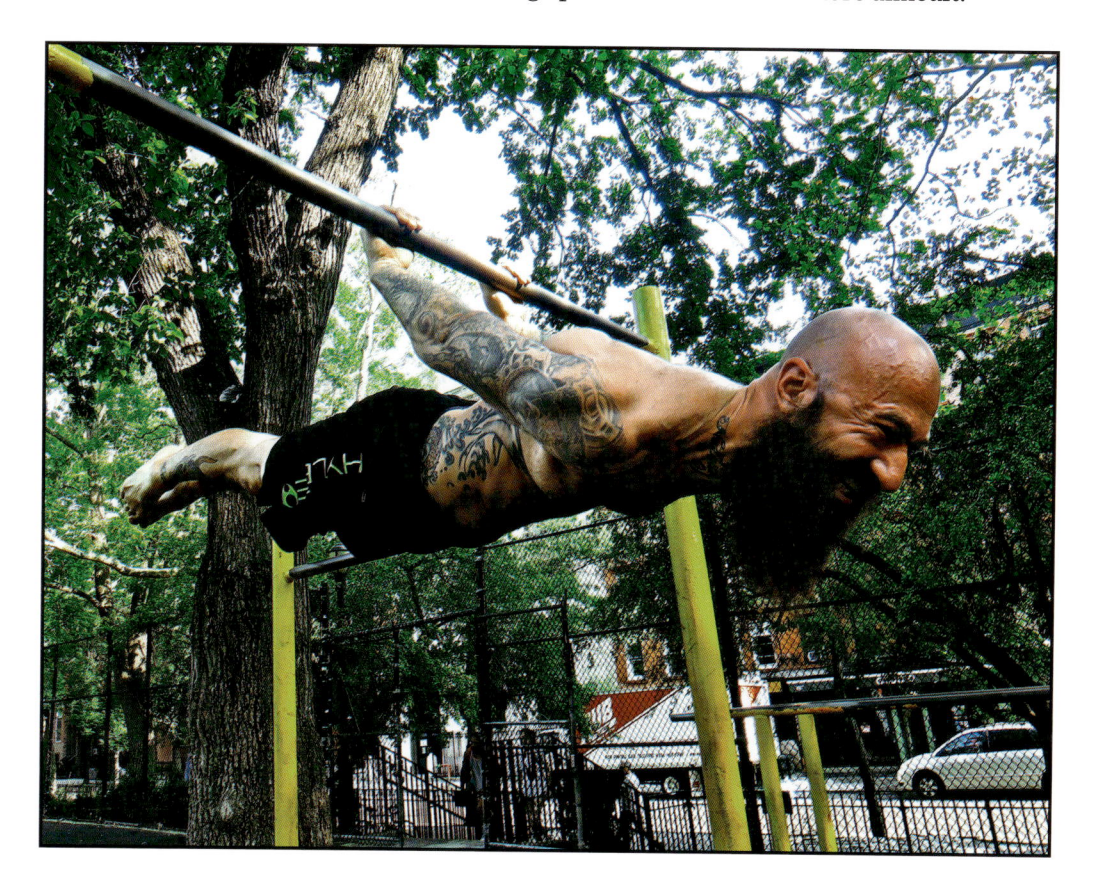

REVERSE GRIP BACK LEVER

Unlike a pull-up, performing a back lever with the palms in a chin-up grip is more difficult than the other way around. Due to the change in arm position, significantly more load is placed on the biceps than in the standard Street Workout style back lever. As such, this variation can be especially stressful on the tendons surrounding the elbow joint. Though this grip is commonly seen when back levers are performed in gymnastics, we recommend learning the Street Workout style back lever first, then going back to the earlier progressions with a chin-up grip in order to build toward this variation. Like the reverse grip muscle-up, you can also experiment with a mixed grip as a transitional step between the classic Street Workout back lever and the reverse grip.

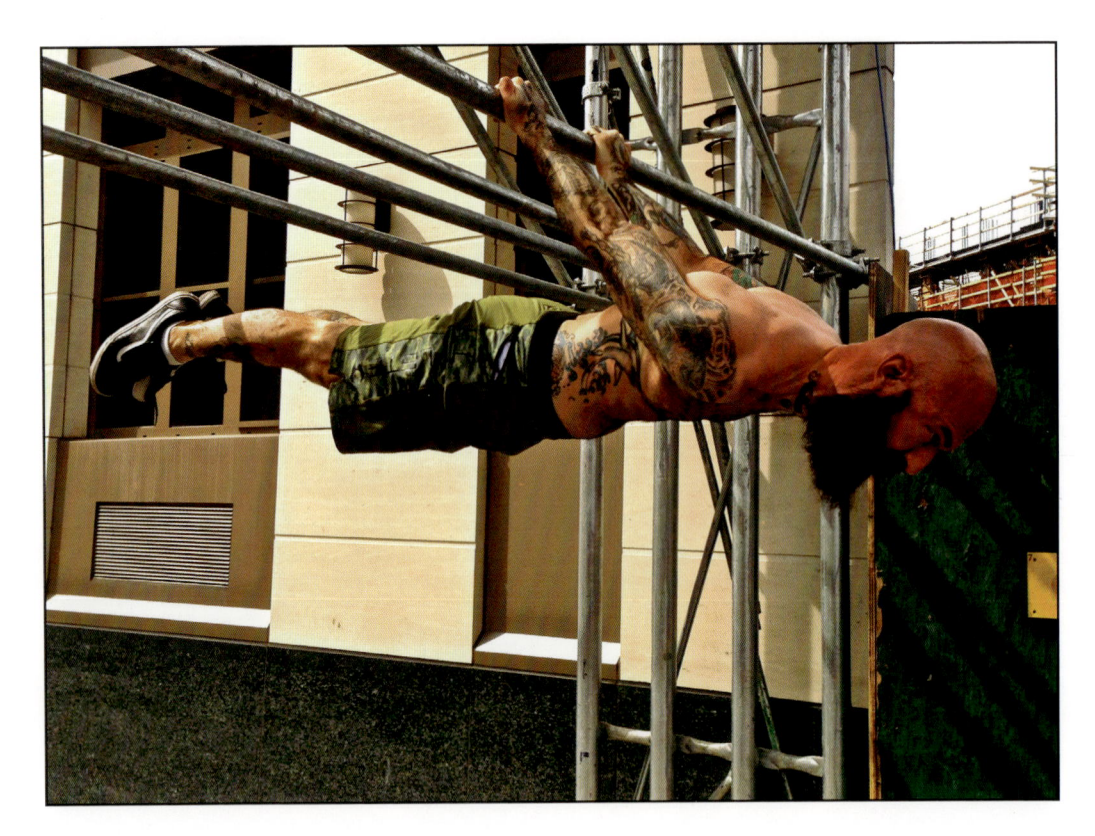

ONE ARM BACK LEVER

The ultimate back lever progression entails holding the pose with just one arm. This move is sometimes referred to as "the shark," due to its visual resemblance to nature's greatest predator as well as its own ferocious bite. Make sure you've got a very solid two arm back lever before diving in!

If you're ready to try it, begin in the standard two arm back lever position, then slowly start shifting your weight toward your primary arm. Before you take your other arm away, it can help to rotate your hips and trunk toward your main arm while reaching your legs behind you for balance. It may help to bend your knees as well. Carefully loosen your grip on the opposite side, ultimately removing that hand altogether when the time comes. Once you take that arm away, reach it overhead, lengthen your whole body and slowly start rotating your body back toward more of a face down position.

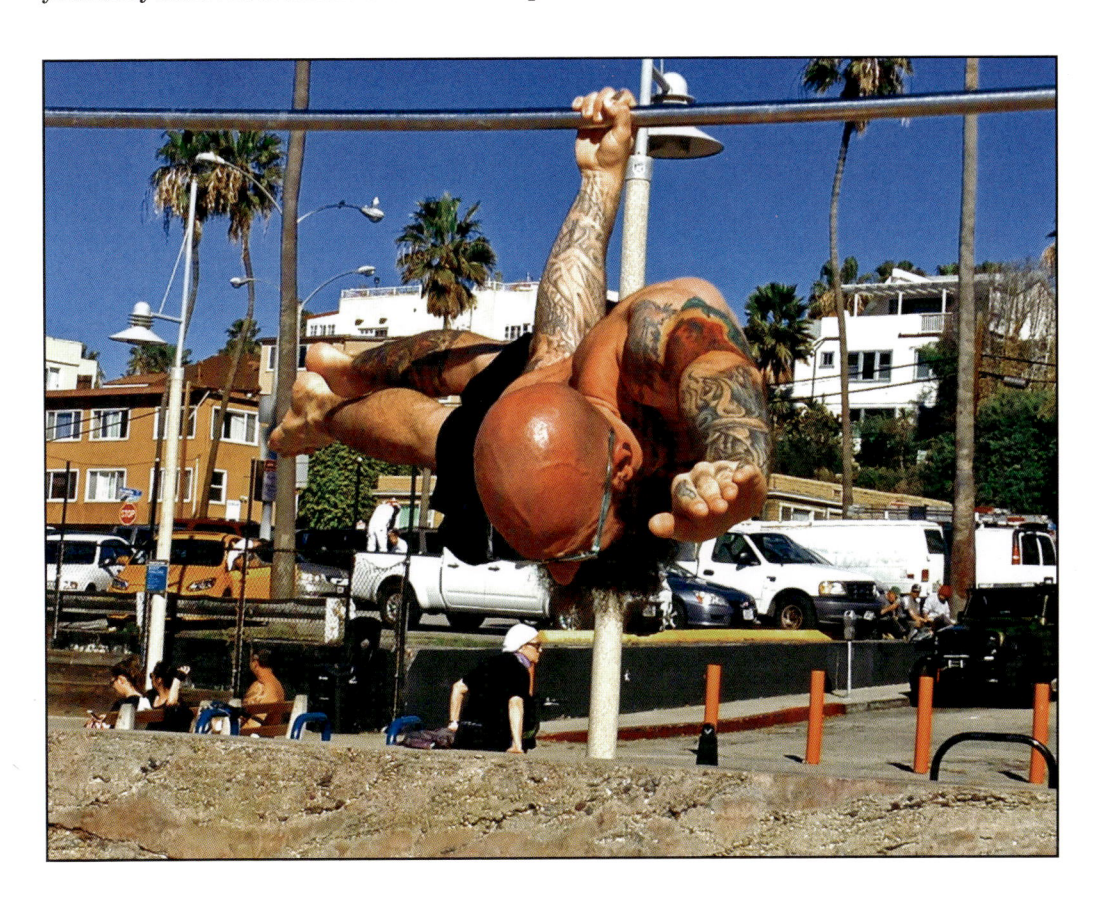

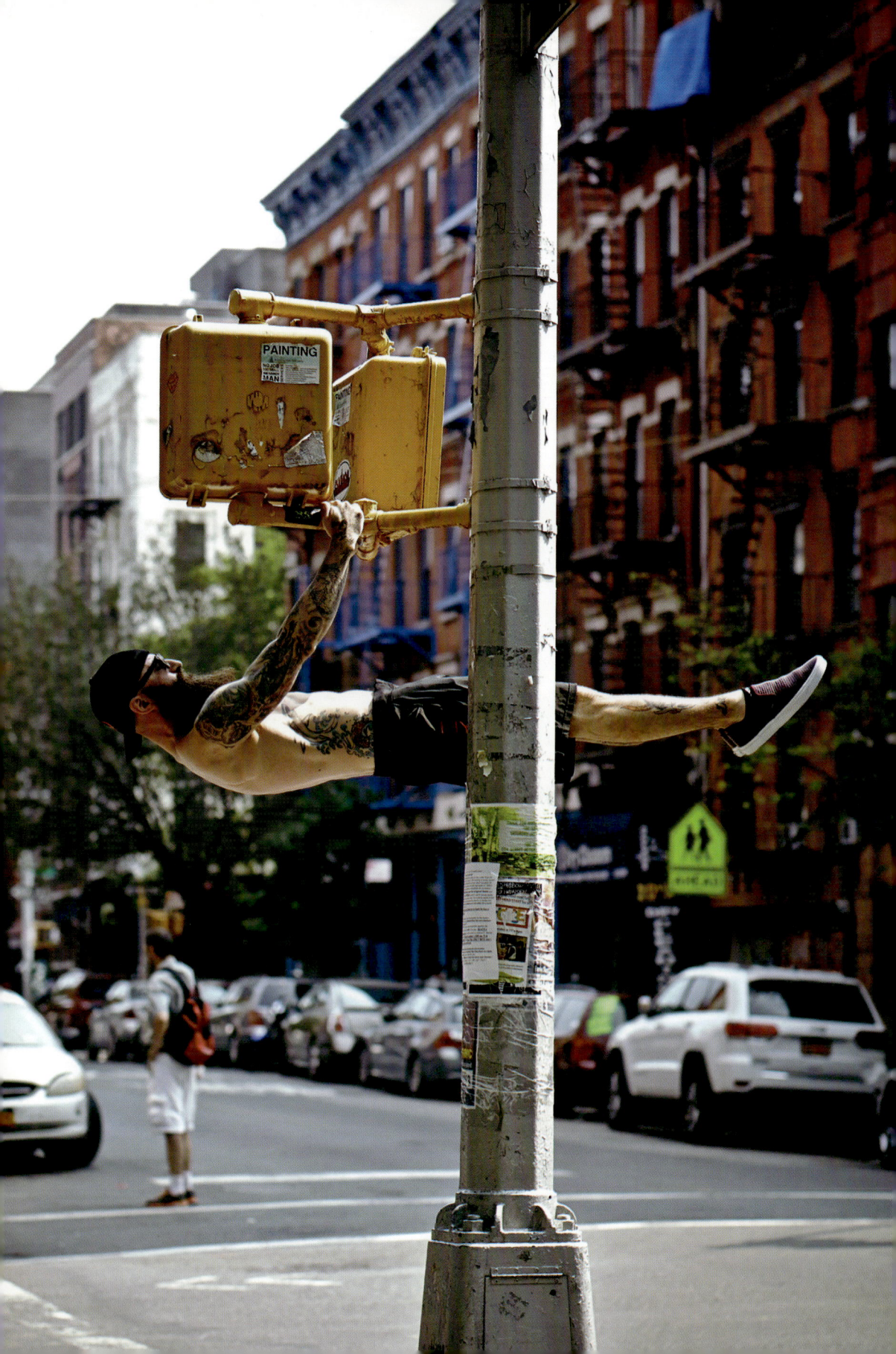

FRONT LEVER PROGRESSIONS

The awe-inspiring front lever is one of the most advanced bar moves in the entire bodyweight empire and one of the most impressive sights you are ever likely to behold. Visually, it's the opposite of the back lever. You are parallel to the ground in both, but this time, you're facing up, like laying down on a bed of air, floating above the world beneath you.

The full expression of the front lever involves keeping your arms locked out at the elbow, with a straight line from your shoulders to your hips to your feet. From a pure strength perspective, the front lever is harder than the back lever. However, it is less spatially disorienting and therefore possibly more accessible for some. The primary muscles involved are the lats and abs, though the entire upper body plays a role, as do the glutes and legs.

Execution of this formidable force is a long road. It can take months, even years, to achieve a full front lever hold for just a few seconds. Train hard, friends!

EXAGGERATED BAR HANG

Remember how we told you to pull your shoulder blades down and back when you do a pull-up? Your very first step toward performing a front lever is simply taking that basic bar hang and cranking it up a notch. For the exaggerated bar hang you are going to lean back, depressing and squeezing your scapulae together as hard as you can. Now begin to think about dragging the bar toward your hips while keeping both arms straight. You may not be able to raise your body very far yet, but practicing this move will start to give you a feel for pulling from your arms without bending at the elbows, which is crucial to performing a front lever.

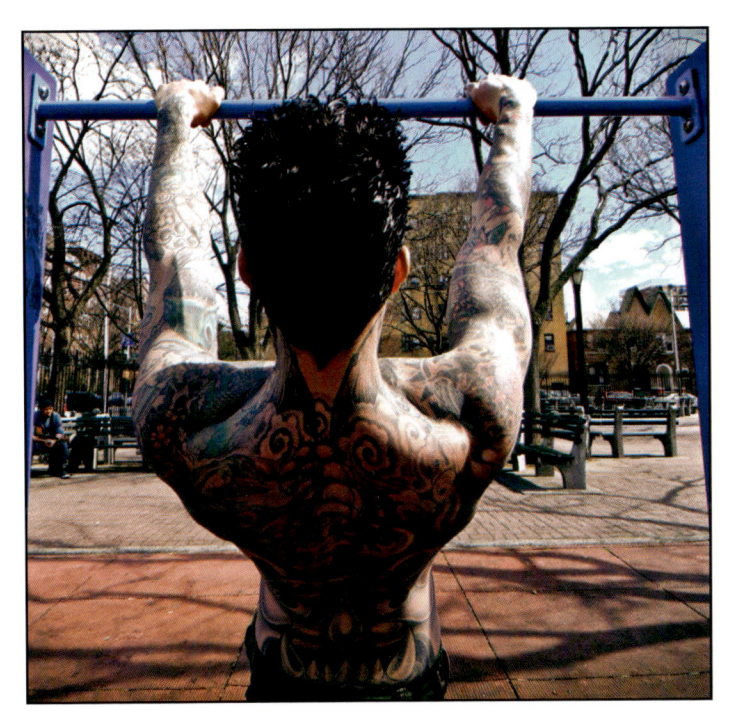

TUCK FRONT LEVER

From the exaggerated bar hang, begin tucking your knees toward your chest just like you were performing a hanging knee raise. When your knees reach the top position, continue pulling your hips up toward the bar until your torso is parallel to the ground. Again, it can help to imagine that you are trying to drag the bar down toward your hips in order to engage your lats.

In the beginning, it's okay to let your lower back round so you can bring your knees close to your chest. The closer your knees are to your chest, the less difficult the hold will be. As such, you can progress this exercise by moving into what you might call an "advanced tuck" position with the lower back completely flat and the knees above the hips, rather than tucked toward the chest.

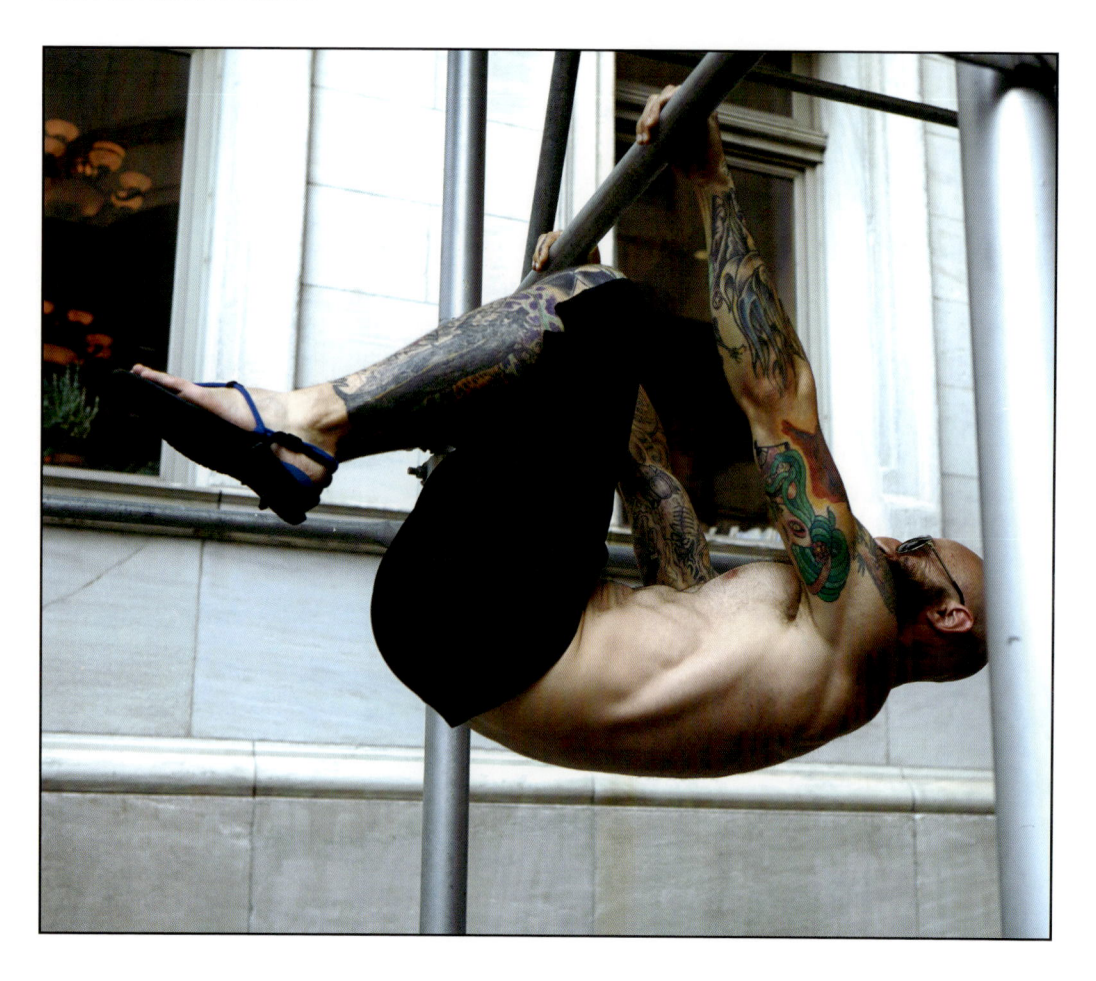

STRADDLE FRONT LEVER

As with the other types of levers, holding a straddle leg position is a helpful progression just before performing the full front lever hold with your body totally extended. Holding your feet apart essentially shortens the body, rendering this exercise more mechanically forgiving than the full front lever.

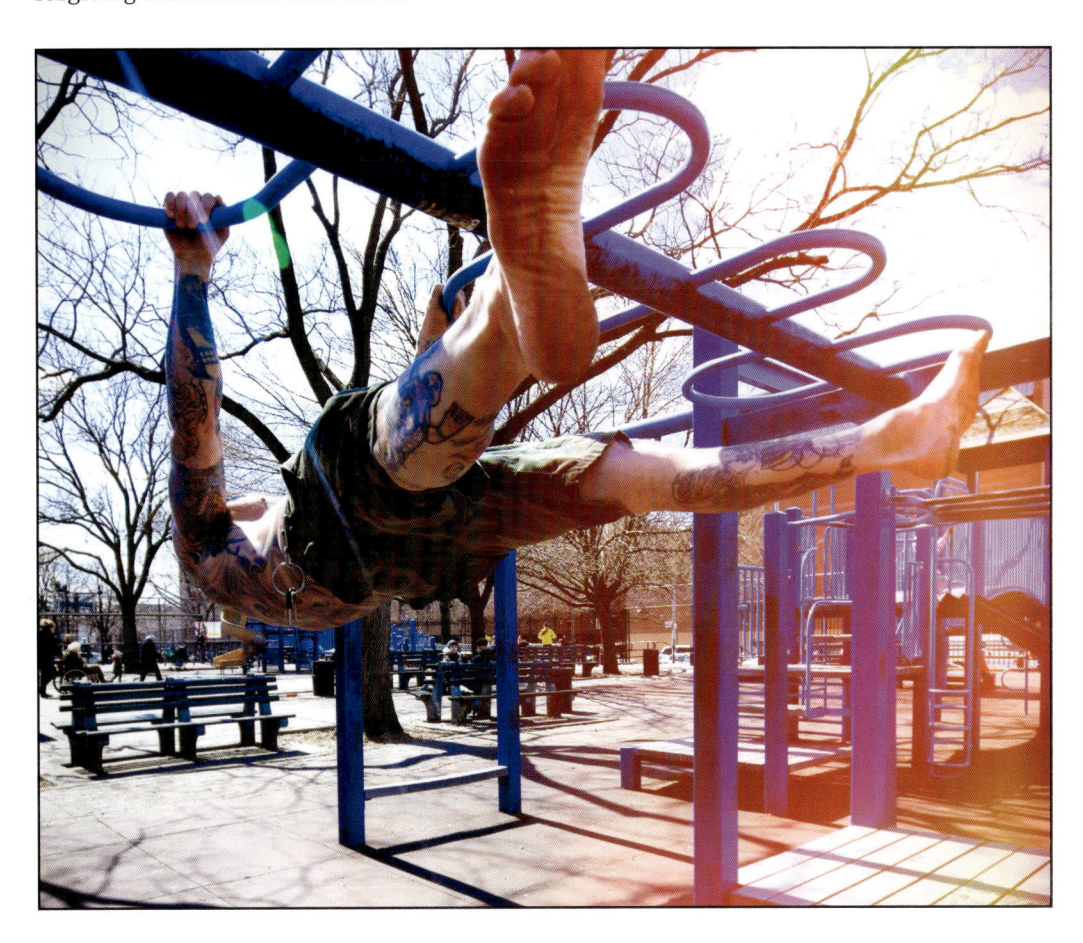

ONE LEG FRONT LEVER

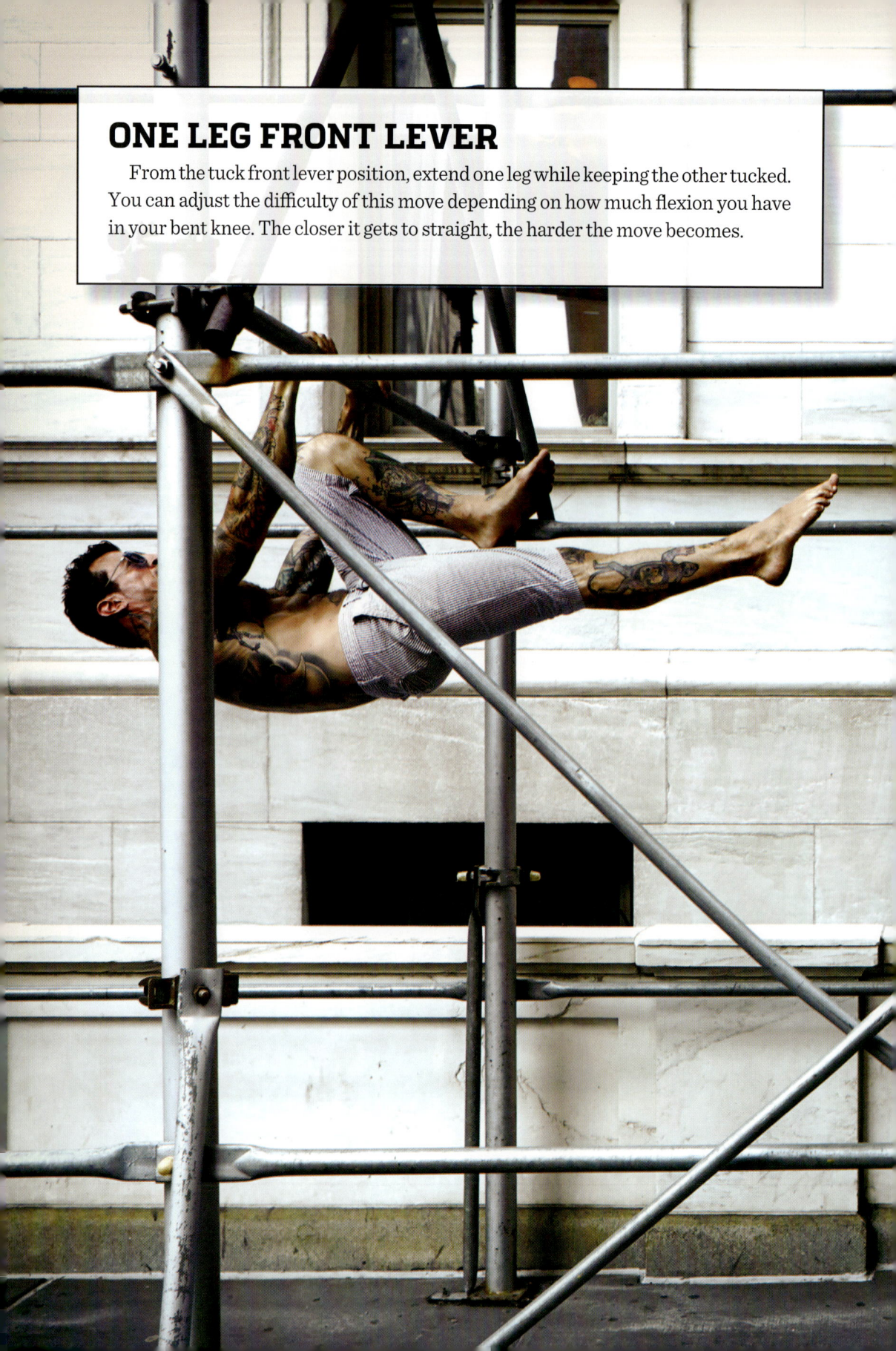

From the tuck front lever position, extend one leg while keeping the other tucked. You can adjust the difficulty of this move depending on how much flexion you have in your bent knee. The closer it gets to straight, the harder the move becomes.

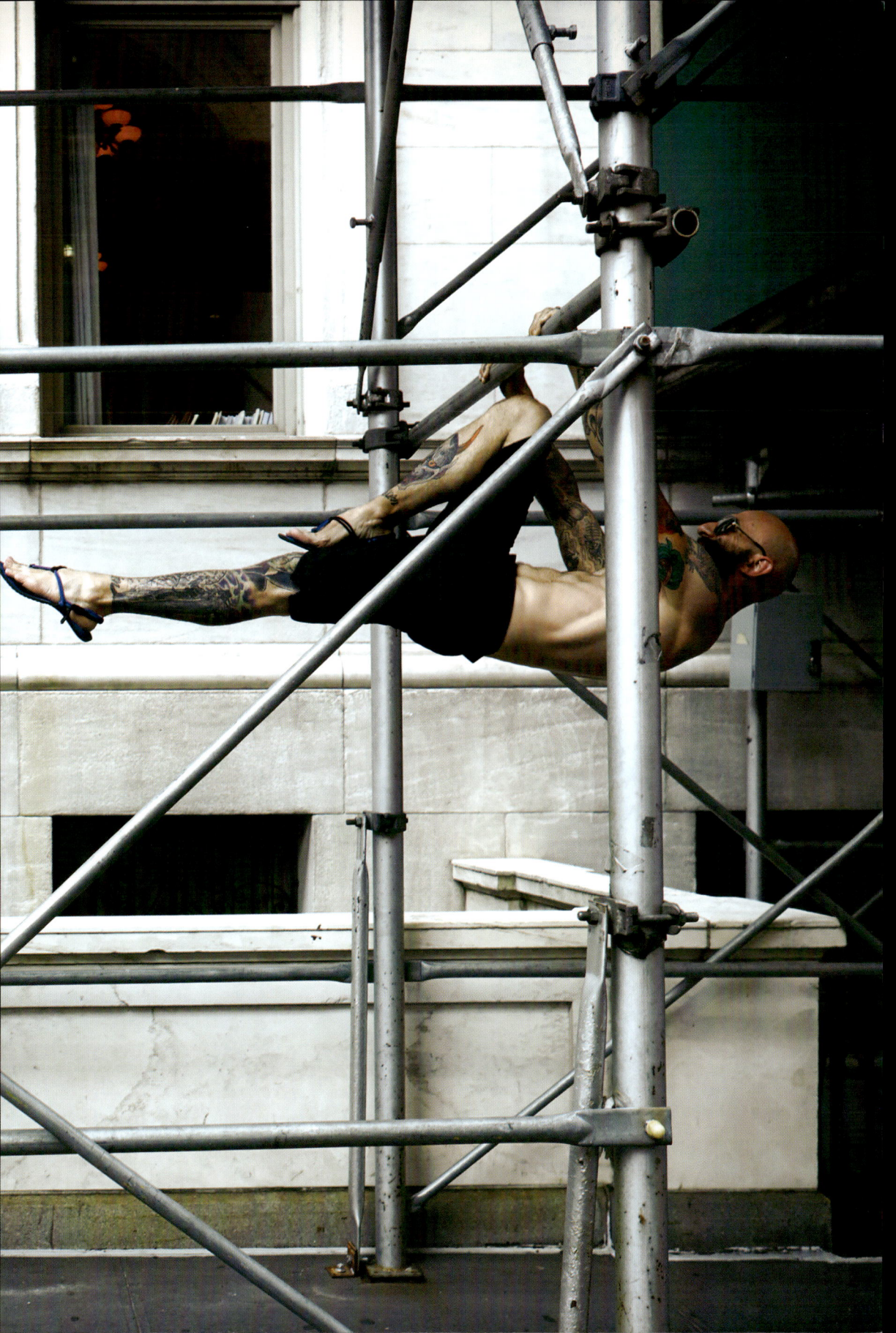

FRONT LEVER

As with the back lever, there are a few ways to approach getting into the full front lever.

The first method involves pulling yourself into an inverted position with your legs above your shoulders and the bar in front of your hips. From here, tense your entire body, then carefully lower yourself into the front lever position. It's helpful to pause every inch or two in order to stay in control. As we've seen before, lowering your body down from an angled position allows you to experience incremental increases in resistance.

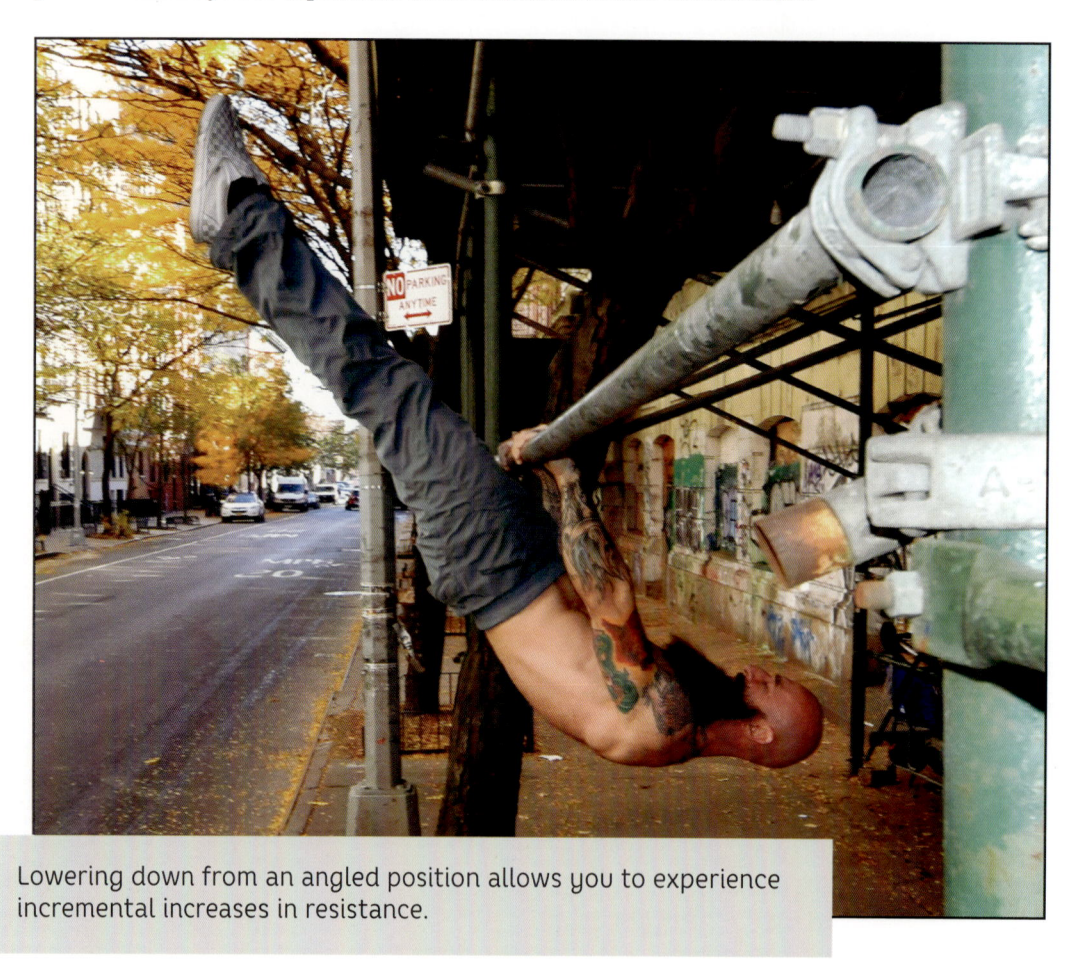

Lowering down from an angled position allows you to experience incremental increases in resistance.

The next method is to start from a tucked front lever, then gradually extend your legs. The straighter your legs get, the more tension you will need to generate in order to hold the position.

The third method is simply to pull yourself into the front lever from a dead hang. This is typically the most difficult (and arguably most impressive) method. It starts out like the exaggerated bar hang but continues until your body is completely parallel to the ground.

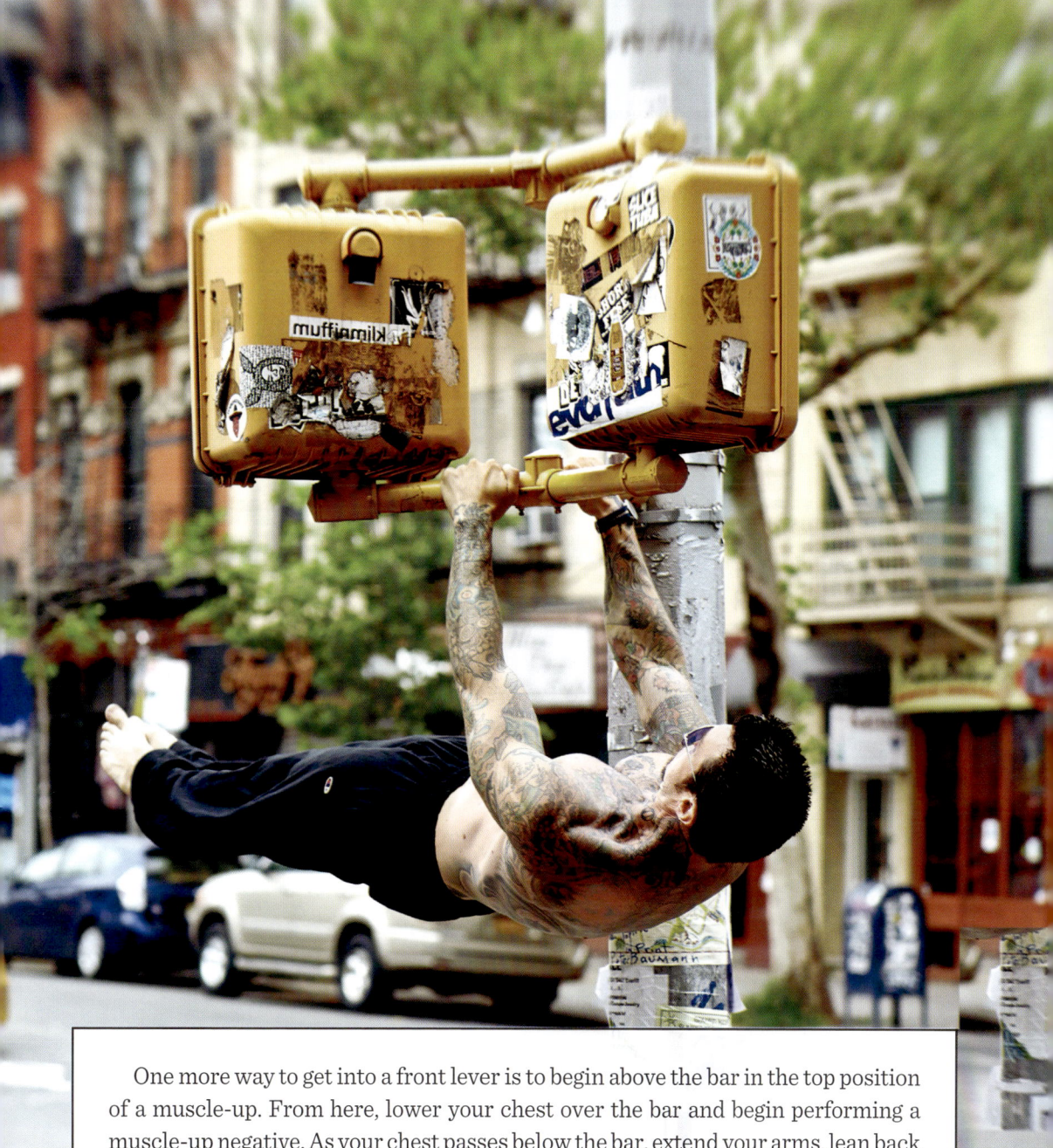

One more way to get into a front lever is to begin above the bar in the top position of a muscle-up. From here, lower your chest over the bar and begin performing a muscle-up negative. As your chest passes below the bar, extend your arms, lean back and reach your legs into the front lever position.

Whichever method you employ, think about contracting every single muscle in your body while using your arms and lats to actively pull the bar toward your hips.

It's very common for people to inadvertently fold at the hips when attempting the front lever. Do your best to avoid this pitfall by looking at your toes to make sure you are maintaining a straight line from shoulders to heels.

FRONT LEVER CURL

Begin by hanging from an overhead bar in a position similar to the headbanger pull-up, with your arms flexed and your head close to the bar. From here, maintain tension in your abs, legs, glutes and shoulders as you extend back into the front lever position, extending your arms while keeping the rest of your body rigid. Pause here briefly then return to the start position and repeat.

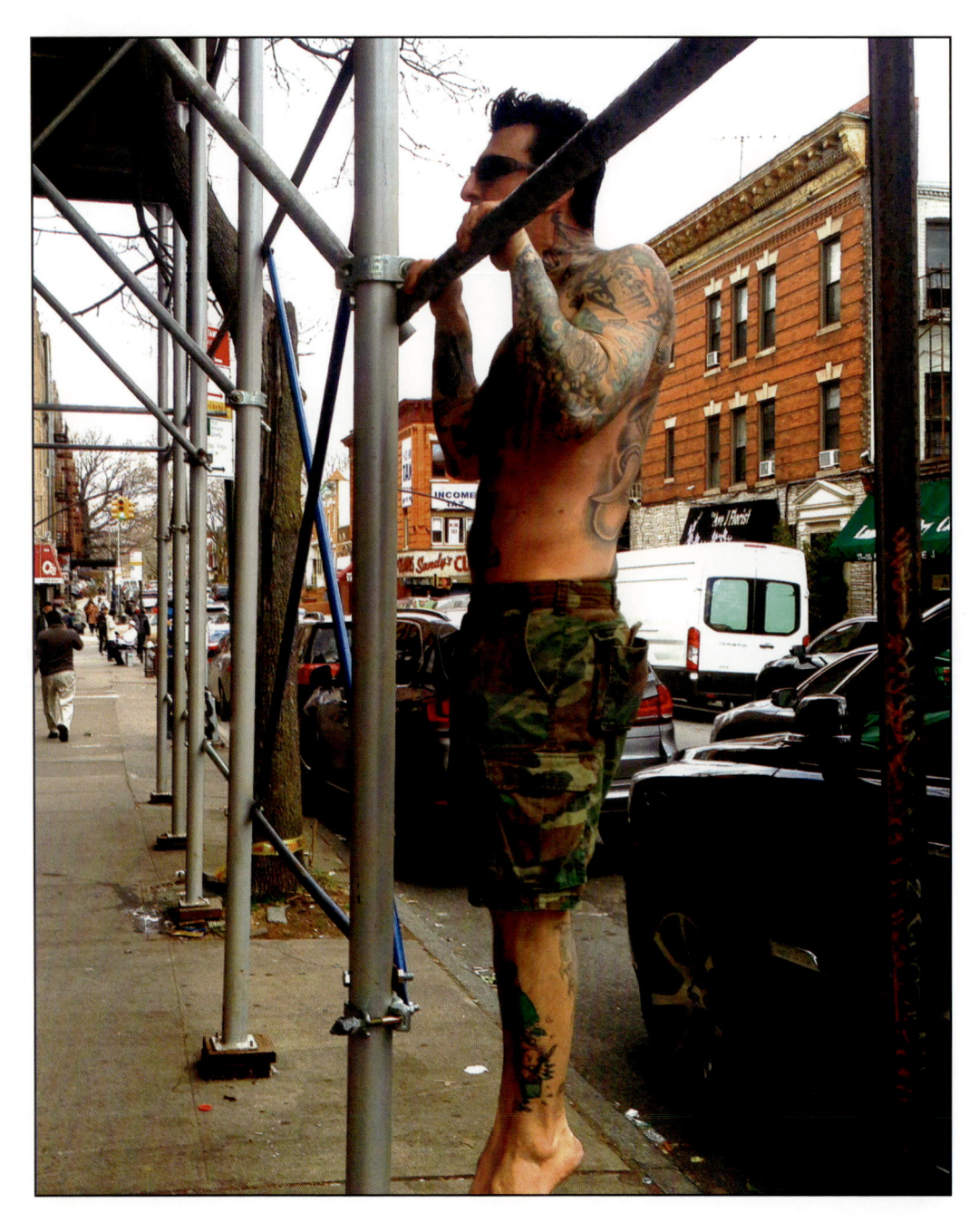

This move, sometimes known as an "ice cream maker," can help you get a feel for the proper alignment of the front lever without having to hold it for very long. As long as you keep your body rigid, using some momentum from the hinging movement at the elbows can help you swing into position, giving you a taste of what holding a front lever feels like.

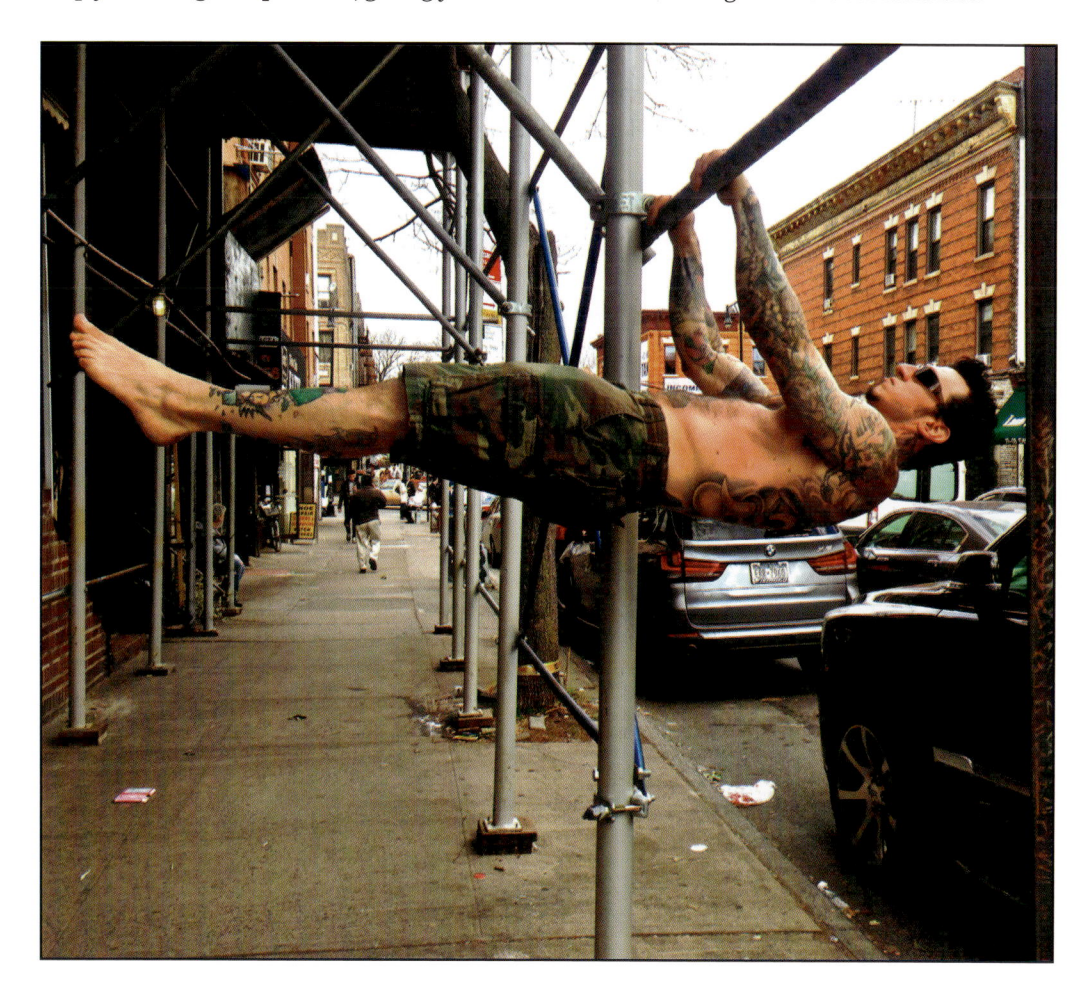

FRONT LEVER PULL-UP

Though a proper front lever is typically performed with the arms straight, hitting a front lever position then pulling your body to the bar with bent arms is a serious and worthwhile challenge. It's almost like an Aussie pull-up with your feet floating in the air.

If you aren't ready for full front lever pull-ups, you can use the tuck, one leg or straddle variations. In fact, these variations can be a helpful accessory exercise on your way to holding a front lever.

When practicing tuck front lever pull-ups, it's helpful to use a parallel bar (neutral grip) set-up like you would for dips. This will allow room for your knees to pass beyond the height of your hands without obstruction.

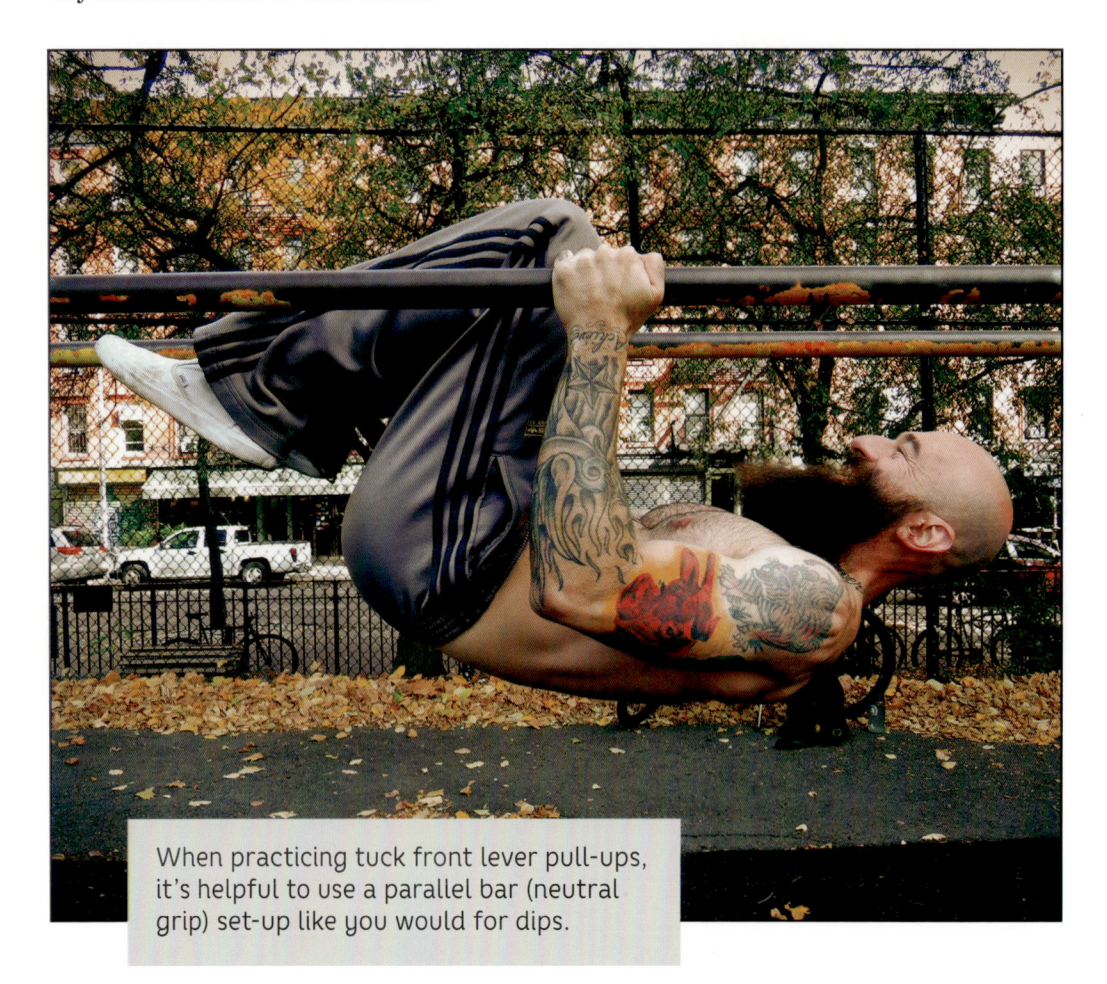

When practicing tuck front lever pull-ups, it's helpful to use a parallel bar (neutral grip) set-up like you would for dips.

THE IMPOSSIBLE POSSIBLE

In the early 20th Century, there was an American Sideshow performer who went by the moniker "The Impossible Possible." He ate fire without getting burned, swallowed swords whole, danced on broken glass and hammered nails into his eye sockets. Sounds impossible, huh?

It wasn't. Nothing is.

In the world of calisthenics, there are some moves that people consider impossible. Exercises that seem to exist in theory only. When folks speak of the "impossible" dip, they are referring to a parallel bar dip, in which the shoulders are stationary, with flexion occurring only at the elbows and wrists. The rest of the body remains perfectly vertical, perpendicular to the ground. The chest does not pitch forward to any degree. The hips do not hinge. The "impossible" muscle-up is a muscle-up also completely devoid of any bending of the body. No maneuvering around the bar; no feet coming out front; no leaning forward at the chest. And the "CTI" or "close to impossible," made famous by legendary calisthenics practitioner Jasper Benincasa, is a bar lever where the performer holds himself upright, away from the bar, arms completely extended and parallel to the ground, straight in front of the body. Although you may never have seen these "impossible" moves in person, does that mean they can't be done?

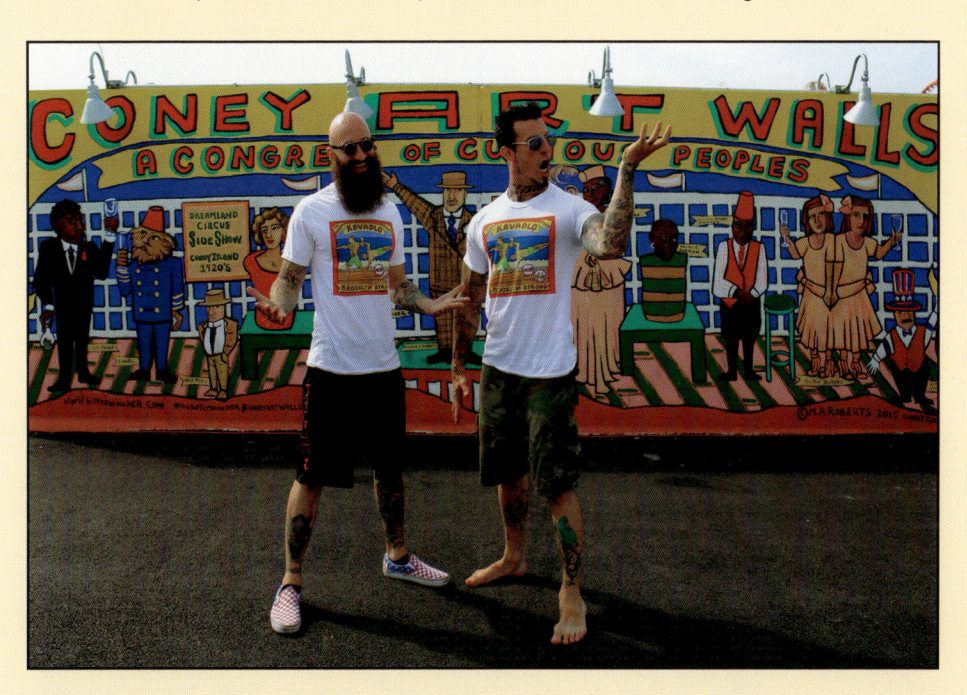

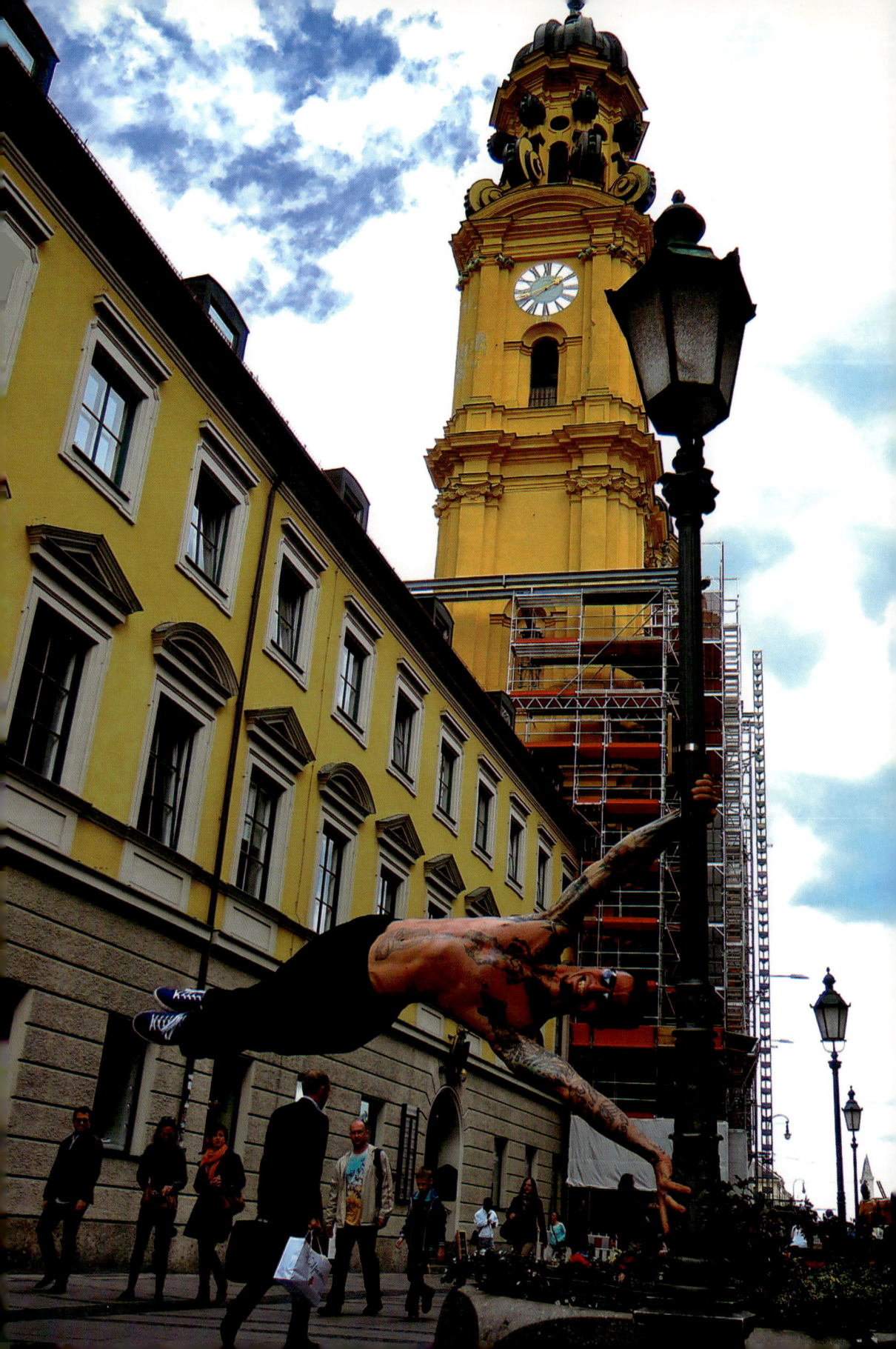

Chapter 11

Human Flag

The full press flag has become synonymous with Street Workout. Try performing it in public and just watch spectators' reactions. Heads spin. Jaws drop. Hearts pound. As anyone who's ever witnessed it knows, nothing attracts a crowd like human flag!

Beyond the amazing visual, there is a tremendous amount of upper body strength needed to perform the numerous types of human flags. Observers often mistakenly think that all the power comes from the lateral chain, but that is far from the truth. Though the sides of the body play a large role in the human flag, beastly arms, shoulders, chest and back are most certainly required, so make sure you have a solid foundation in push-ups, pull-ups and dips. Additionally, the glutes, abs and legs have to work harder than one may think. The flag is also an enormous proprioceptive challenge.

Do you have what it takes?

CLUTCH FLAG PROGRESSIONS

Between the elbow lever and the press flag lies the mighty clutch flag. When you perform a clutch flag, your arms are not over your head; they are clutching the pole against your chest, as you leverage against your elbow. Therefore, the length of your body is shorter than in a full press flag, due to the fact that your head and shoulders are on the other side of the pole.

Although these clutch flag variants are considered to be progressions leading up to the full human flag, as they prime the body in terms of muscular loading, spatial awareness and neurology, the clutch flag is a legitimate force in its own right.

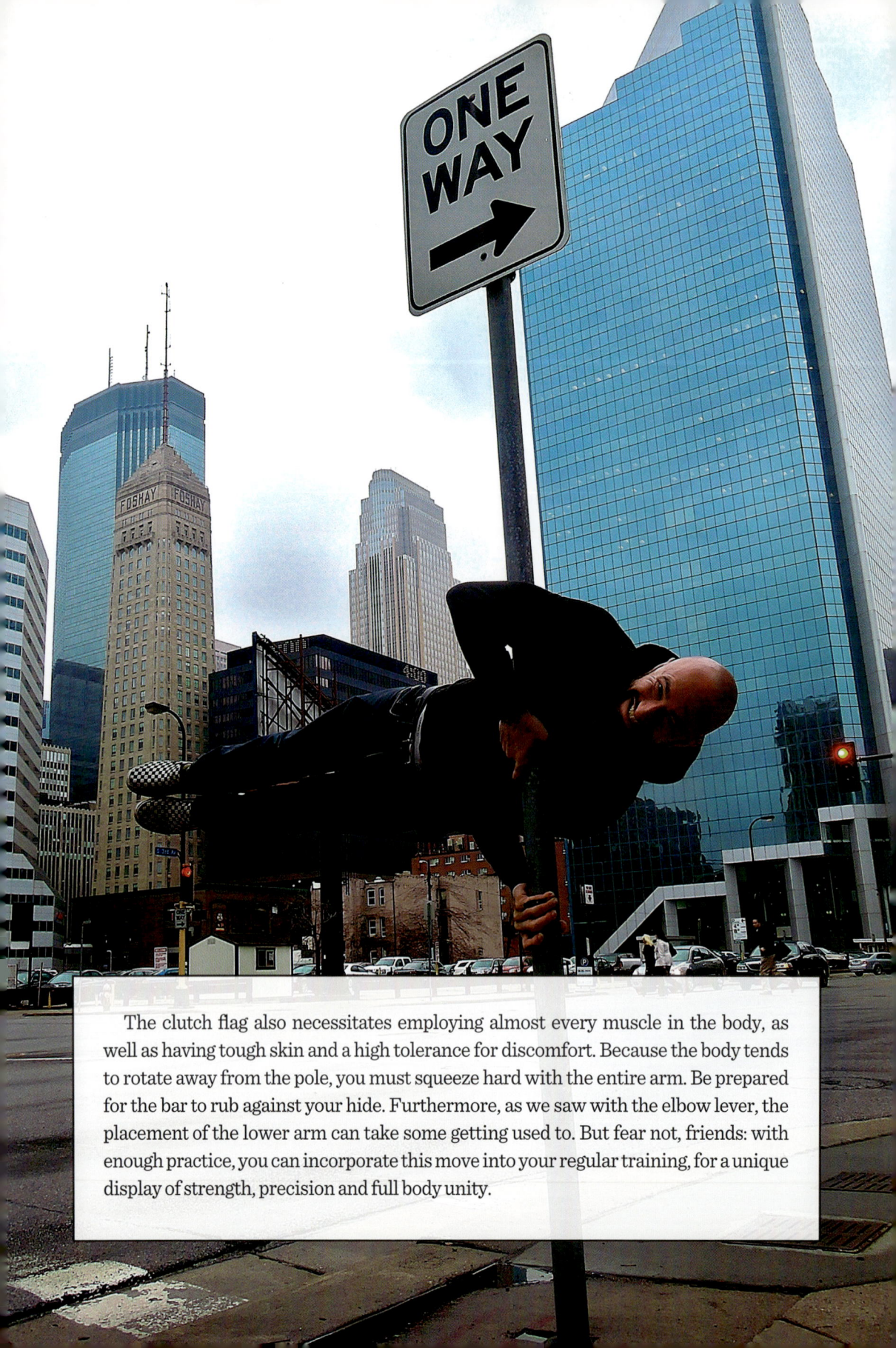

The clutch flag also necessitates employing almost every muscle in the body, as well as having tough skin and a high tolerance for discomfort. Because the body tends to rotate away from the pole, you must squeeze hard with the entire arm. Be prepared for the bar to rub against your hide. Furthermore, as we saw with the elbow lever, the placement of the lower arm can take some getting used to. But fear not, friends: with enough practice, you can incorporate this move into your regular training, for a unique display of strength, precision and full body unity.

SIDE PLANK

The very first step toward performing a human flag is holding a basic side plank. Get into a standard push-up position and begin shifting all of your weight onto one hand. Rotate your body so that your chest faces sideways instead of toward the ground, stacking your feet, ankles and legs as you remove the opposite hand from the ground and reach it into the air. This is a great way to begin training to tense your body in a lateral position.

To make the move more difficult, you can elevate your feet, thus placing more weight in your hand as well as increasing the workload for your trunk by placing your body in a fully horizontal position.

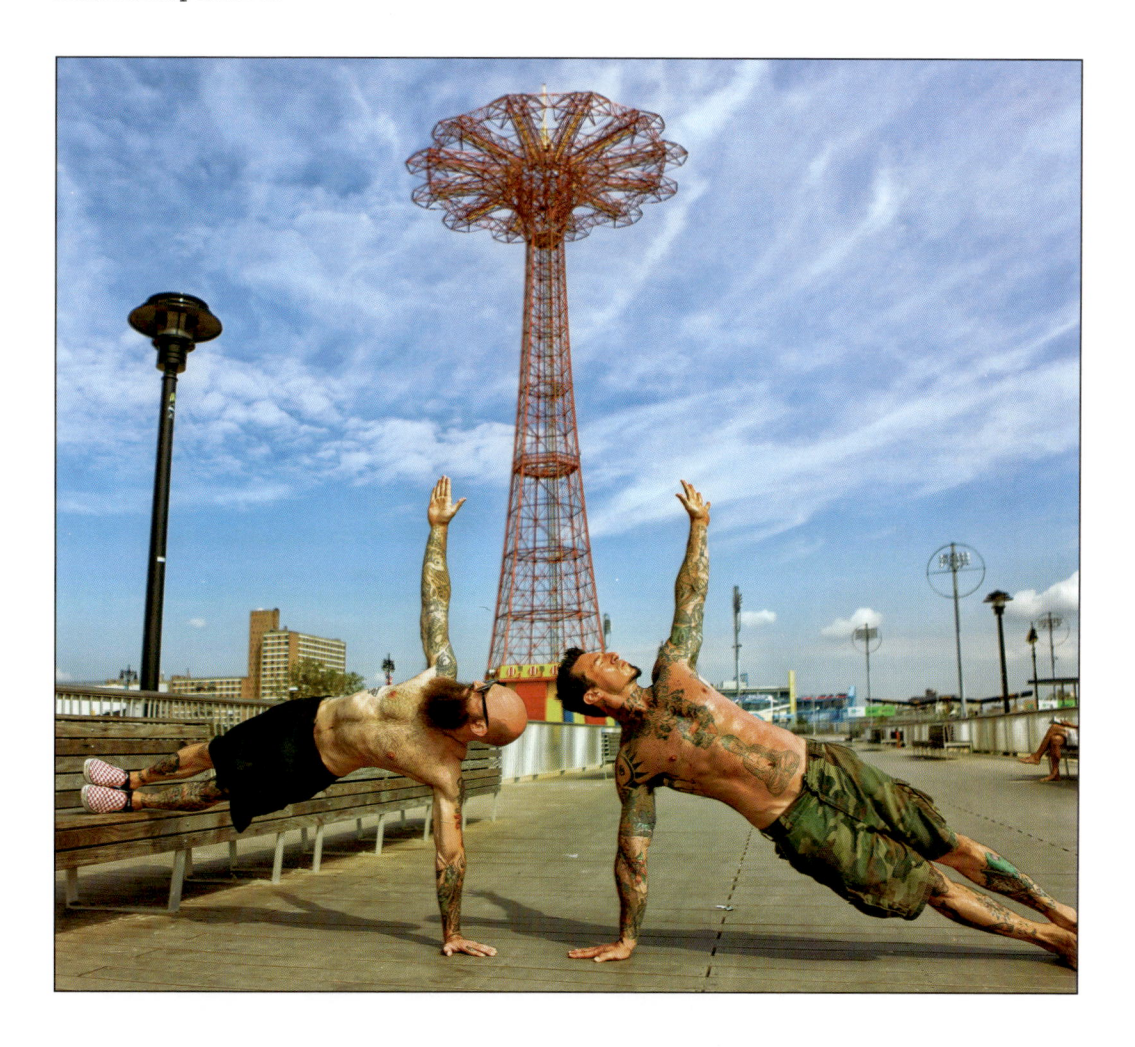

STREET WORKOUT

CLUTCH FLAG ARM SETUP

The following three clutch flag variants all share the same arm set-up, which is crucial for generating the leverage needed to perform the exercise correctly.

Grasp a vertical pole just below waist height using an underhand grip so your elbow points down. Now bend that arm and bring your hip bone to rest on your bottom elbow, similar to how you would for an elbow lever. Reach your top arm around the pole so it winds up in your armpit, keeping your elbow above your shoulder, with your thumb facing down.

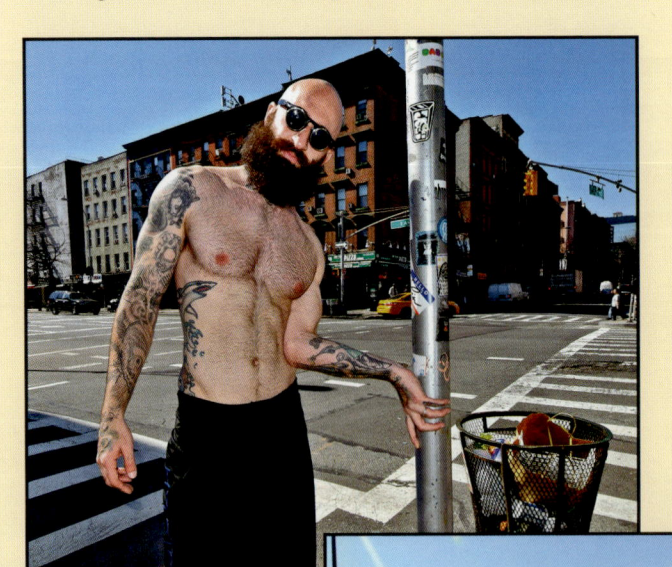

As with the elbow lever, the rotational flexibility needed to get the bottom elbow into the proper position will be a challenge. Use the same "bound eagle" stretch discussed in the elbow lever section to work on this crucial aspect of the move.

LOW HANGING CLUTCH FLAG

Once you've established your arm position, squeeze the pole firmly with both hands. Turn your chest toward the pole and begin shifting your weight off your feet and into your hands. Make sure to maintain contact between your hip and your bottom elbow so you can leverage your torso against your arm. The aim here is simply to get your feet of the ground with your legs hanging low. Knees bent is okay here as well.

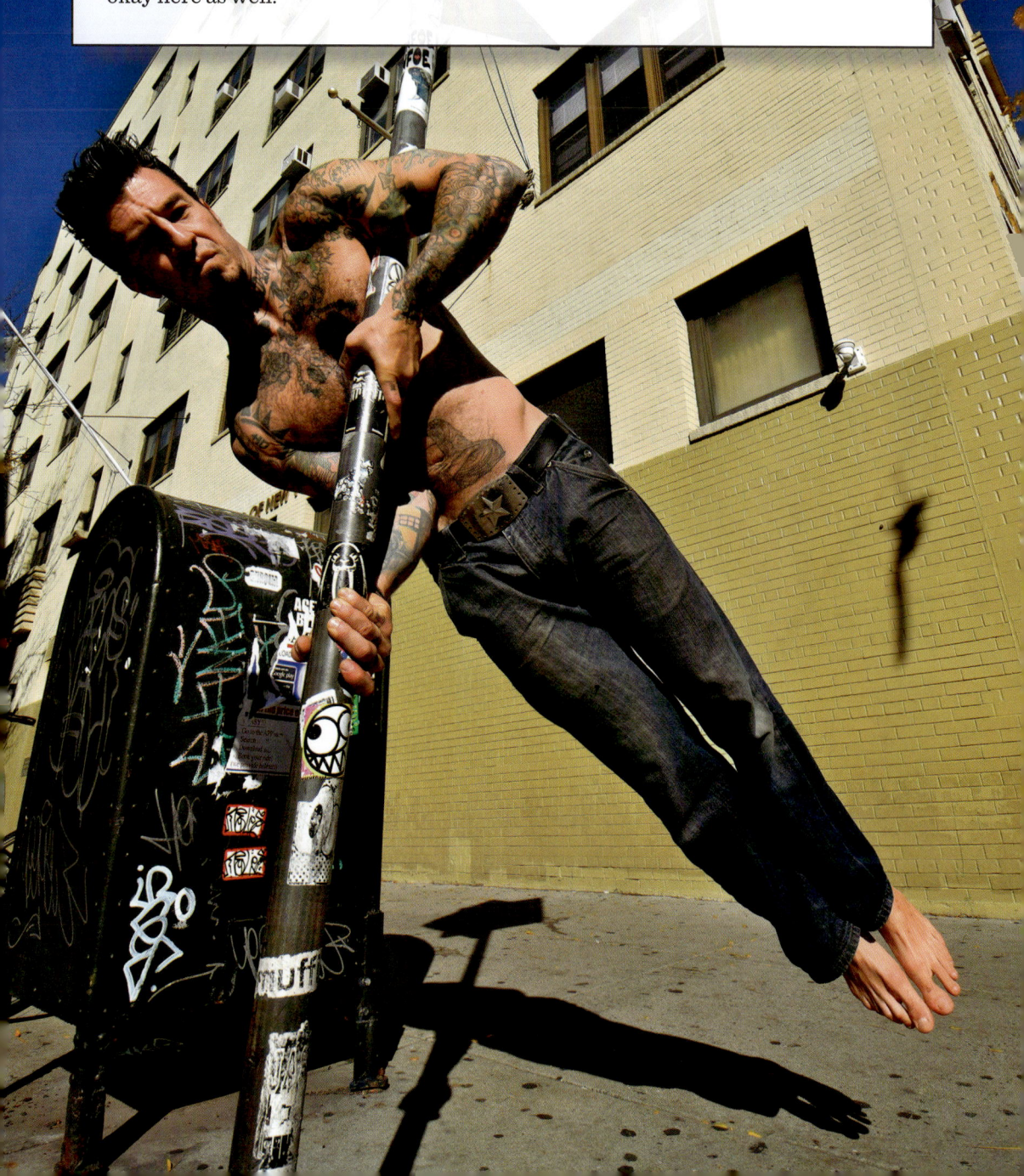

TUCK CLUTCH FLAG

Begin in a low hanging clutch flag, then lift your hips to shoulder level as you tuck your knees toward your chest. By shortening the length of your legs you'll make the move less difficult. The tuck clutch flag is a great way to get a feel for holding your torso completely sideways without having to overcome as much resistance as you need to for a full clutch flag.

Once you get a feel for holding the clutch flag with both legs tucked, you can begin to extend one leg, which is a great intermediate step toward the full expression of the exercise.

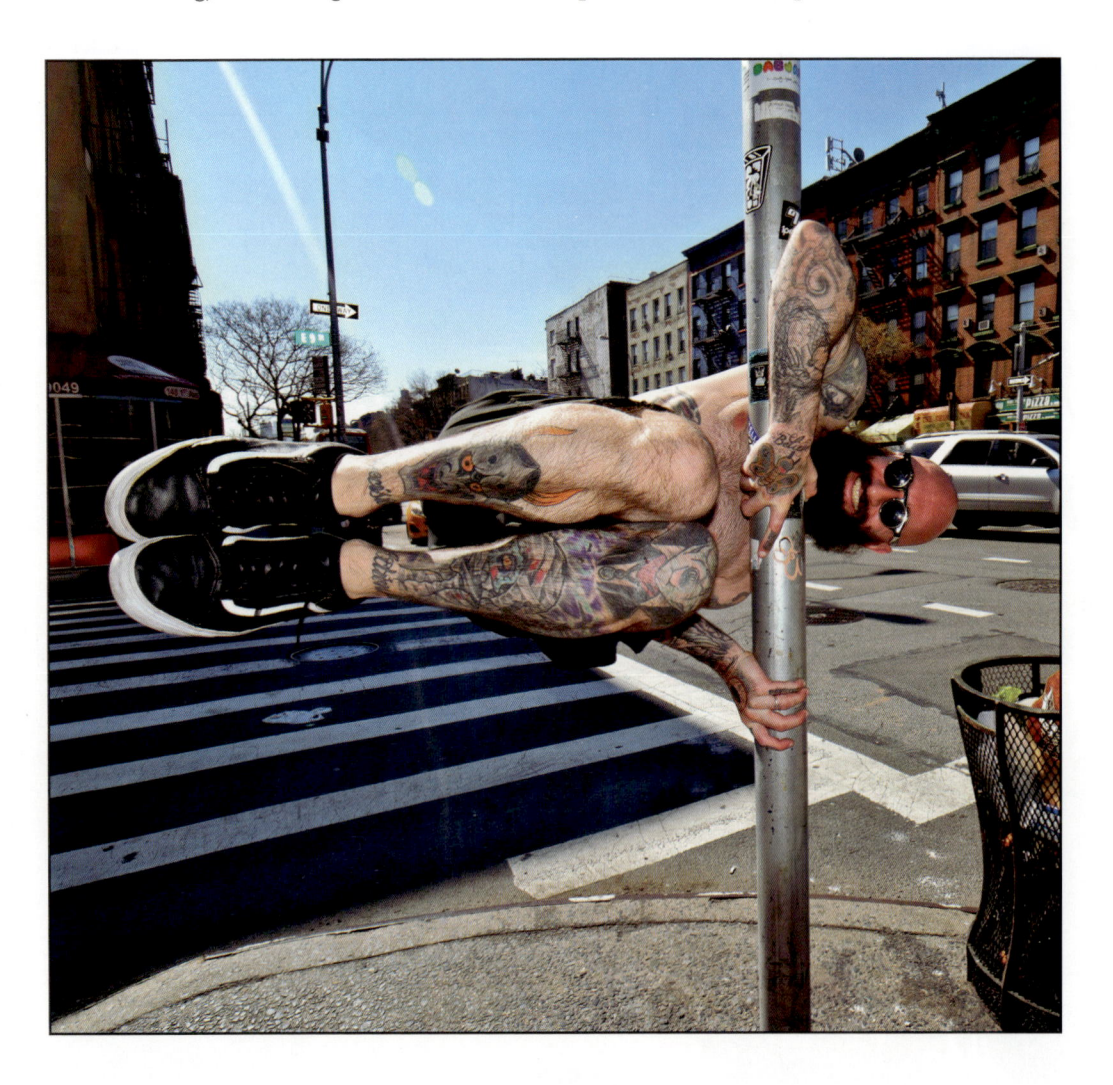

CLUTCH FLAG

Set up your arms as described earlier. Then tense your entire body, shift your weight onto your bottom elbow and squeeze the pole as hard as you can. Focus on keeping your body tense and completely sideways, being mindful not to face downward. This is where the previously discussed shoulder mobility can be an issue. Aim for the pole to wind up pressed flat against your upper chest. Remember to squeeze your glutes and legs.

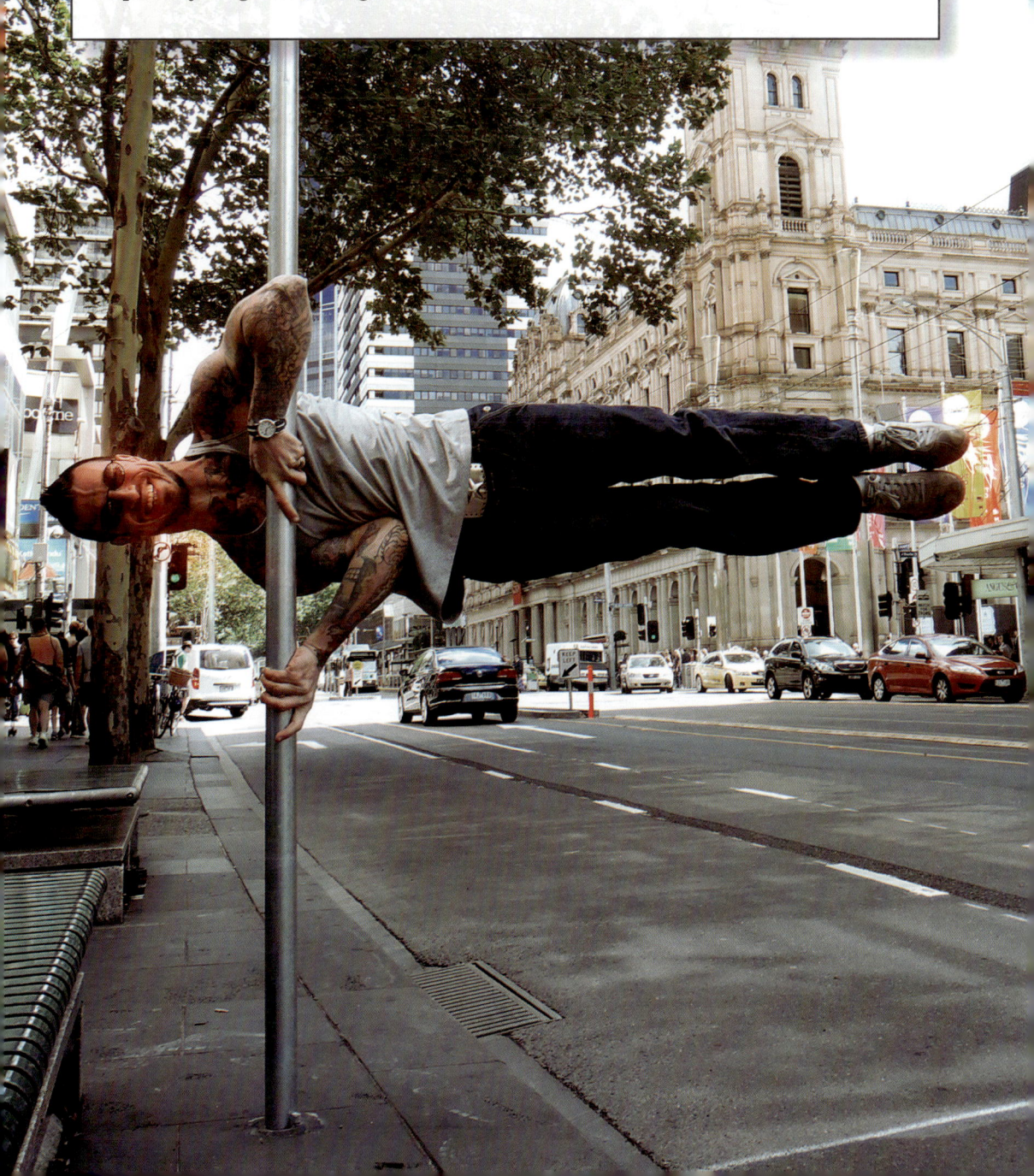

CLUTCH LEVER

You can think of this exercise as a hybrid between a clutch flag and a front lever. Grasp a vertical pole at chest height and reach your opposite arm behind your back, gripping the pole just outside your hip. Squeeze tightly with both hands and lean your trunk back, using your forearm beneath you for support as you lie back into a horizontal position. Allow your top arm to extend as you lean back; feel free to experiment with varying degrees of elbow flexion. Make sure to maintain tension through your entire body and be careful not to lean your weight too much toward the pole. Doing so can cause you to spin out and lose control.

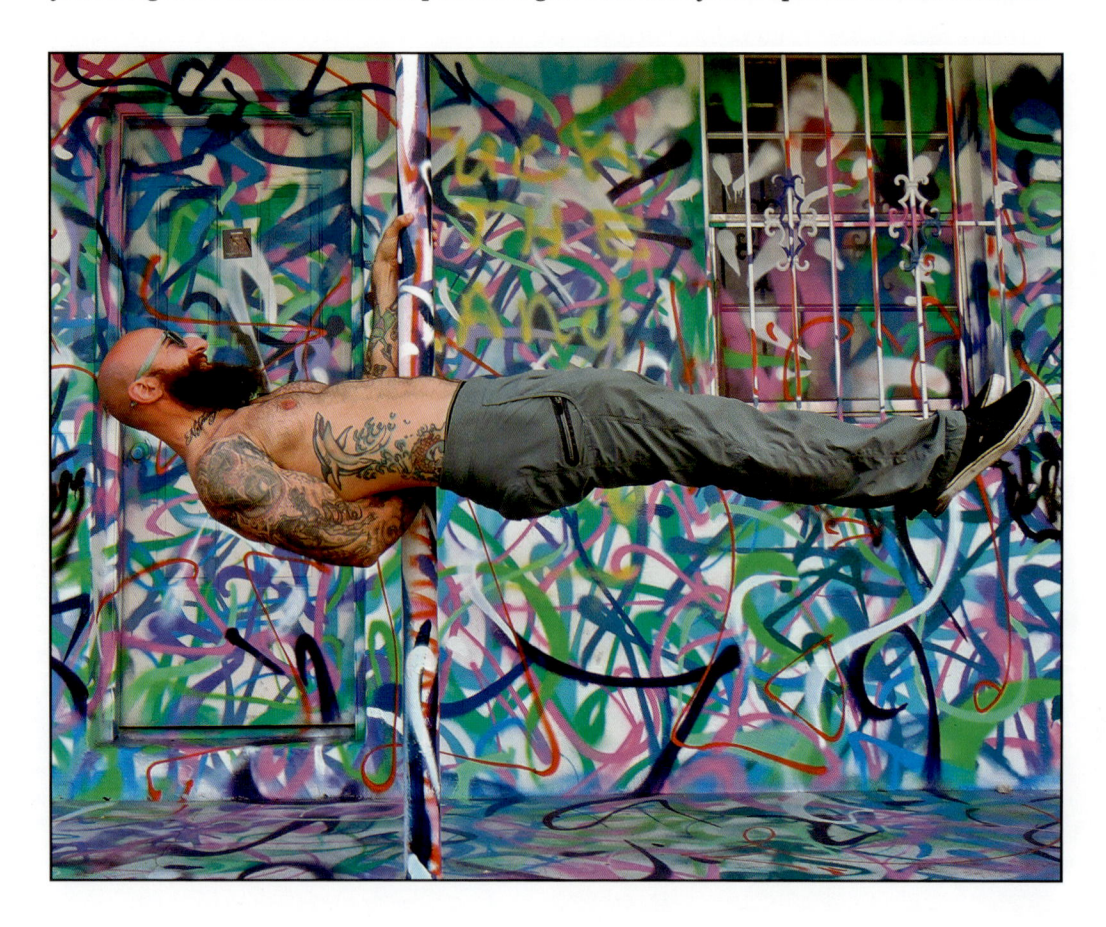

X CLUTCH FLAG

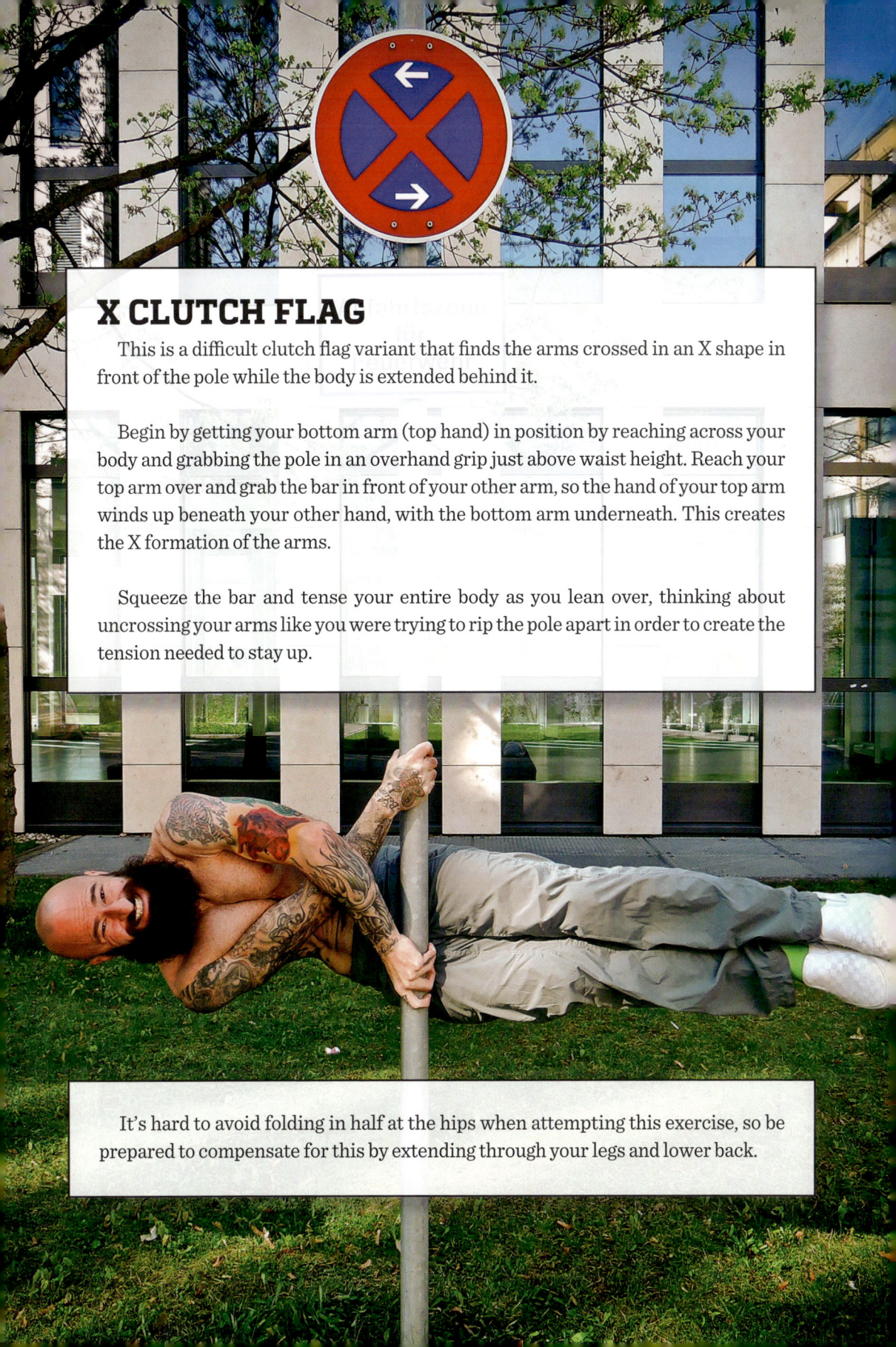

This is a difficult clutch flag variant that finds the arms crossed in an X shape in front of the pole while the body is extended behind it.

Begin by getting your bottom arm (top hand) in position by reaching across your body and grabbing the pole in an overhand grip just above waist height. Reach your top arm over and grab the bar in front of your other arm, so the hand of your top arm winds up beneath your other hand, with the bottom arm underneath. This creates the X formation of the arms.

Squeeze the bar and tense your entire body as you lean over, thinking about uncrossing your arms like you were trying to rip the pole apart in order to create the tension needed to stay up.

It's hard to avoid folding in half at the hips when attempting this exercise, so be prepared to compensate for this by extending through your legs and lower back.

ALTERNATIVE GRIPS

As is often the case with Street Workout, the possibilities are endless when it comes to the clutch flag. Practicing on unique objects and with creative hand positions calls upon your ingenuity and imagination in unexpected ways. Leave it to your environment and your own sense of adventure to continually keep the clutch flag fun and interesting.

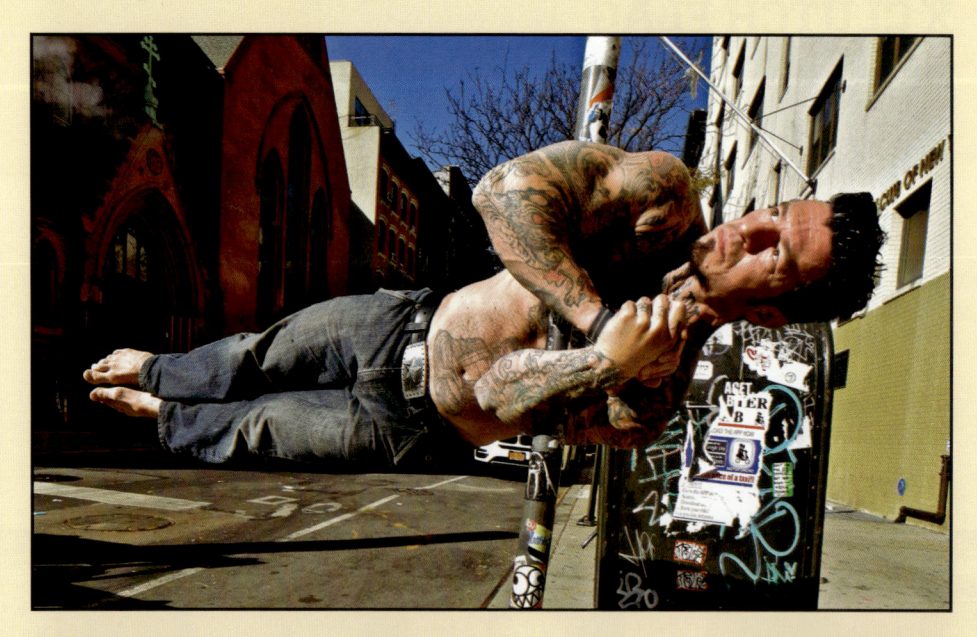

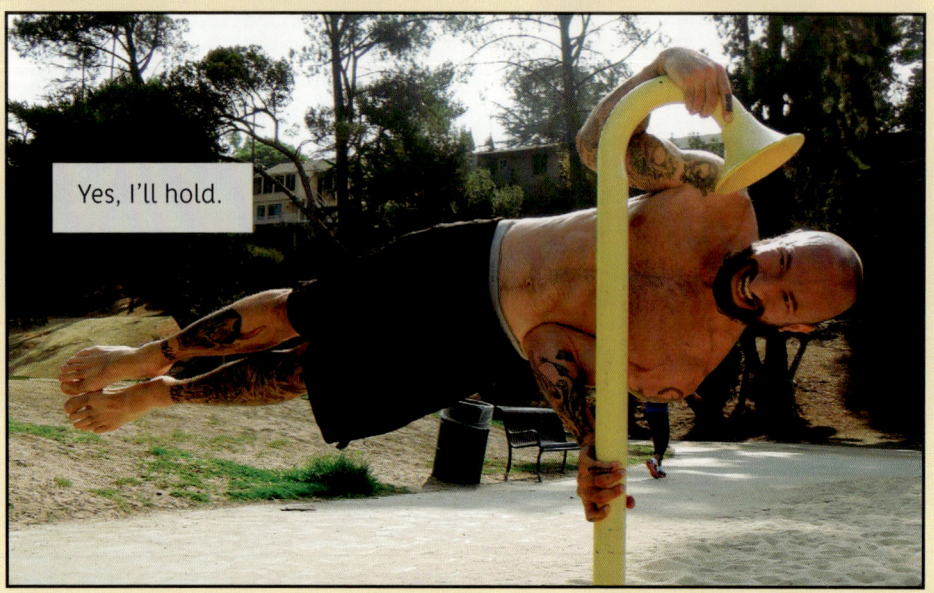

Yes, I'll hold.

PRESS FLAG PROGRESSIONS

Picture a human being suspended sideways on a vertical pole, completely parallel, elbows locked, with no points of contact other than their own two hands. Mind-blowing. Riveting. Spellbinding. Whether you saw it at the playground or on YouTube, no one can forget the first time they witnessed this feat of super-human strength. The combination of power, precision and control never fails to leave an indelible impression.

Spatially, the press flag is entirely its own entity, so be prepared for some trial and error. Though the idea is to perform the press flag as a static hold, you will have to overcome many opposing forces. The body doesn't just move up and down or front to back. It actually rotates against the pole. This torqueing or twisting of the flagger himself is a challenge in its own right. Counter this by squeezing the pole extra tightly and maintaining tension in your entire body including your abs, glutes and even your legs, not just the upper body. You must learn to use every muscle together. Take your time with these progressions. The human flag can take years to attain and a lifetime to master. Train hard and have fun with it. Get ready to let your freak flag fly!

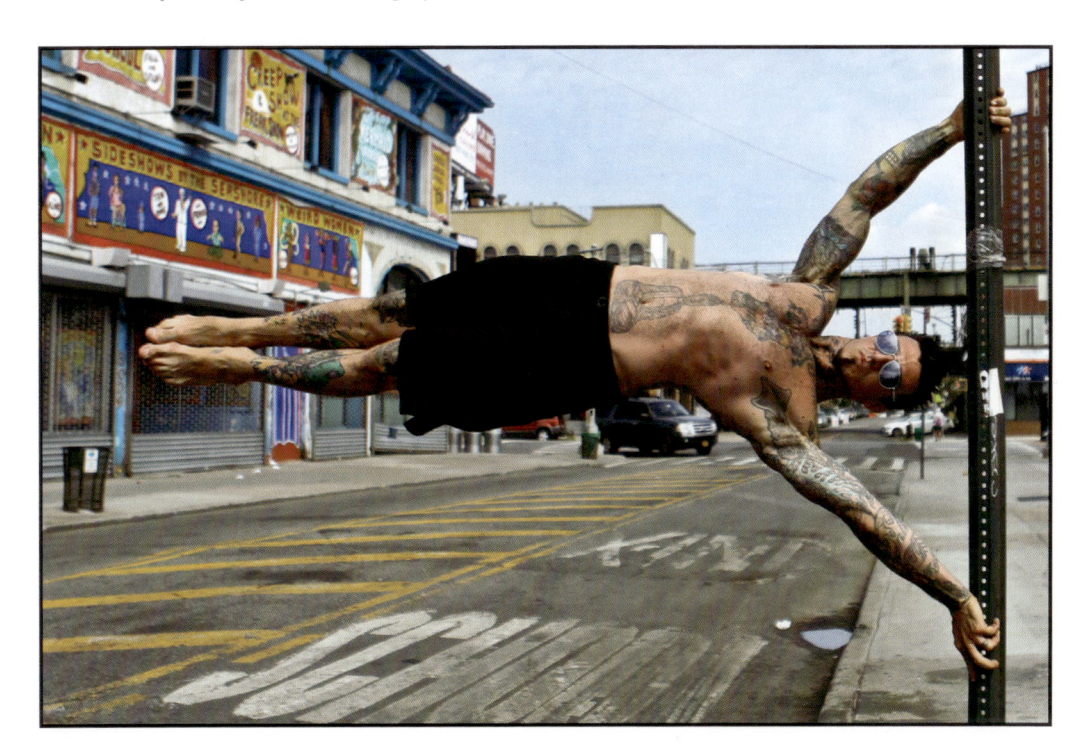

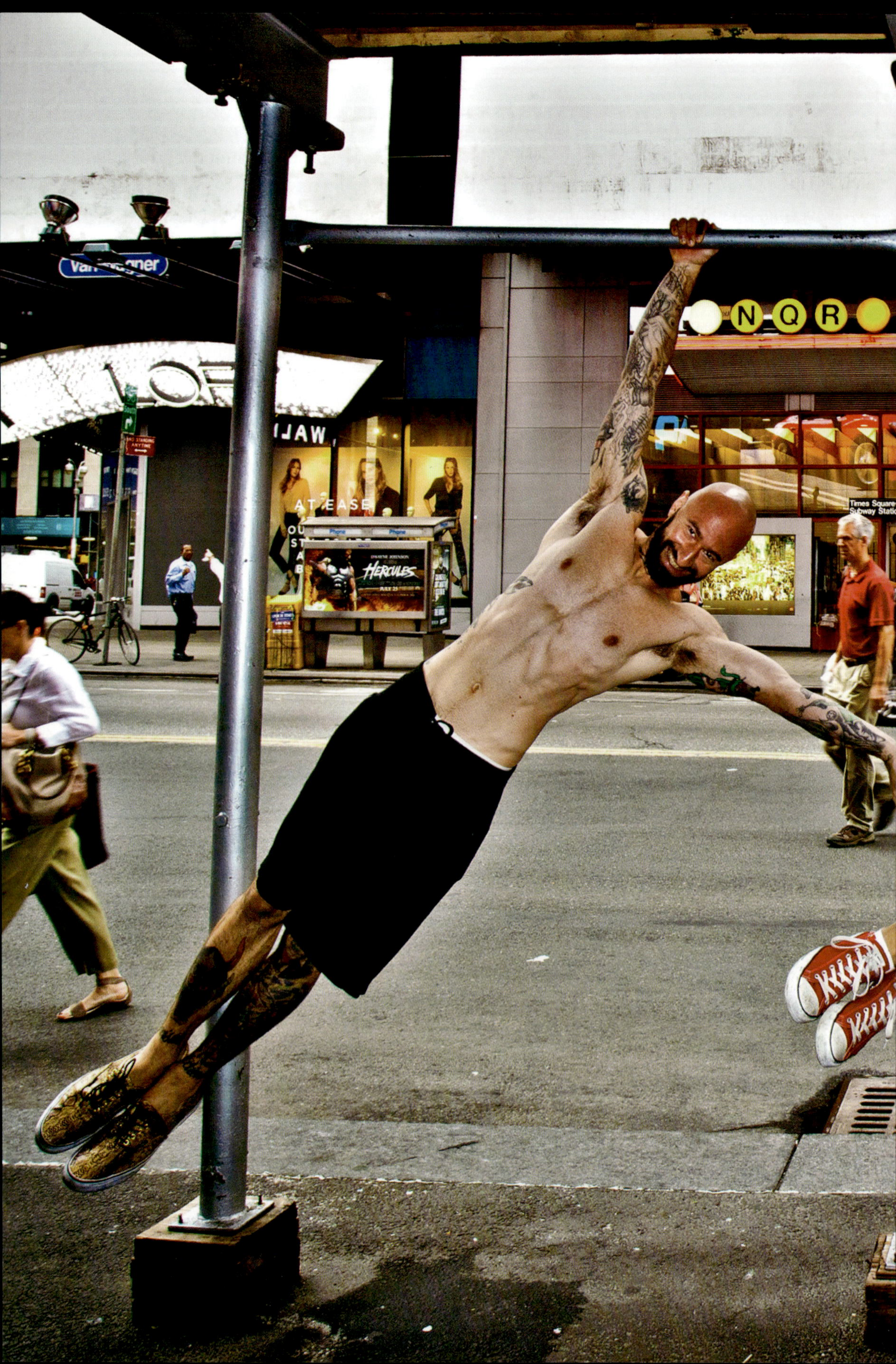
N Q R
Times Square
Subway Station
AT EASE
Phone
HERCULES

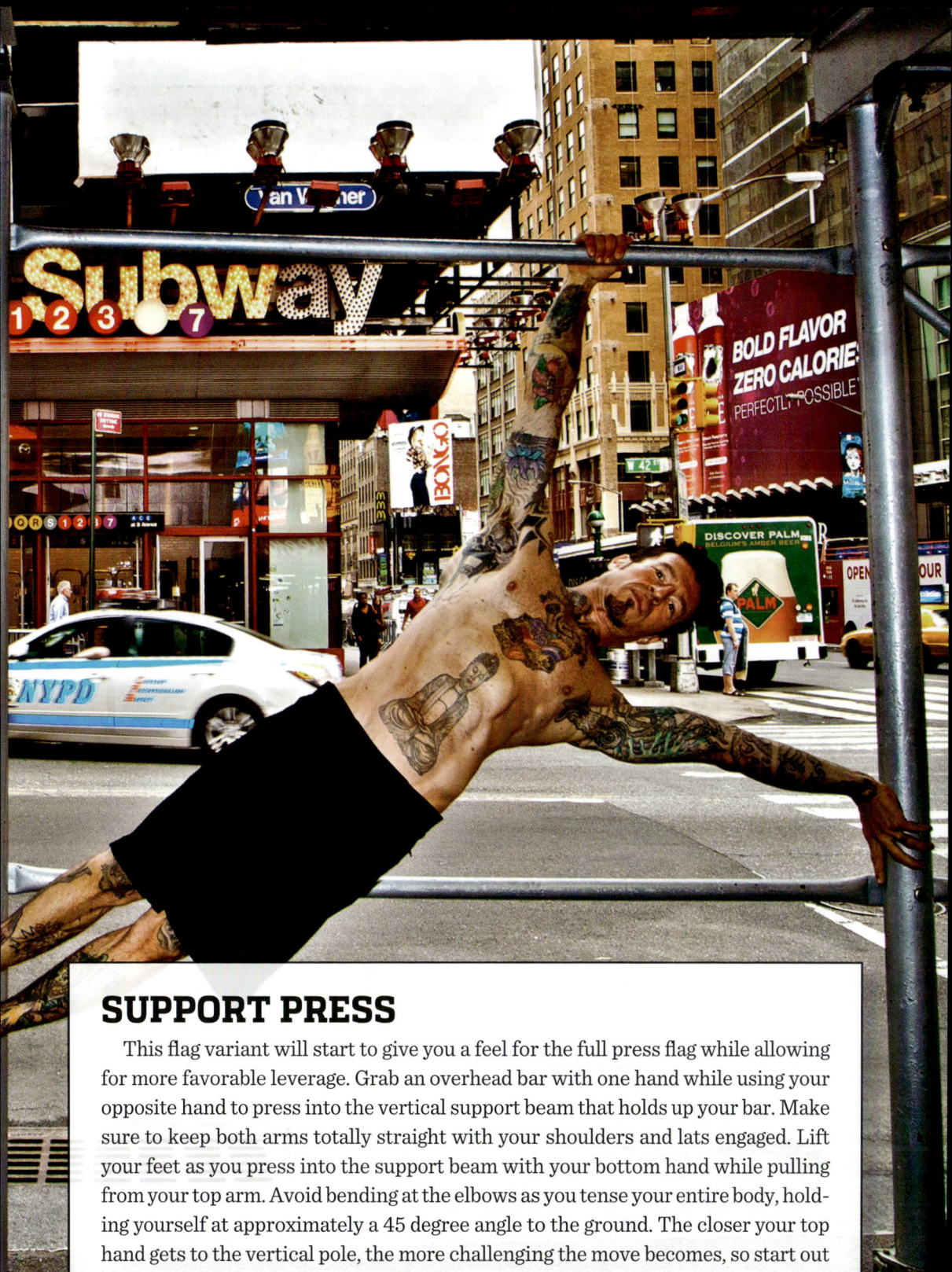

SUPPORT PRESS

This flag variant will start to give you a feel for the full press flag while allowing for more favorable leverage. Grab an overhead bar with one hand while using your opposite hand to press into the vertical support beam that holds up your bar. Make sure to keep both arms totally straight with your shoulders and lats engaged. Lift your feet as you press into the support beam with your bottom hand while pulling from your top arm. Avoid bending at the elbows as you tense your entire body, holding yourself at approximately a 45 degree angle to the ground. The closer your top hand gets to the vertical pole, the more challenging the move becomes, so start out by placing it fairly far away and gradually work toward getting it closer.

PRESS FLAG ARM SETUP

Most of the following human flag variants will involve using the same grip. Grasp a vertical pole with your top hand in an overhand grip and your bottom hand turned under facing the opposite direction. The bottom arm will be positioned so that the elbow faces downward. This is the foundation of the human flag. The bottom arm's job is to support most of your body weight. To do this, you're going to have to press into the pole as hard as possible. Aim to fully extend your elbow and keep it locked out. It is essential to have a solid grip in order to execute the move properly.

Try to maximize the amount of contact between your hands and the bar. It may be helpful to point your index finger down depending on wrist mobility and bar thickness. Squeeze the pole tightly and straighten both arms.

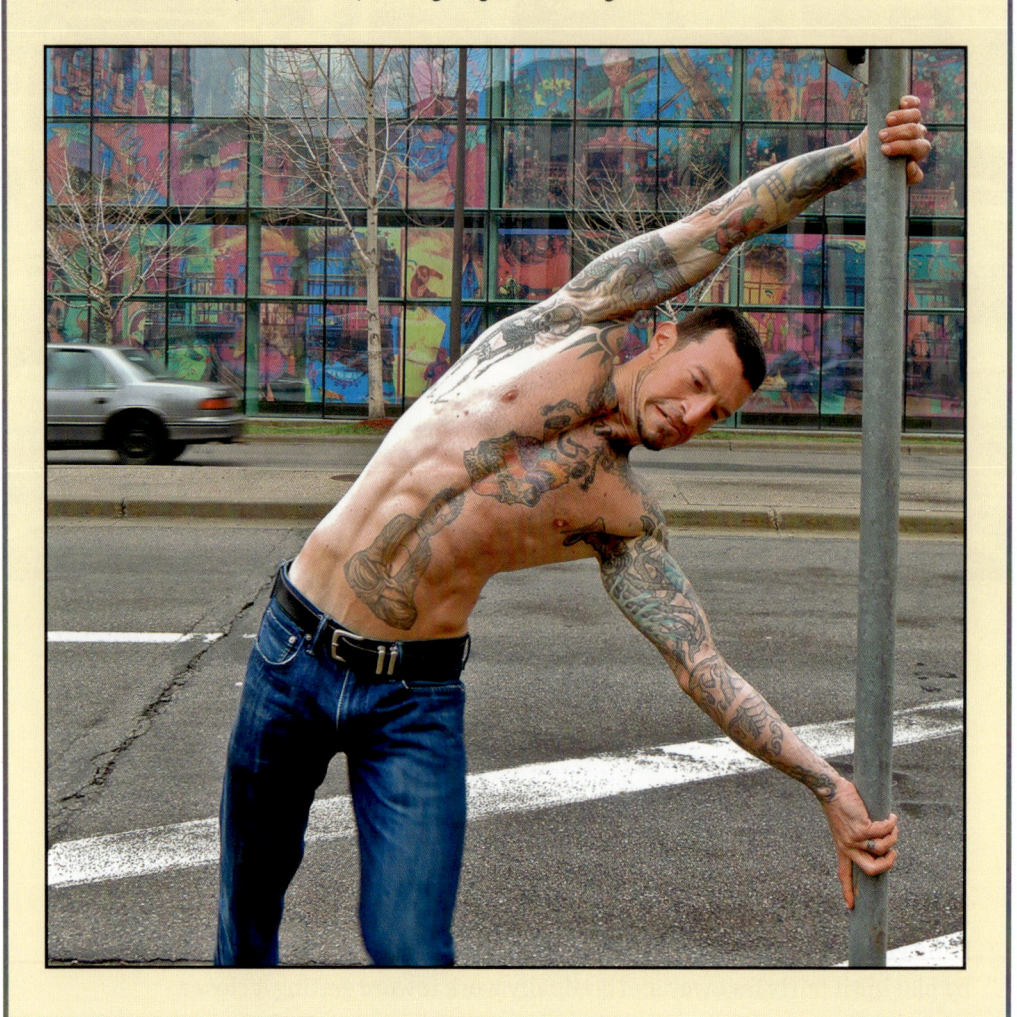

KEEP IT WHEEL

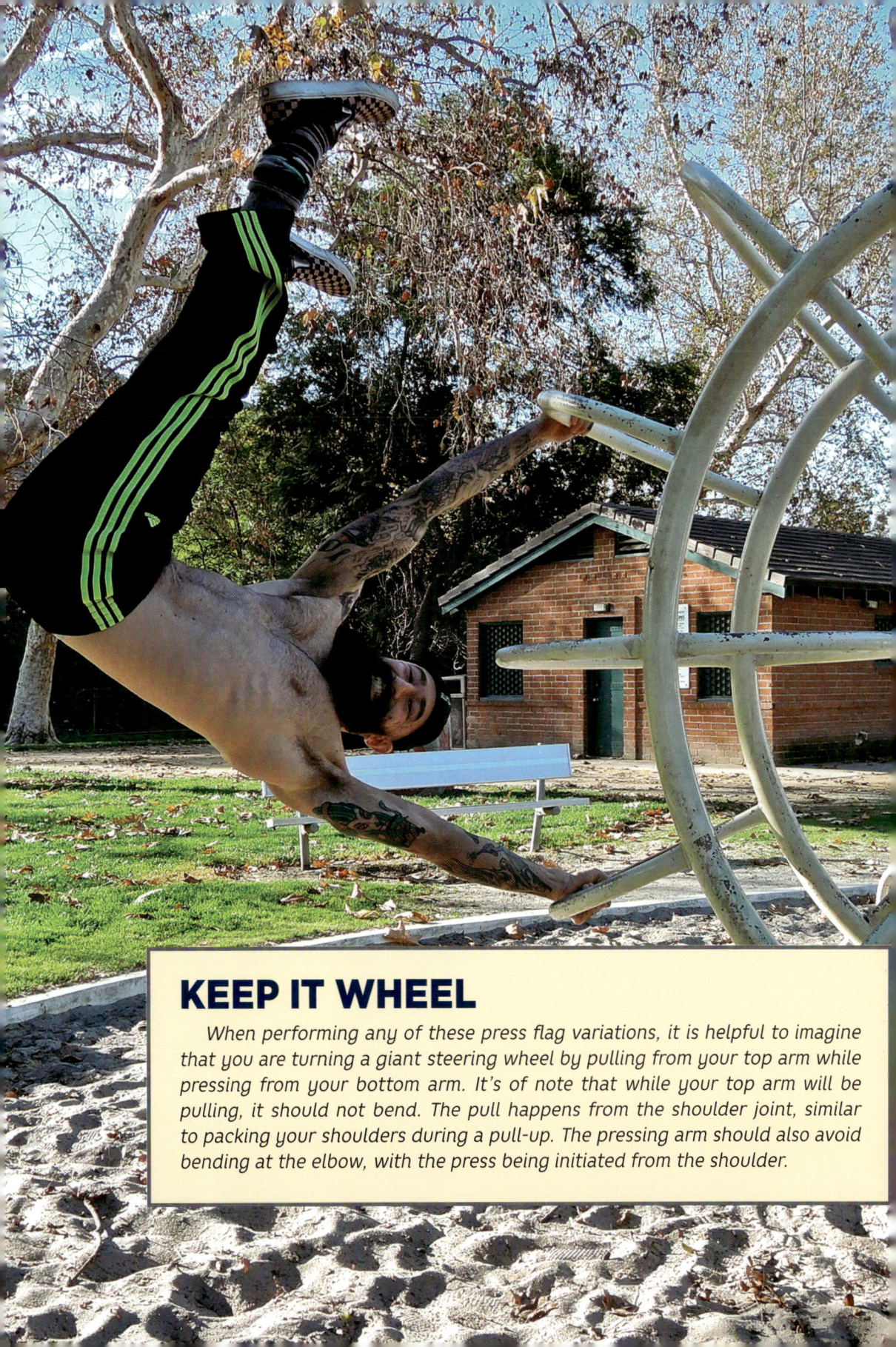

When performing any of these press flag variations, it is helpful to imagine that you are turning a giant steering wheel by pulling from your top arm while pressing from your bottom arm. It's of note that while your top arm will be pulling, it should not bend. The pull happens from the shoulder joint, similar to packing your shoulders during a pull-up. The pressing arm should also avoid bending at the elbow, with the press being initiated from the shoulder.

CHAMBER HOLD

Once you're able to comfortably hold the support press for several seconds, you can begin the transition to practicing with both hands on a vertical pole. As the leverage here becomes significantly more difficult than the support press, we'll be elevating the hips above the shoulders and bending both legs to compensate. Changing the angle and shortening the length of your body will allow you to get a feel for holding yourself sideways against a vertical pole without having to overcome your entire body weight. In the beginning, you'll need to learn to jump and kick your legs to get your hips up, which can take some practice. It's helpful to aim to overshoot the kick up when starting out, as it's higher than it often seems.

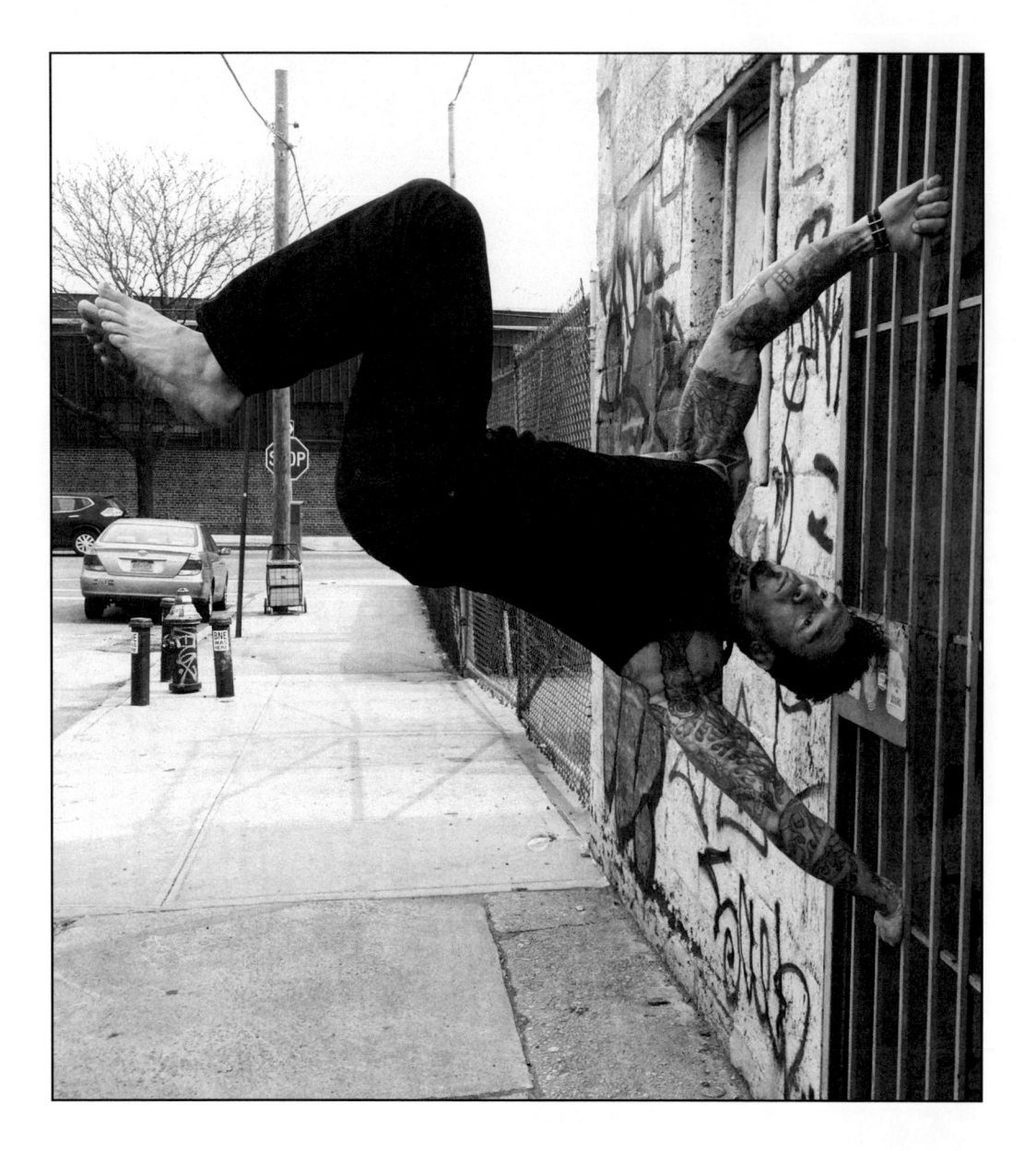

VERTICAL FLAG

After establishing a solid chamber hold, you can begin lengthening the legs to prepare for what it will feel like to move toward a full press flag. For this variant, keep your body closer to vertical than horizontal, almost like a crooked handstand. We'll also allow some leeway here with the elbow position. In other words, if you need to bend your top arm a bit, it's okay in the beginning. The vertical flag requires less strength than a full press flag but starts to give you a taste for the full expression of the move.

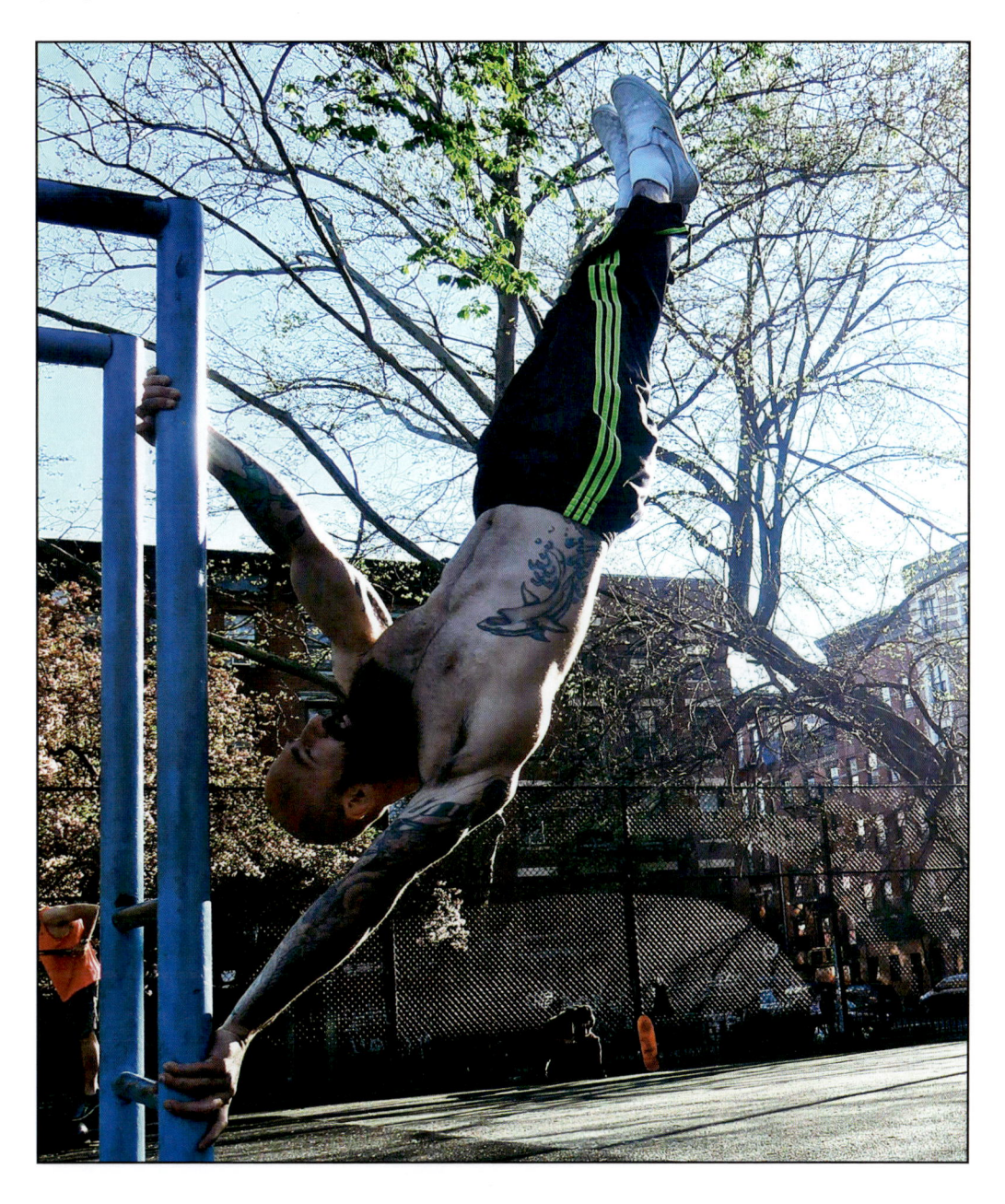

LOW HANGING FLAG

The low hanging flag is a nice step to practice concurrently along with the chamber hold and the vertical flag. Some people may find it less difficult; others may find it to be more difficult. Progressions are not always experienced in the same linear fashion by all.

Just as the vertical flag is less difficult than the full human flag, a low hanging flag incorporates the same principle, only with the legs below horizontal rather than above. Either way, you are closer to the pole, which allows for more favorable leverage. Get your hands in position as previously described, then tense your entire body as you lift your legs, allowing them to hang down while your hips stay below shoulder height.

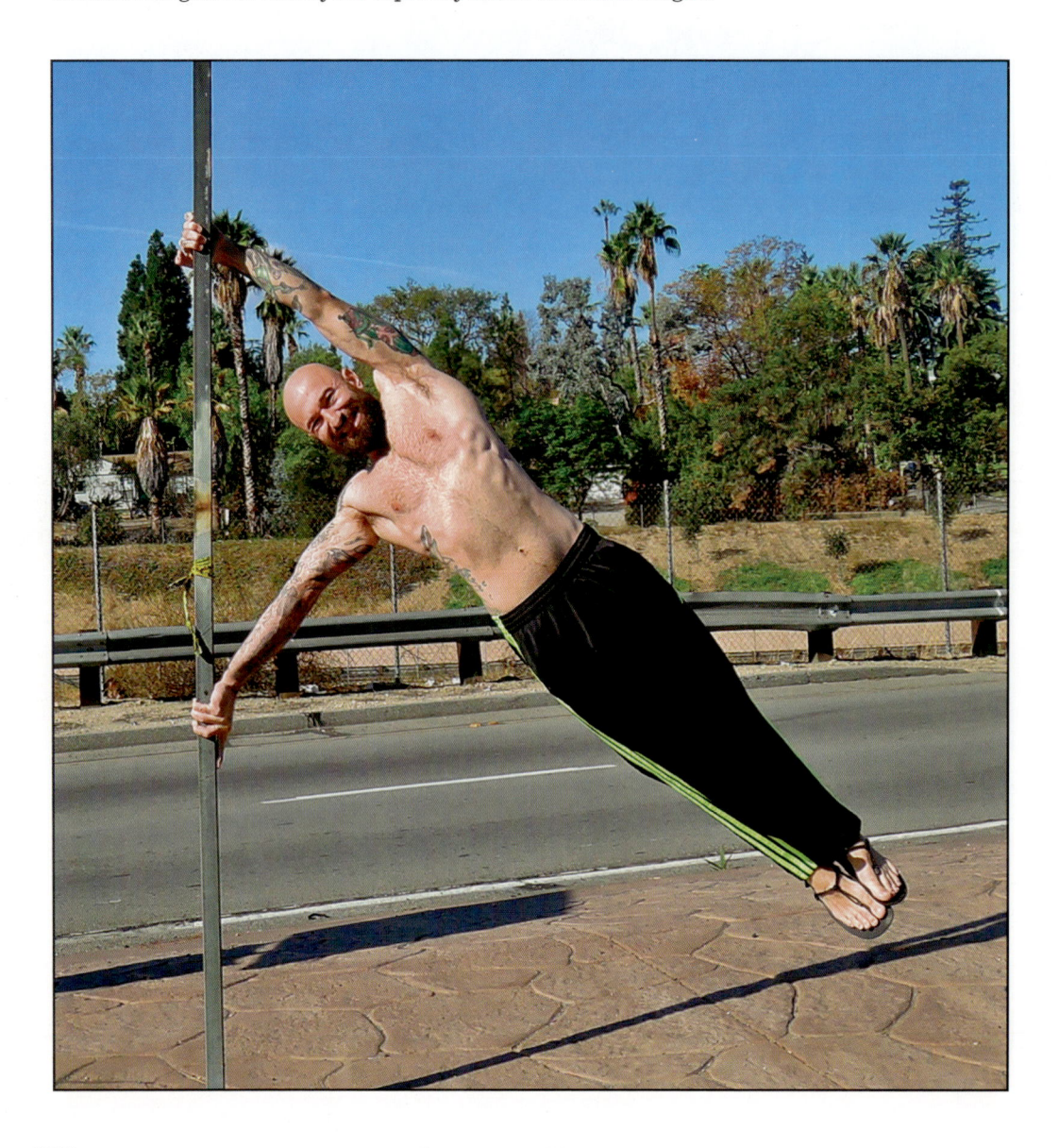

HIGH ANGLED FLAG

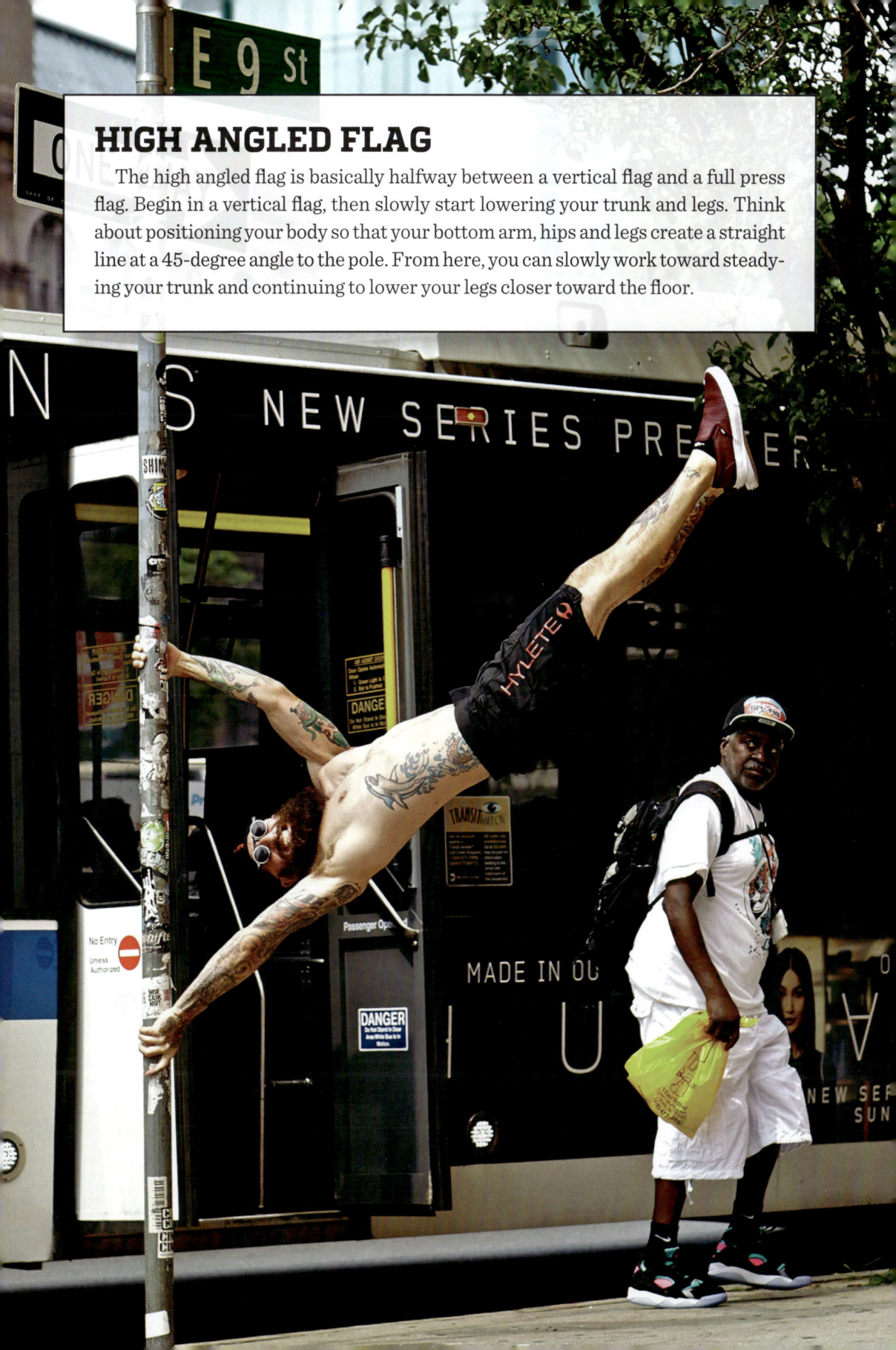

The high angled flag is basically halfway between a vertical flag and a full press flag. Begin in a vertical flag, then slowly start lowering your trunk and legs. Think about positioning your body so that your bottom arm, hips and legs create a straight line at a 45-degree angle to the pole. From here, you can slowly work toward steadying your trunk and continuing to lower your legs closer toward the floor.

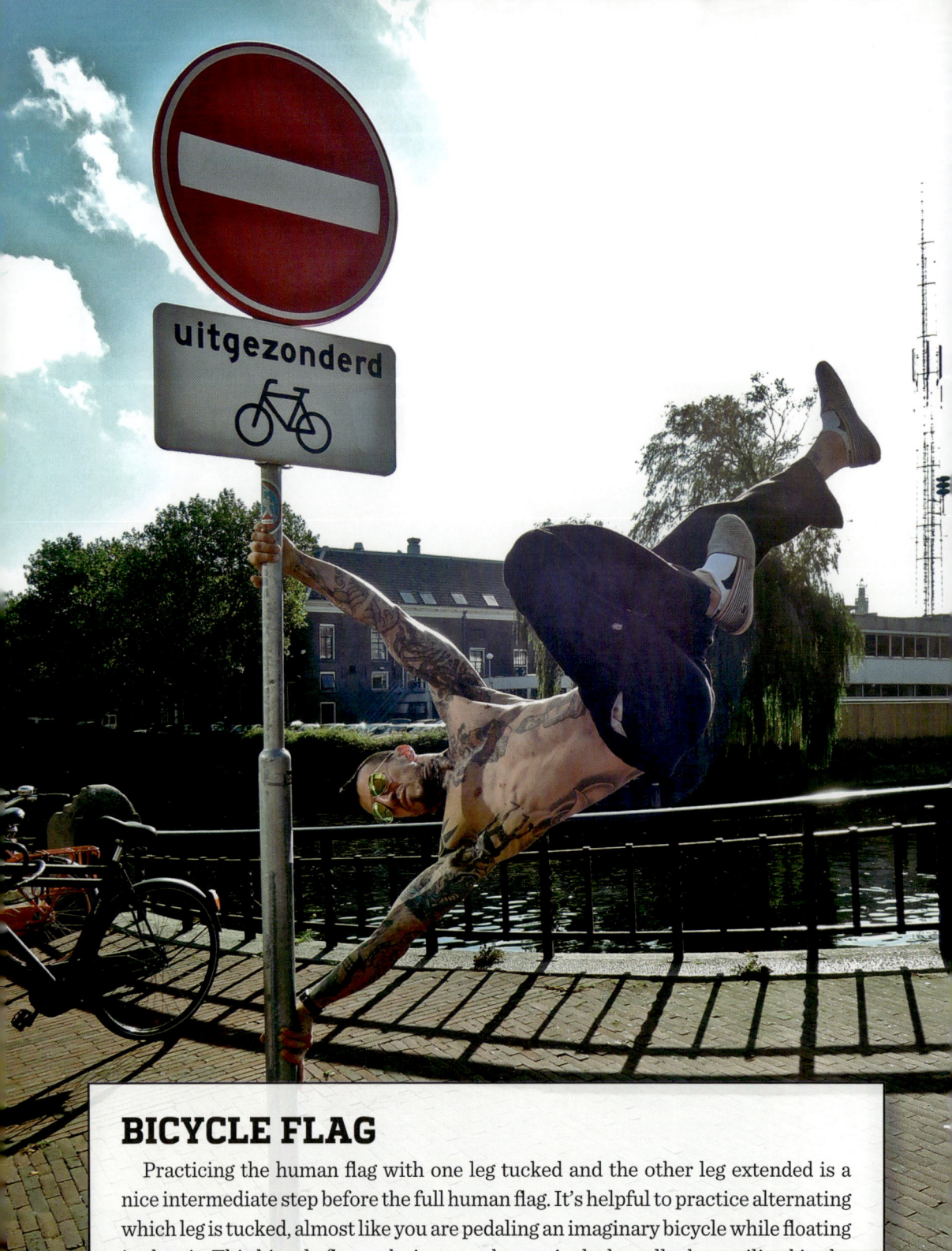

BICYCLE FLAG

Practicing the human flag with one leg tucked and the other leg extended is a nice intermediate step before the full human flag. It's helpful to practice alternating which leg is tucked, almost like you are pedaling an imaginary bicycle while floating in the air. This bicycle flag technique works particularly well when utilized in the angled position.

STRADDLE FLAG

By straddling your legs during a human flag, you can essentially shorten your body length, which will improve your leverage, making the move less difficult. It's a nice in-between step after you can hold an angled flag but before you are ready to move onto the full human flag.

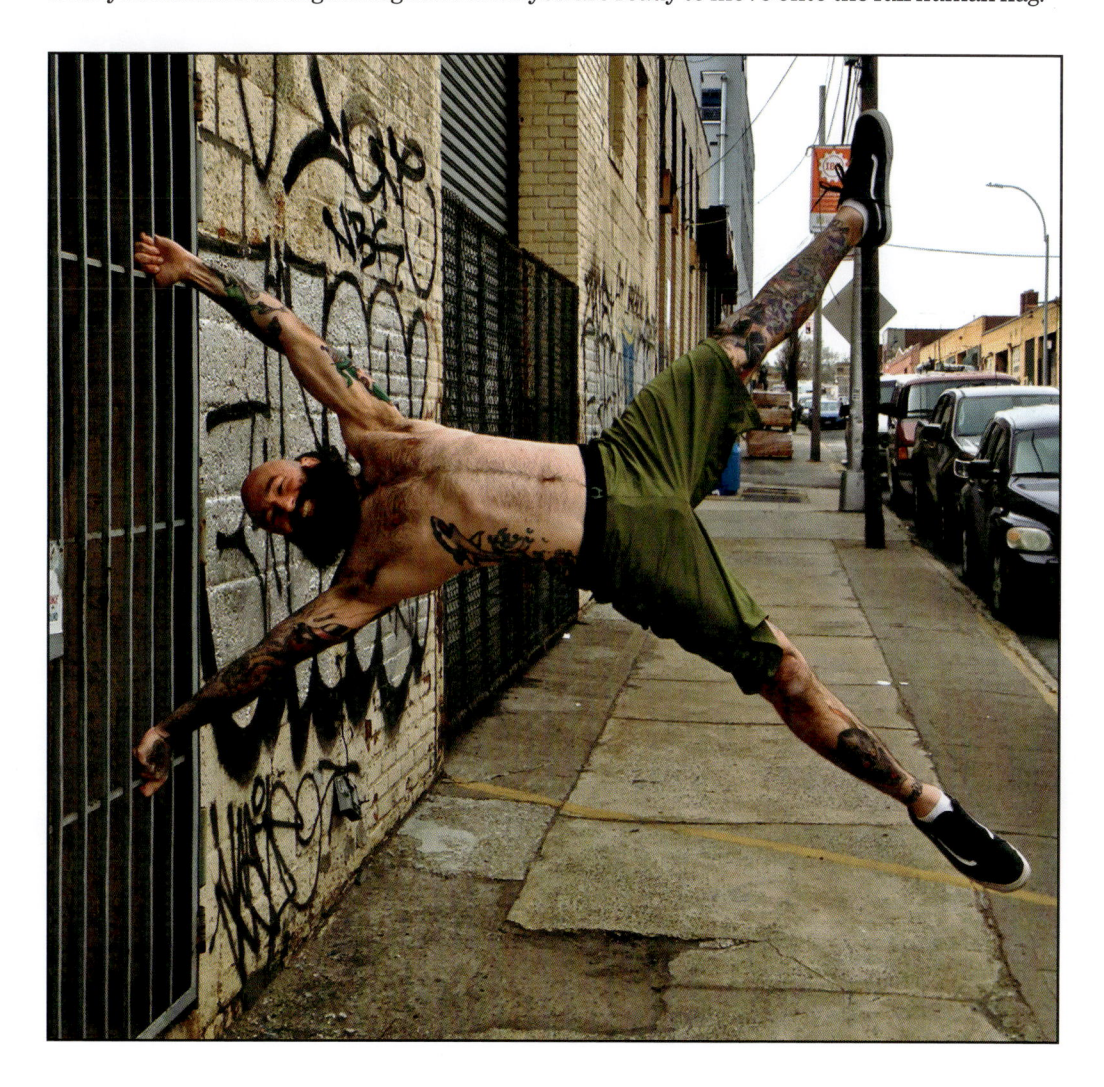

HIGH SUPPORT PRESS

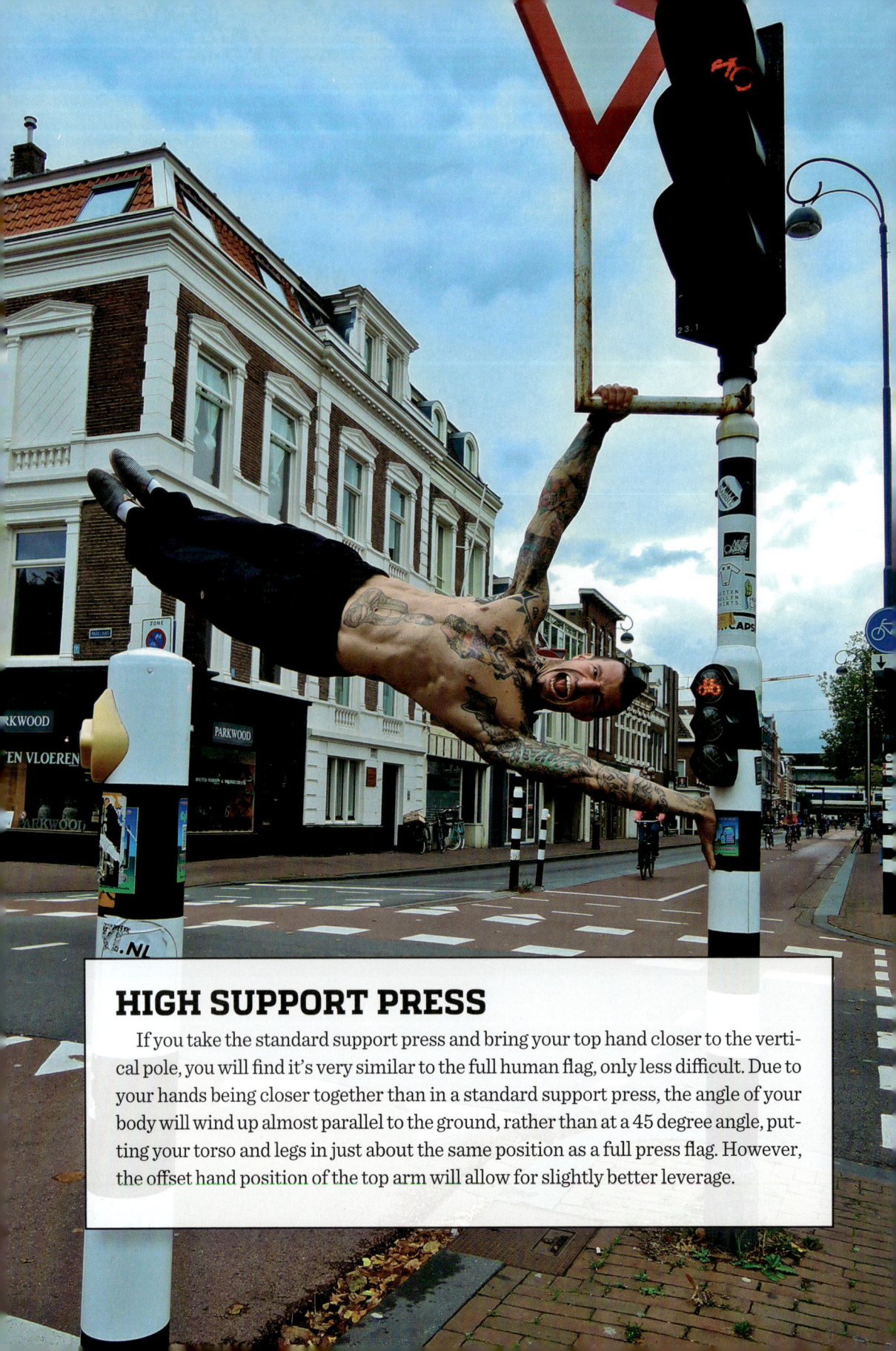

If you take the standard support press and bring your top hand closer to the vertical pole, you will find it's very similar to the full human flag, only less difficult. Due to your hands being closer together than in a standard support press, the angle of your body will wind up almost parallel to the ground, rather than at a 45 degree angle, putting your torso and legs in just about the same position as a full press flag. However, the offset hand position of the top arm will allow for slightly better leverage.

PARALLEL BAR FLAG

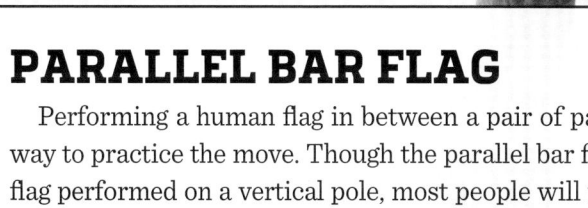

Performing a human flag in between a pair of parallel bars is another fantastic way to practice the move. Though the parallel bar flag appears similar to the press flag performed on a vertical pole, most people will find this variation less difficult. A more stable foundation can be achieved due to the fact that the hands face each other in a neutral grip. Make sure your hands are stacked directly above one another, however, as a staggered hand placement can cause you to spin out of control.

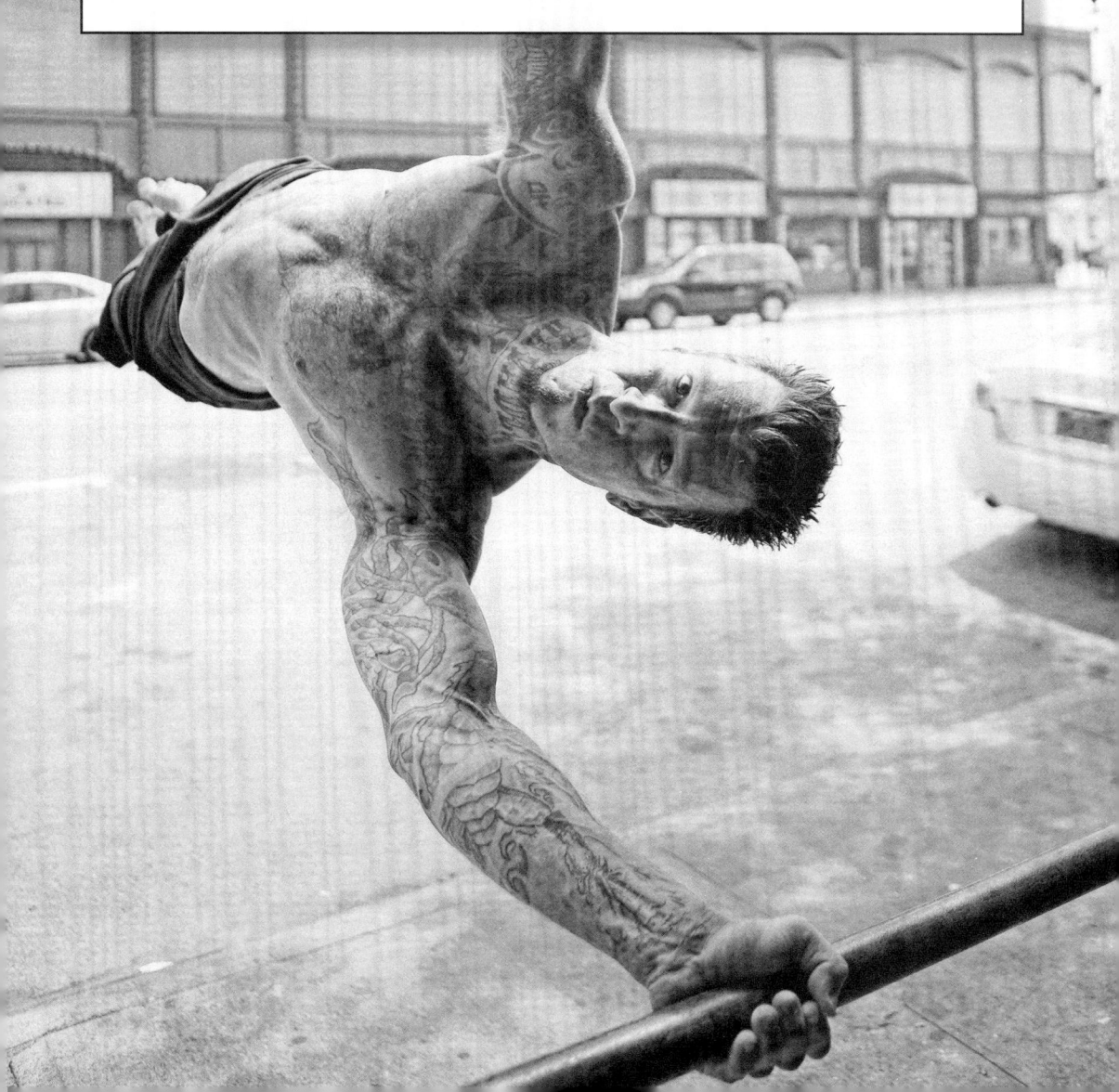

PRESS FLAG

There are essentially two ways of getting into position for your human flag: from the bottom up, and from the top down. For the top down method, which is generally less difficult, kick into a vertical flag, then slowly transition into an angled flag, then a straddle flag, finally closing your legs together after you're locked in position. The idea behind the top down method is to gradually increase the load on your body so that you can prime your neurological system for the full weight of your body being supported by just your two hands on a vertical pole.

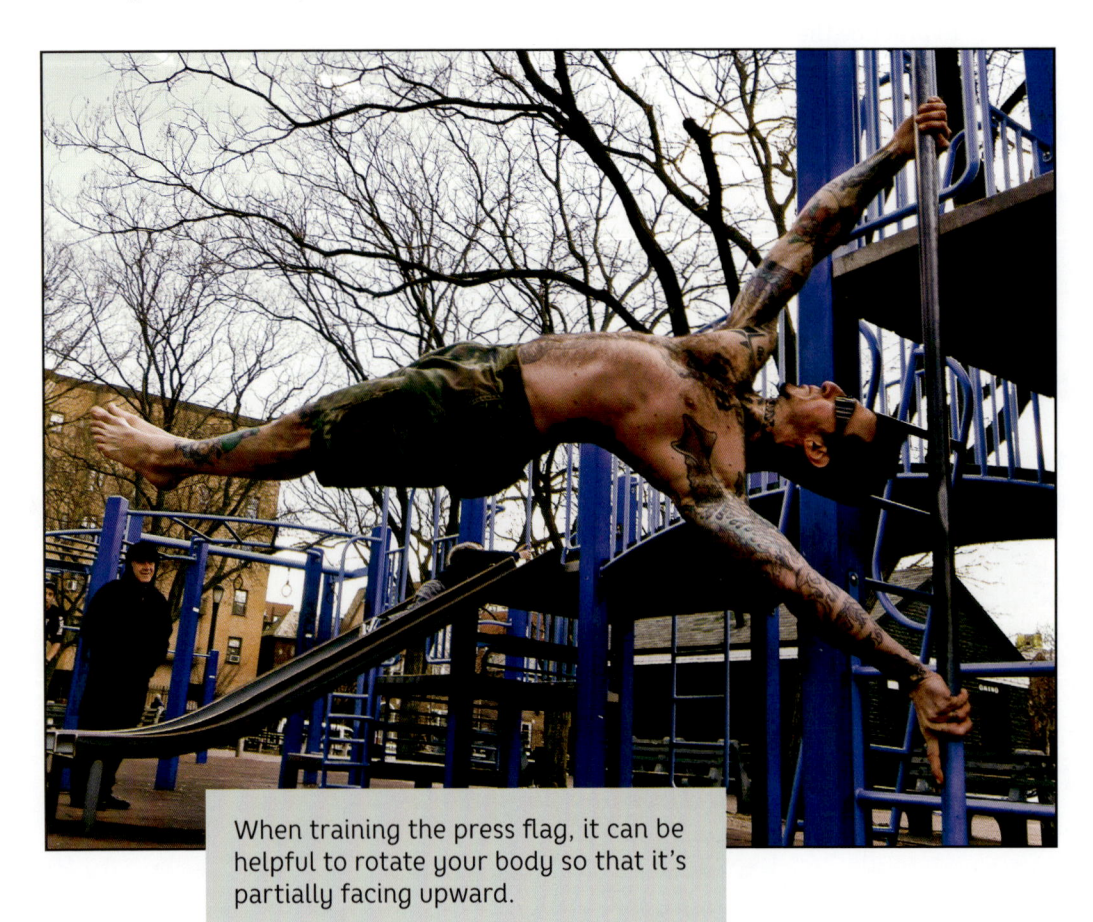

When training the press flag, it can be helpful to rotate your body so that it's partially facing upward.

The bottom up method is more difficult as it involves pressing yourself up into the horizontal position from the floor. Get your grip, then lift into a low hanging flag. From here, lift your hips, pull from your top arm and press from your bottom arm to lift yourself into the horizontal position, keeping your trunk actively engaged the entire time.

When training the press flag, it can be helpful to rotate your body so that it's partially facing upward. This will give you greater support from your spine. In time and with practice, you can work toward holding your flag in the full sideways position.

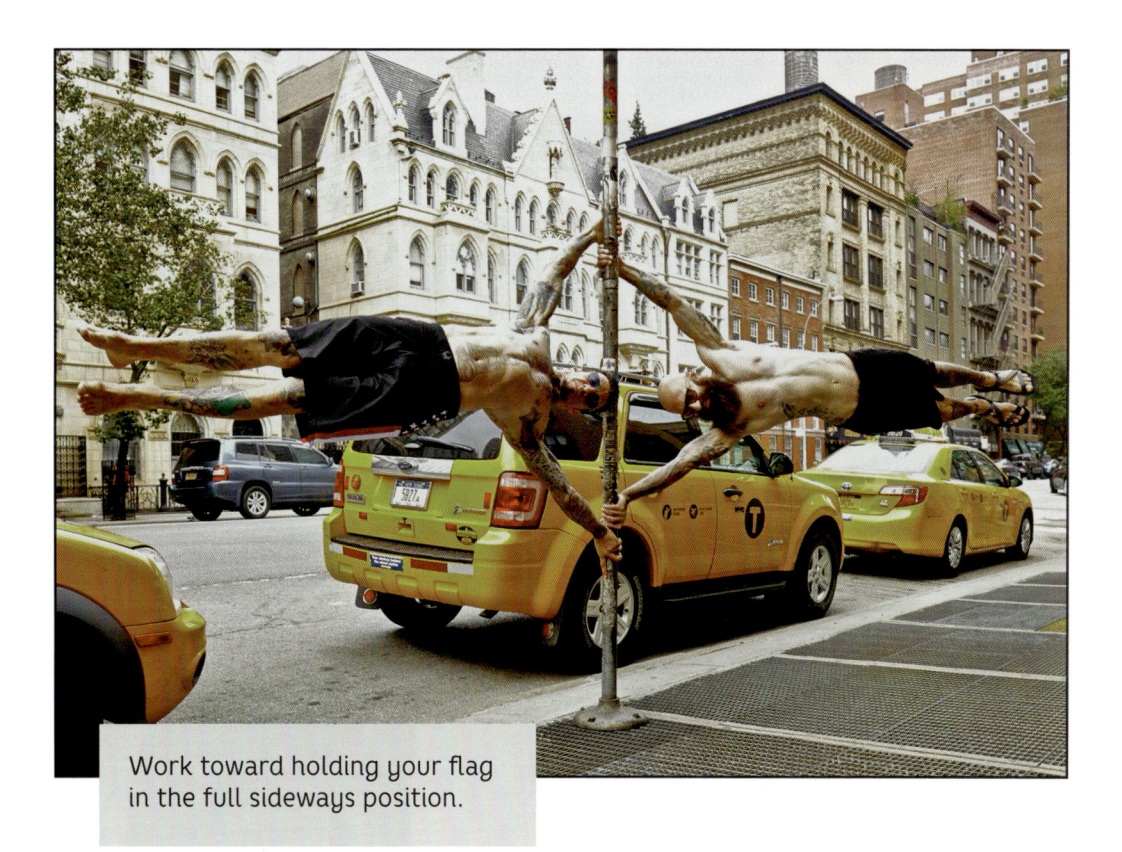

Work toward holding your flag in the full sideways position.

HOOK HAND/FLAT PALM FLAG

This fun variant on the standard human flag is helpful for flagging on many unconventional surfaces. This particular grip not only involves an altered top-hand placement, but also an adjusted lower-hand position. When performing a traditional flag, you use your top hand to grab the pole as you would if you were grabbing a pull-up bar. This time, however, your fingers must hook over the top in a neutral grip, rather than around the pulling surface.

While the hook hand (top hand) requires extra grabbing from the fingers, the flat palm (bottom hand) eliminates any gripping at all. But that doesn't mean it's easier. The lack of grip from the bottom hand can force you to press even harder and tense your body even tighter.

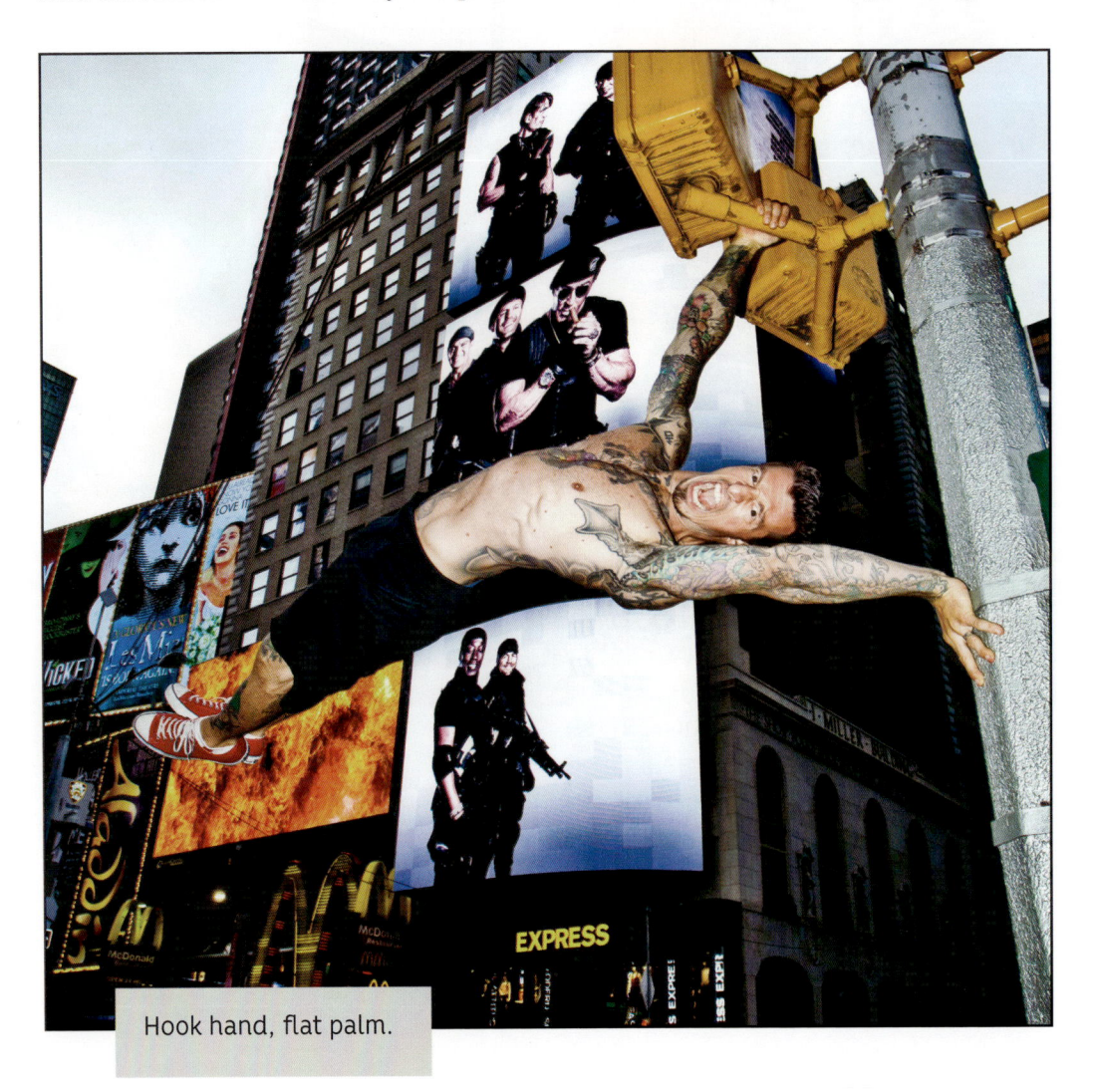

Hook hand, flat palm.

You can further increase the difficulty of this variation by performing it on the ground, placing your flat palm on the floor instead of on a vertical object. The farther your flat palm hand gets from your hook hand, the more difficult it becomes (almost the opposite of the support press). Depending on the surface employed, some kinking at the top arm may be unavoidable.

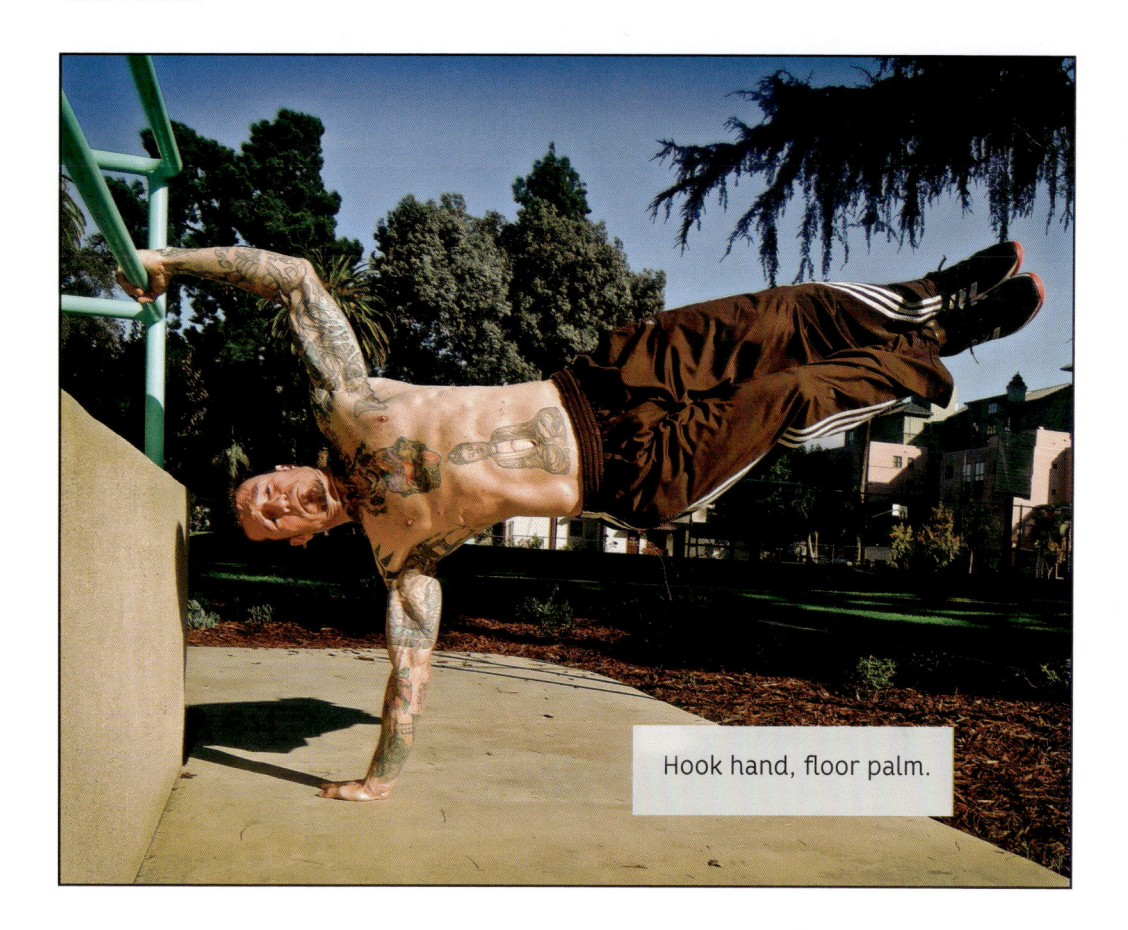

Hook hand, floor palm.

SHOULDER FLAG

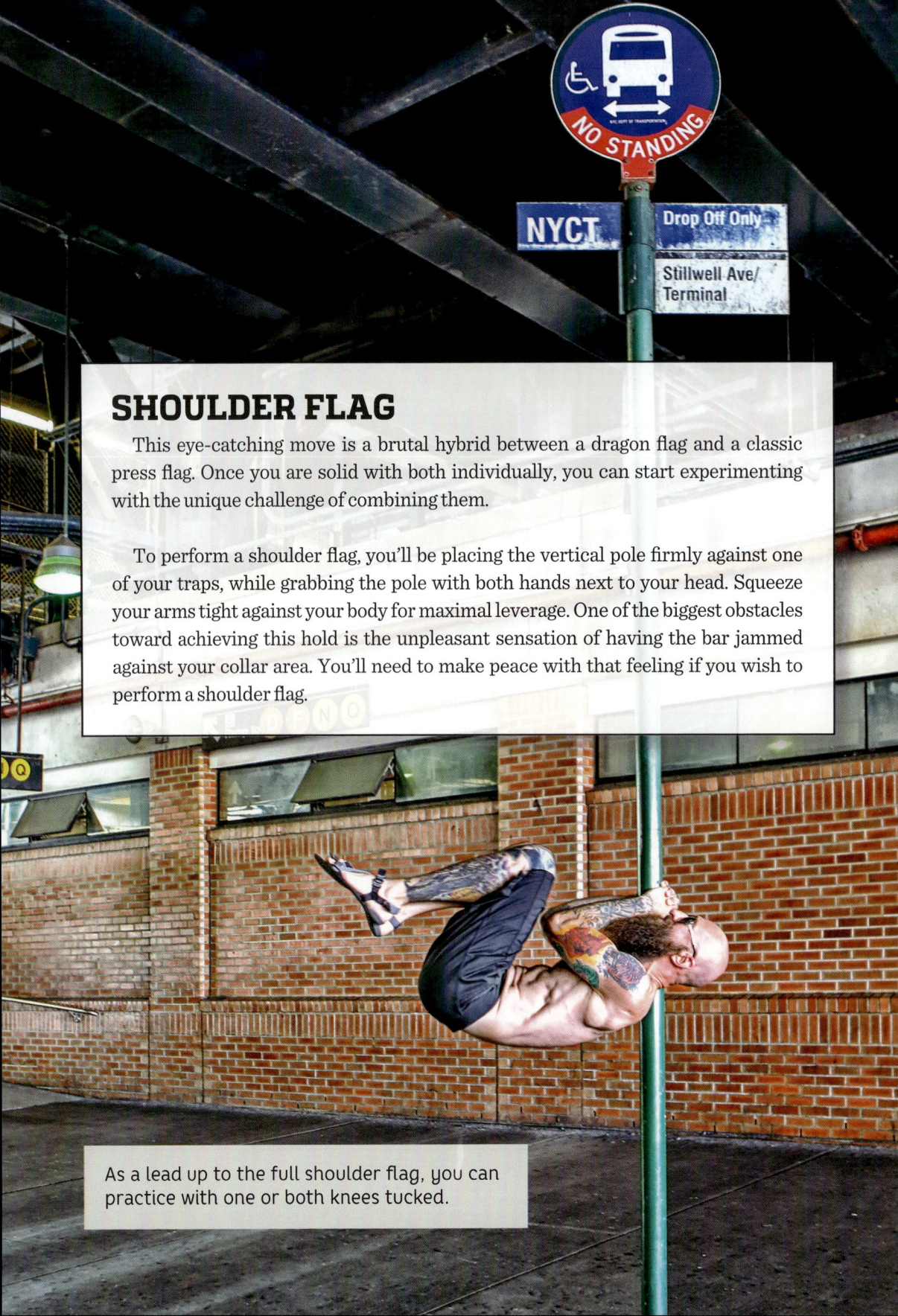

This eye-catching move is a brutal hybrid between a dragon flag and a classic press flag. Once you are solid with both individually, you can start experimenting with the unique challenge of combining them.

To perform a shoulder flag, you'll be placing the vertical pole firmly against one of your traps, while grabbing the pole with both hands next to your head. Squeeze your arms tight against your body for maximal leverage. One of the biggest obstacles toward achieving this hold is the unpleasant sensation of having the bar jammed against your collar area. You'll need to make peace with that feeling if you wish to perform a shoulder flag.

As a lead up to the full shoulder flag, you can practice with one or both knees tucked.

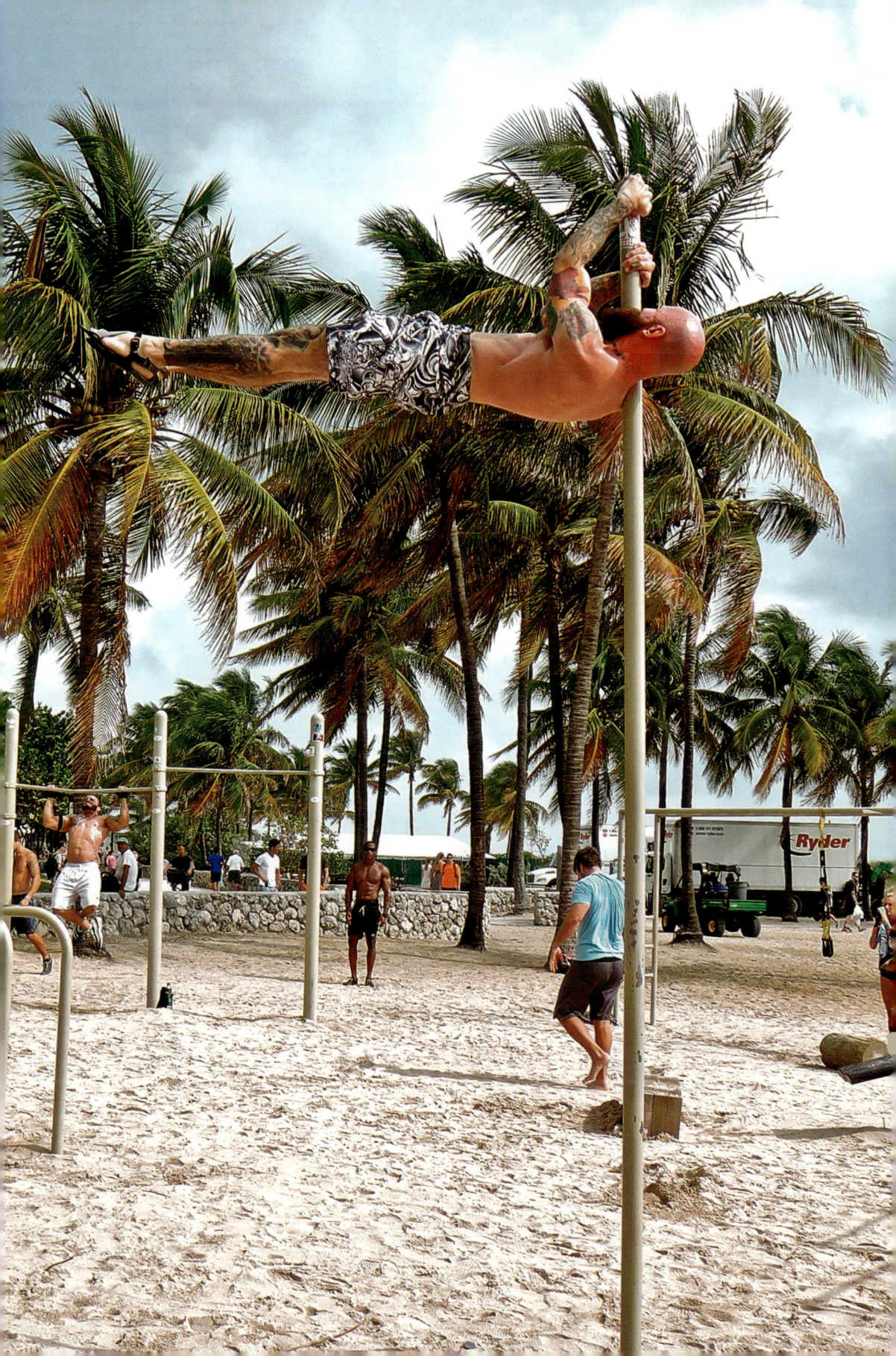

SWITCH GRIP FLAG

If you have good wrist mobility you can try a switch grip (aka pole dancer's grip) on the vertical pole. This involves rotating the top hand all the way around so that your thumb points up instead of down. Get your top arm in place first by reaching behind your back. Then turn your body to get into position, as you grip the pole with the bottom hand in the same fashion as a classic press flag. Though many will struggle with the rotational mobility needed from the top arm, those who are able to do so may find this hand position allows for better leverage, while also helping to keep the top arm from bending.

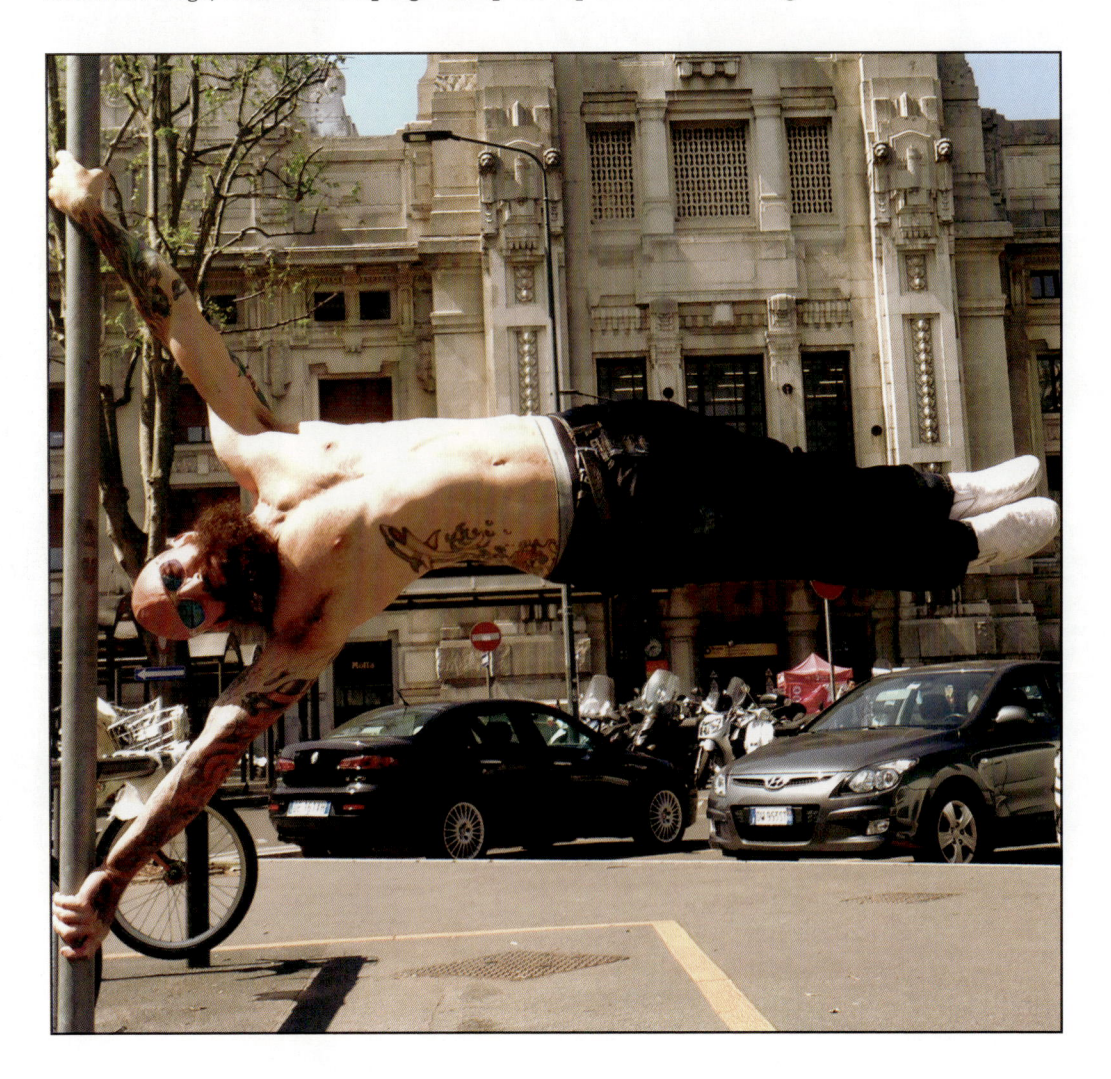

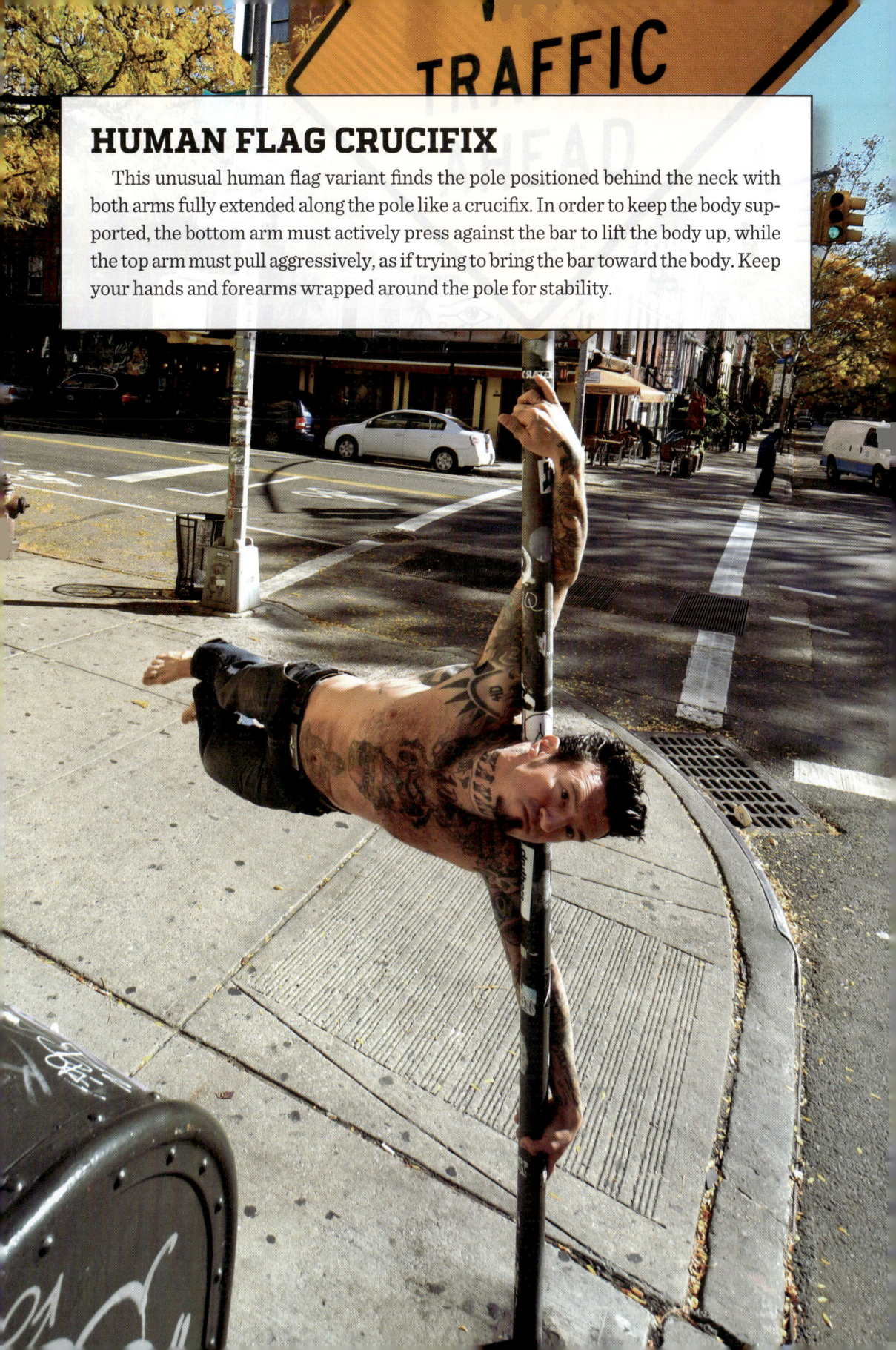

HUMAN FLAG CRUCIFIX

This unusual human flag variant finds the pole positioned behind the neck with both arms fully extended along the pole like a crucifix. In order to keep the body supported, the bottom arm must actively press against the bar to lift the body up, while the top arm must pull aggressively, as if trying to bring the bar toward the body. Keep your hands and forearms wrapped around the pole for stability.

ONE ARM FLAG

The one-arm flag takes tremendous neck strength and full body power to execute, as your head will be placed against the flagging surface instead of your bottom arm. It's not enough for the head simply to support the body, however. You must actively press it into the surface from which you are flagging. (We recommend wearing a hat.) It is also worth mentioning that this progression cannot be performed on a pole, since a flat area for your head is required.

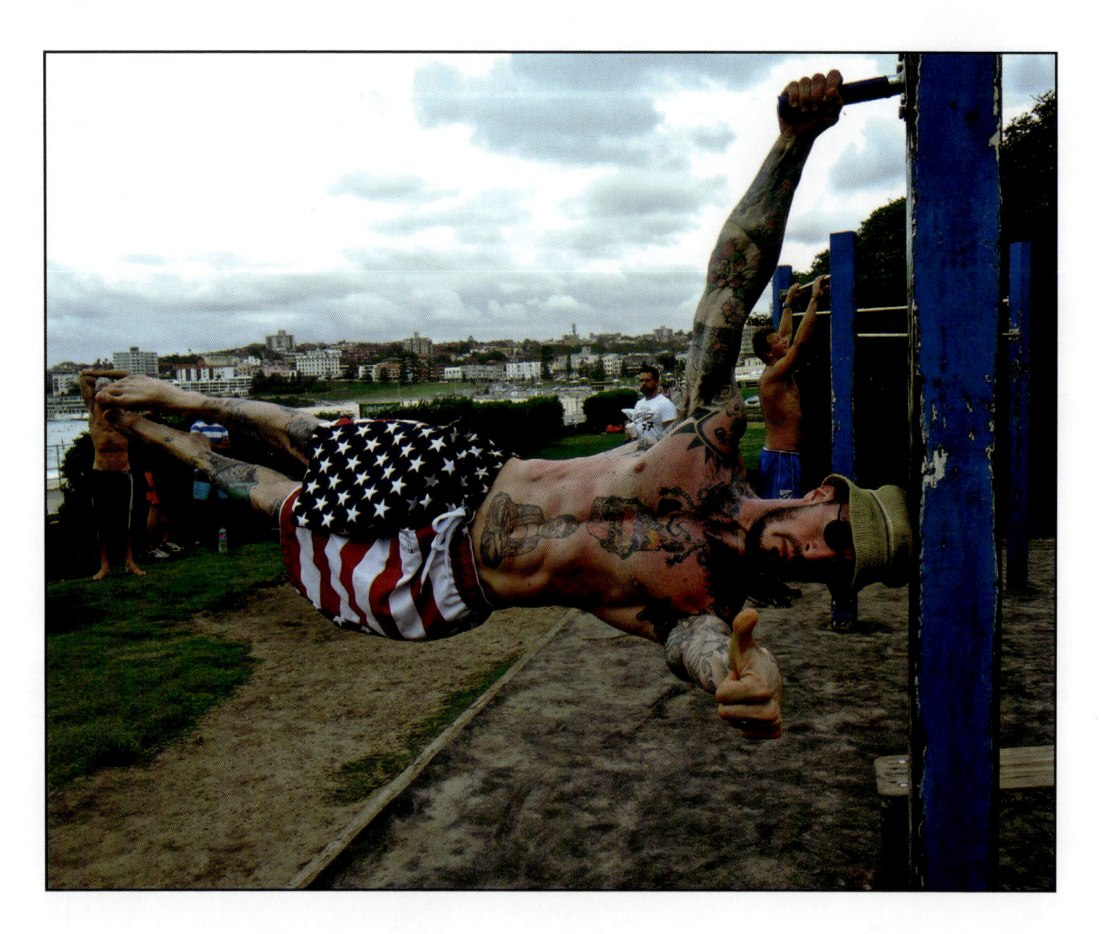

HUMAN FLAG AND HUMAN FLAG POLE

The human flag is impressive enough when performed on a steel pole, but when it's performed on another human being it is even more amazing!

At first glance, it's easy to discern that the flagger has some extra work on his hands. Obviously, no one's skin is completely taut, no matter how hard they train, so the flagger must constantly adjust his grip—and many other nuances—to the uncontrollable wavering of his partner's skin.

The flagger must also be extremely conscious of where he places his hands. The lower hand must be placed close to the foot to maximize stability. If you put it too high, not only will you put yourself in a mechanically disadvantageous position, you may snap your partner's shinbone!

The partner being flagged upon (the human flag pole) faces an enormous task as well. First of all, you've got to be as solid as a rock—both physically and in your mental focus—for someone to flag off of you. Secondly, be prepared to subtly lean away from the flagger as they lift their feet off the ground to get into position. Failure to counter the flagger's weight will result in both of you toppling over. It may be helpful to extend your free arm to help strike a balance.

As with any partner workout, communication is key. It took us plenty of time and practice to finally nail it.

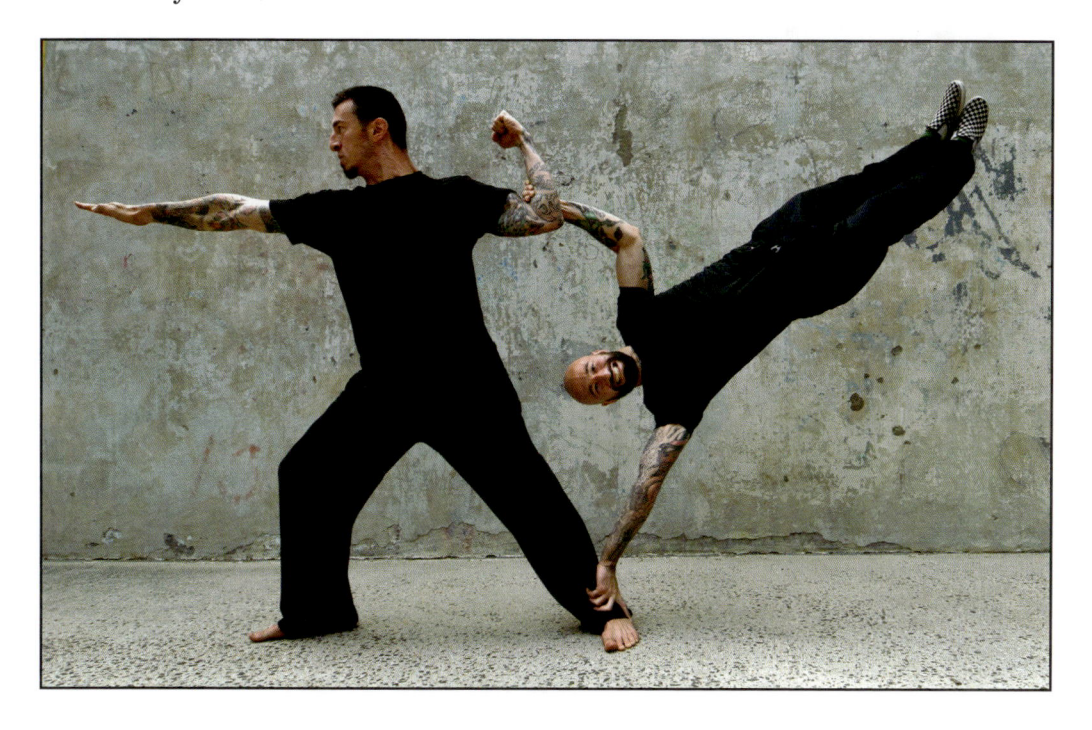

ALTERNATIVE GRIPS

The human flag can be progressed in ways that move past the pole itself. Whether you're flagging on a rock formation, subway station, tree or fence, many objects lack something obvious to grab onto in the first place.

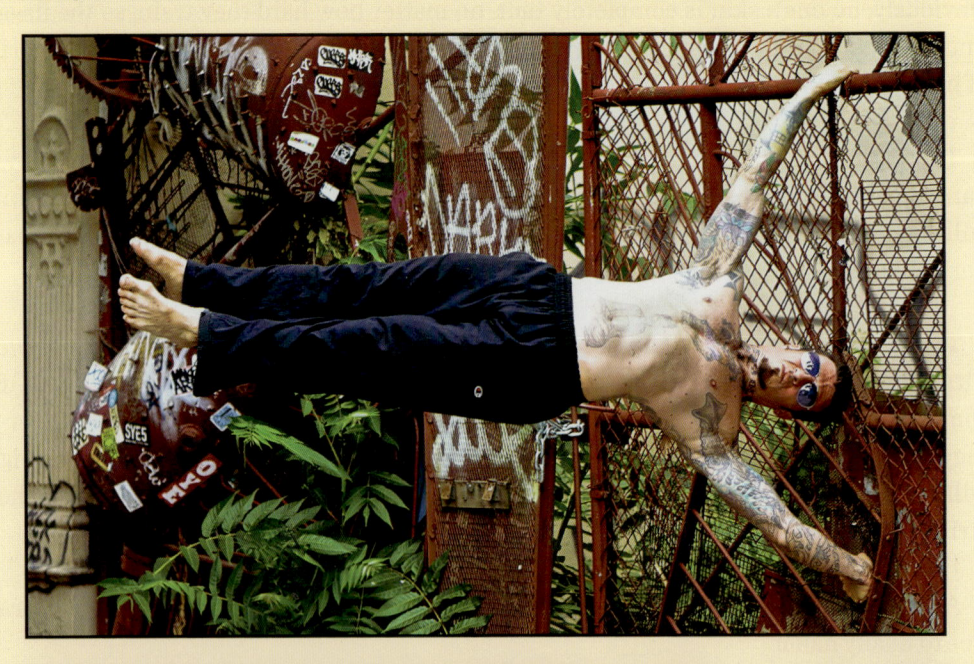

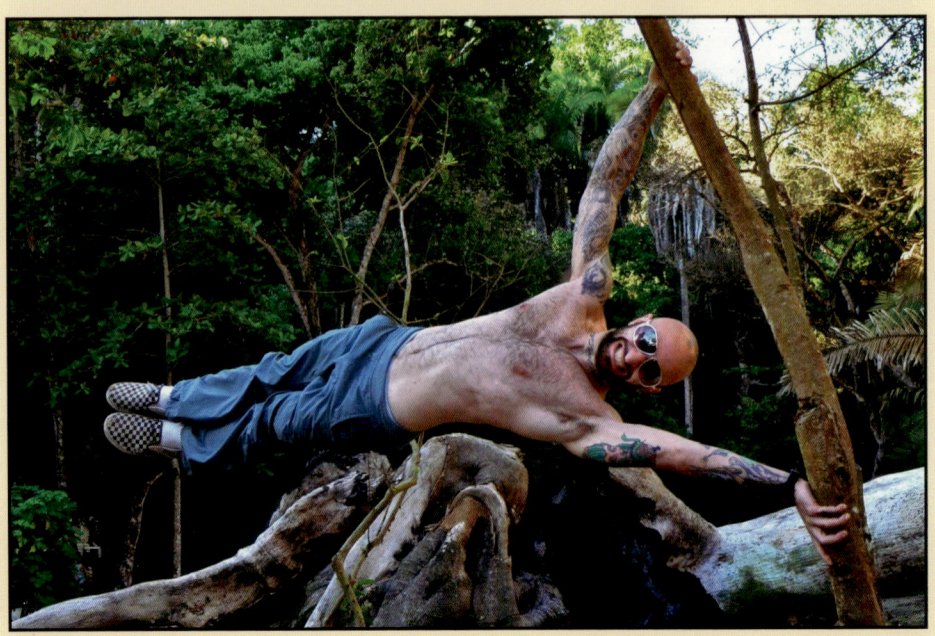

Employing odd surfaces, uneven grips or staggered hand patterns for your flagging purposes not only takes your training over the edge, but also gets your creative juices flowing! One of the core philosophies of Street Workout is not only to accept, but to embrace, the fact that we must improvise. Sometimes the rulebook has to go out the window.

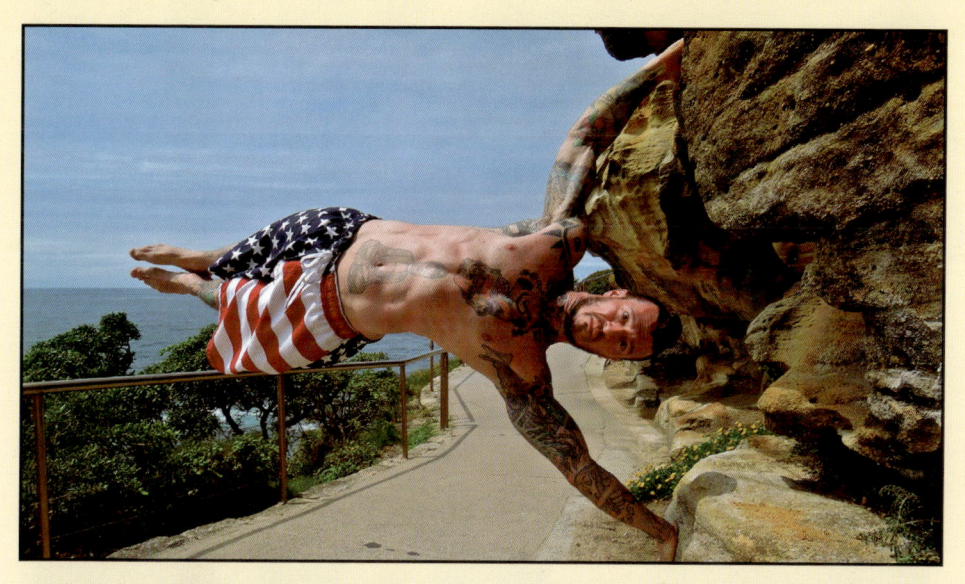

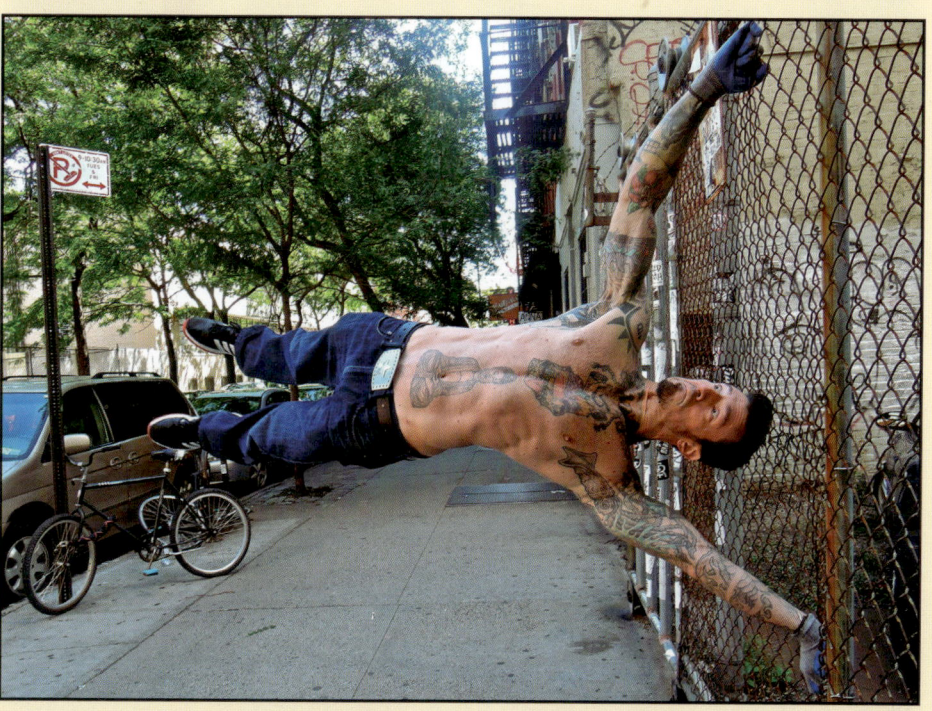

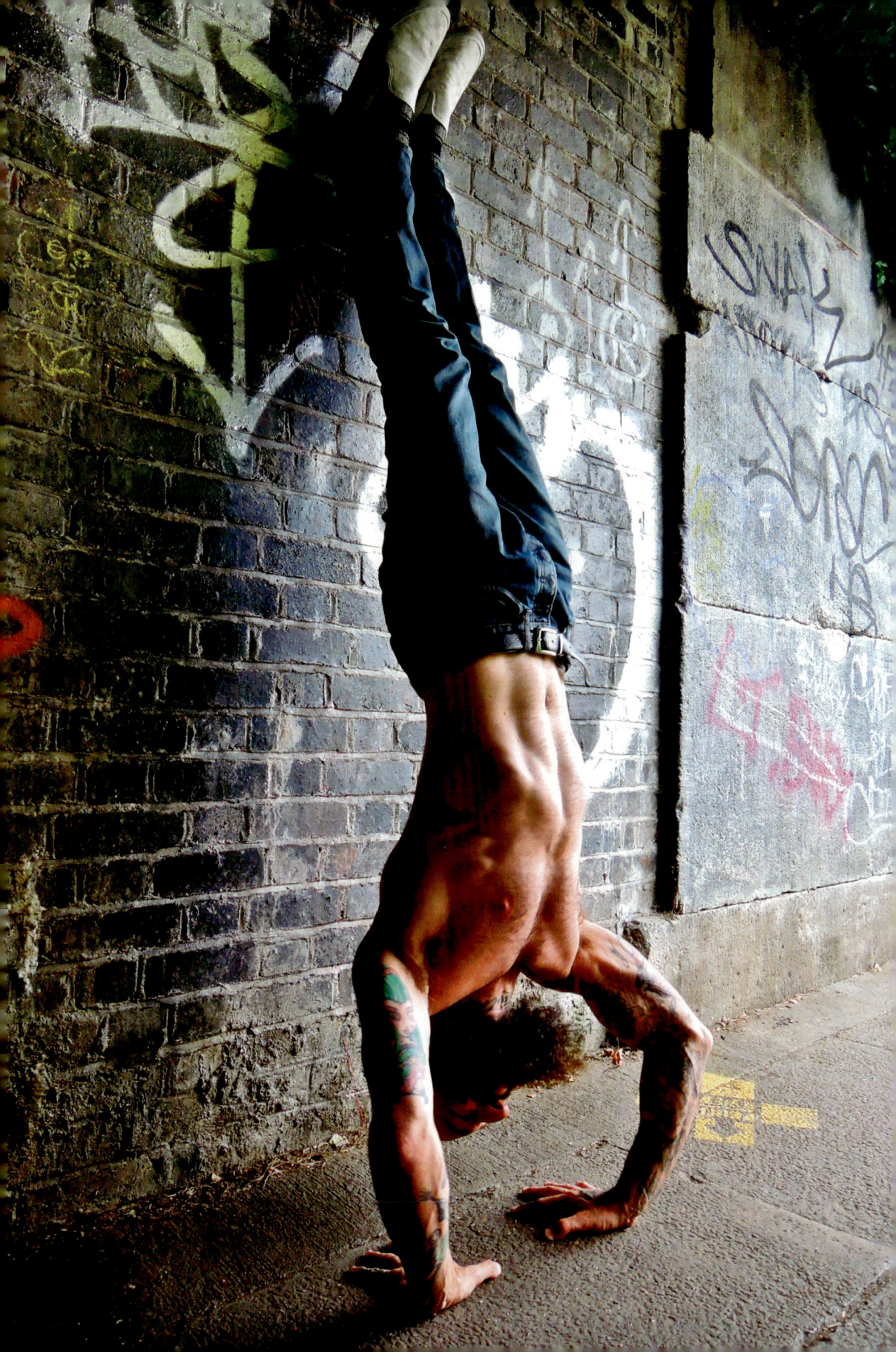

IV
Programming

When it comes to programming, there are many options. Full body workouts, split routines, circuits, pyramid sets and more all have their place in the world of strength training. Yet there is no method that is universally the best for all people and all goals. Though it's nice to have a guideline, we encourage you to use the following assessments, templates and workouts as a starting point, rather than the final verdict.

Oftentimes in the fitness world, the tendency is to overanalyze programming. While it is an important aspect, you sell yourself short if you underestimate the power of observation and the value of improvisation. Don't be afraid if you need to make changes in the moment or deviate slightly from the plan. The truth is that any program will work if you're prepared to work hard over an extended period of time.

Strength training makes you stronger.

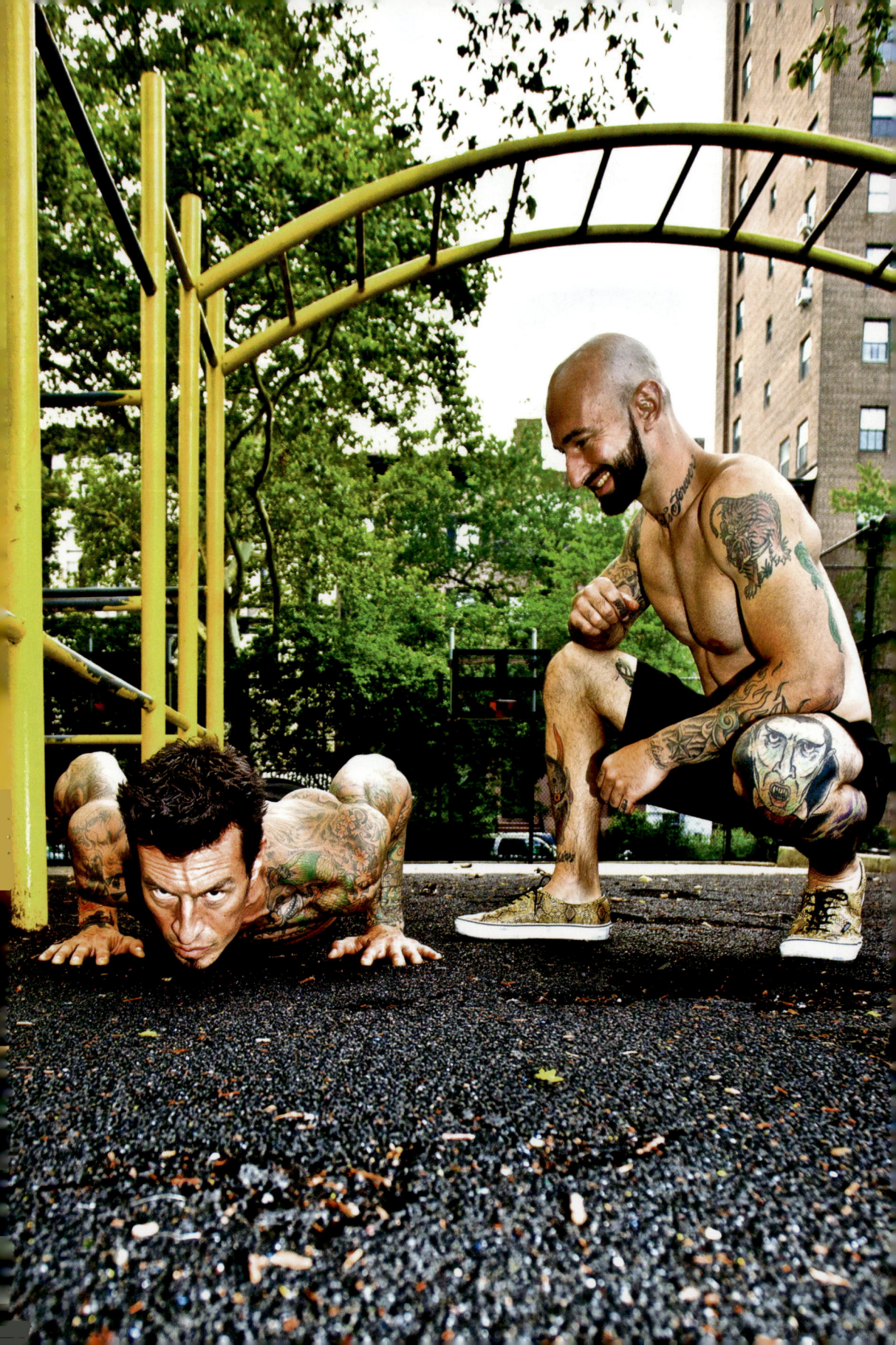

Chapter 12

Assessments

Dying to know where you stack up against the best of the best in the bodyweight kingdom? The following charts can help you assess your calisthenics competency across a broad array of classic street workout exercises. These charts can also serve as a guideline to help you determine when it is appropriate to move onto harder exercises.

There is one chart for dynamic exercises (those that you perform for reps) and another for isometric exercises (those that you hold for time). In both cases, the exercises are listed in approximate order from least difficult to most difficult. Each includes a baseline standard, an advanced standard and an elite standard.

The numbers in the first chart refer to reps performed in one continuous set. In the second chart, the numbers refer to how many seconds the position is held. Strict form must be adhered to in all cases.

The baseline number represents what can potentially be achieved within your first 6-12 months of consistent training, while the advanced figure can take years to achieve. As for the elite standard, well, just keep training hard and keep the dream alive!

This stuff has to be earned the old fashioned way, and that's the beauty of it. Depending on where you are starting from, your personal journey may take more or less time. Additionally, different individuals may find that they progress quicker with certain exercises than others. Again, this is part of the beauty of the Street Workout phenomenon.

Dynamic Exercises

Exercise	Baseline	Advanced	Elite
Squat	40	100	200
Push-up	30	60	100
Hanging Knee Raise	20	40	60
Aussie Pull-up	20	40	60
Pike Press	20	40	60
Parallel Bar Dip	15	30	50
Pull-up	10	20	30
Hanging Leg Raise	10	20	30
Handstand Press	1	10	20
Pistol Squat	1	10	20
Shrimp Squat	1	10	20
Muscle-up	1	10	20
One Arm Push-up	1	5	10
One Arm Pull-up	–	1	5

Isometric Exercises

Exercise	Baseline	Advanced	Elite
Headstand	60	120	240
Crow Hold	60	120	240
Back Bridge	60	120	240
L-sit	20	60	120
Elbow Lever	20	60	120
Freestanding Handstand	20	60	120
Tuck Back Lever	10	30	60
Clutch Flag	10	30	60
Tuck Front Lever	10	30	60
Tuck Planche	10	30	60
Back Lever	–	5	10
Press Flag	–	5	10
Front Lever	–	5	10
Planche	–	3	5

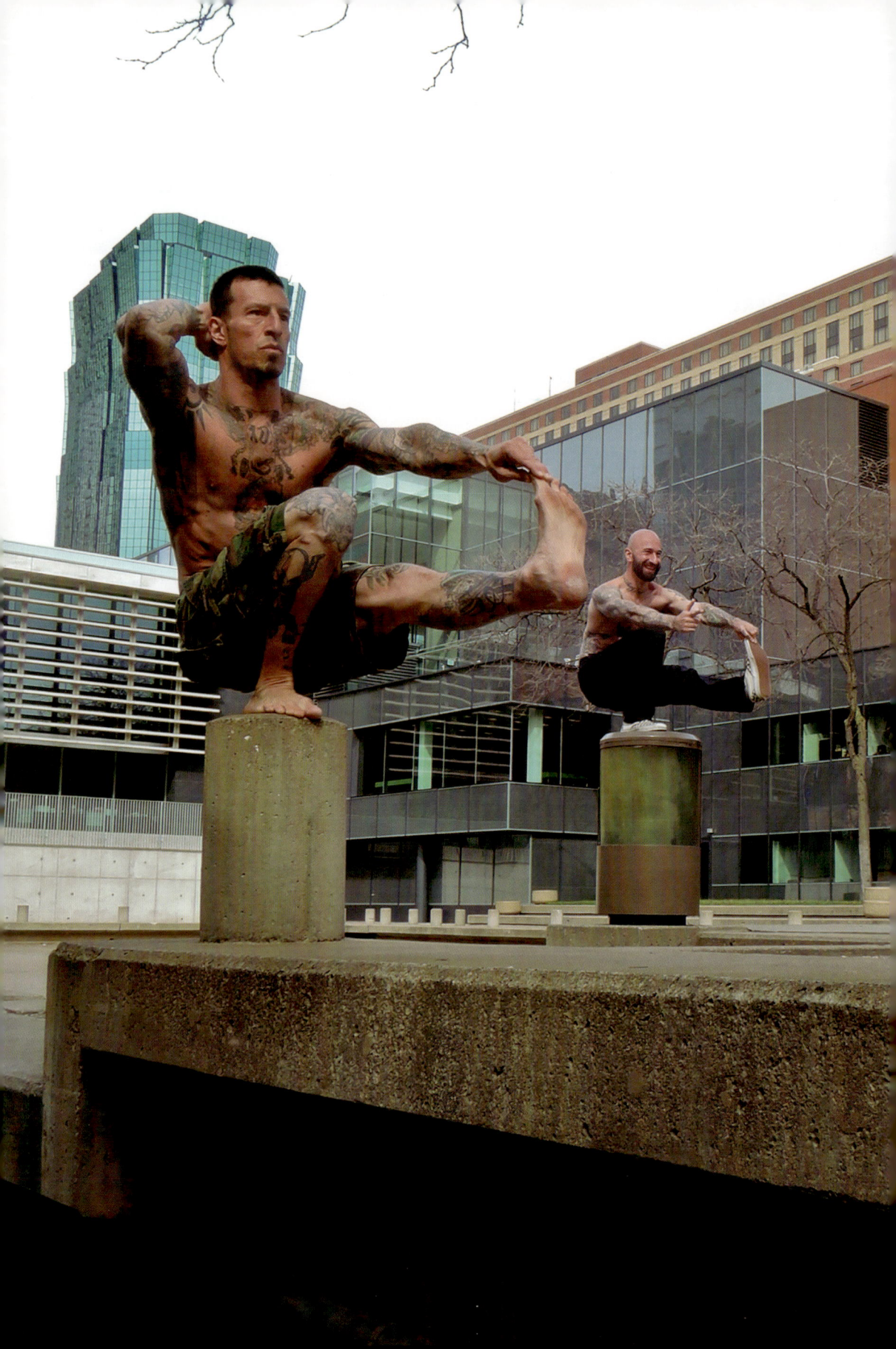

Chapter 13

Street Workouts

Here are sample workouts that give you a good overview of different ways that you can approach your training. Perform them as written or modify them as you see fit.

As you will see, there are various templates that your workouts can follow. Which one is the best? Try them all and see what works best for YOU!

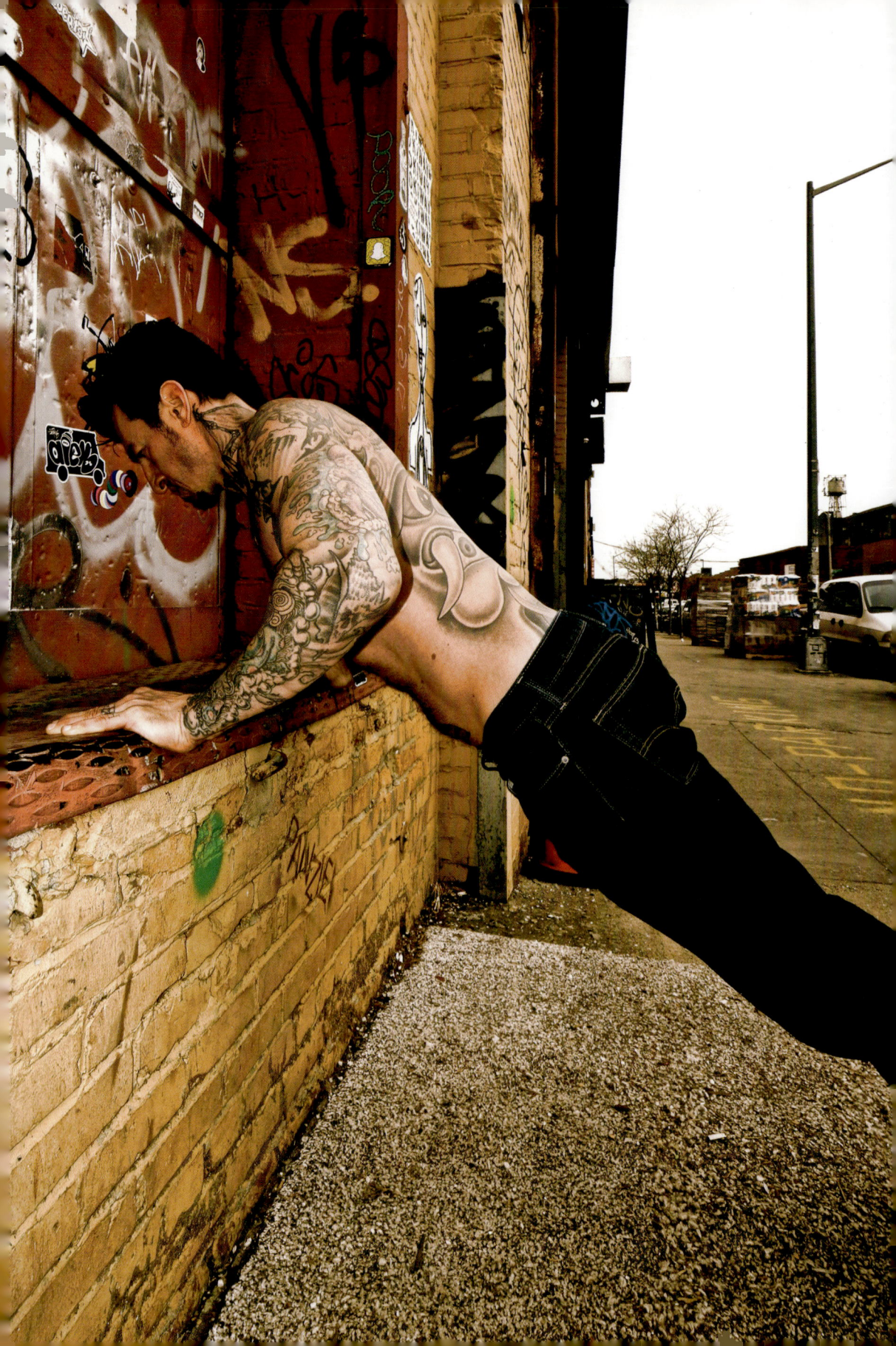

START ME UP

As the name implies, this beginner workout is the perfect place to get started if you are new to strength training. Start Me Up is a compilation of all the major foundational strength movements put in a capacity that the starting practitioner will find accessible.

When you begin, rest as much as you need in between sets, completing all reps of each exercise before moving onto the next. Once this becomes comfortable, try not to rest for more than 1-2 minutes in between sets.

As your conditioning improves, you can mix it up by performing the workout as a circuit. Do one set of each exercise in succession. Then repeat them all until you've done three sets of each. This method employs active recovery and can prevent your training from growing stagnant.

After several workouts, you can progress to full push-ups, unassisted squats and straight leg Aussies.

3 sets of 10 Hands Elevated Push-ups

3 sets of 10 Bench Assisted Squats

3 sets of 10 Bent Knee Aussie Pull-ups

3 sets of 10 Lying Bent Knee Raises

3 sets of 10 Hip Bridges

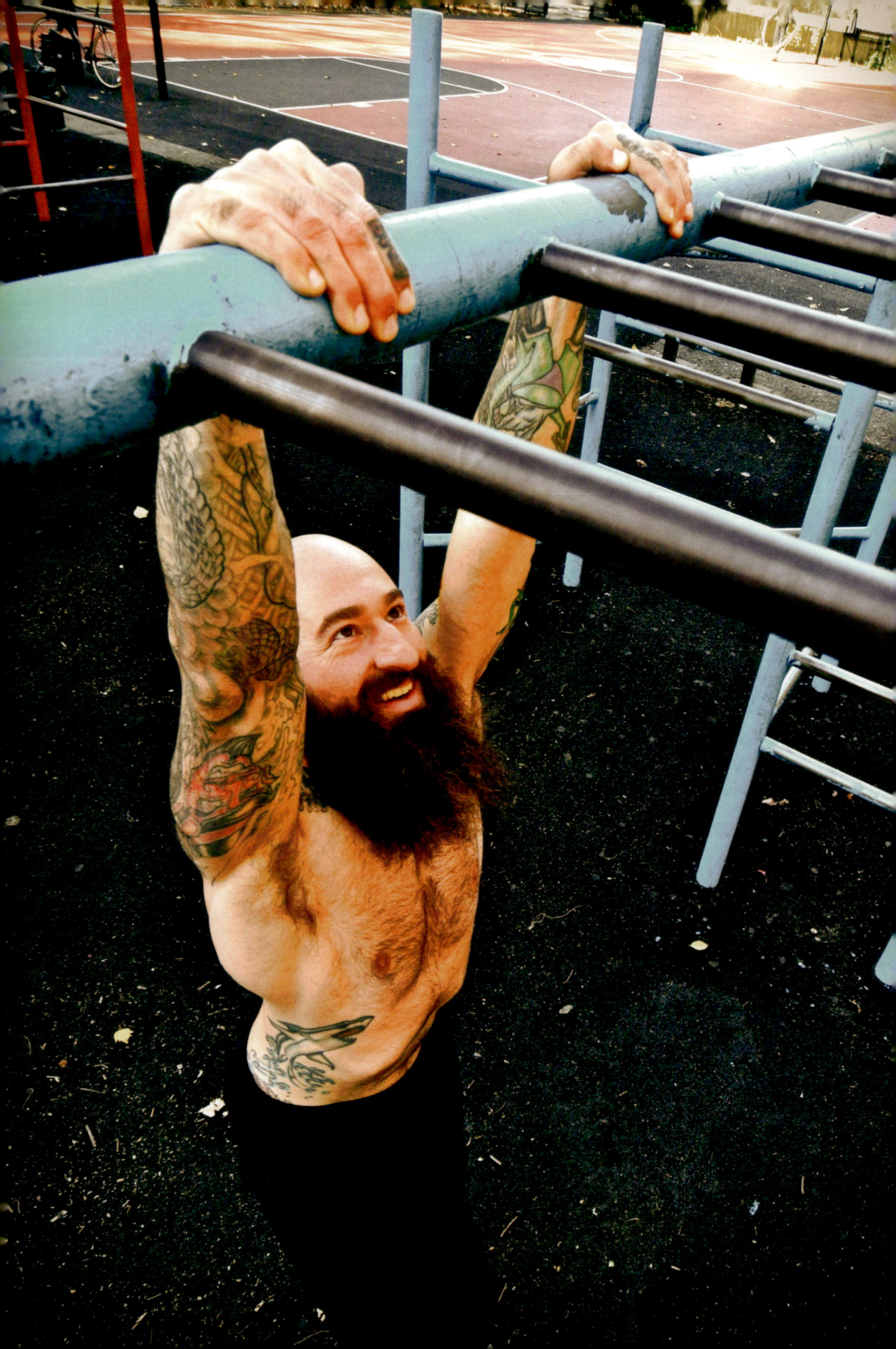

50 REP CHALLENGE

The 50 rep challenge consists of doing 50 reps of a fairly difficult exercise in one workout, no matter how many sets it takes. Even if it means you are doing sets of one rep by the end.

For example, you might start out with a set of 10, followed by a set of 8, followed by a set of 7, then 2 more sets of 5, 3 sets of 3, 2 sets of 2, and end with a couple sets of 1. This could take a while at first, but over time the amount of sets that you can do this in should decrease.

Choose an exercise that you can do between 5-15 of reps in one set, and focus on keeping your form clean and avoiding failure. You can take as long of a break between sets as you need. In fact, you are encouraged to take long breaks. Stretch. Breathe. Ponder the beauty and simplicity of Street Workout.

This method is a fantastic way to increase your maximum reps on basics like squats, push-ups or pull-ups, though advanced trainees can use it for more difficult exercises like muscle-ups and pistol squats as well. Make sure to do both legs!

At first we recommend doing this only once a week per body part, as it can be a bit of a shock to your system. Eventually, however, you can condition yourself to doing this regularly.

Additionally, if 50 reps is just not realistic for you right now, pick a smaller number (maybe 30?) and build up from there.

When 50 is no longer a challenging number, pick a harder exercise or raise the total reps to 100 or more.

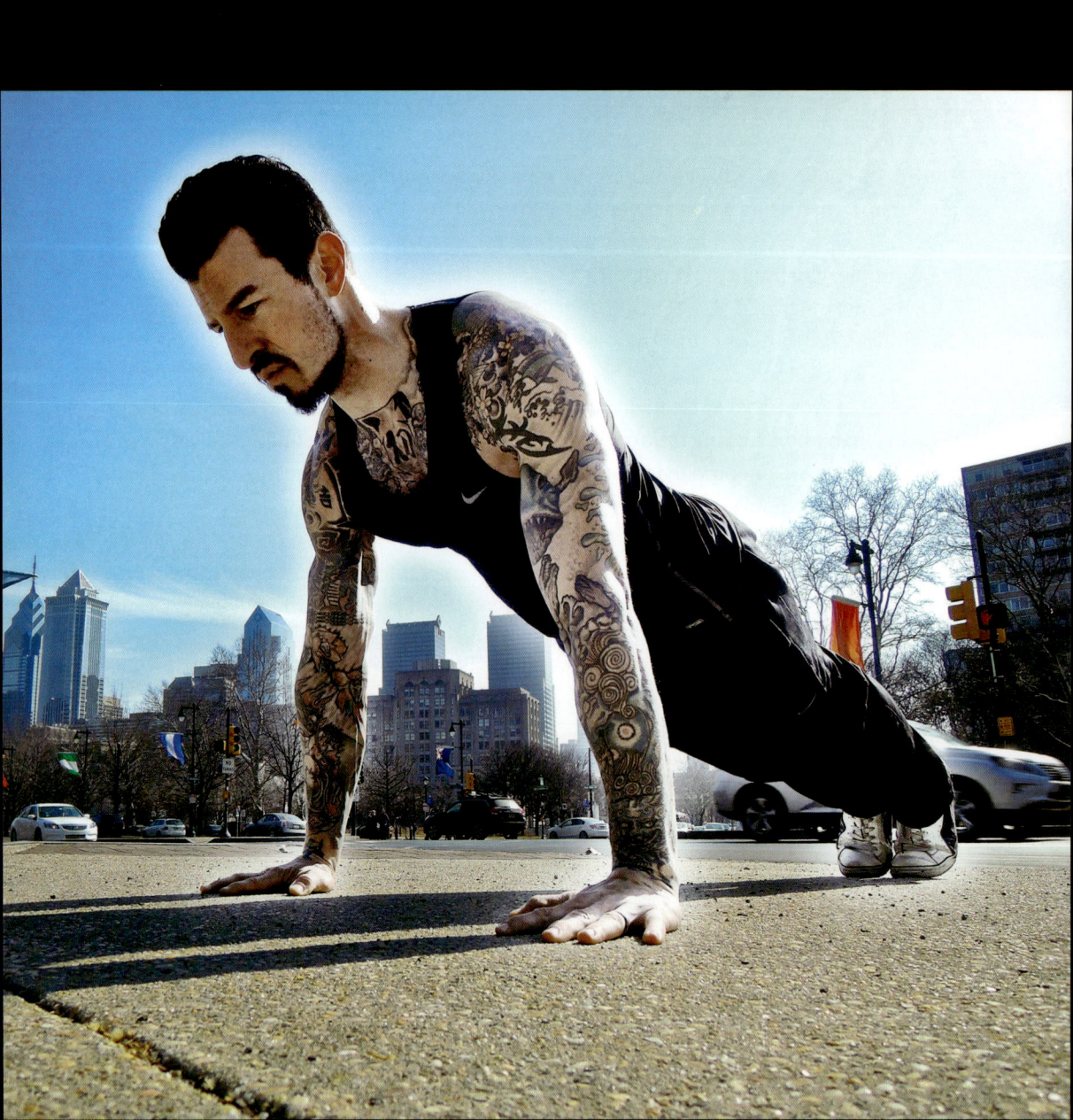

THREE AMIGOS

This is a very simple workout based on a pyramid training protocol that will work every single muscle in your body—including your heart!

Start by performing one squat, then immediately grab an overhead bar and do one pull-up, then drop down and do a push-up. Next do two squats, two pull-ups and two push-ups. Continue to add one rep to each exercise until you fail to get through the circuit. Then start taking one rep away and work your way back down.

Aim to keep breaks to a minimum, but rest enough to maintain strict form. If you're not strong enough to do full push-ups or pull-ups, substitute knee push-ups and Aussie pull-ups in their place.

1 Squat

1 Pull-up

1 Push-up

2 Squats

2 Pull-ups

2 Push-ups

3 Squats

3 Pull-ups

3 Push-ups...

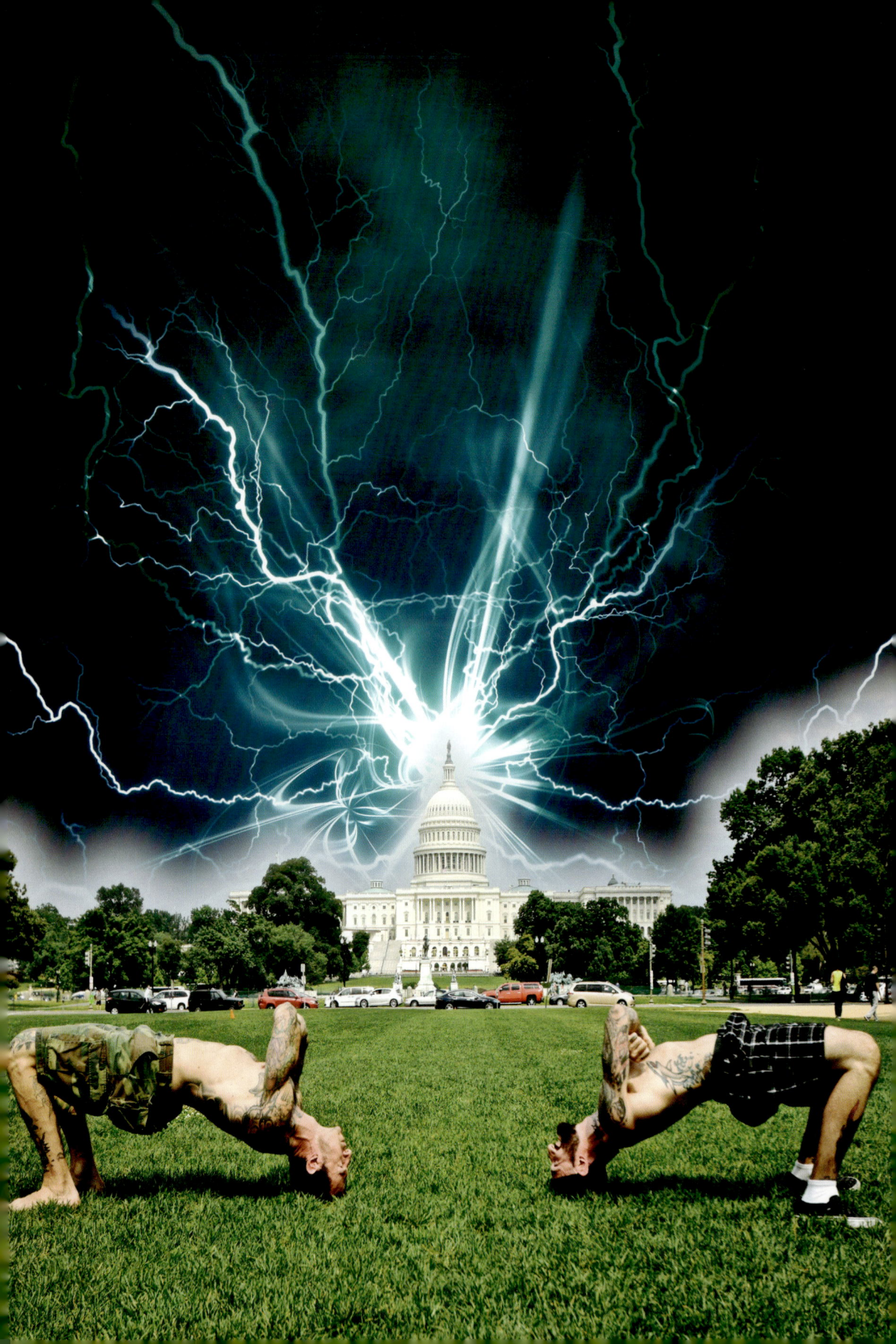

STATIC ELECTRICITY

This isometric workout infuses strength and skill training into a diverse collection of static holds. It is likely that different individuals will have various strengths and weaknesses amongst this group of exercises. For any exercise that you cannot hold for the suggested amount of time, we recommend breaking it up into several smaller sections. For example, if you can hold an L-sit for only ten seconds, then perform four 10 second holds.

Many of these exercises have a mobility component in addition to the strength and skill factors. If you have limitations that prevent you from performing the full expression, then use one of the earlier progressions. For example, if the neck bridge is inaccessible, you can substitute a hip bridge.

Plank (90 seconds)

Side Plank (30 seconds per side)

Crow Pose (90 seconds)

Elbow Lever (40 seconds)

L-Sit (40 seconds)

Neck Bridge (90 seconds)

Wall Handstand (90 seconds)

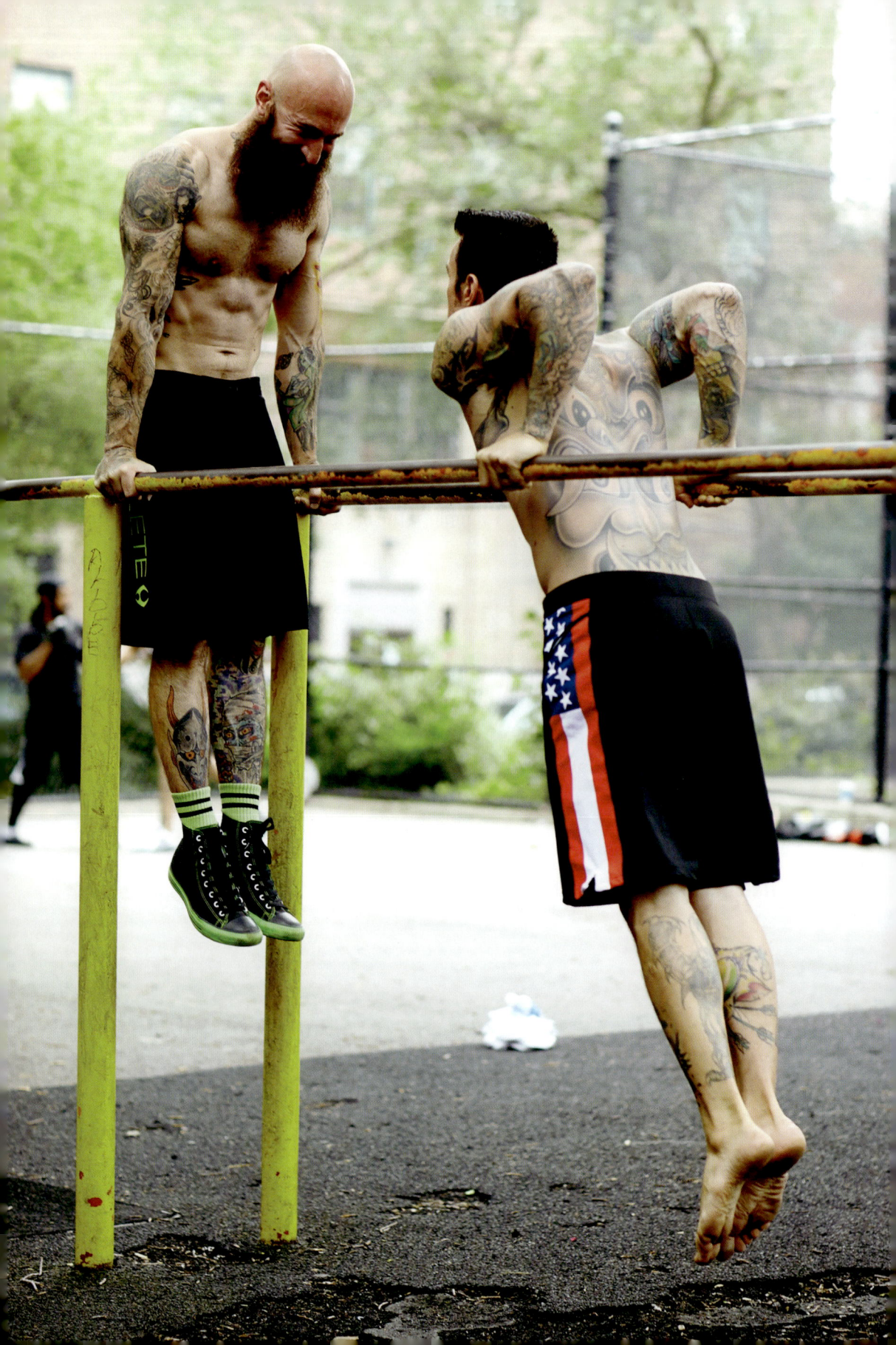

UP ABOVE

While the advocacy of full body training is a principle we stand behind, using a split routine is also a viable way to train, provided your schedule allows for it. After all, you can't go for full body exhaustion every day. Furthermore, changing up your system can be a valuable training tool. This is a basic upper body workout that will leave you in stitches.

The workout is divided into two rounds, focusing on the same movement pattern with slight alterations to target the muscles differently.

Round 1:

2 sets of 20 Push-ups

2 sets of 8 Pull-ups

2 sets of 15 Parallel Bar Dips

2 sets of 10 Wide Aussie Pull-ups

2 sets of 10 Hanging Knee Raises

Round 2:

2 sets of 15 Wide Push-ups

2 sets of 8 Chin-ups

2 sets of 15 Feet Elevated Bench Dips

2 sets of 10 Narrow Aussie Pull-ups

2 sets of 10 Twisting Hanging Knee Raises

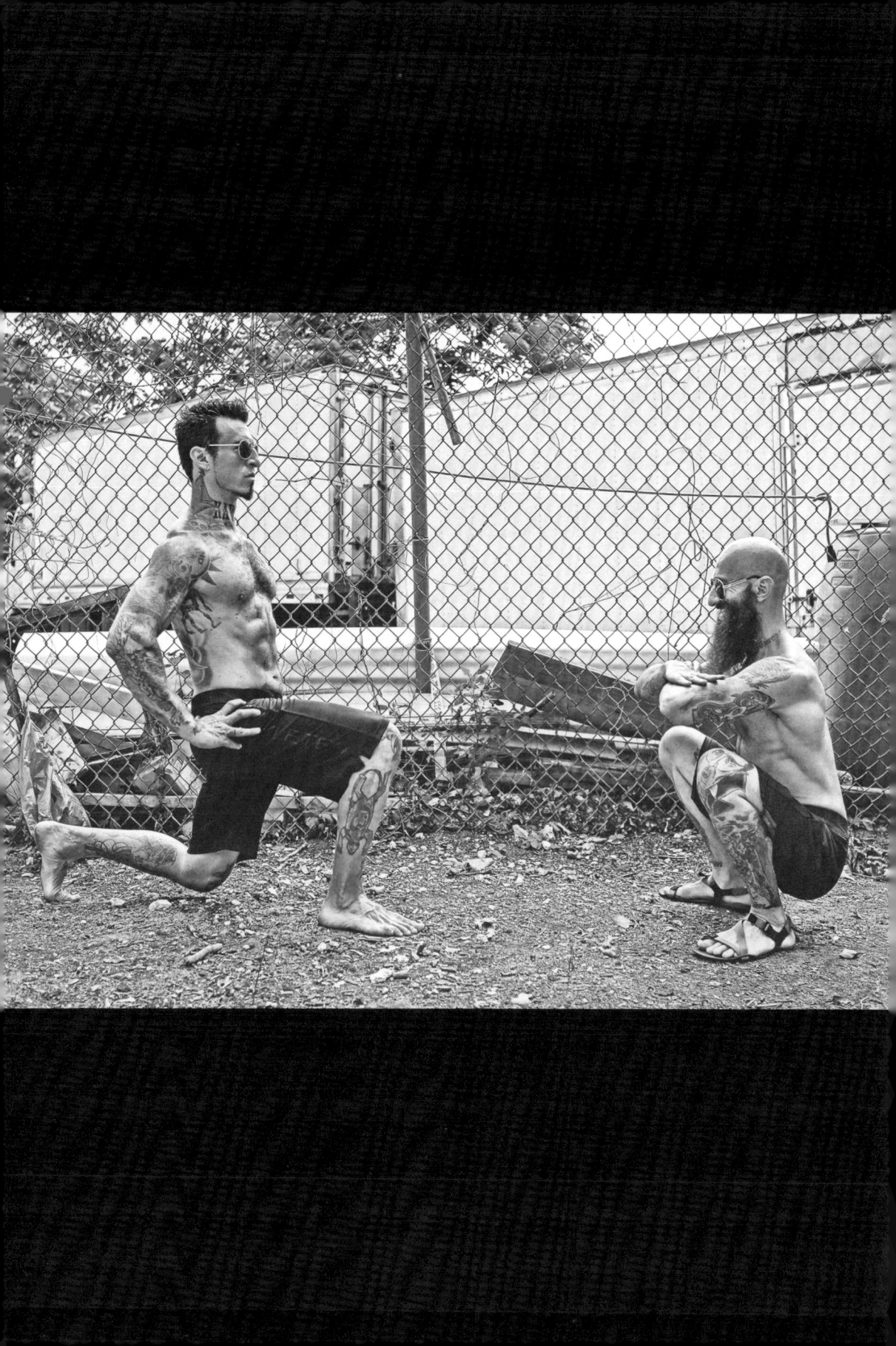

DOWN BELOW

This is a general lower body workout that incorporates several basic movements. The first exercise is a lower body "push" where you remain in a stationary place as you press your feet against the ground beneath you, while the following two exercises incorporate movement patterns which demand that you travel either linearly or up and down. Next, we emphasize some often overlooked lower body muscles that tend to get neglected. And finally, the last movement is a pull or "hinge," as well as an exercise in balance, which perfectly complements the start of the workout. This versatile workout is sure to get you going. Legs do it!

2 sets of 20 Squats

2 sets of 20 Walking Lunges (per leg)

2 sets of 20 Step-ups (per leg)

2 sets of 20 Drinking Birds (per leg)

2 sets of 20 Calf Raises

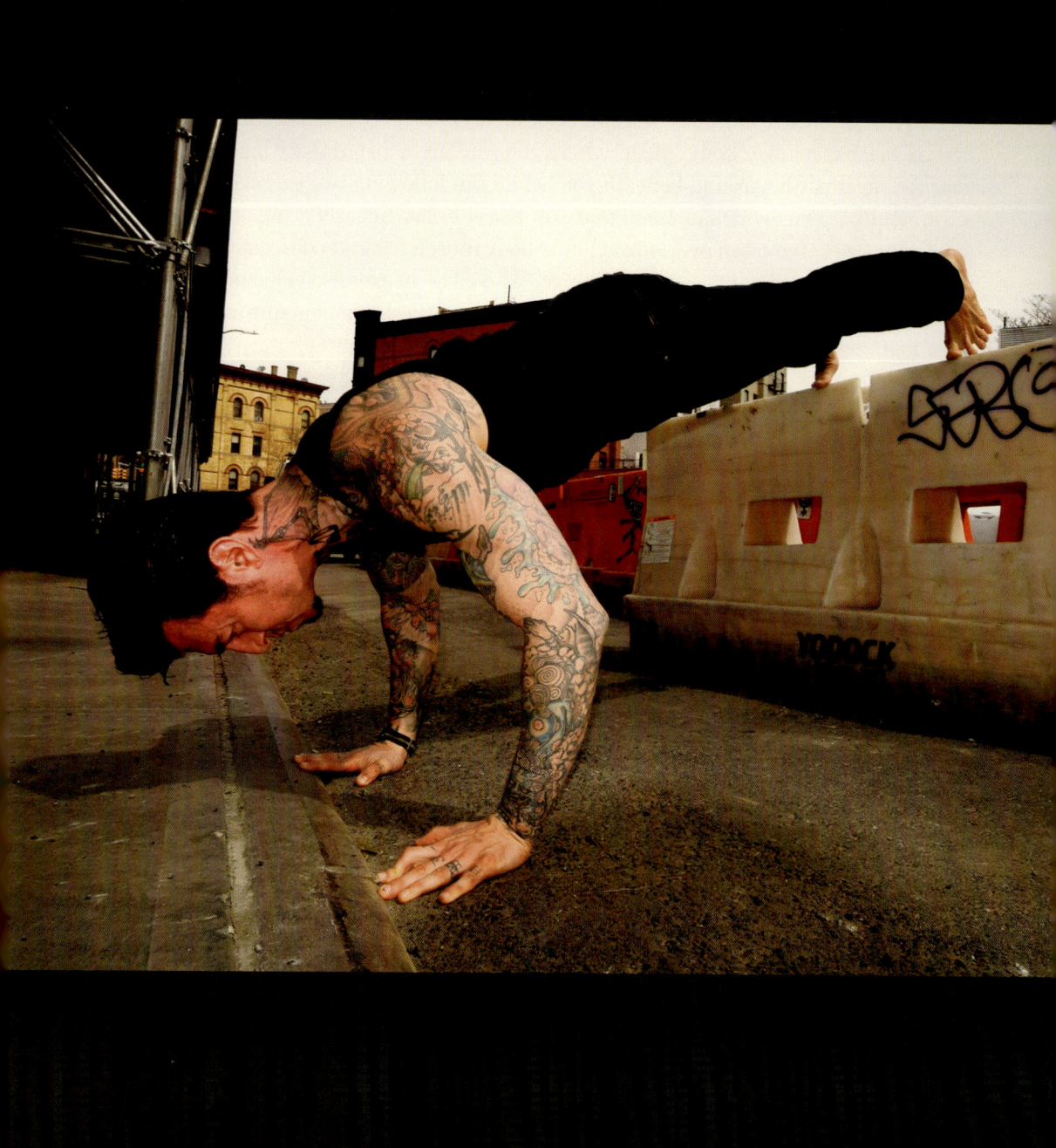

FULL FRONTAL

This intermediate workout focuses on the anterior chain of the body, including the quadriceps, chest, abs and shoulders. While it is of note that several of the exercises included will require a degree of stability from the rear muscles, particularly the low back and hamstrings, the front muscles are preeminent.

3 sets of 20 Narrow Squats

3 sets of 10 Bulgarian Split Squats (per leg)

3 sets of 15 Wide Push-ups

3 sets of 15 Feet Elevated Push-ups

3 sets of 10 Pike Press-ups

3 sets of 15 Hanging Leg Raises

3 sets of 20 Grounded Windshield Wipers (10 per side)

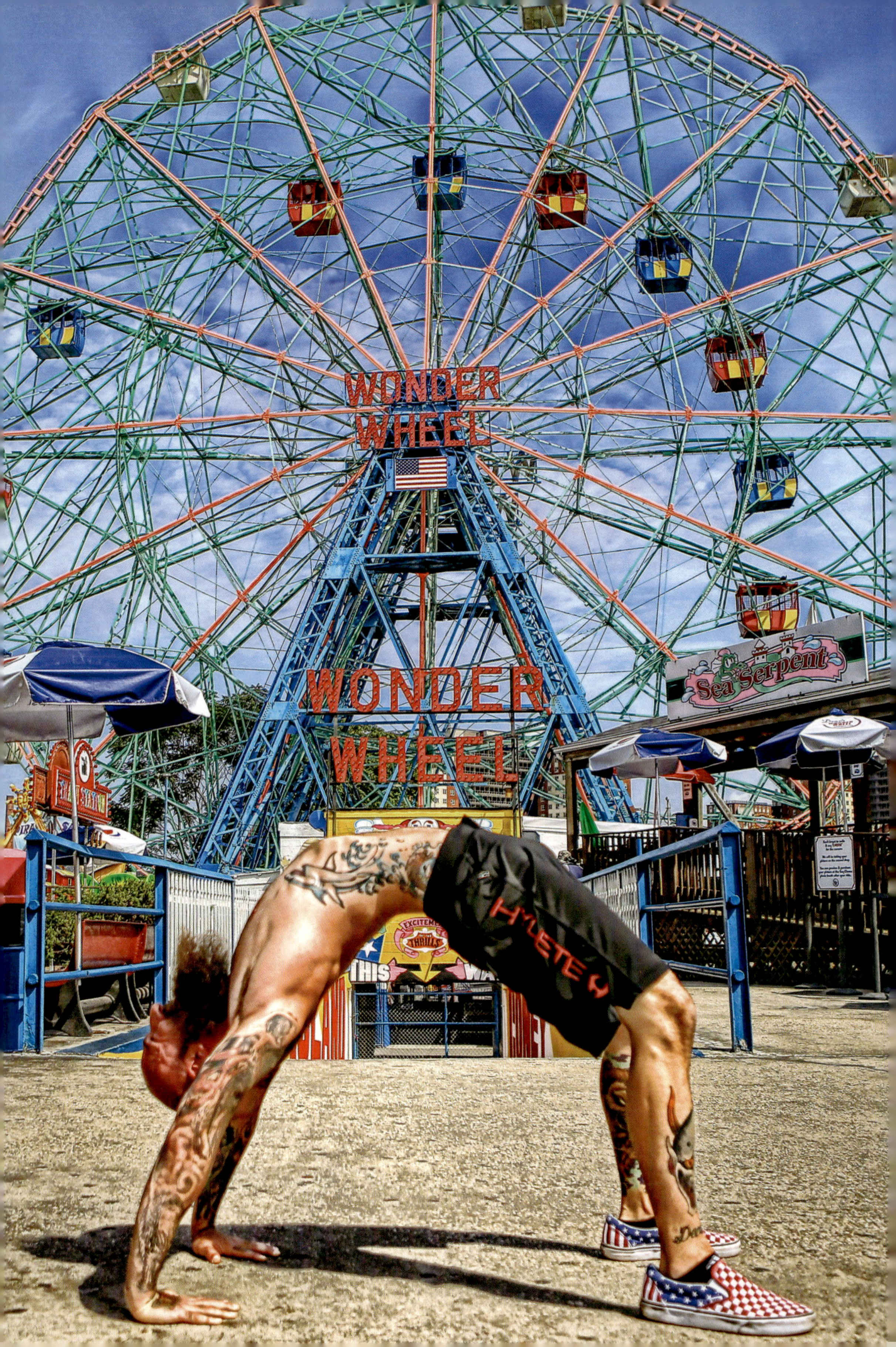
WONDER
WHEEL
WONDER
WHEEL
Sea Serpent

BACK FOR MORE

As we know by now, the posterior muscles of the body often go neglected in our culture, which prioritizes looking good in a mirror (or a selfie) over full body holistic health. This workout is designed to combat that by focusing primarily on the muscles on the back of the body, such as the lats, back, hamstrings and glutes. Be prepared to exert hard as you may be forced to emphasize some muscles that you may not be used to employing.

The first four exercises are to be performed for sets and reps, while the last three are static holds. For these holds, please feel free to break them up into multiple sets if you are incapable of holding them for the full duration. For example, three full bridge holds of 20 seconds each will work in place of one 60 second hold if that is what your skill level dictates. Do the best you can. Back it up!

3 sets of 10 Wide Grip Pull-Ups

3 sets 10 Wide Grip Aussies

3 sets of 10 Candlestick Bridges (per leg)

3 sets of 10 Drinking Birds (per leg)

Tuck Back Lever (20 second hold)

Neck Bridge (60 second hold)

Full Bridge (60 second hold)

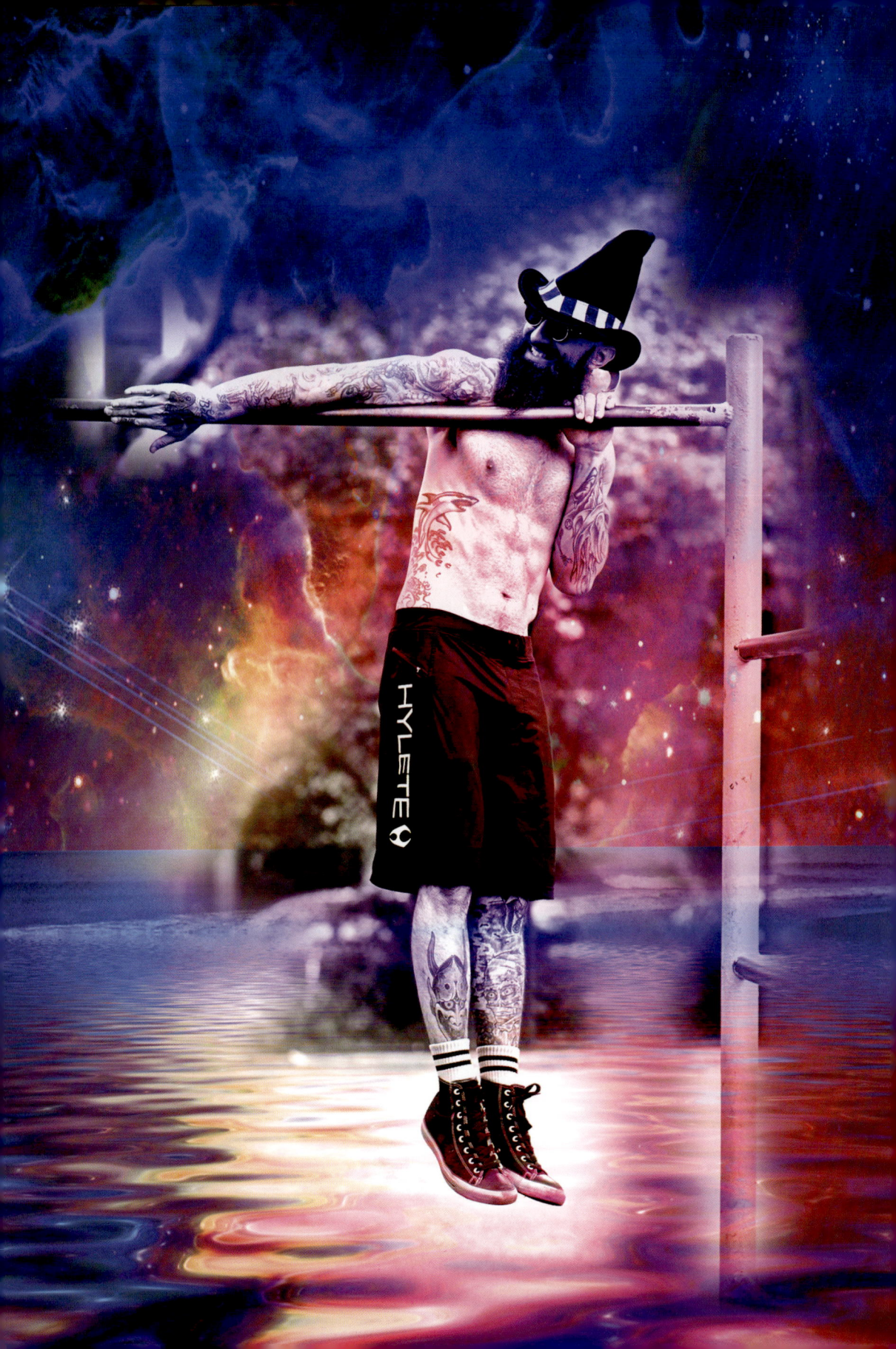

WIZARD'S CAULDRON

This intermediate/advanced level workout uses a little calisthenics magic by pairing each primary exercise with a regressed version of the same movement pattern. By warming up with the less difficult exercise, you can prepare your muscles and nervous system to activate more powerfully and get maximal strength gains when you crank it up a notch for the working sets. As this template is designed to get the highest possible strength yields, we recommend taking long breaks in between sets. Anywhere from 2-4 minutes is fair game if you need it, particularly as the workout goes on.

Warm Up: 20 Walking Lunges (per leg)

Work Sets: 3 sets of 5 Pistol Squats (per leg)

Warm Up: 20 Narrow Push-ups

Work Sets: 3 sets of 3 One Arm Push-ups (per arm)

Warm Up: 10 Pull-ups

Work Sets: 3 sets of 3 Archer Pull-ups (per arm)

Warm Up: 10 Hanging Knee Raises

Work Sets: 3 sets of 5 Toes-to-Bar Leg Raises

Warm Up: 10 Hip Bridges

Work Sets: 3 sets of 3 Wall Crawls

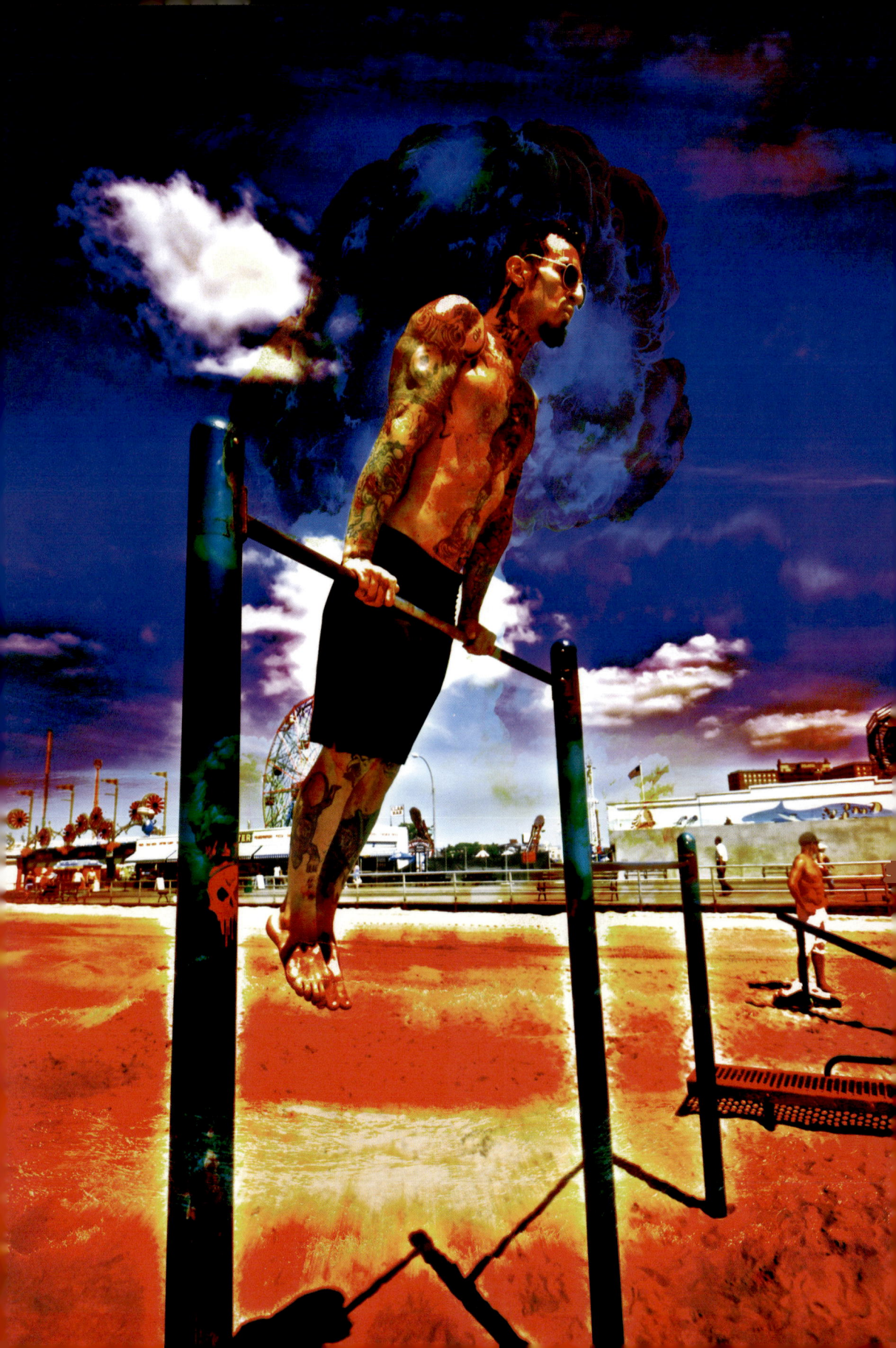

DANNY'S INFERNO

This is an elite upper body bar workout. Though Danny's Inferno is extremely quick, it's also incredibly intense. You will get maximum efficiency in minimal time. Be sure to put in your hours on the pull-up bar before embarking down this road.

Perform all exercises without coming off the bar. After all 25 reps are completed, come off the bar, rest 2-3 minutes and repeat. Aim to repeat the entire circuit 3-5 times. Feel the burn!

5 Muscle-Ups

5 Straight Bar Dips

5 Front Lever Curls

5 Pull-Ups

5 Toes To Bar Leg Raises

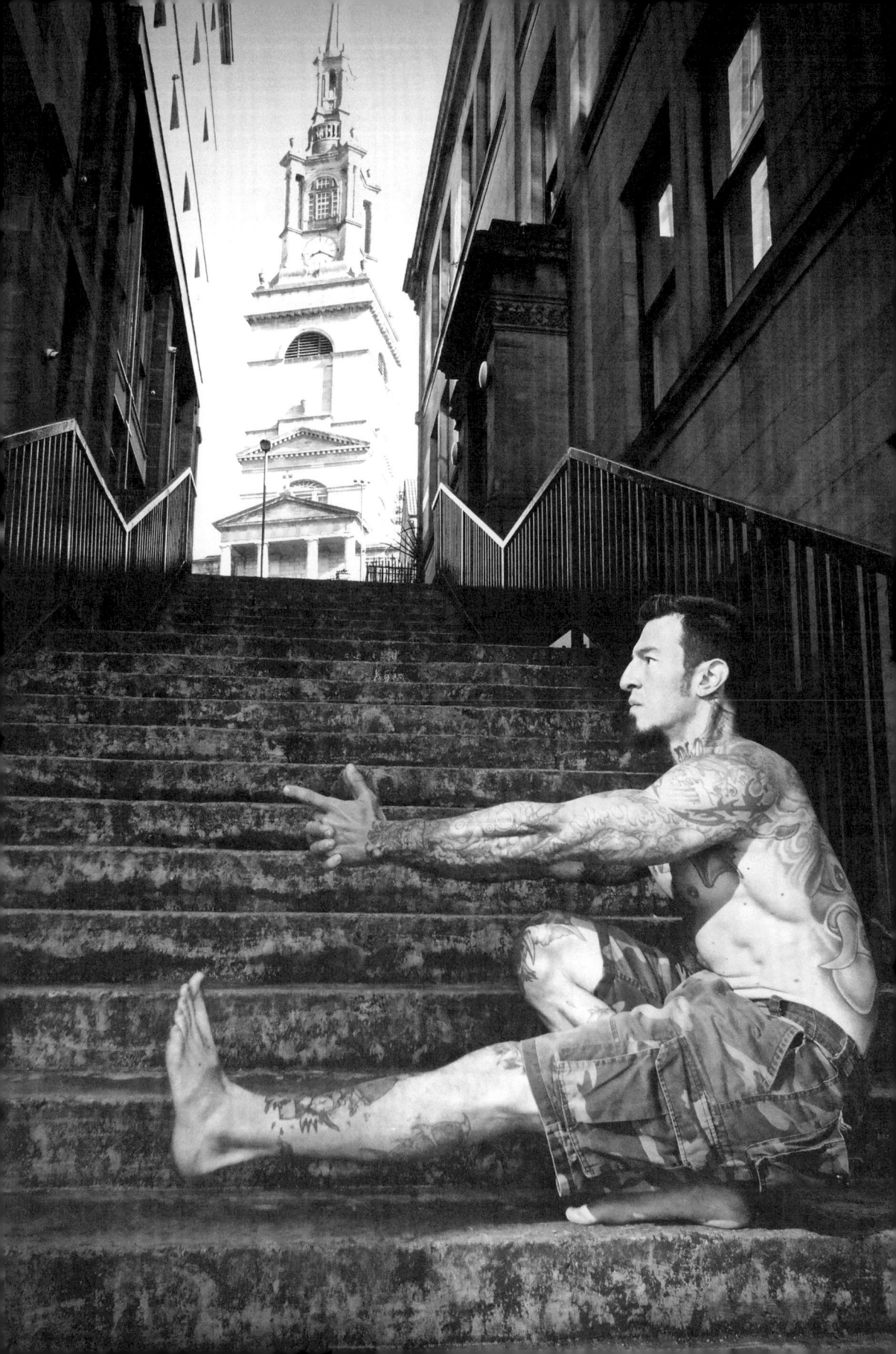

LEG DAZE

The following lower body workout is a brief but powerful way to smoke your legs when time is of the essence. Leg Daze begins with a warm up of 3 progressive exercises. It is to be performed once at the start of the workout to prepare your legs on a muscular and neurological level for what is to follow. The workout set consists of a total of fifteen reps per leg of three different exercises. After completing each leg, rest 3 minutes before repeating. Shoot for a total of 3-5 rounds, depending on your strength level.

Warm Up:

1 set 20 bodyweight squats

1 set of 15 split squats (per leg)

1 set of 10 archer squats (per leg)

Workout (repeat 3-5 times):

5 pistols (per leg)

5 shrimp squats (per leg)

5 Hawaiian squats (per leg)

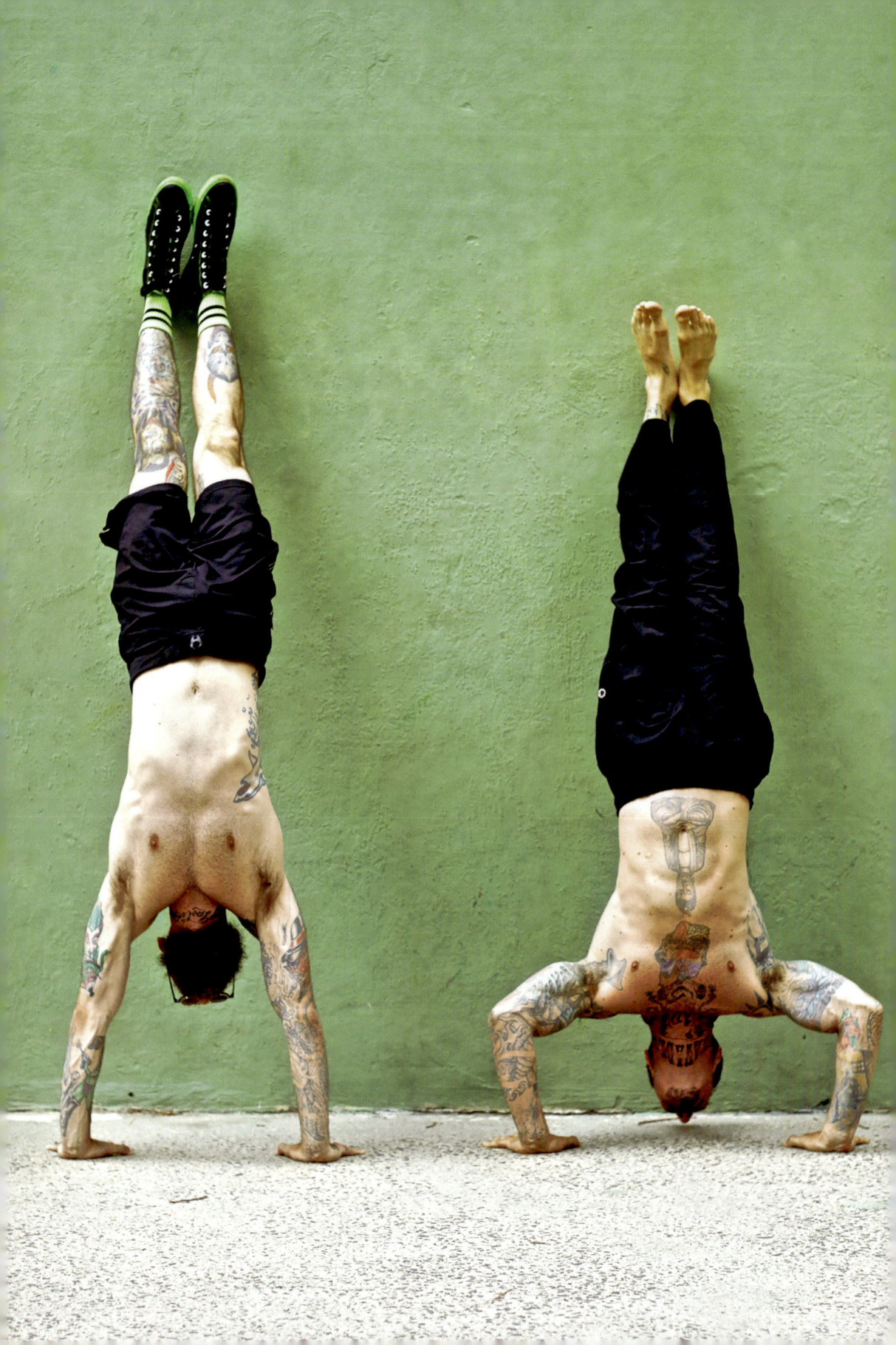

DESTROYER OF WORLDS

This workout is not for the faint of heart! Aim to complete each exercise in as few sets as possible, while adhering to strict form. A truly devoted Street Workout warrior can eventually train to perform each exercise in a single unbroken set with little to no rest between exercises, but you should definitely plan to give yourself several breaks during your first attempt. Make sure you take at least one rest day both before and after attempting this grueling workout for the first time.

100 Squats

50 Push-ups

20 Pull-ups

10 Pistol Squats (per leg)

30 Dips

20 Aussie Pull-ups

10 Hanging Leg Raises

5 Handstand Press-ups

5 Muscle-ups

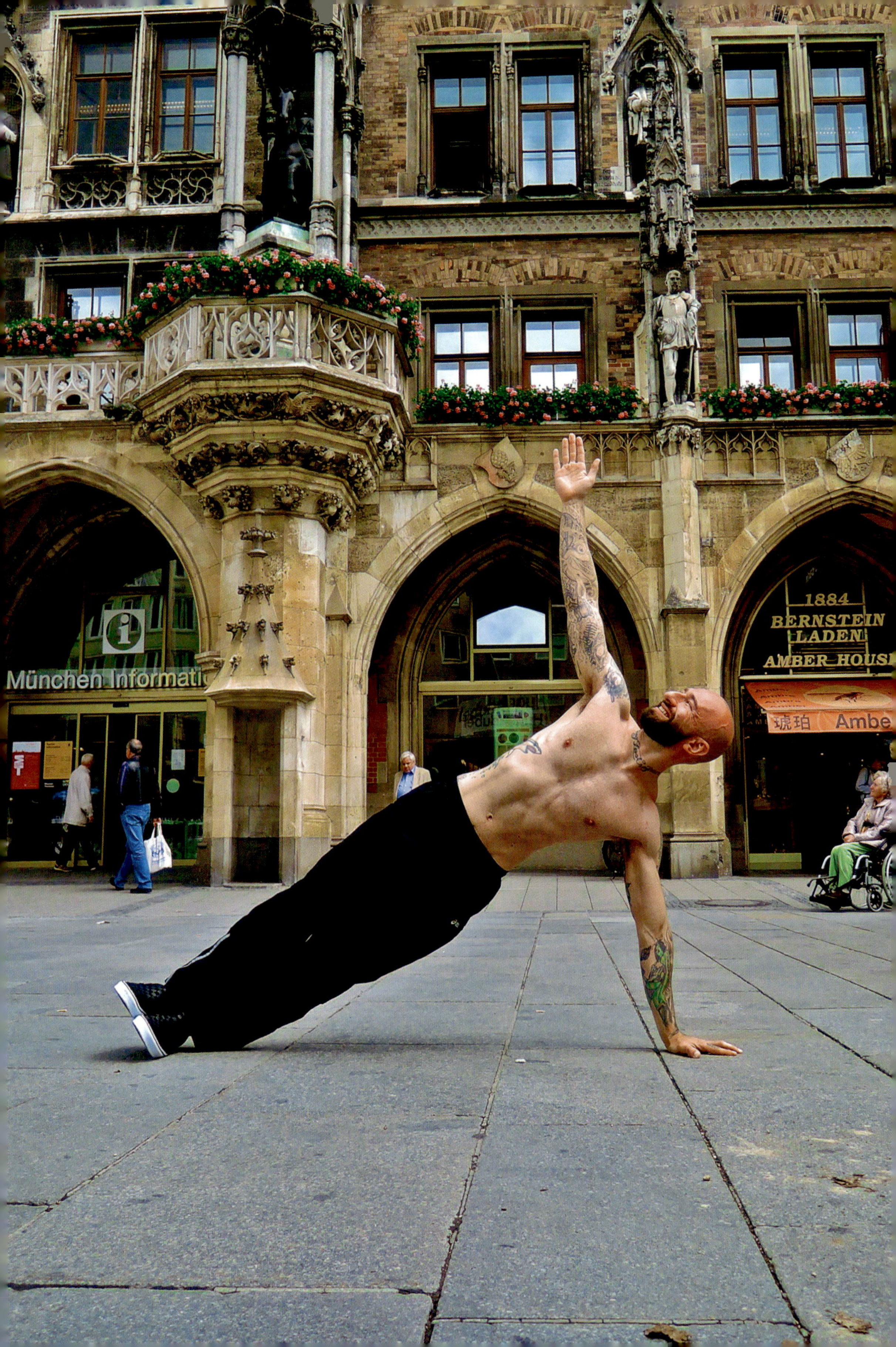
München Informati
1884
BERNSTEIN
LADEN
AMBER HOUS
琥珀 Ambe

Chapter 14

Training Templates

Here are some sample training templates that you can incorporate into your programming. They serve as examples of how you can approach your routines. On some days, full body strength workouts are suggested. On others, we propose a program that emphasizes certain muscle groups or physical skills. Finally, certain days are reserved for rest and recovery.

Full body training is a great way to train. It involves working the whole body as a cohesive unit and does not separate it into components. On these days, because you will be training just about every part of your body, it is not generally suggested that you do every exercise to absolute exhaustion; there is a need for muscular recovery at times. This is not to say that you should not work hard: quite the contrary. In fact, you will not get results without hard work. We simply wish to assert that working every single muscle to complete exhaustion is an unrealistic plan when you train them all with great frequency.

For that reason, sometimes split routines are devised. Split routines play on the principle of active recovery, meaning that while certain muscles bear the brunt of the workout, the muscles that play a less substantial role can recover. It's of note that in the world of Street Workout, a split routine focuses on *one section* of the body per day (as opposed to *one muscle* per day, which is sometimes the case in other disciplines). In other words, even in a split routine, we stress the notion of "emphasis" over "isolation," and still encourage various muscles and muscle groups to work in harmony.

Upper body/lower body splits are common in all worlds of strength training. The term upper body refers to training exercises where the primary movers are above the waist. This includes all forms of push-ups, press-ups, dips, all bar work and more. Lower body incorporates leg exercises such as squats, lunges, calf raises and drinking birds.

A front/back (sometimes called a "push/pull") split is another fantastic way of using active recovery. Front exercises emphasize (though they do not isolate) the muscles found on the anterior of the body—the ones you see when you look in the mirror. These include push-ups, press-ups, all abs flexion, front lever progressions and most squatting patterns. Back exercises are the ones that emphasize the posterior chain, such as pull-ups, Aussie pull-ups, drinking birds, back lever progressions and bridge variations.

On the days that are designated for skill, we propose that you work on those exercises that have a greater technical element than strength component. As we've stated earlier in these pages, all Street Workout exercises require some level of both skill and power, but for the exercises to be performed on these days, finesse is a greater priority than force. Such exercises include hand balancing, headstands and elbow levers. It can be helpful on these days to think in terms of "practice" rather than "training."

Like all programs, these splits are suggestions, devised to serve as examples, but still subject to interpretation. That goes for your rest days, too. The term "rest" does not mean that we advise you to sit on the couch all day, with your most strenuous activity being flipping the channels on your remote control. No. You can still take a bike ride, jog or work on flexibility. It's okay to be on your feet and active. On the other hand, there are times when we train harder than we perceive at the time. If this is the case, then taking it easy is most certainly an option. You may need to recover for two days at times, even if the template suggests only one. Let your own experience dictate.

All of the exercises in this book can be incorporated into your program. Your fitness and skill level will dictate which specific moves are appropriate for you. You can use the same templates indefinitely, so long as you switch out the exercises for harder ones when called for. Remember, in each section exercises are presented in approximate order of least to most difficult. For example, a beginner who starts out doing hands elevated pushups can eventually progress to classic push-ups, feet elevated push-ups and ultimately one arm push-ups.

Template A: Old Faithful

DAY 1	Full Body
DAY 2	Rest
DAY 3	Full Body
DAY 4	Rest
DAY 5	Full Body
DAY 6	Rest
DAY 7	Rest

Template B: Terminator

DAY 1	Full Body
DAY 2	Rest
DAY 3	Upper Body
DAY 4	Lower Body
DAY 5	Rest
DAY 6	Skills
DAY 7	Rest

Template C: Terminator II

DAY 1 Full Body

DAY 2 Rest

DAY 3 Front

DAY 4 Back

DAY 5 Rest

DAY 6 Skills

DAY 7 Rest

Template D: The Gauntlet

DAY 1 Upper Body

DAY 2 Lower Body

DAY 3 Rest

DAY 4 Front

DAY 5 Back

DAY 6 Skills

DAY 7 Rest

Template E: Mad Skills

- DAY 1 Full Body
- DAY 2 Rest
- DAY 3 Skills
- DAY 4 Full Body
- DAY 5 Rest
- DAY 6 Skills
- DAY 7 Skills

Template F: Sharpshooter

- DAY 1 Upper Body
- DAY 2 Lower Body
- DAY 3 Skills
- DAY 4 Upper Body
- DAY 5 Lower Body
- DAY 6 Skills
- DAY 7 Rest

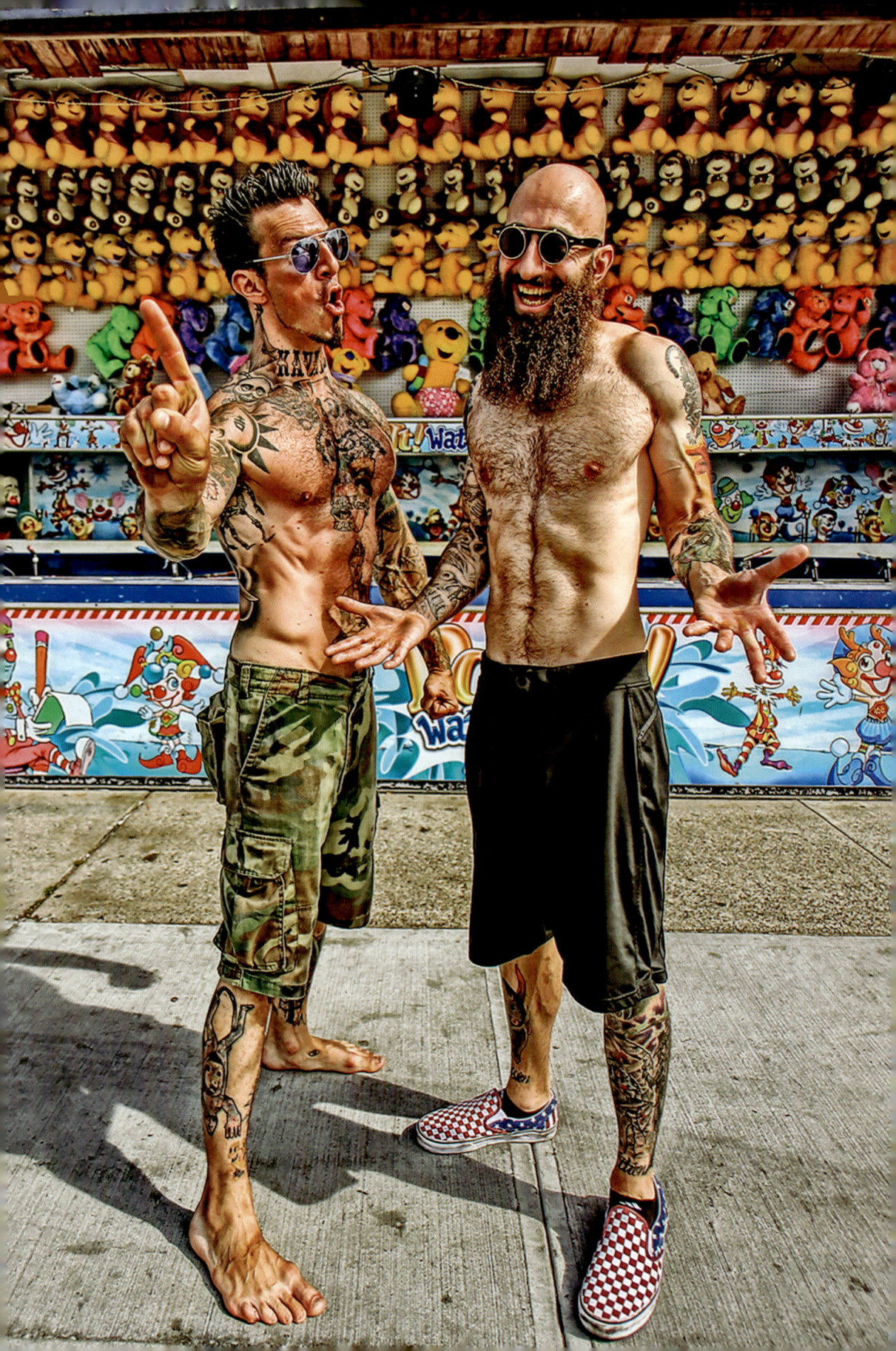

V
Bonus Section

Beyond the moves and past the programming, there is still so much more to discuss. Transcending the text is where your journey truly begins. Once you take that first step, you will see that there are aspects of Street Workout that defy standard categorization, as well as unanswered questions, unresolved issues and other proverbial stones that remain unturned.

How do we take what we've learned and put it to action?

What happens when we encounter unforeseen obstacles?

How can we apply our newfound skills to various real world situations?

In the following pages, we'll show you how to put it all together and start getting stronger right now. Be it in your very own backyard jungle gym or in the urban jungle outside your front door, here's the real deal on how to maximize these training tactics. The world is your playground.

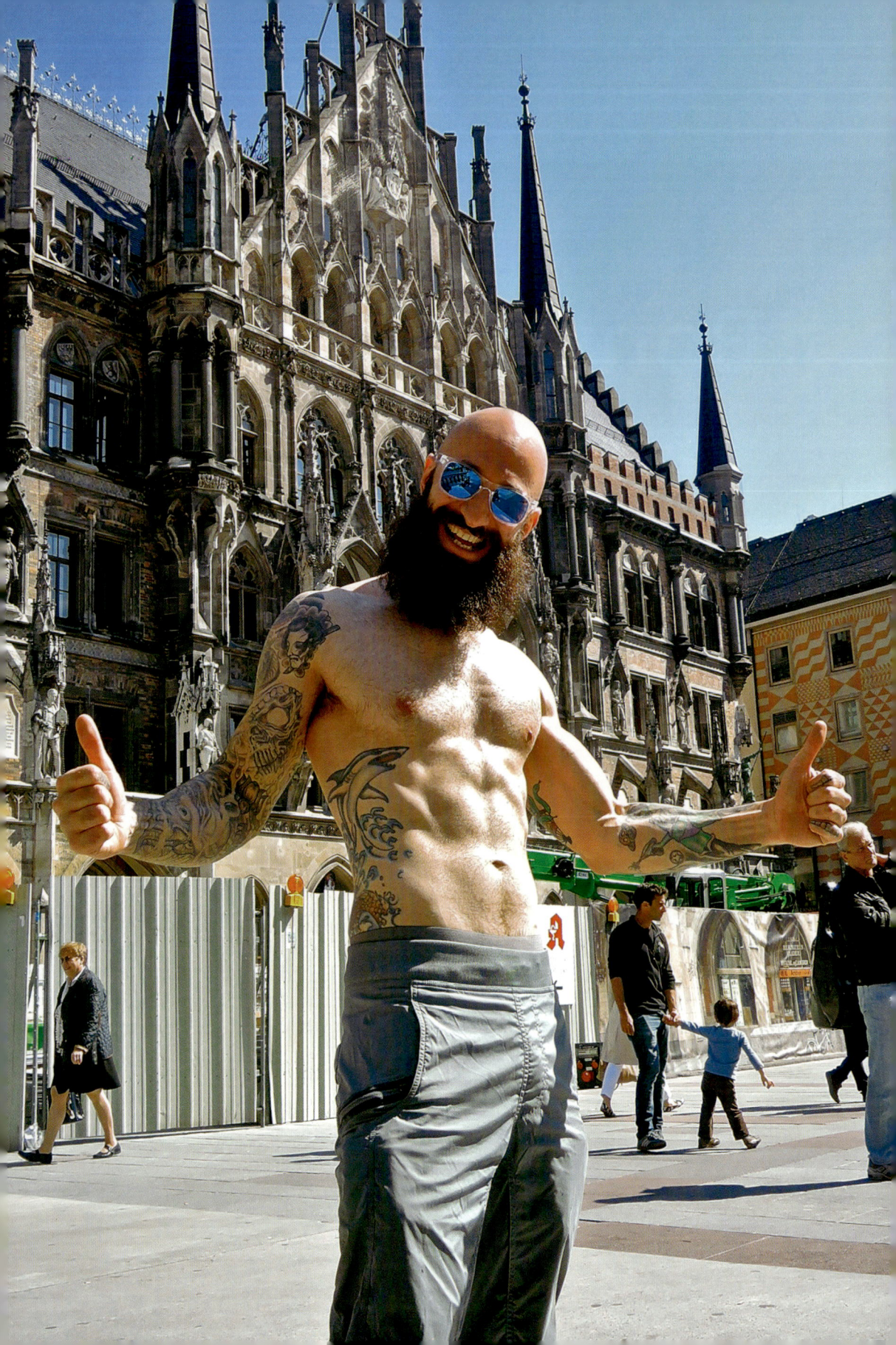

Chapter 15

Ask Al

I get asked a lot of questions! What follows are some of the most common ones I've gotten throughout my career as a fitness trainer, along with the most pragmatic answers I can give. A lot of them are about my observations as a personal trainer, while others are about my own personal training. Chances are that most questions you have are already answered here, though they may be phrased slightly differently in your head. Hopefully you will be able to apply these general answers to your particular situation. If not, that's okay. You can always drop me a line on Facebook or Instagram.

> Dear Sir,
> I am in Ghana - West Africa. A 31 year old man who weighs 58kg. I am very slim. I got hold of your book pushing the limits and I love it. How can I do the push ups well? Having practice in my lifetime before. Thank you

> Bro give advice! Amounted to exercise program on a lot but don't fit in 45 minutes, exercises can't be deleted because they complement each other. If you break it into parts, to do all that time for 40 minutes and the rest to finish before bedtime. What do you think?

> hey hey hey , Al when we see your vidios we feel like you were a good friend for a long time thanks for your great works and also i must say you looks very friendly and nice with your long beard you are lucky man

What is your diet like?

I don't really follow any diet. My only rule is to avoid heavily processed fake foods and to keep my portions from getting out of control. I don't count calories and I don't concern myself with food groups, fats, proteins or carbohydrates. I usually get most of my calories in the second half of the day, but that's just when I tend to get hungry.

Do you take any supplements?

No, I do not take any powders, pills, or other supplements of any kind.

But what about...

No Supplements. No creatine, no glutamine, no BCAA's, no fish oils, or anything else. I don't take any exercise/dietary supplements whatsoever. None.

Ok, I get that you don't use supplements. But what about protein powder?

Noooooooo!!!!!!!!

Do you lift weights?

No. Though I did lift during my teens and early twenties, weight training has not been part of my lifestyle for over a decade. On occasion if I'm in a gym I might pick up a weight just for the heck of it, but that is a rare occurrence.

Contrary to what some people will tell you, however, I have nothing against weight training. I fully acknowledge that lifting weights is an effective way to build strength and muscle. It's just not my thing.

What about adding weights to calisthenics exercises, like wearing a weighted vest for push-ups?

Again, not my thing, but if that's what you're into, then don't let me stop you. You don't have to add weights. Just look for a harder exercise. We've got a lot of them in this book.

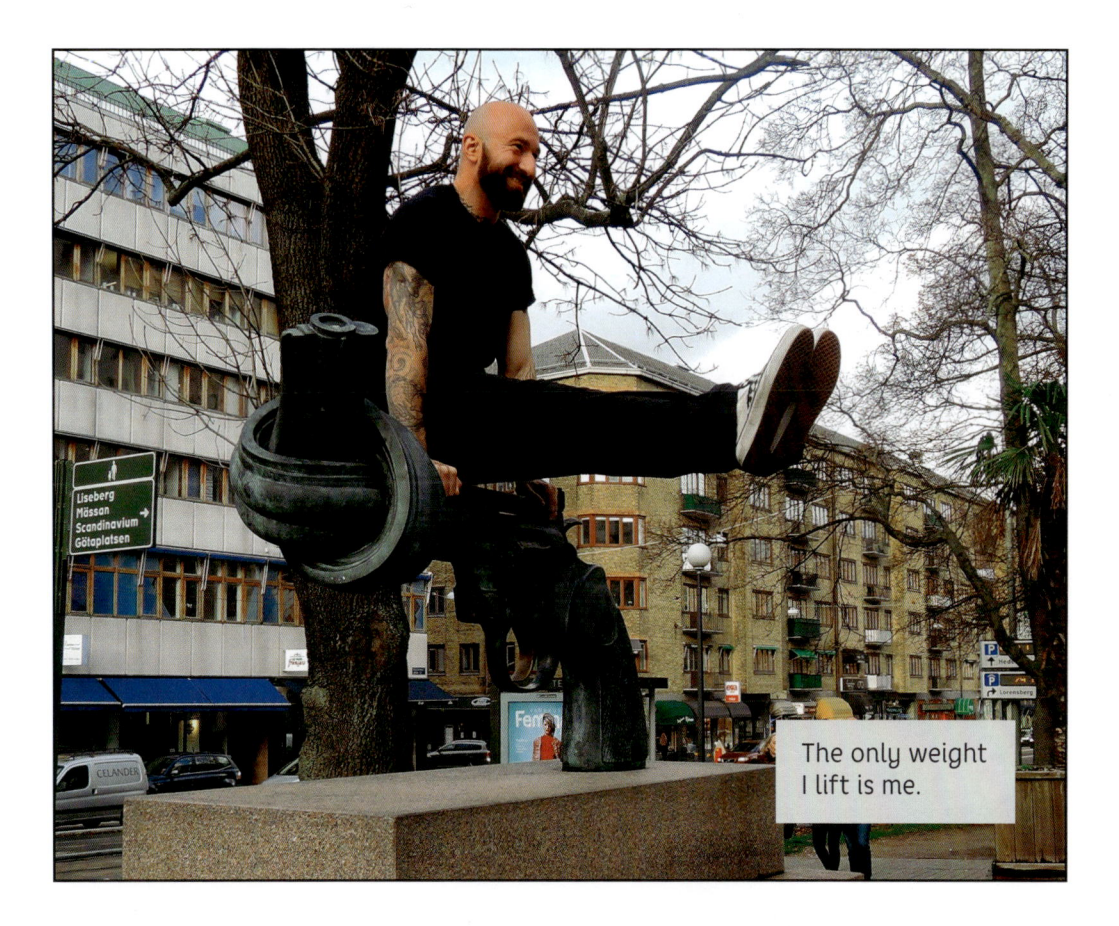

But what if I want to get big? Don't I need to lift?

For the last time, no, I don't believe weights are necessary to gain muscle mass. If you want to gain mass, do lots of sets and reps of the basics (4-5 sets of 10-20 reps per exercise) and eat a lot of clean food. Also be aware that individual genetics will play a factor. Check out my friend Coach Wade's book C-Mass if you want more info on gaining mass with calisthenics.

Can I combine weights and calisthenics in the same program?

For sure! Just because I don't, doesn't mean that you can't. Do whatever you like!

What about cardio?

I like to go for a run or jump rope from time to time, but I don't do it for weight loss, I do it for fun!

But don't I have to do cardio to get ripped?

No. If you want to be well-rounded in your fitness, I recommend you get some cardiovascular exercise, but if you just want to get strong and look good with your shirt off, strength training is far more effective than cardio. If you need to lose fat, changing your eating habits will do more for you than any workout.

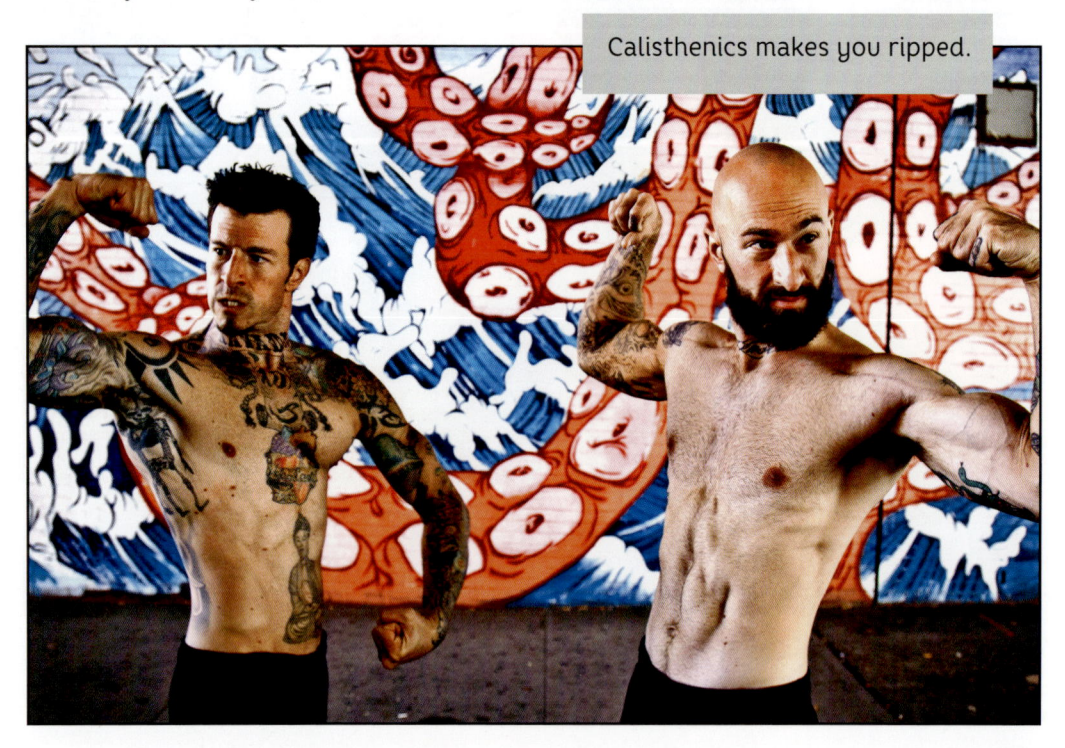

Calisthenics makes you ripped.

What do you think of Crossfit/P90X/Zumba/etc?

I am a fan of anything that inspires people to exercise, which all of those brands have successfully done. That's the most important thing. There is no best program and all of them will work if they are implemented with consistency and intensity, so pick something that appeals to you and stick with it. Obviously, the exercises in this book are my favorites. That's why they're here! But all forms of exercise are beneficial.

I heard isometric holds are better than reps, but then I read that someone else said the opposite. Who's right?

It's great to practice both isometric holds like planks and L-sits as well as rep out on moves like push-ups and pull-ups. The two complement each other very nicely and practicing both will help you develop better body control than just practicing one or the other.

Why am I better than my friend at some exercises, but my friend is better than me at others?

Though some people have more natural aptitude than others in certain areas, we all get better at the things we practice consistently. So if your friend is better than you at pull-ups, practice more pull-ups and you'll get better. If you struggle to hold a handstand, spend time practicing your handstand. Work on the stuff you need to work on and you'll get better at everything.

Do you wear gloves when you work out?

The only time Danny or I wear gloves when we train is if we would be wearing them anyway. If you're worried about getting callouses on your hands, Street Workout is not for you. If there's snow on the bar, however, that's a different story.

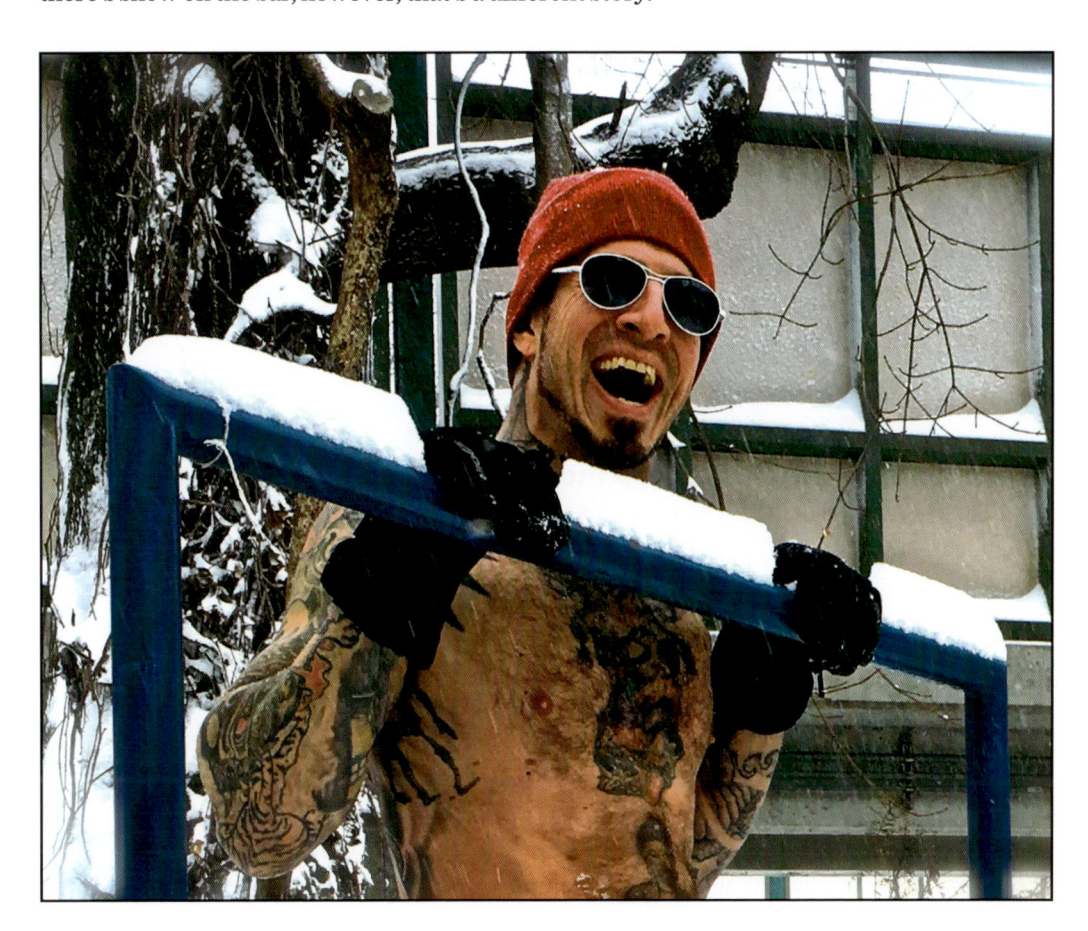

Do you still train outdoors in the rain/snow/cold? If so, what modifications do you need to make?

I prefer outdoor workouts over training indoors, but sometimes being warm and dry is a higher priority, so I do train at home or in a gym sometimes. The great thing about working out in the cold, however, is that if you wear enough layers and keep moving, eventually you won't notice that it's cold out. Then it starts to feel really good!

As for modifications, when I train in the cold, I tend to focus on exercises that I can perform more reps of, so I won't need to take as much rest. I will also often do circuit workouts where I alternate between upper and lower body exercises. Both of these things allow me to keep moving, which helps me keep warm. Isometric holds like planks and L-sits also help generate body heat. I recommend wearing several layers to start, so as you warm up you can begin to remove some clothing. Moves that require extreme mobility or place a great deal of emphasis on a single joint (like the back bridge and one arm pull-up, respectively) are better kept to warmer circumstances.

Do you ever get scared that you are going to fall and get hurt when practicing moves like elevated handstands, human flags, etc?

If my instincts tell me not to try something, I'll usually listen. Then I'll look for something similar that's less intimidating and try that first. Once I've done the less-scary move a few times, I might be able to go back to the original challenge with newfound courage. Sometimes that confidence even starts to extend into other aspects of my life.

What's better: high reps at a moderate intensity or fewer reps at a higher intensity?

Both of these training methods will make you stronger and promote muscular growth, but the emphasis will be slightly different. Conventional wisdom says that performing 5 sets of 5 reps at a higher intensity will place more of an emphasis on strength, while performing 3 sets of 15-20 reps at a moderate intensity is better for growth. However, the strongest, most muscular people tend to be able to perform well across the board. The idea that strength and endurance are on opposite sides of the spectrum is not always applicable in the world of calisthenics. I assure you, the same folks who are performing one arm pull-ups and human flags are also capable of 20 pull-ups in a single set. In short, it doesn't matter much which type of program you use, just as long as you train hard and are consistent with your workouts.

Street Workout takes big balls.

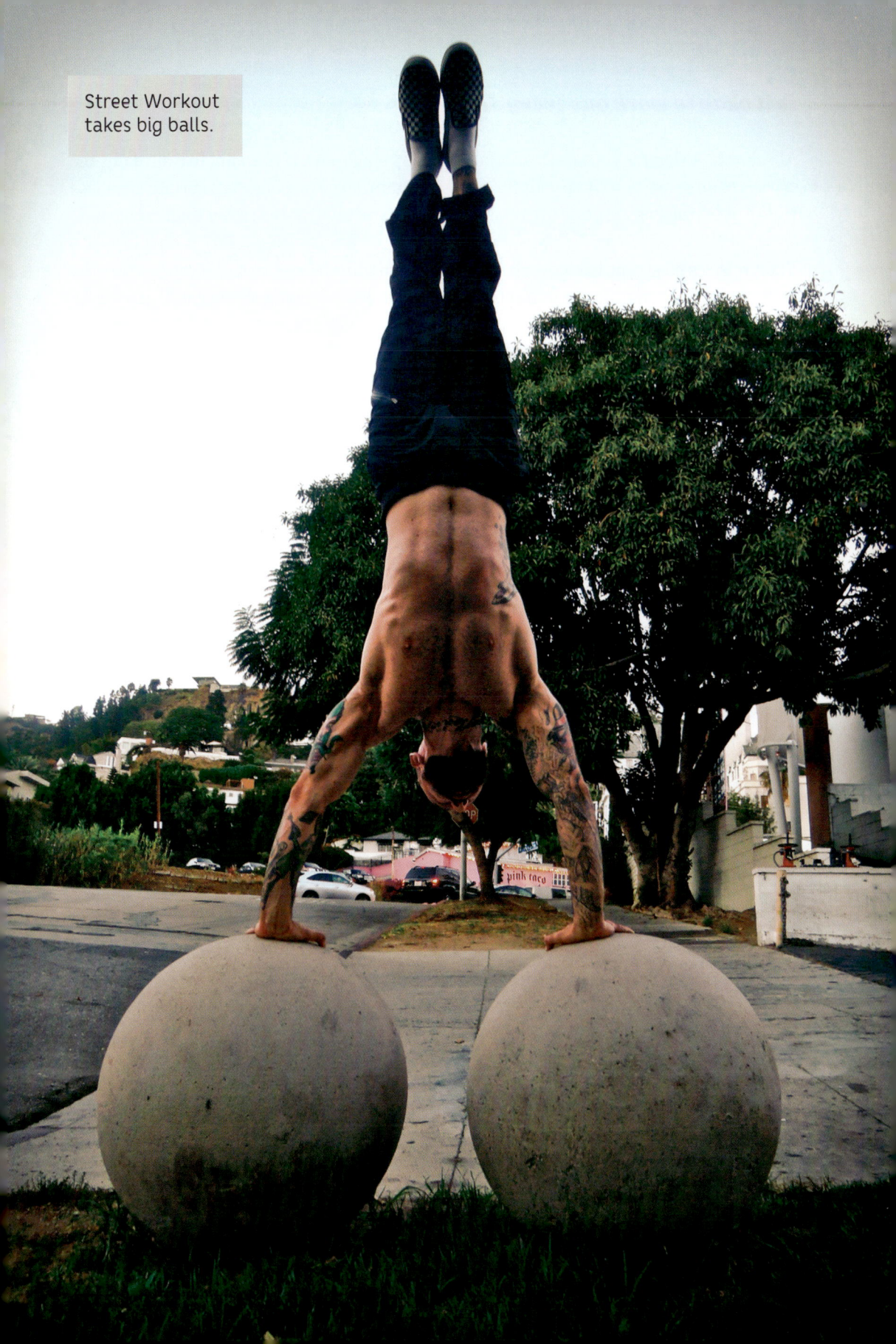

Is it okay to work out every day?

Absolutely. As long as you aren't going all out every single day. If you want to train daily, the best ways to do so are to split up your training so certain days are focused on certain exercises or to do a quick full body routine every day that leaves you invigorated rather than exhausted.

Your muscles need time to recover between strength training sessions, so if you feel sore the next day after your training, it can be best to give yourself a day off, but you can also practice "active recovery" if you don't like taking rest days. This simply means that you do some form of physical activity on the days that you are not strength training. This can be jogging, swimming, hiking, cycling or any other low-to-moderate level physical activity of your choosing.

How do I know when I am ready to move onto harder progressions?

As a general rule, get comfortable with the basic versions from each family of exercises before you move onto more advanced exercises. This book is laid out in such a way as to guide you through the progressions, with the more difficult moves toward the end of each section, but it's ultimately up to you to control your destiny. How hard you work is going to be the most important factor that determines your progress. Having said that, take your time and embrace the process.

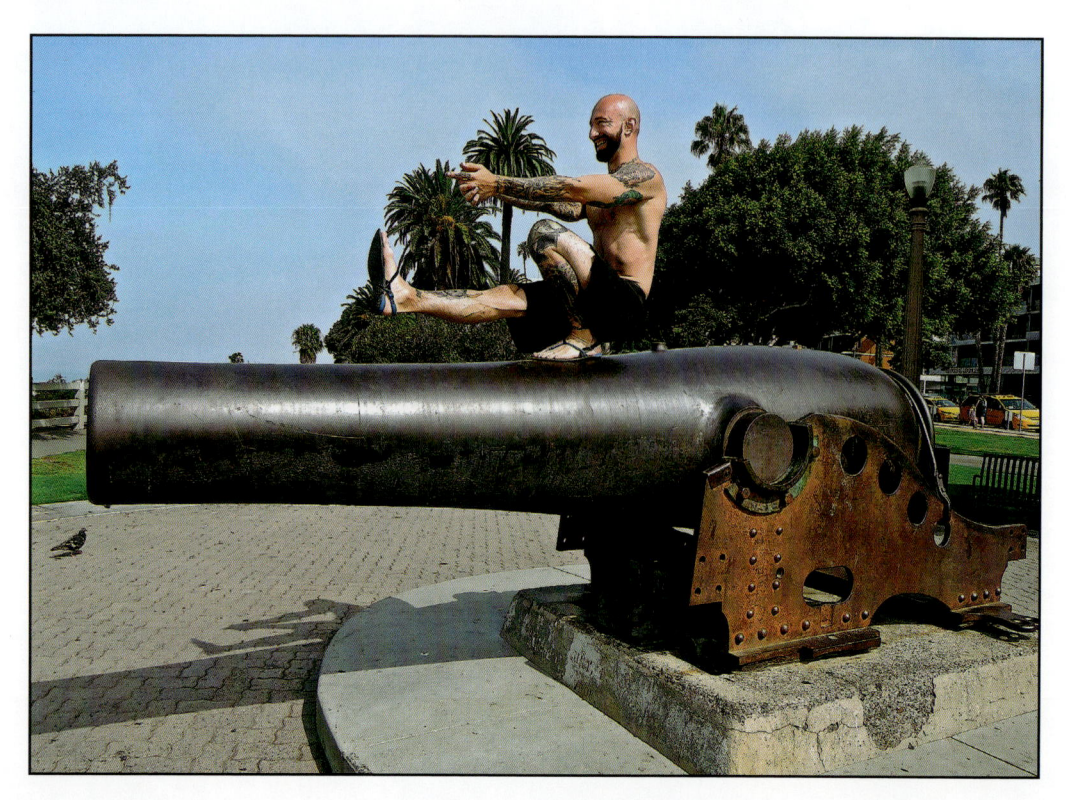

How long is it going to take before I can do a pistol squat/muscle-up/human flag/etc.?

It depends on a lot of individual factors, so I can't give a definite timeline that will be accurate for everyone. As a general rule, however, it's important to make sure you have a solid foundation in the basics before you attempt advanced moves. If you are new to strength training, be prepared to spend at least six months working on things like push-ups, pull-ups, dips, squats and lunges before moving onto anything advanced. For many people it will be much longer. Take your time. There is no rush!

I train karate/wrestling/football/etc. Which exercises should I be doing to get stronger at my martial art/sport?

The best thing you can do to improve at any martial art, sport or other discipline (other than developing the skills specific to that sport, like kicking or throwing) is to get stronger. General strength training exercises like push-ups, pull-ups and squats are ideal for this.

You will not magically become better at your sport because you learned to do an elbow lever, but getting stronger will make you better at everything (including elbow levers).

How can I further develop my upper chest, lower chest, biceps peak, calves or other body part?

If there is a specific body part that you feel is lagging behind the others, you can try to target that body part by doing additional exercises, sets or reps of moves that emphasize that area. For example, you could do more push-ups if you feel your chest is lagging or do additional chin-ups to target your biceps.

It's important to remember, however, that individual genetics are a huge factor that affects all of our physical appearances. While you can change the size of your muscles with strength training, you can't do much to change the shape of your muscles. Some people have a natural peak on their biceps, while others do not. Some of us have crooked abs, while others have boxy abs. Some people's chest tends to develop more in certain places than others. It's just like how some people have brown eyes and others have blue eyes. Do the best with what you got and try not to obsess over your perceived imperfections. Regardless of where you are at today, you can still improve and expand your physical capabilities.

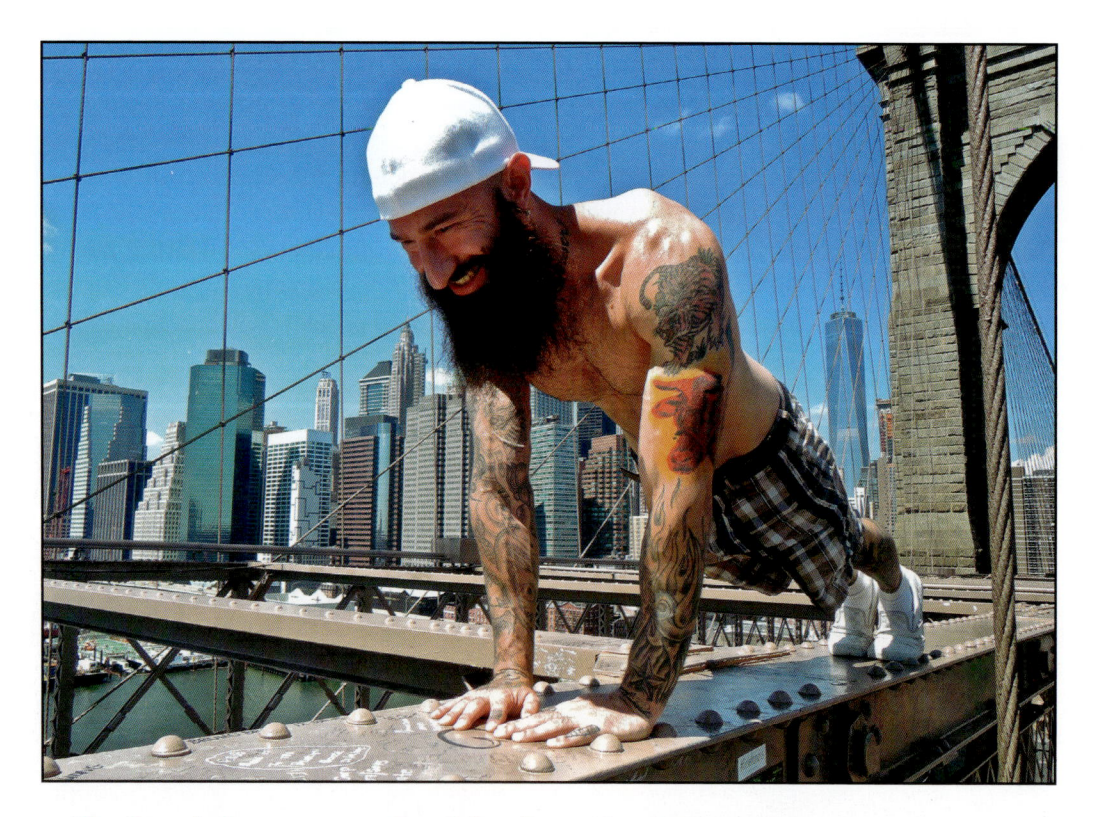

I had an injury to my shoulder/knee/wrist and it hurts to do squats/push-ups/pull-ups/dips/etc. What should I do?

It's impossible to give one-size-fits-all rehab programming because each injury is unique. The best thing I can tell anyone who wants to train while healing an ailment is to avoid anything that feels like it is exacerbating the situation.

That said, do whatever you can do without causing pain. If you can't work your upper-body for a little while, then focus on your legs. If you've got a busted ankle, then focus on pull-ups. If all you can do is walk, then walk. If you can only do push-ups on your knuckles, then so be it. There is always something productive you can do no matter the situation.

My friend/trainer/someone on the internet says pistols squats are bad for your knees/bridging is bad for your back/muscle-ups are bad for your shoulders/etc. Is that true?

The wrong exercise for the wrong person can be detrimental. Is a 500 pound deadlift bad for you? No, not if you're strong enough to handle it. But if your grandma tried to lift that much she might break her back. The same is true for advanced calisthenics: Try to do too much, too quickly, and you could run into a problem. Furthermore, employing poor technique can potentially lead to mishaps. However, if you are smart about building up to advanced moves, there is very little risk involved.

Keep in mind that no matter what exercise you choose, someone on the internet has probably written an article about how it is going to kill you. That's just the world we live in. There is a lot of fear mongering in this world, but we're here to empower you. In the end, it's up to each individual to use their own common sense and make their own decisions.

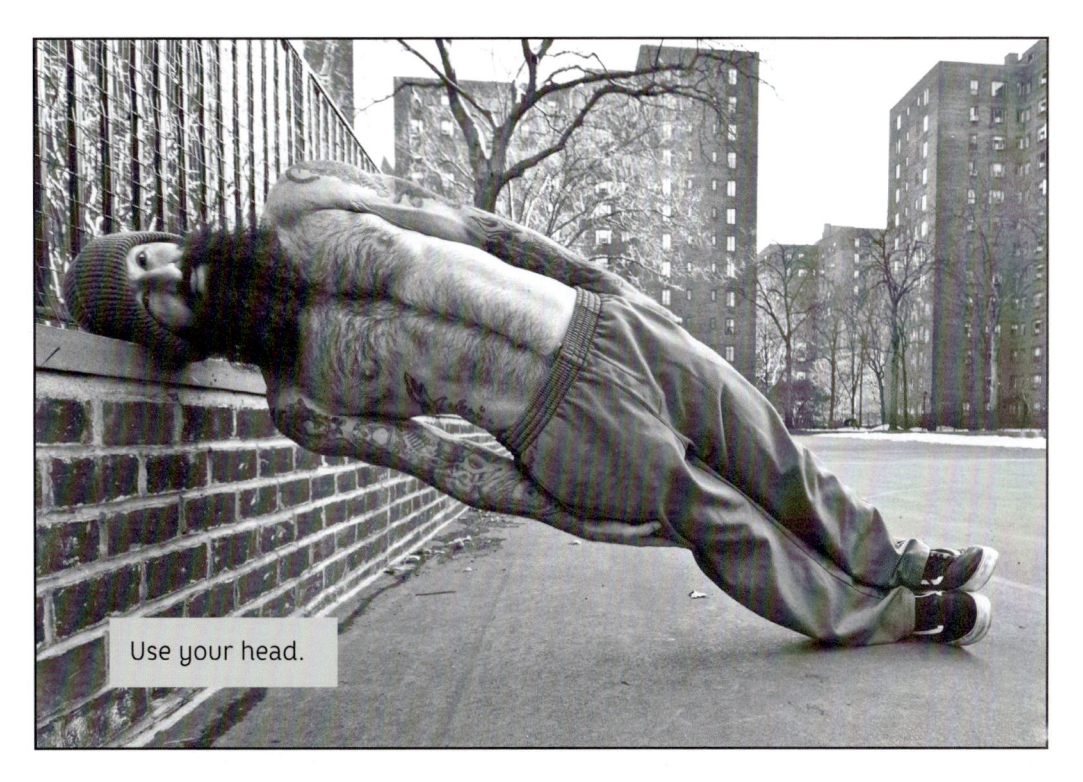

Use your head.

It hurts when I do a push-up/pull-up/bridge/etc. Should I keep doing it anyway?

No. Pain is a signal from your body that whatever you are doing is causing harm. However, a burning sensation in your muscles (and/or lungs) is to be expected, though it should not be mistaken for pain.

If you are experiencing actual pain (it shouldn't be too hard to tell the difference), then you are likely performing an exercise incorrectly, attempting an exercise that is outside of your current capabilities and/or you may have an injury/ailment that is causing the problem. Do your best to make adjustments accordingly. If you are unable to find a solution, seek the help of a medical professional.

I read the whole book and I still don't know what to do. There's so many different exercises in here! What should I do?

Start wherever you are and do whatever you can. We have done our best to give you the tools to build the body you always wanted, but you have to take action. Use the workout plans in this book as a guide, but make whatever adjustments you have to. Focus on consistent training more than the details of said training, and be honest with yourself. You reap what you sow.

I really want to start training, but I think I need to get in better shape first. What should I do?

If you're looking for an excuse not to train, you'll always be able to find one. But the truth is, it doesn't matter where you are starting from, it only matters that you start.

But I'm too old to start now, right?

I've heard the "I'm too old" excuse from folks as young as 20 years old. I've also met fit individuals who didn't begin training until well after their retirement. It's never too late to start, and there's no better time than right now. Let's do it.

We're Working Out!

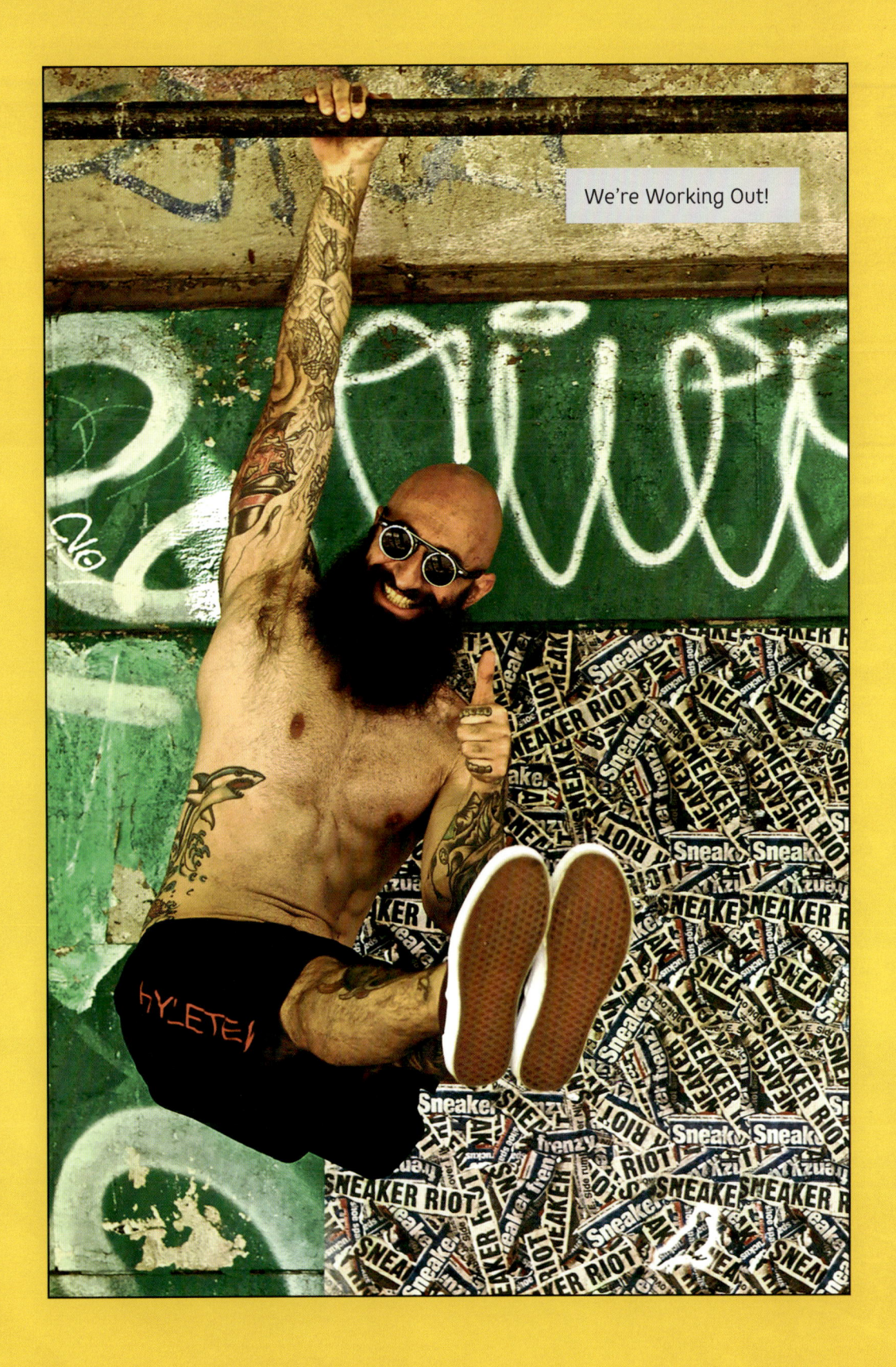

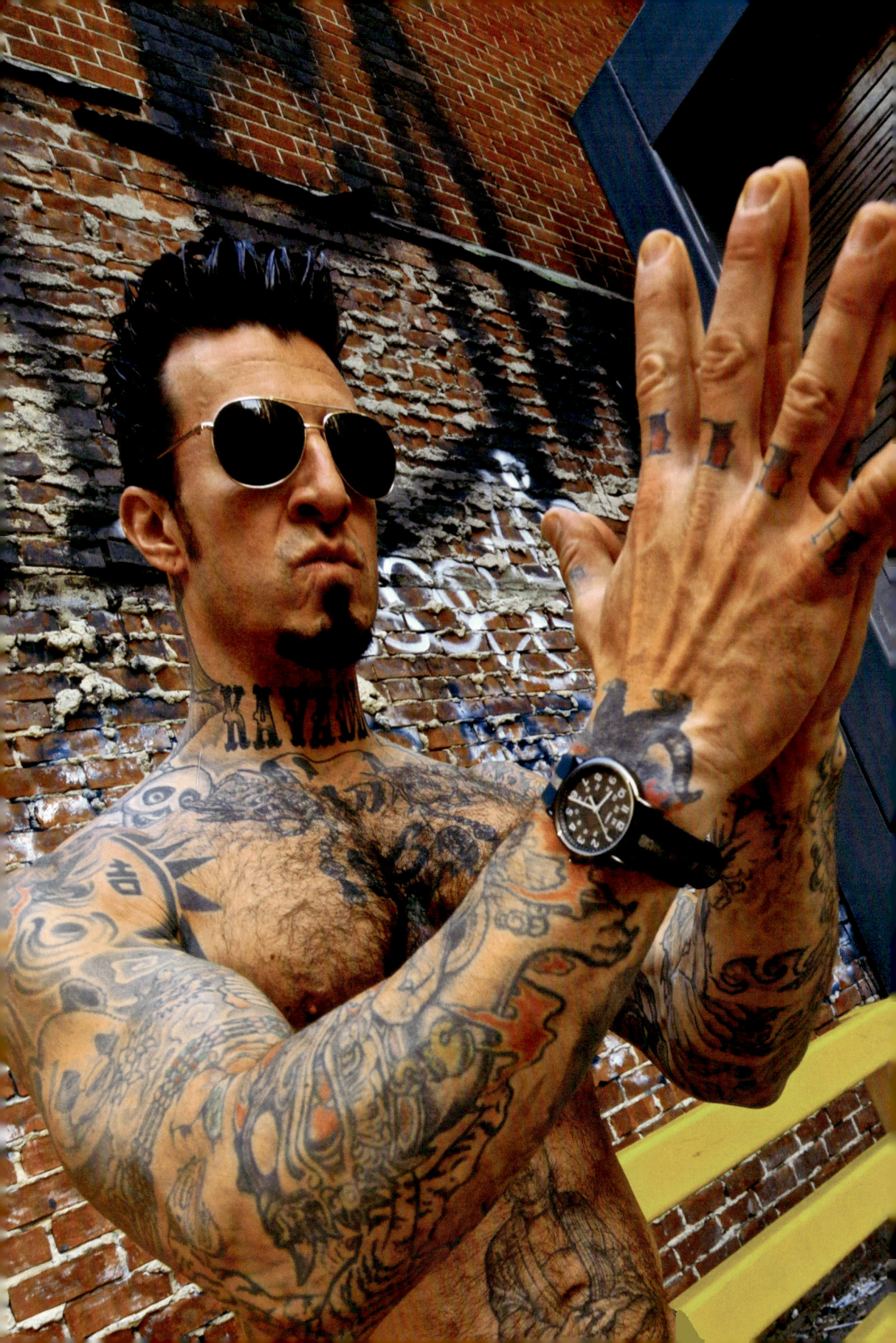

Chapter 16

Danny's Dos and Don'ts

1. DO WORK HARD.

If your training doesn't feel strenuous, then it isn't. And it's probably not working. Sweat, muscular soreness, and an accelerated heart rate are all byproducts of exercise. In life and fitness, results do not often come without hard work. It's not supposed to be effortless. By the same token, be weary of fitness claims that boast of easy, proven methods. No matter what anyone says, fitness must be earned. Almost everything worthwhile does.

In other words, you gotta try. When I say that, I do not mean acting out a half-hearted attempt at something special. I don't mean simply showing up and going through the motions. That is not trying. I am referring to effort and hours and elbow grease. Be honest and don't kid yourself. Hell, even if you're good at exercise and in shape, you still have to work hard to make improvement. That's the beauty of it.

You see, ambition wins over talent every time. No matter what situation you were born into, or even earned, you cannot excel without drive and motivation. Put in the time. Make the effort. Be consistent and accountable.

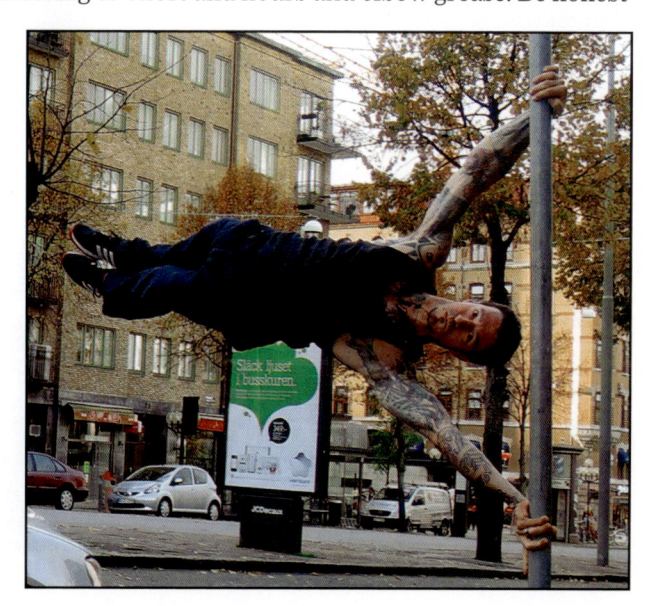

2. DO SET REALISTIC GOALS.

There are long term goals and there are short term goals. Be realistic about your timeline. If your goal is to do a muscle-up, but you cannot do one proper pull-up, then the muscle-up should probably be a long term goal.

On that note, if your goal is to do a muscle-up in *two weeks* (or any other short, absolute time frame), but you are incapable of doing ten proper pull-ups right now, then you are setting yourself up for disappointment. Perhaps a better goal would be to train toward a muscle-up four days a week, long term, without a perceived date of execution.

On the other hand, sometimes you do set a viable goal and it is still not met. I know this can be disappointing, but understand that this is not always a bad thing. Goals are organic; they change. The turnout may not be what was initially anticipated, but that doesn't mean you should reject all possible outcomes. Let's say you set out to lose twenty pounds. In the process, you change your lifestyle, start eating right and begin training consistently. After several weeks, you feel more alive than ever, you are stronger than before and your clothes fit better. But you only lost fifteen pounds.

So what? You did good, kid. The destination you reached may not have been the target you set, but it was the pursuit that got you there.

To go back to the previous example of training for the muscle-up: perhaps it doesn't happen in the timeframe you planned, *but your pull-up count increases from ten to twenty*. Even though you did not get the muscle-up, you still made great progress.

Setting a goal does not necessarily mean achieving it. It means embarking on the struggle to attain it and seeing where that takes you. Progress means moving forward.

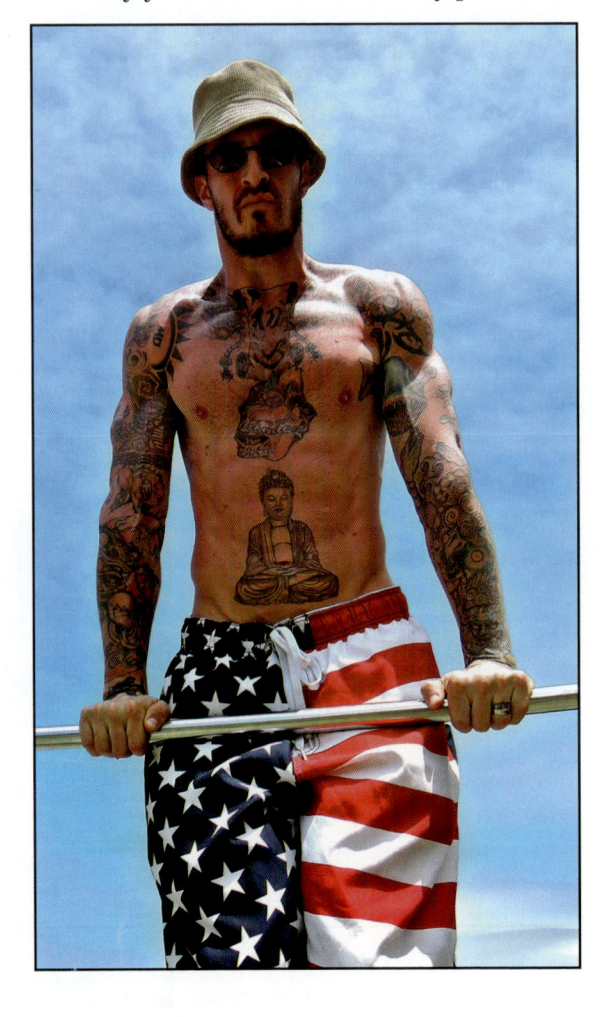

3. DO BELIEVE IN YOURSELF.

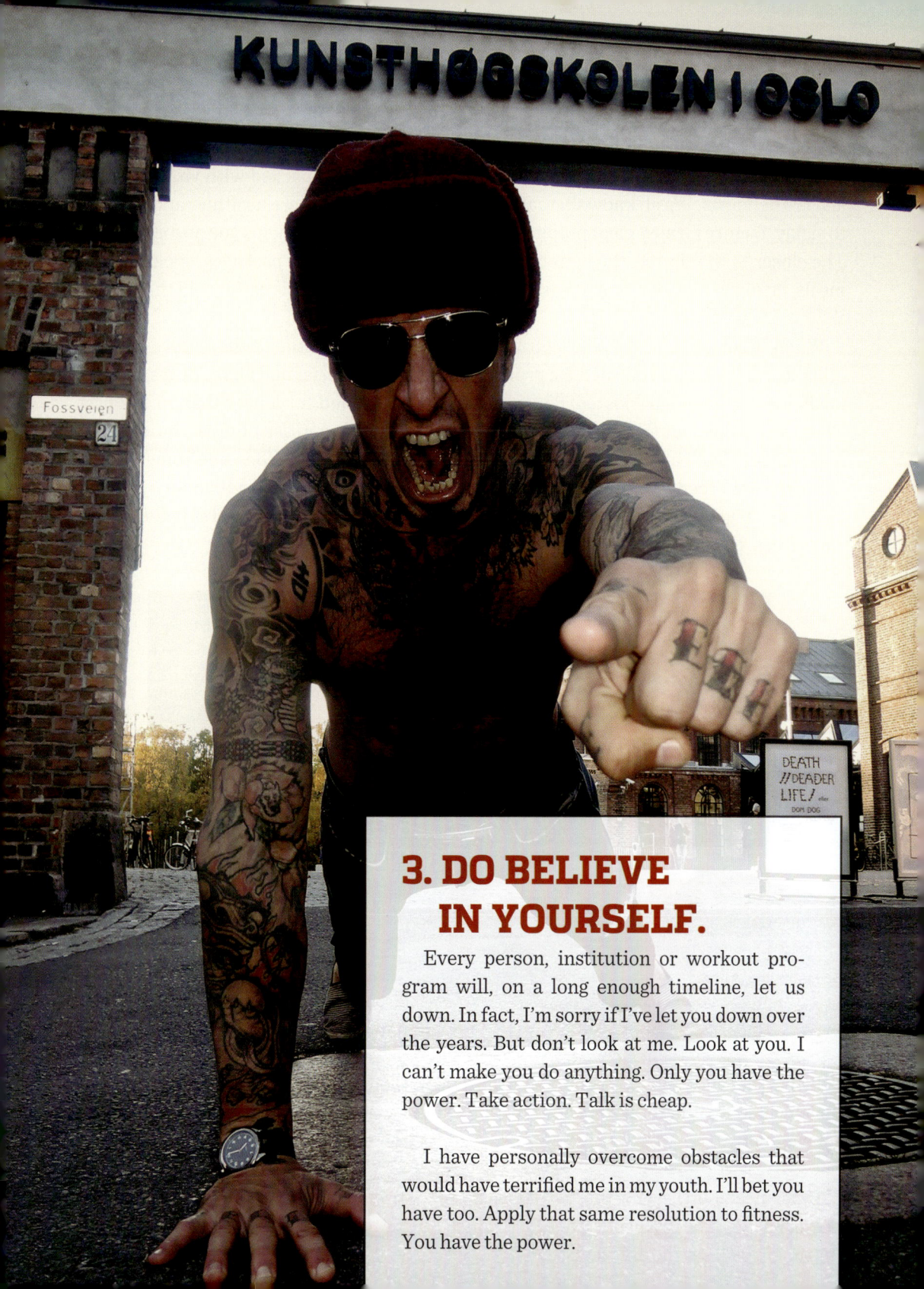

Every person, institution or workout program will, on a long enough timeline, let us down. In fact, I'm sorry if I've let you down over the years. But don't look at me. Look at you. I can't make you do anything. Only you have the power. Take action. Talk is cheap.

I have personally overcome obstacles that would have terrified me in my youth. I'll bet you have too. Apply that same resolution to fitness. You have the power.

4. DO PUT GOOD THINGS IN YOUR BODY.

We find ourselves telling our kids the same things our parents told us. Fruits and vegetables are good for you. They make you lean and strong, are packed with vital nutrients and are delicious. We all know that farm raised animal proteins are healthier and superior to sickly, factory farmed meat products. Fish is brain food. Fiber helps you absorb vitality. The closer to the source, the better. I advise eating out of fewer packages, cooking more meals, drinking more water and having less sugar. For many, this is easier said than done.

When it comes to health, our culture focuses more on treatment than prevention. In other words, by employing medical procedures, gastric surgeries and lots of drugs, modern medicine can keep our bloated, flaccid bodies above ground for longer than in the past. There are people out there who would rather take large quantities of prescription pharmaceuticals than eat a salad every day. Others would choose to consume some strange "Frankenstein food" mechanically rendered to simulate meat, rather than enjoy a farm raised pig. If you are someone who prefers a handful of multivitamins and supplements to some fresh, cold-pressed juice, then you've missed the point.

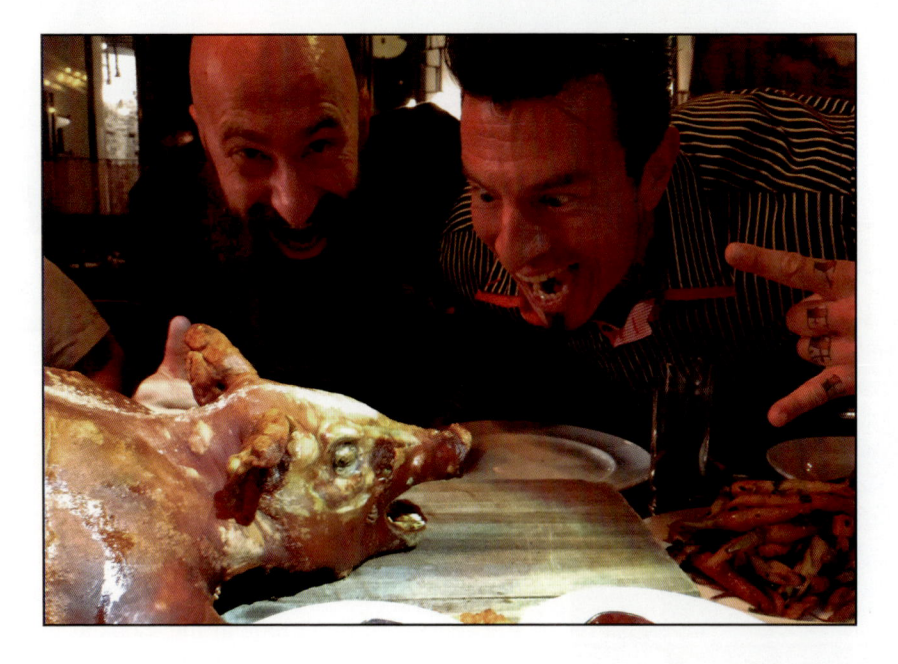

By putting pure and unadulterated things in our bodies we can prevent disease, rather than have to treat it. By getting our nutrients directly from the source, there is no need to supplement.

By no means am I saying that we must adhere to strict dietary procedures every moment of every day for the rest of our lives. Far from it. But try to eat clean and naturally 80-90% of the time. You'll see the difference.

5. DO TREAT YOURSELF RIGHT.

You work hard. Don't forget to reward yourself, too. Having said that, a reward does not have to be in the form of an ice cream cone or ten cocktails (at least not every time). It can be a fun excursion, a new life experience or even just a little downtime. Sure we gotta pay our dues, but it's important to love life too. Enjoy the ride.

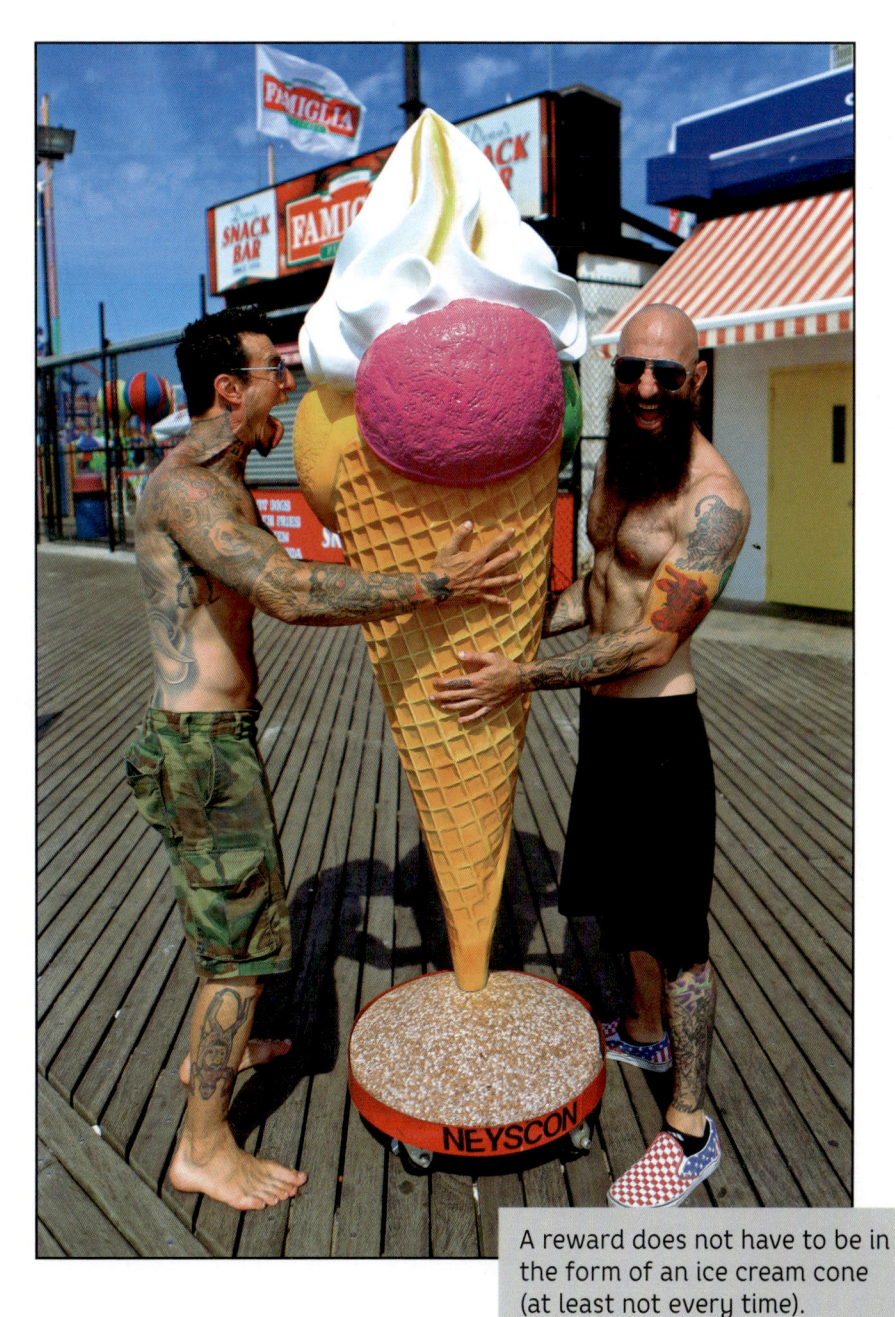

A reward does not have to be in the form of an ice cream cone (at least not every time).

STREET WORKOUT

6. DON'T BE AFRAID TO SEEK HELP WHEN NEEDED.

In 1967, underrated Beatle Ringo Starr sang the words "I get by with a little help from my friends." As much as we are tempted to do everything on our own, there are times when the help of others is invaluable.

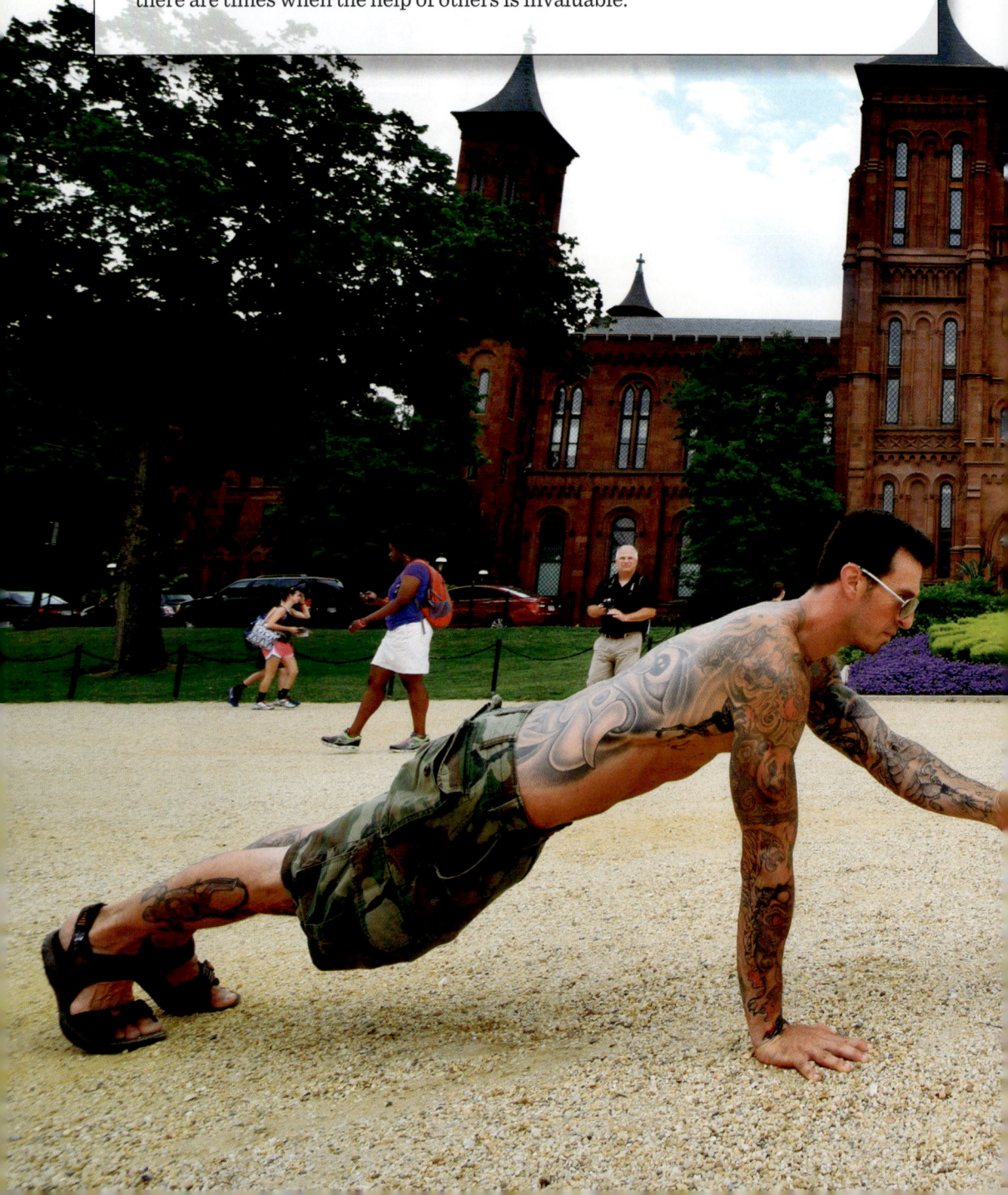

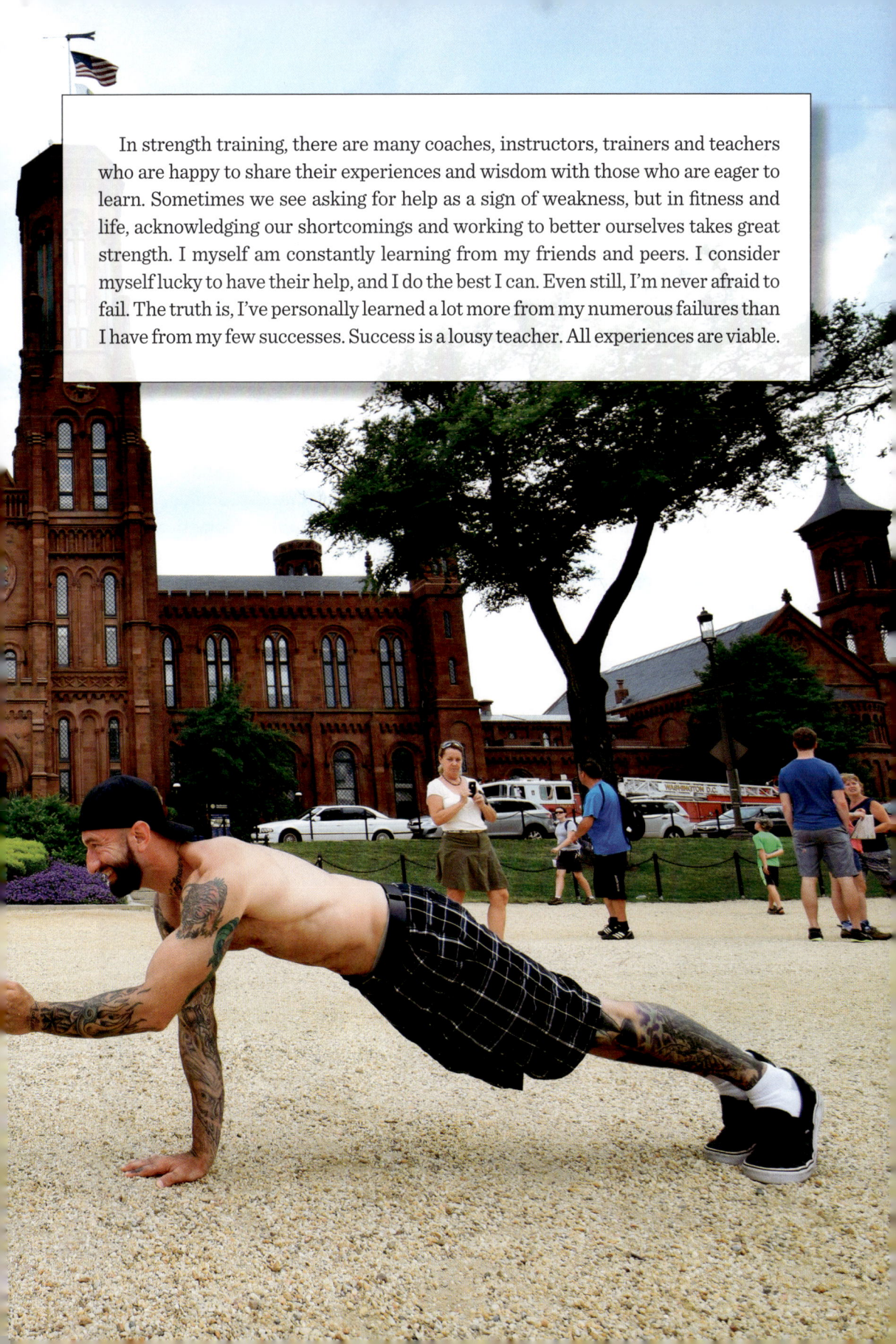

In strength training, there are many coaches, instructors, trainers and teachers who are happy to share their experiences and wisdom with those who are eager to learn. Sometimes we see asking for help as a sign of weakness, but in fitness and life, acknowledging our shortcomings and working to better ourselves takes great strength. I myself am constantly learning from my friends and peers. I consider myself lucky to have their help, and I do the best I can. Even still, I'm never afraid to fail. The truth is, I've personally learned a lot more from my numerous failures than I have from my few successes. Success is a lousy teacher. All experiences are viable.

7. DON'T MAKE PHYSICAL FITNESS YOUR WHOLE LIFE.

Diversity is key. Many people assume that all Al and I do is train, eat, sleep and talk about training. While there is no doubt that we choose to prioritize training, it is not the be-all and end-all. Far from it. I don't have a train "all day, every day" mentality.

I cook. I write. I draw. I play music. I go to the beach.

Training is not the only thing that makes my life worth living: Gangster movies, rib-eye steaks, poetry and prose, tattooing, rock 'n' roll music, the Simpsons and summer barbecues, among many other things, all give my life meaning.

Some people think that if they acknowledge that anything besides the pull-up bar brings them joy, that they are somehow invalidating their passion for fitness. Gimme a break! Life is a broad, bold, beautiful trip. Unless you are a competitive athlete (something I am certainly not), then training should enhance your life, not take it over. Inspiration comes from different places. Sure it can be a workout video on YouTube, but it can also be a song on the radio or a piece of art.

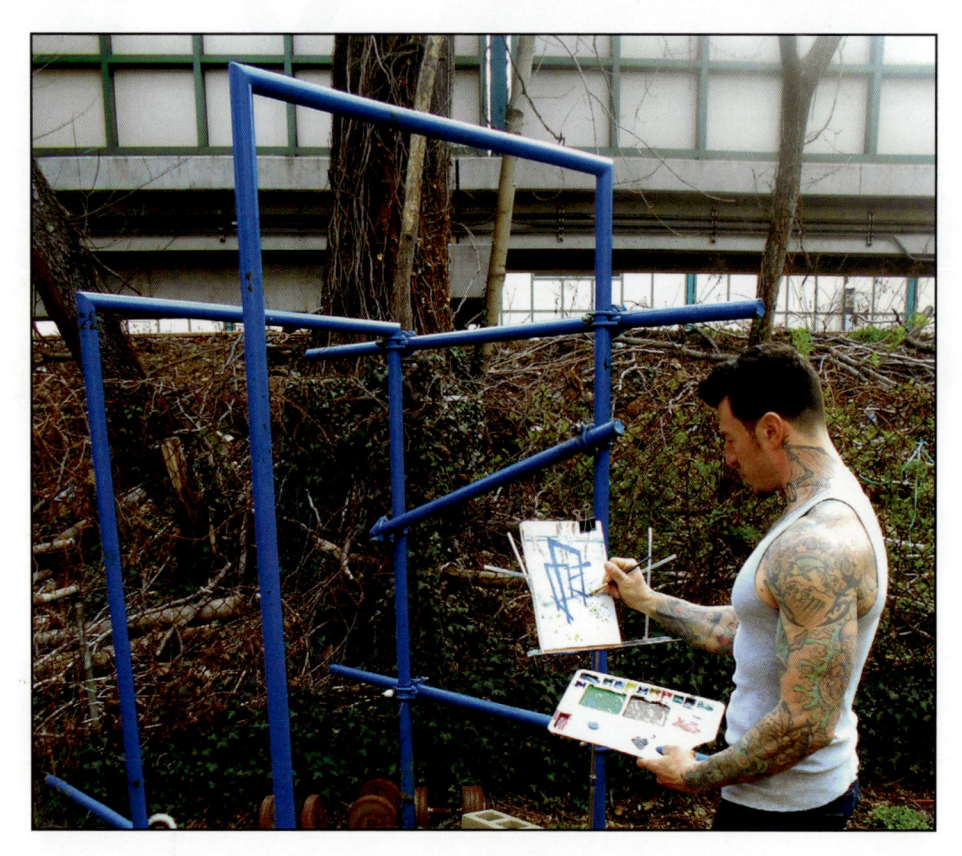

8. DON'T FOLLOW THE LATEST TRENDS.

In life and fitness, there are many paths to take. There will always be a new product, study or scientific experiment, each with the supposed "expert" testimony to back it up. Many of these products and systems were designed by people who do not even work out in the first place.

The methods that are most effective were not just discovered last week. They have stood the test of time. Bodyweight strength training pre-dates any of the new "revolutionary" products on the market. For that matter, calisthenics even came ahead of other classic methods (that work) like barbells, sandbags and kettlebells.

The basic movement patterns, when progressed appropriately, will produce results. We don't need an infomercial to tell us that.

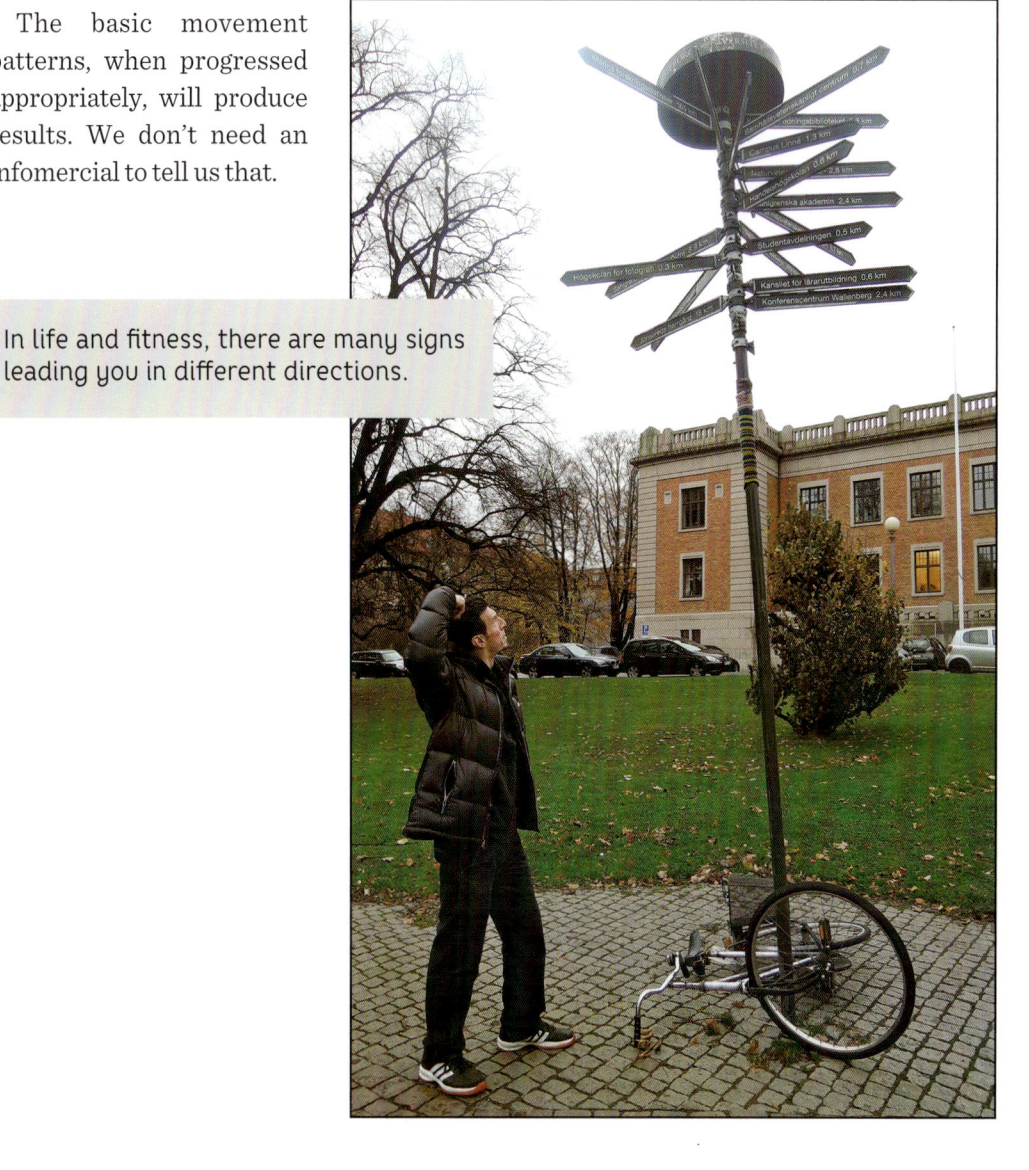

In life and fitness, there are many signs leading you in different directions.

9. DON'T EXPECT CHANGE TO HAPPEN OVERNIGHT.

If you're forty years old and haven't done a push-up since high school, then don't expect to do fifty today. If it took you 20 years to put on superfluous body weight, then don't expect it to come off right away. If you've never done an elbow lever before, it is unlikely you'll get it your first time. Transformations do not happen instantly, despite the fact that we're often told the opposite. It's what we spoke about earlier in regards to consistency and effort toward the task at hand. Over time, with attention and hard work, results will come. Our jobs, lifestyle and other obligations consume time. This is not a bad thing. If anything, this *adds* value to the time that you do have. The busiest people are the ones who train. They find the time, as we all can.

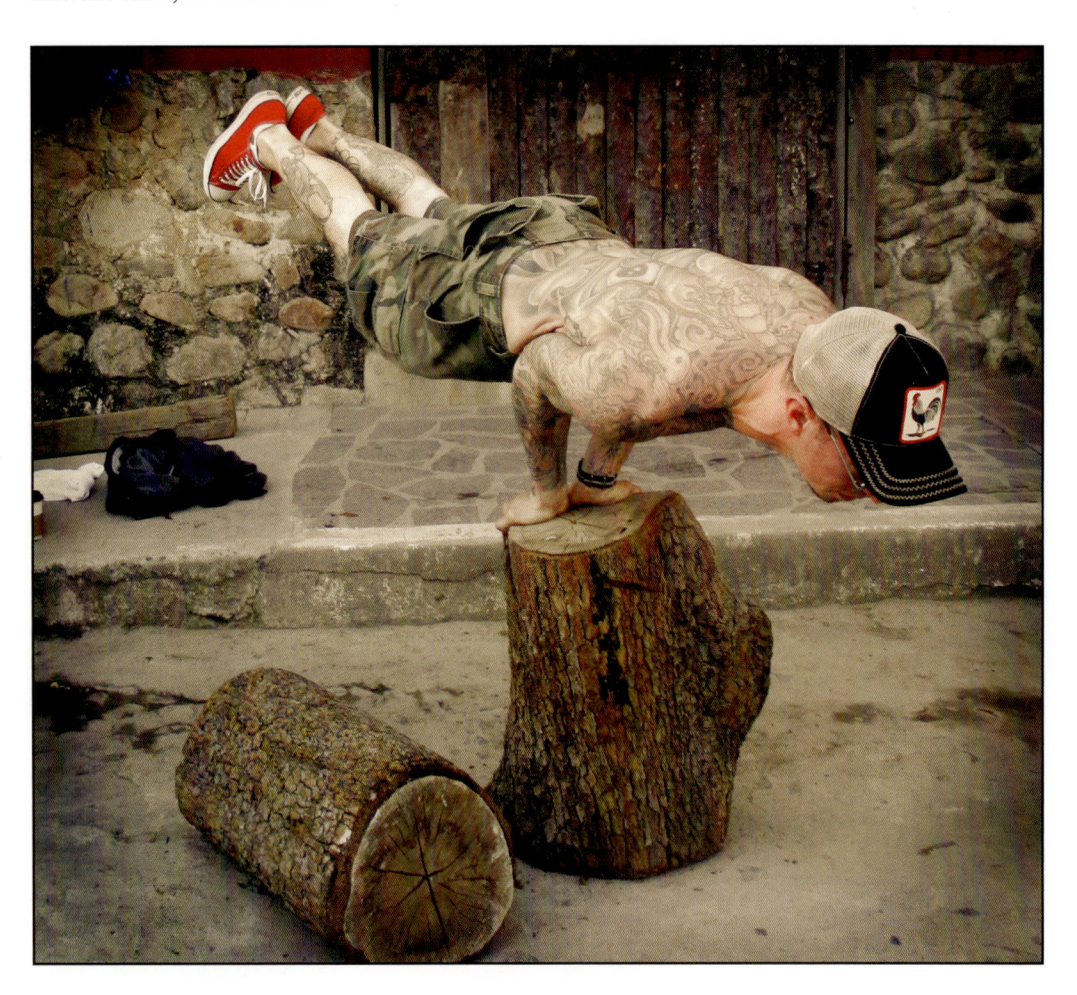

10. DON'T BELIEVE EVERYTHING YOU READ.

When we were kids, in order for information to be presented on a large level, someone would have to follow the scientific method, hypothesize, do the research, come up with findings, compose it and find an investor to publish it. These days, anyone can come across as an authority if they know how to make a nice website and rack up a lot of views. A website's attractiveness does not validate its content, nor does the forcefulness with which some forum poster or author phrases their point of view. No, when it comes to fitness, the only thing that makes something true is if it works for you. To succeed, you will have to experiment for yourself, taking care to employ your own reason and common sense. Don't believe everything you read—not even if I wrote it—unless it makes sense and works for you.

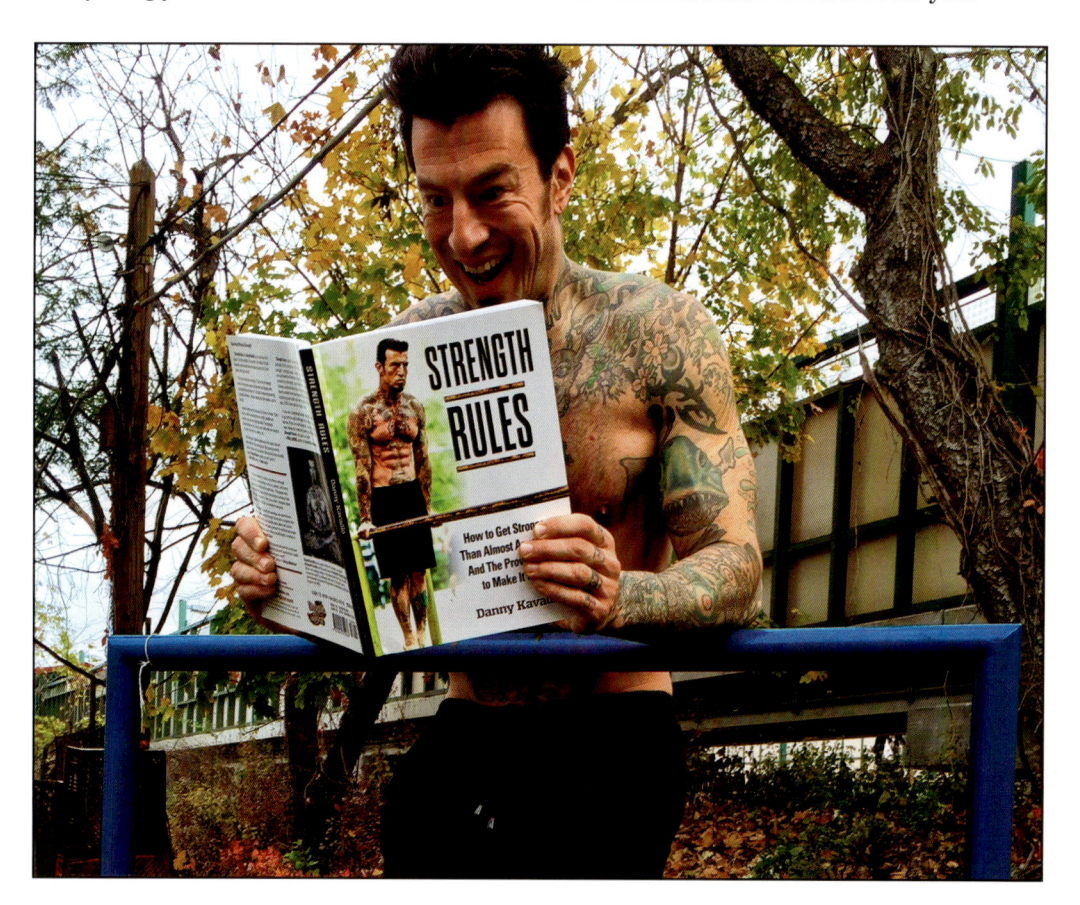

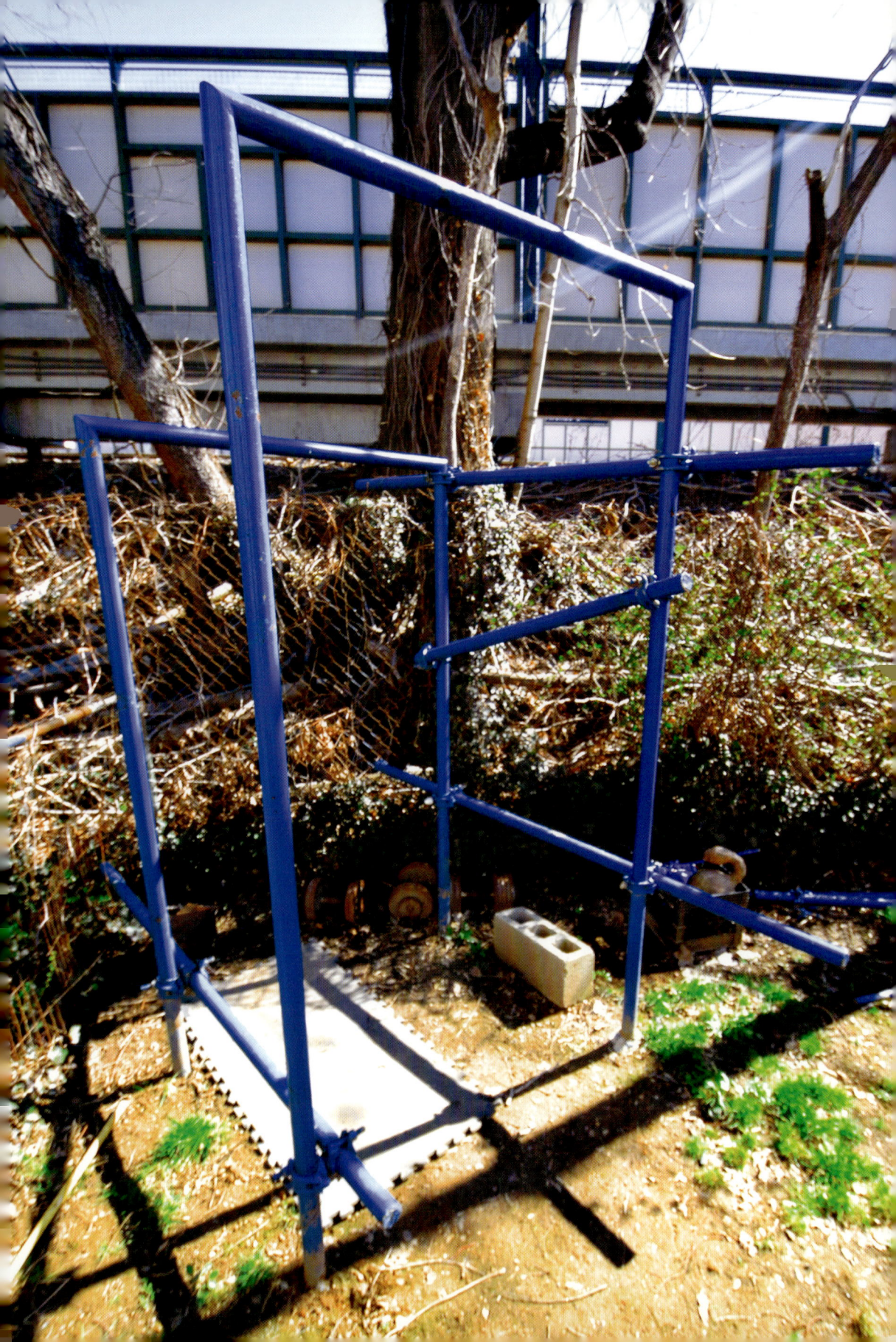

CHAPTER 17

Building A Backyard Pull-up Bar

There are many paths one can take when putting together a home gym. In our lives, we've owned barbells, dumbbells, benches, medicine balls and door-frame pull-up bars. Many things have come and gone. As we progress in this journey of fitness and life, our goals can change. So do our needs.

Obviously the main point of working out is to stimulate the body, but the mind and spirit need to be challenged as well. It behooves the soul to use your creative forces and make something from nothing. So when the itch to create a home gym struck again in 2010, it was a no-brainer: a backyard pull-up bar was the only way to go!

WHY A BACKYARD PULL-UP BAR?

Practicality. To be honest, a door-frame or stand up (power-tower) design simply would not have met our needs. We required something not only capable of withstanding hundreds of pounds of explosive pulling force, but also sturdy enough to bear the weight of multiple practitioners at the same time.

For our training style, this was clearly the sensible solution. In terms of pure function, nothing else would have come close.

PROGRAM DESIGN

The basic design of a backyard pull-up bar is a horizontal bar supported by two vertical posts dug deep in the ground. The main thing is that the unit needs to be SOLID. Our plan was to use 12' posts, leaving 7 1/2' of pole above ground and 4 1/2' below. The idea was that this would give us plenty of height *and* stability. But even within that simple layout, there were many choices to make.

WOOD POSTS VS. METAL POSTS

If you are working with wood posts, a 2×4 is not going to cut it. Don't go any smaller than 6×6. Be sure to use "treated" wood (it's the one at Home Depot with the green tint). It's worth the extra money to have something that will stand up to the elements. When using wood posts, you'll have to purchase circular metal flanges to affix the bar to the wood. These flanges range from $8-$25 depending on the style. The advantages to wood is that it's cost efficient, solid and visually compelling, but we looked forward to practicing moves like the human flag and clutch lever on these bars. For that reason, our posts had to be metal.

Generally, plumbers' galvanized 2" pipe is about $7 per foot at a commercial realtor. However, you can't get anything larger than 8' at most hardware stores, even giants like Home Depot or Lowes. To make 12' posts, you'd have to buy two 20' pipes directly from a supplier, pay for each one to be cut and then buy 90 degree fittings (also about $8-$25) to attach each of the posts to the pull-up bar.

Instead, we took the path of least resistance and contacted a local gate manufacturer who fabricated the initial design for $180. It consisted of two 12' iron posts welded to a 4' bar up top. There was also another 4' bar welded 3 1/2' from the bottom—this lower bar gets buried for stability.

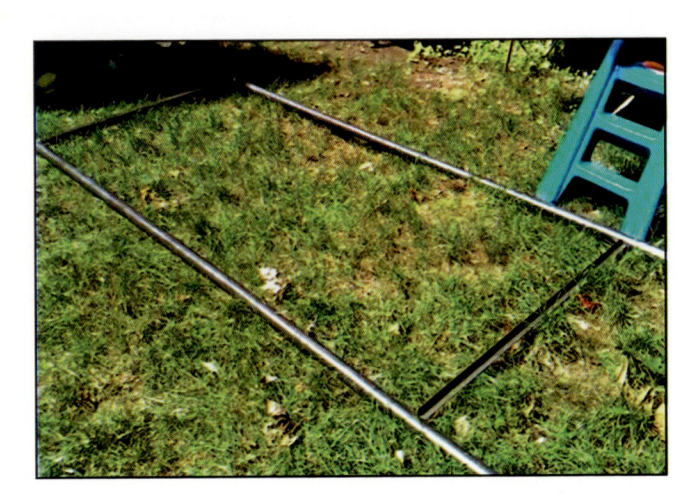

Another factor influencing stability is the amount of concrete used in the foundations. In most of the articles and blogs we consulted prior to this endeavor, the authors expressed remorse about not using enough cement. We decided to avoid that problem by using 2,000 lbs. of cement. We were planning on getting downright aggressive on that bar!

THE BAR ITSELF

A standard pull-up bar is usually 1/2"-1 1/2" in diameter and 2-3' in length. To get the most out of ours, we did 2" diameters and 4' across. The 2" grip makes for a much tougher workout and is excellent for building grip strength. We train hard in Brooklyn!

Be aware that raw metal bars are open on the ends. You'll need to seal them so they don't get rusty from the inside. We filled the ends of the exposed bars with cement and painted over them, but you can use nylon or rubber stoppers instead if you choose.

ADDITIONAL CONSIDERATIONS

Aside from the posts and bars, you'll need the following when constructing a backyard pull-up bar:

- Post Hole Diggers
- Shovel
- Cement (we used twenty-five 80 lb. bags)
- Something to mix it in (You don't need a wheel barrow. We got a huge planter for $15 and grew fresh herbs in it the next summer.)
- Leveler
- Six 2×4's and some screws (for building a temporary support frame)
- Oil-based enamel for metal posts or lacquer for wood posts

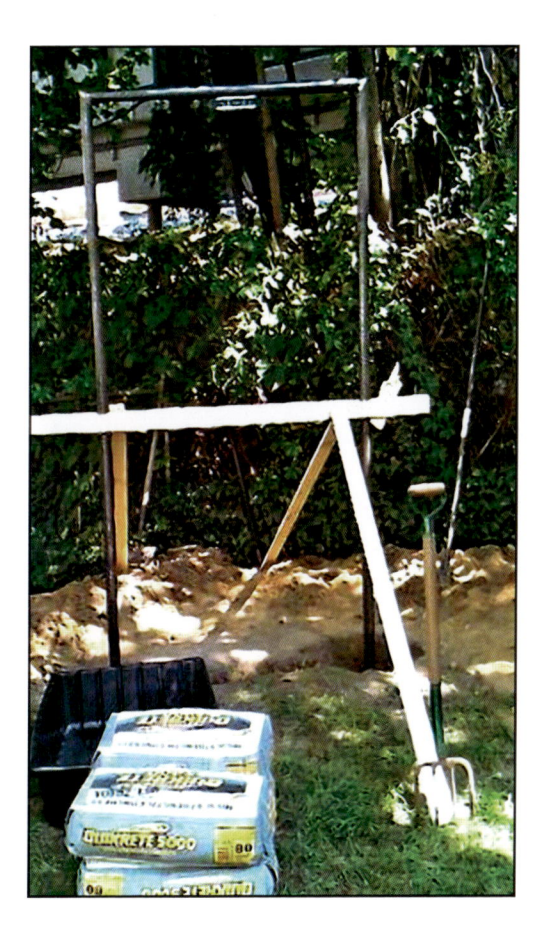

BUILDING YOUR BAR

Make sure you have plenty of space. You'd be surprised at how much room the building process demands, so do it in a nice, open area. Our bar was 4' in length so we set the holes 4' apart. We dug the holes about 12" in diameter at the bottom of the hole and 18" on top. Because our bar was fused at the metal shop with a low support bar close to the bottom of the posts, we also dug a trough about 18" deep from one post to the other. (When filled with cement, the low bar was covered.) Even with post-hole diggers, digging holes that are 4 1/2' deep is extremely challenging. It made for a great workout!

Each post has to go in perfectly straight. If there is a bar connecting them (as was the case with our piece), it must be level. This needs to remain the case until the concrete sets. The best way to ensure this is to build a wooden frame out of 2×4's around the structure before you put the concrete in. Take your time. This step is important and will require a lot of trial and error. You do *not* want an un-level bar.

Once the structure is level, straight and properly framed in wood, fill the holes with concrete. When the concrete dries, remove the frame and you've got the home gym of your dreams!

Almost...

A NEW LIFE

Even with four and a half feet in the ground and (literally) a ton of cement, explosive muscle-ups caused the backyard pull-up bar to vibrate more than we wanted. It was just a tiny bit, really, but that wasn't part of the vision. Changes had to be made. The bars needed diagonal support. Vertical and horizontal were not enough.

We decided that in making it more stable, we'd change the whole shape and make it better! We had a smaller post/bar combo fabricated and set it up 4' behind the initial one. This one was 10' high; we buried just shy of 4' of it. The second unit had to be parallel to the first structure, as well as level with the ground. Once it was in the ground, we used four 7' cross beams mounted diagonally to hold the two structures together using standard scaffold clamps. (We got them used for about $10 each.) We made sure it was level and filled the holes.

Finally, when the concrete dried and the smoke cleared...**THIS BABY WASN'T GOING ANYWHERE!**

The best part of this new design was that it wasn't limited to pull-ups, muscle-ups, and flags. With the second bar, it could accommodate Aussie pull-ups, dips and an unlimited variety of grips. At the end of the day, the backyard pull-up bar wound up different than we planned, yet exceeded even our most fantastic expectations!

In this world, things don't always go as you planned. Sometimes you set a goal and the outcome turns out differently than you had imagined. But when we move forward and roll with the changes, we may find ourselves grateful for the unexpected. That's part of what makes life beautiful. Now let's do some pull-ups!

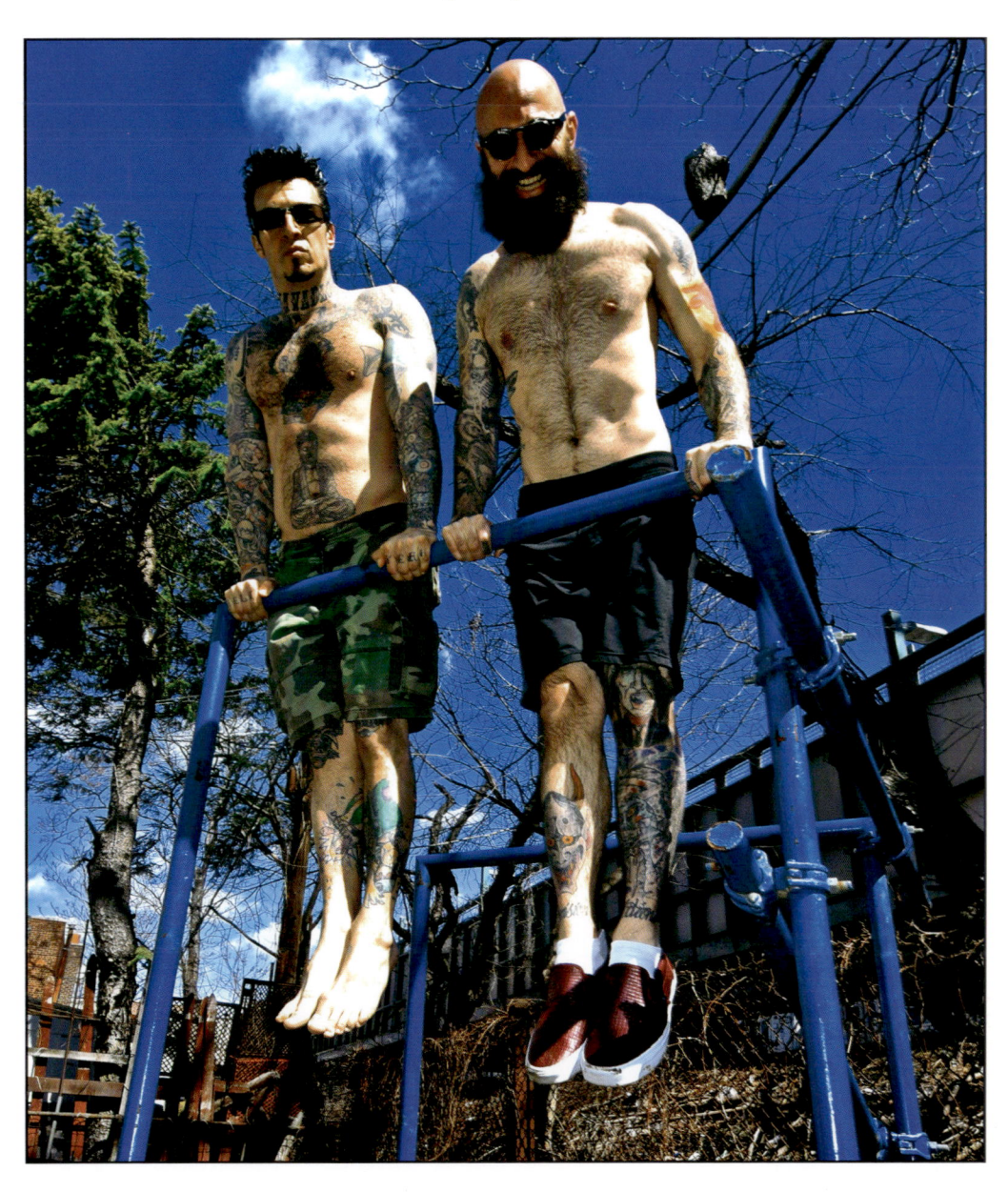

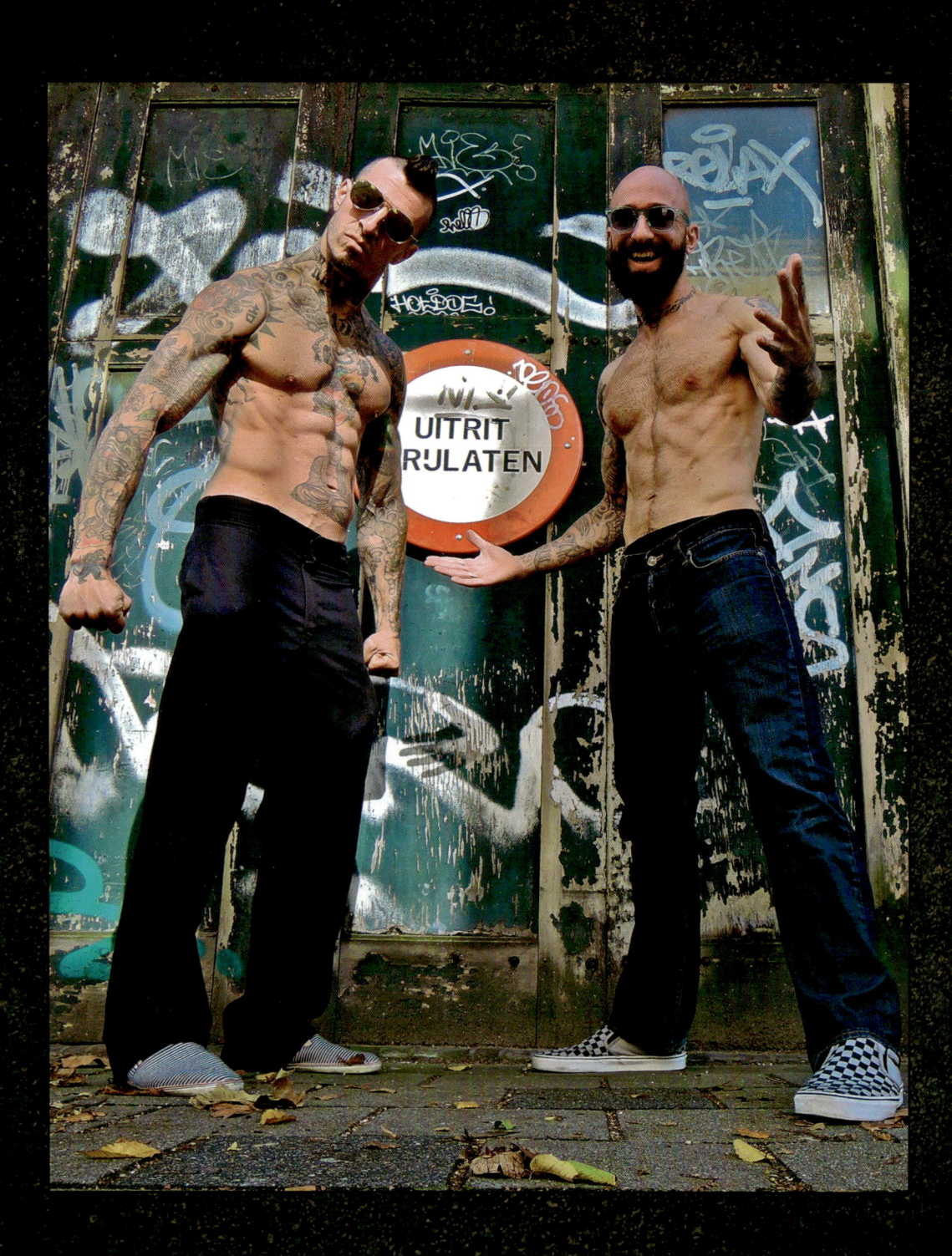

CHAPTER 18

Taking It To The Streets

When you do Street Workout, the world becomes your gym. Don't be afraid to get creative and try different things. What follows is a small sample of some of the many ways you can utilize whatever you may encounter in your surroundings to perform various exercises. The possibilities are endless!

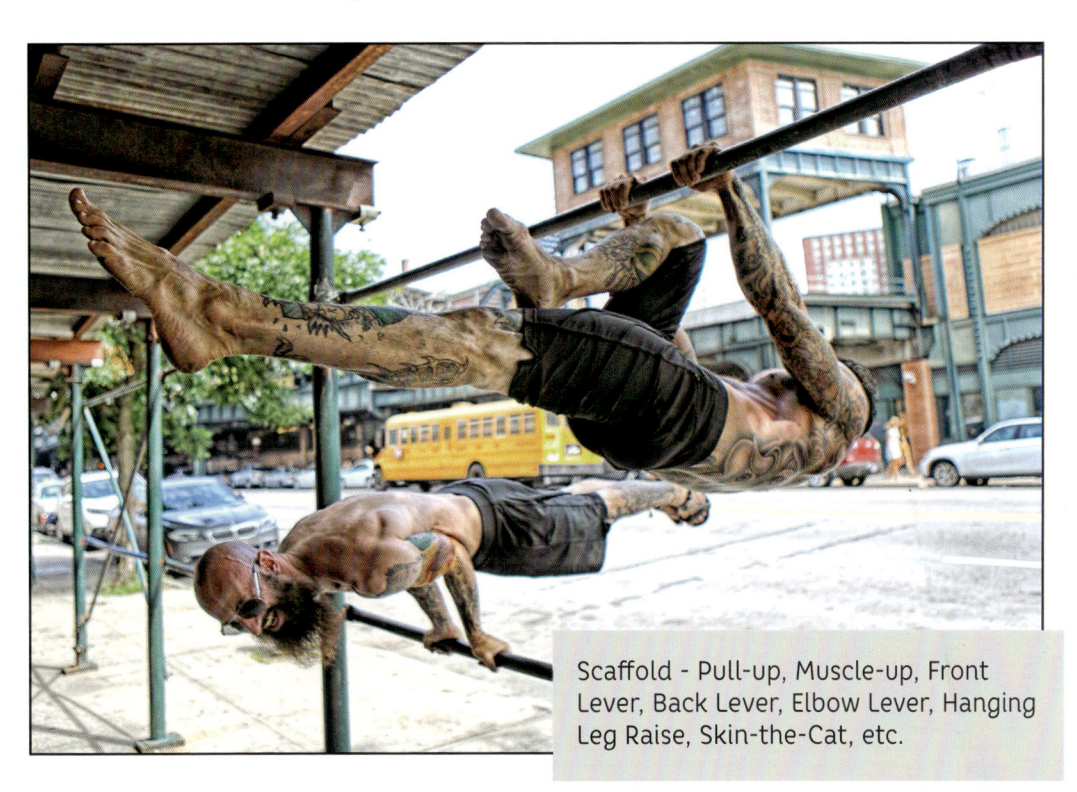

Scaffold - Pull-up, Muscle-up, Front Lever, Back Lever, Elbow Lever, Hanging Leg Raise, Skin-the-Cat, etc.

STREET WORKOUT

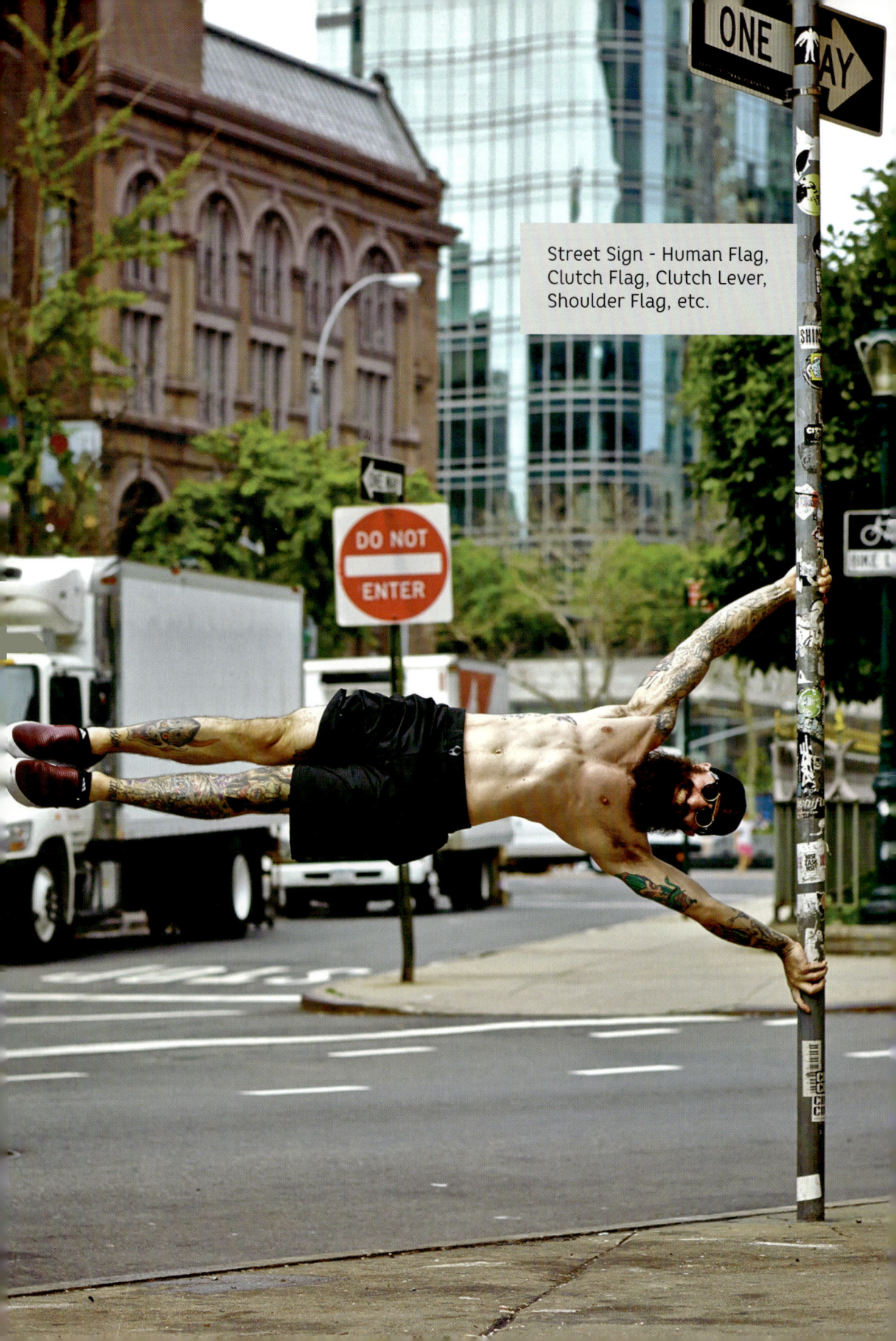

Street Sign - Human Flag, Clutch Flag, Clutch Lever, Shoulder Flag, etc.

Rail - Elbow Lever, Rail Pistol, Iguana Push-up, etc.

Taking it to the street... Literally!

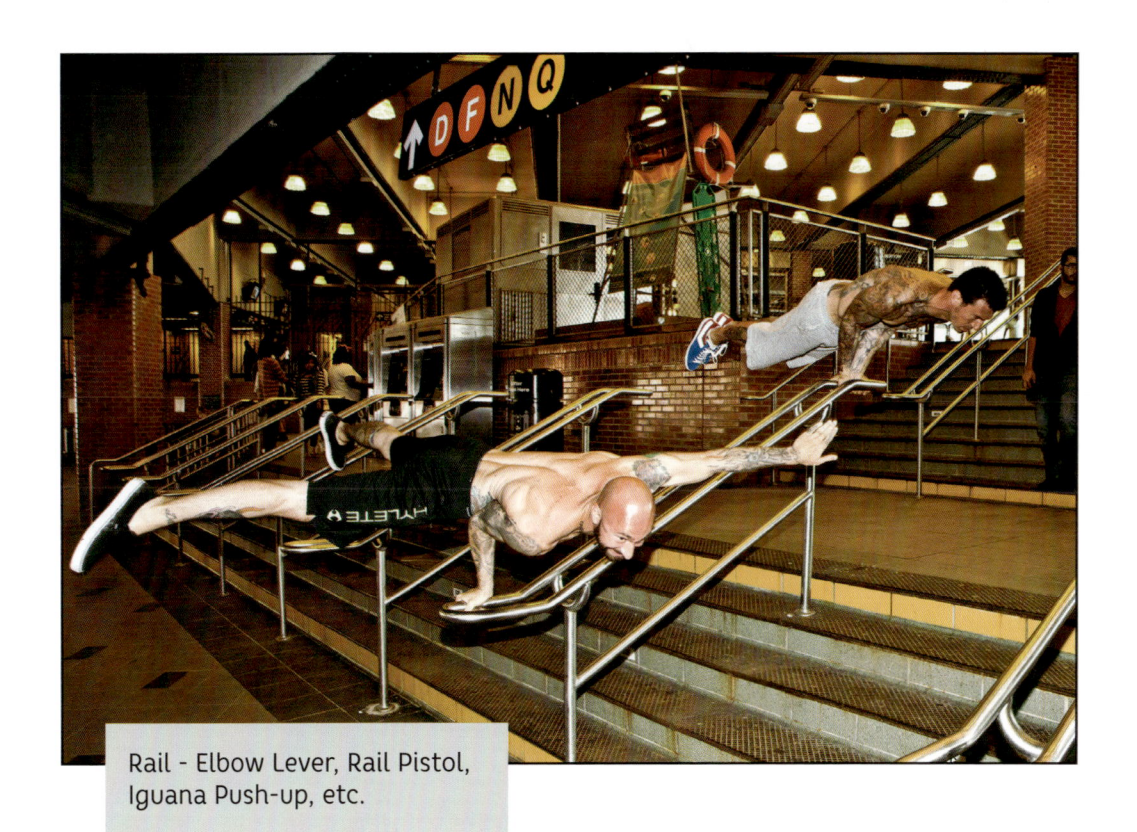

STREET WORKOUT

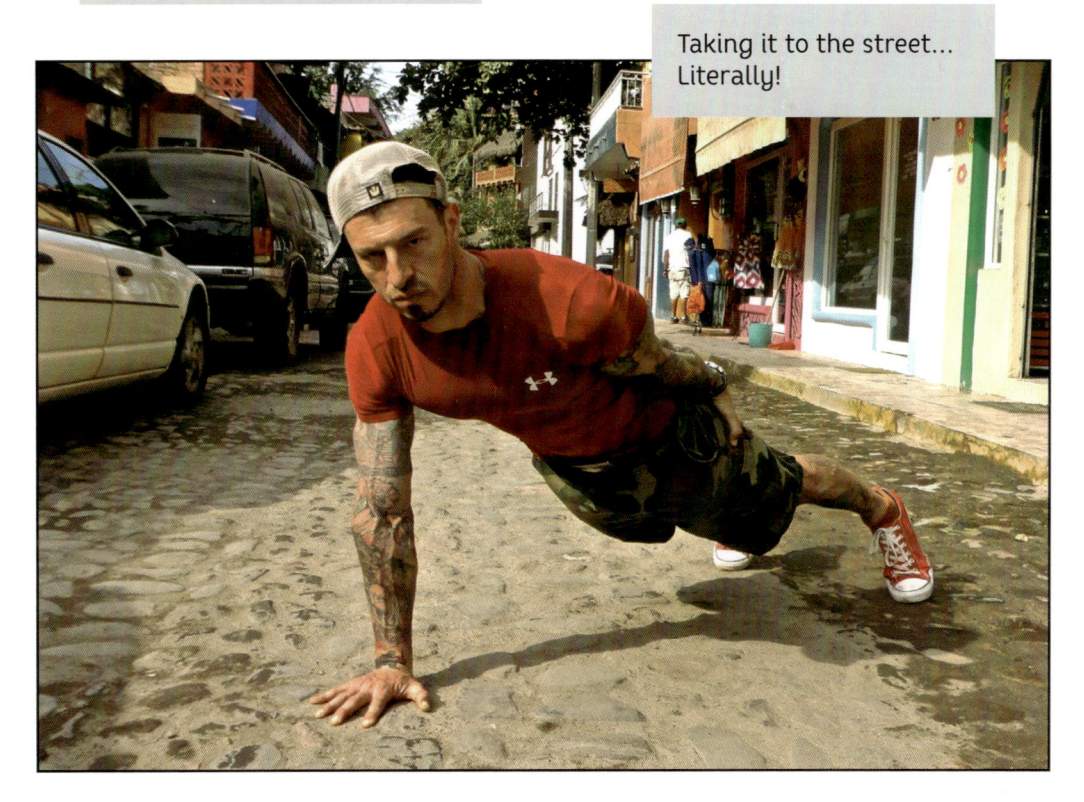

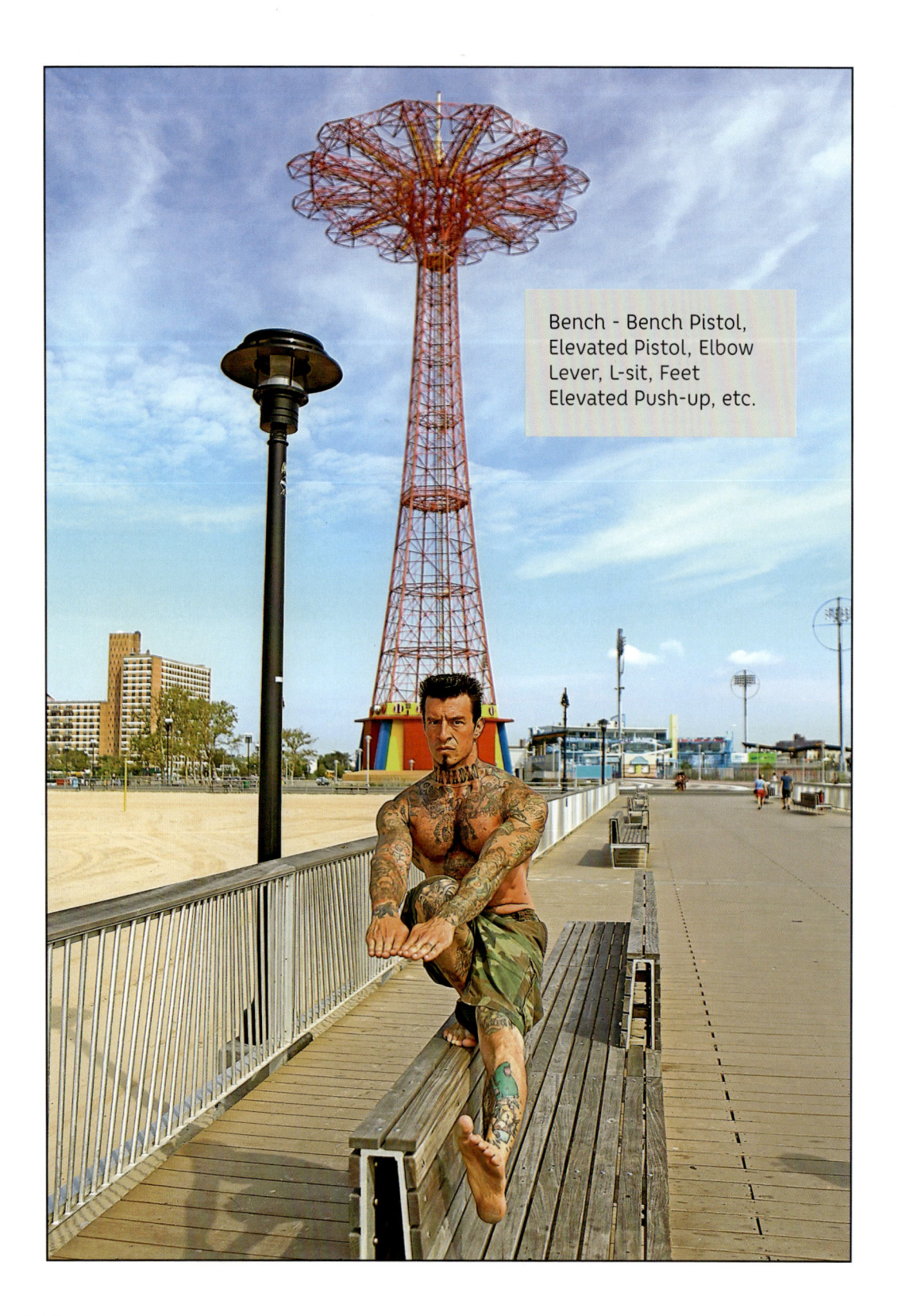

Bench – Bench Pistol, Elevated Pistol, Elbow Lever, L-sit, Feet Elevated Push-up, etc.

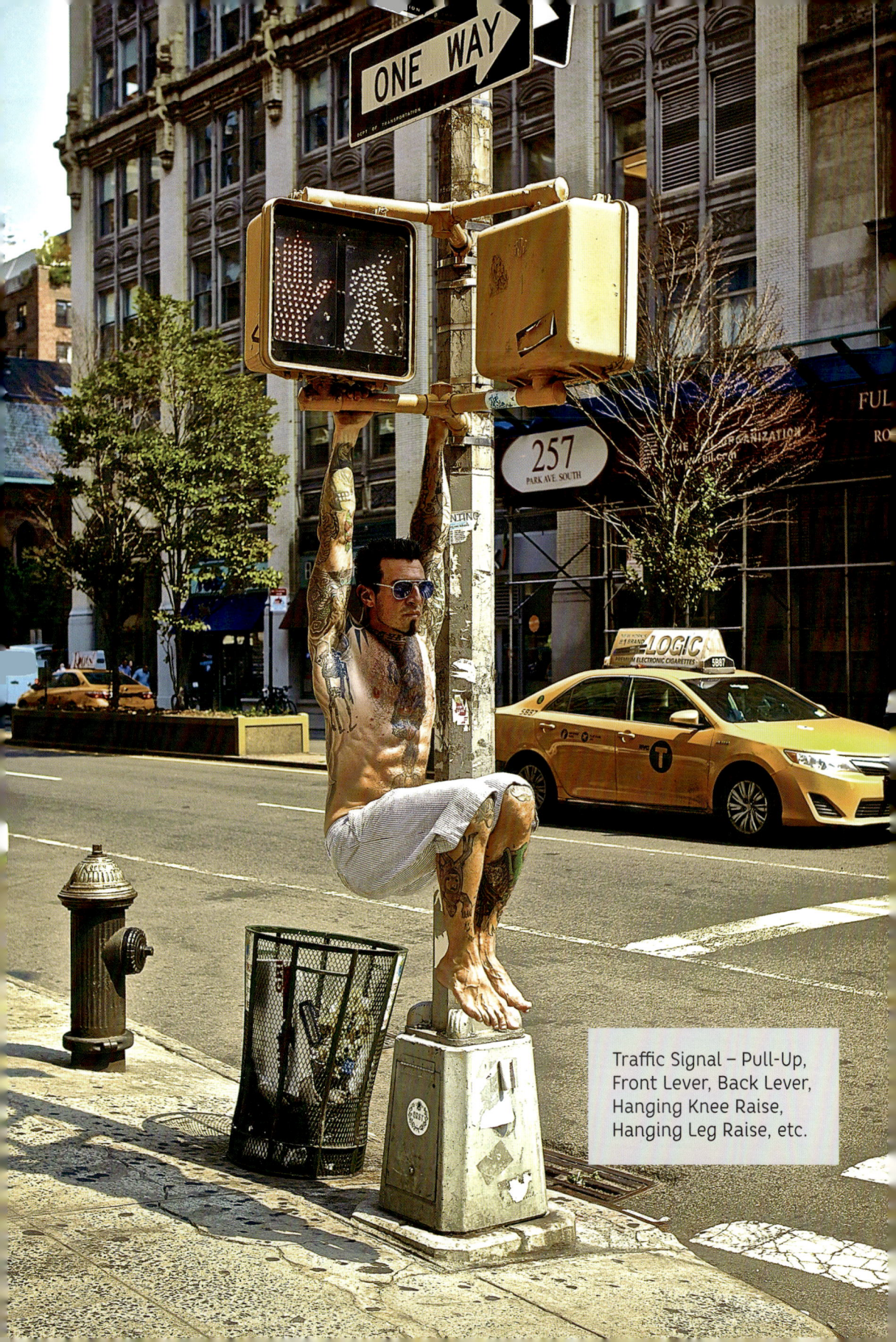

Traffic Signal – Pull-Up, Front Lever, Back Lever, Hanging Knee Raise, Hanging Leg Raise, etc.

One finger pull-up!

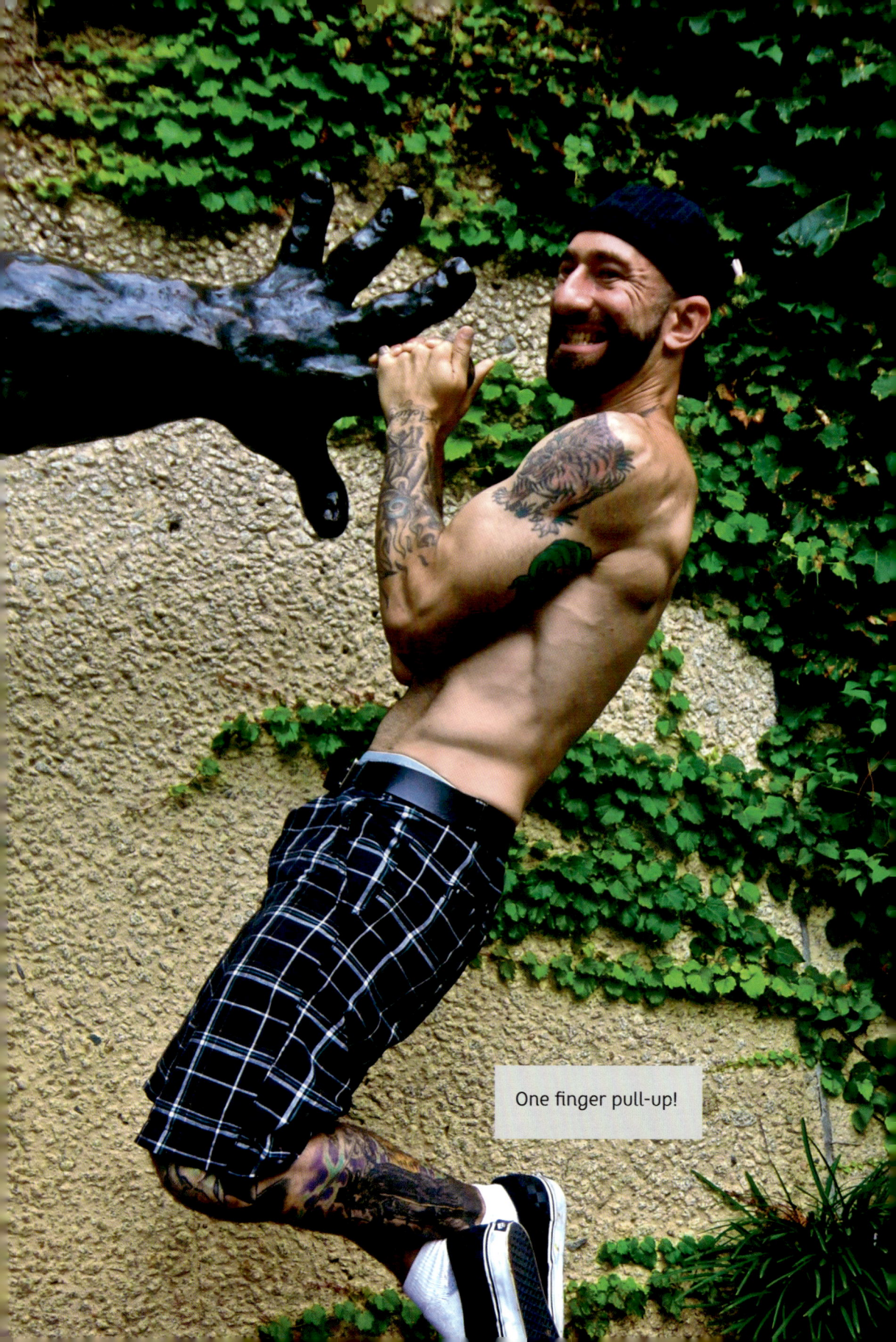

Tree - Pull-up, Hanging Leg Raise, Human Flag etc.

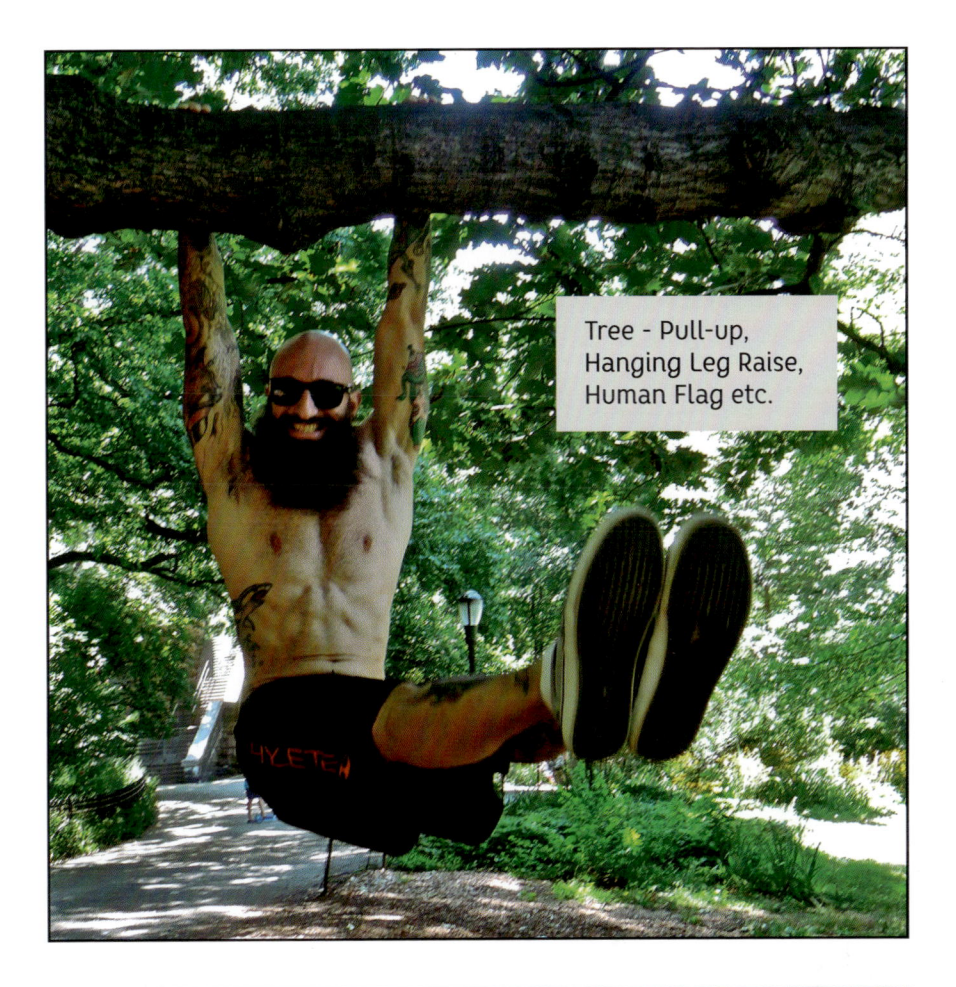

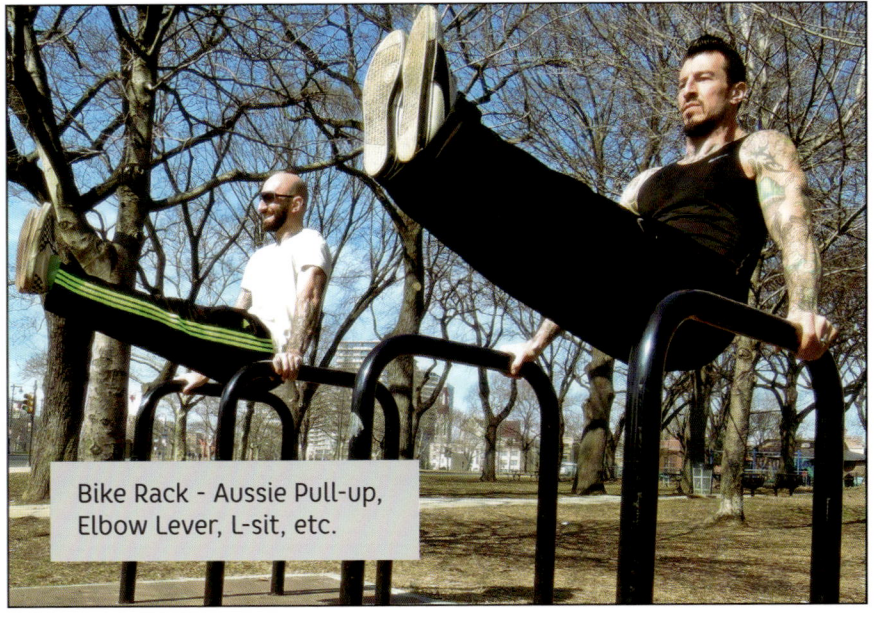

Bike Rack - Aussie Pull-up, Elbow Lever, L-sit, etc.

STREET WORKOUT

REMEMBER WHERE YOU CAME FROM

Long before we were trainers, we worked at a little restaurant in NYC called Live Bait, shucking clams and delivering food on a bicycle. It was not the most exciting or pleasant job. We've been struck by taxis, berated by customers and we always came home smelling like shellfish. But because we worked so hard to get where we are now, we appreciate it that much more. We've been hustlin' since way before anyone knew the name Kavadlo!

Here we are paying tribute—Street Workout style—to that early job which helped to instill the work ethic that allows us to continue to thrive. Remember, there is no such thing as overnight success. Nothing worthwhile will come without hard work.

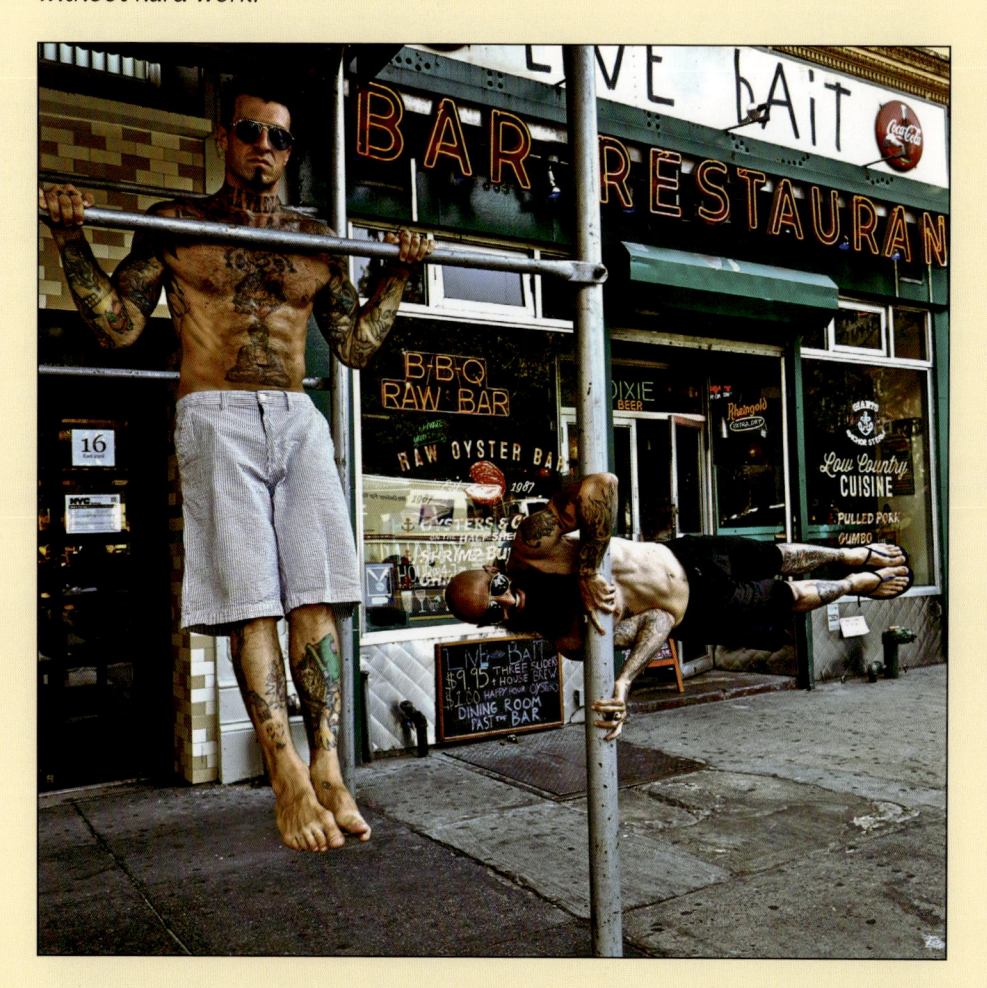

TRAIN

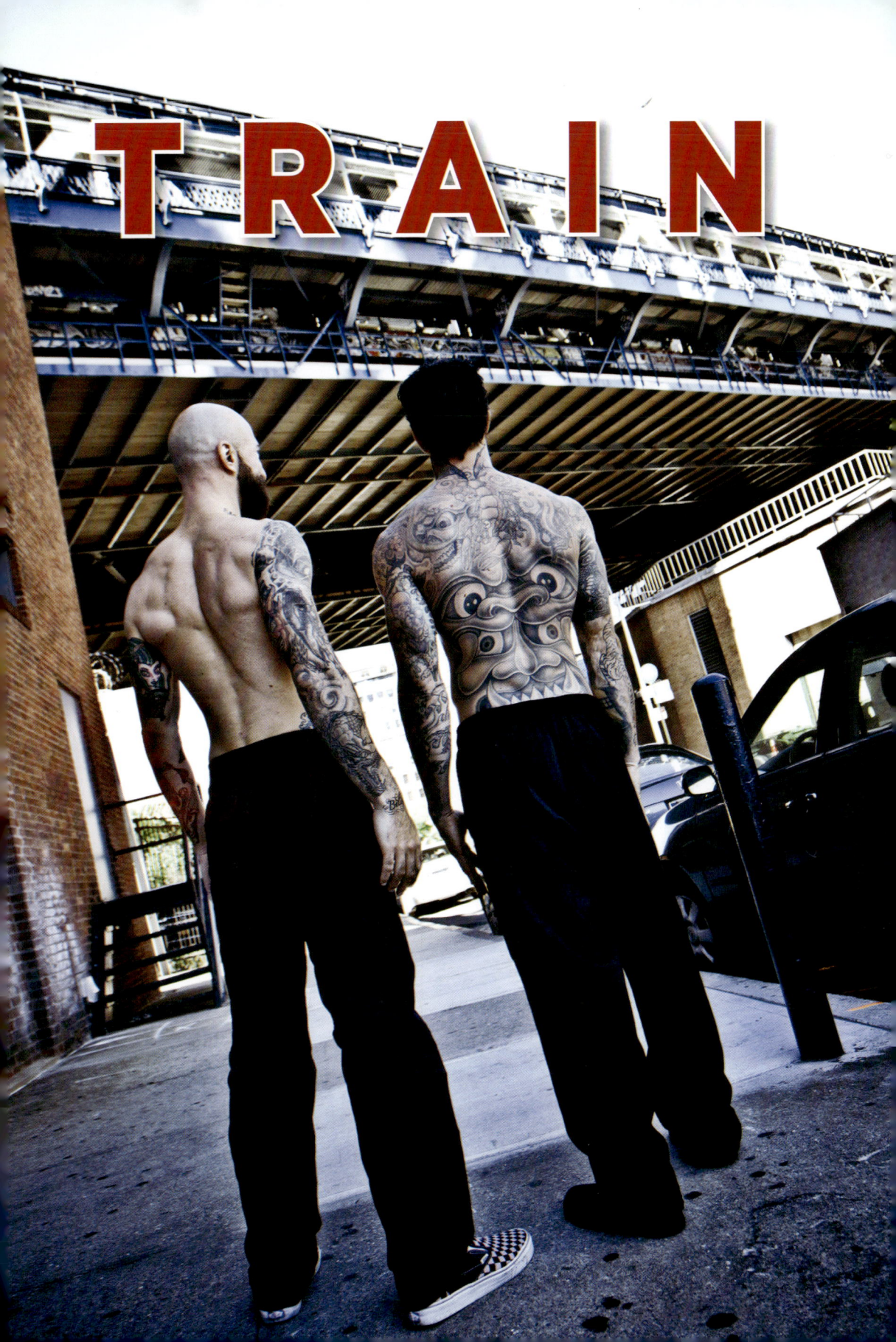

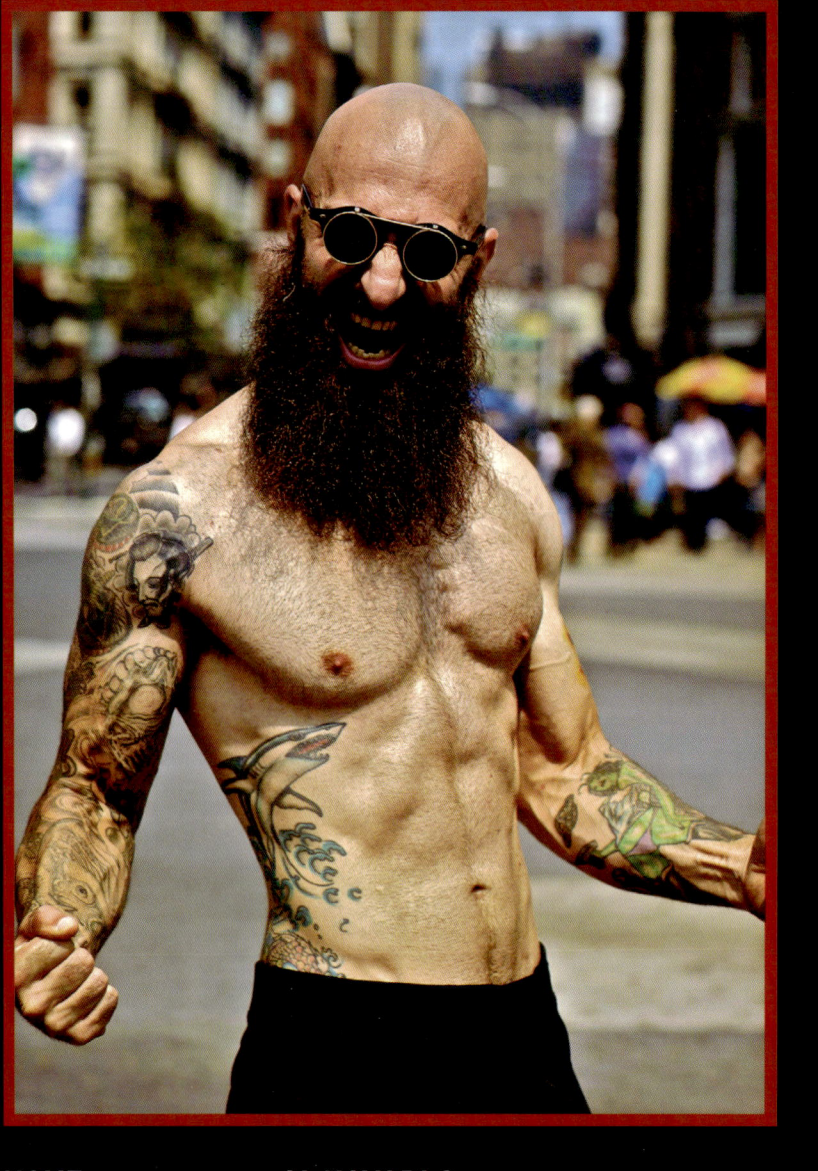

NAME: AL KAVADLO

BIRTHDATE: SEPTEMBER 1, 1979

HEIGHT: 5'11"

WEIGHT: 160 LBS.

SIGNATURE MOVE: MUSCLE-UP

CATCH PHRASE: "HEY, HEY, HEY! WE'RE WORKING OUT!"

NAME:	DANNY KAVADLO
BIRTHDATE:	AUGUST 9, 1974
HEIGHT:	6' 0"
WEIGHT:	180 LBS.
SIGNATURE MOVE:	HUMAN FLAG
CATCH PHRASE:	"KEEP THE DREAM ALIVE!"

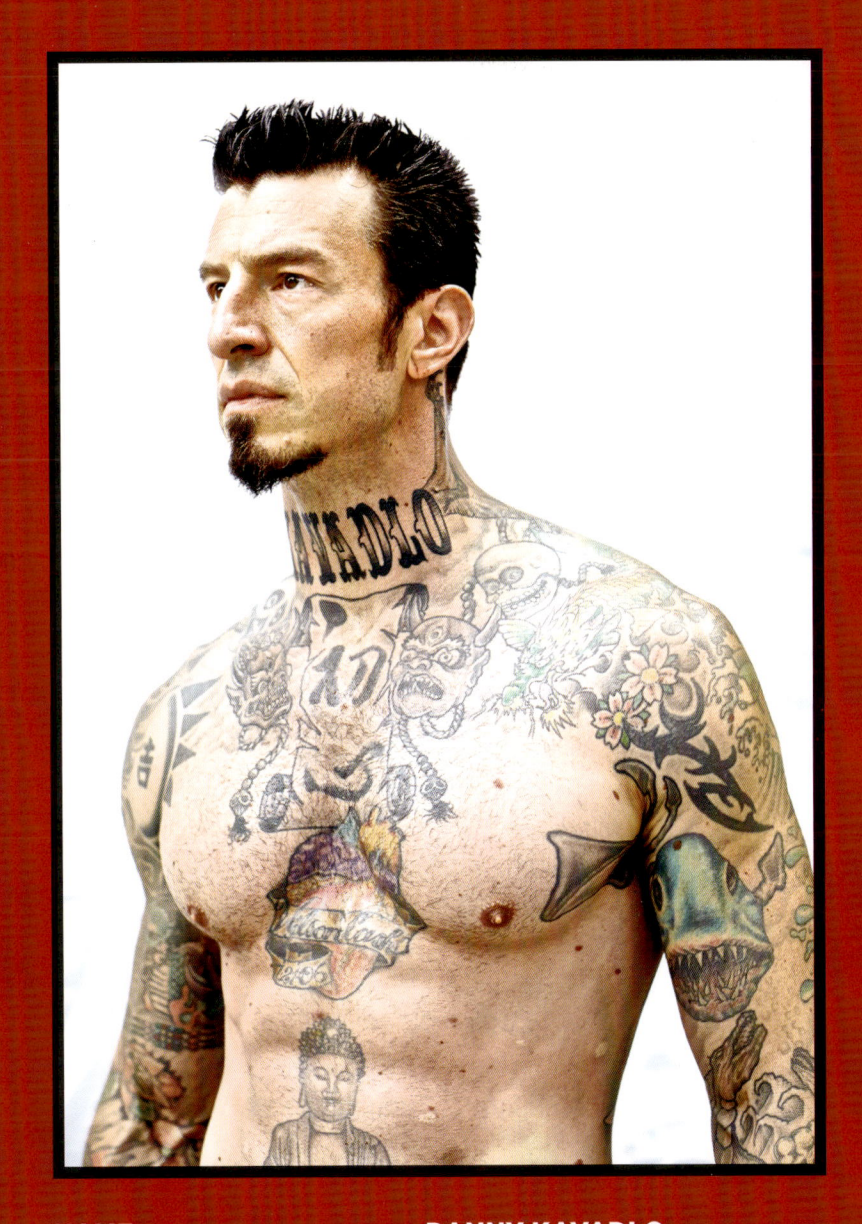

—Acknowledgments—

Al wishes to thank his wife Grace and their dogs, Weezer and Puffy.

Danny wishes to thank Wilson Cash Kavadlo, Mike Anderson and Annie Vo.

Additional special thanks to Rosalie & Carl Kavadlo, John Du Cane, Paul "Coach" Wade and Derek Brigham.

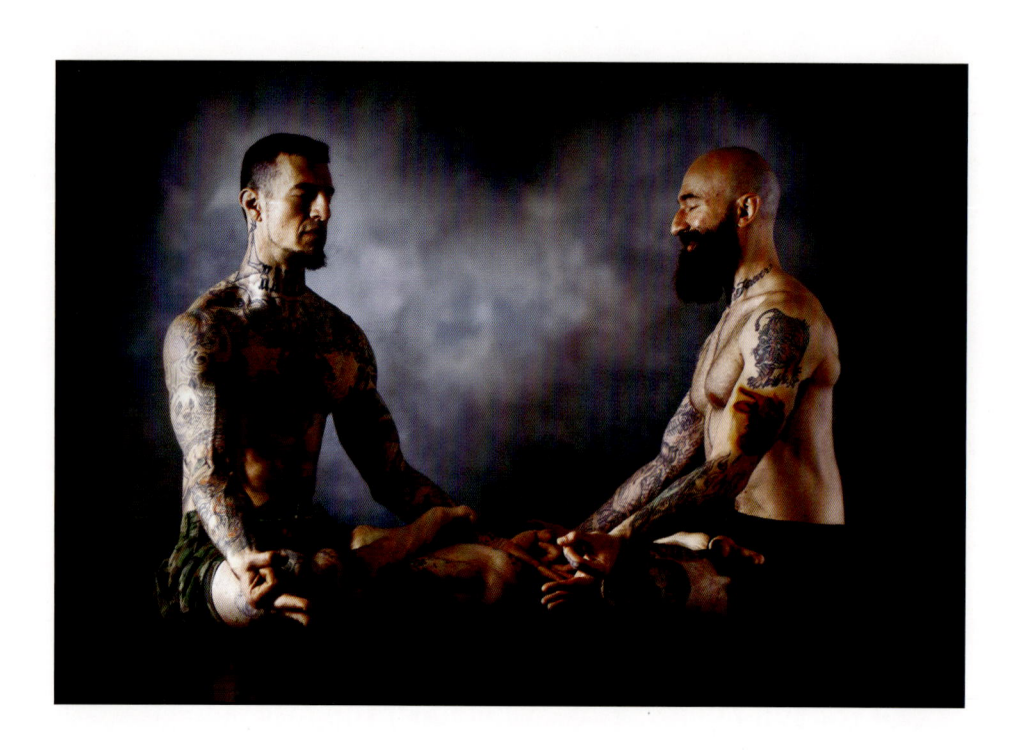

—About The Authors—

Al and Danny Kavadlo are two of the world's leading authorities on calisthenics and personal training. The Kavadlo brothers have authored several internationally-acclaimed, best-selling fitness books. They have appeared in numerous publications including The New York Times and Men's Health, and are regular contributors to Bodybuilding.com and TRAIN magazine. As Master Instructors for Dragon Door's Progressive Calisthenics Certification, Al and Danny travel the world teaching bodyweight strength training to athletes, professional trainers and fitness enthusiasts from all walks of life.

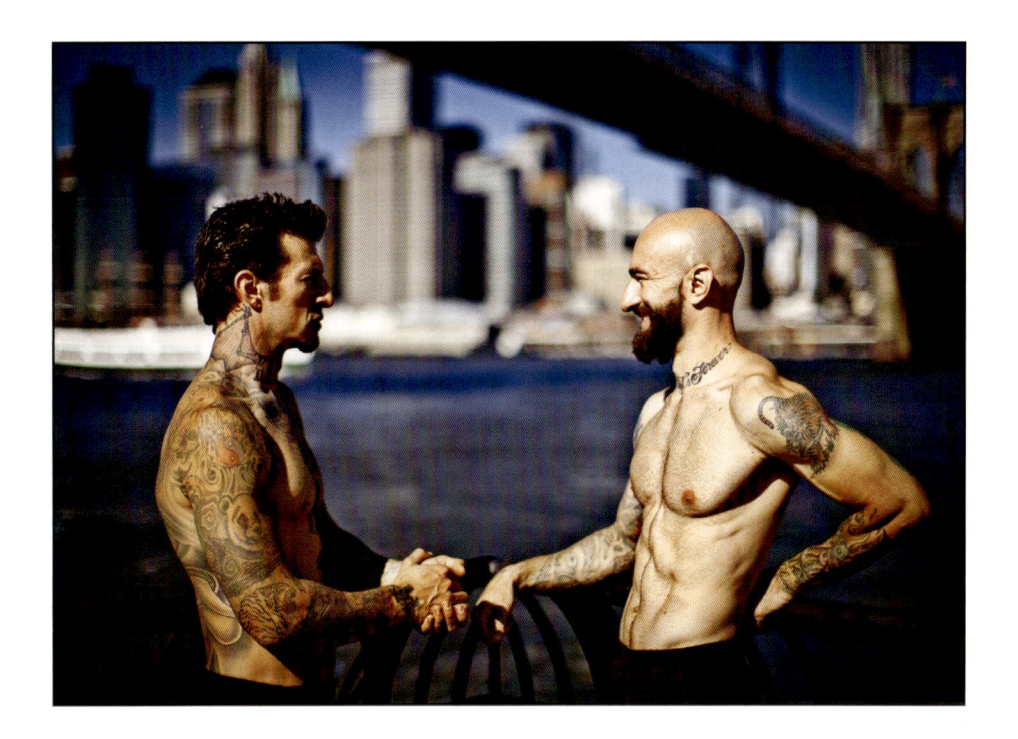

—Index of Exercises—

Advanced One Arm Elbow Lever 206
Advanced Pistol 115
Advanced Shrimp 119
Archer Aussie 66
Aussie Pull-up 60
Archer Pull-up 83
Archer Push-up 36
Archer Squat 104
Back Bridge 160
Back Lever 228
Bar Hang 71
Behind The Neck Pull-up 81
Bench Assisted Pistol 110
Bench Assisted Squat 92
Bench Dip 50
Bent Knee Aussie 61
Bent Knee Hold 131
Bicycle Flag 264
Bridge Rotation 164
Bulgarian Split Squat 101
Calf Raise 103
Candlestick Bridge 156
Candlestick Straight Bridge 157
Chamber Hold 260
Chin-up 73
Claw Push-up 33
Closed Umbrella 199
Clutch Flag 251
Clutch Flag Arm Setup 248
Clutch Lever 252
Commando Pull-up 78
Crane Pose 174
Crow Hold 173
Dragon Flag 136
Dragon Pistol 116
Drinking Bird 108
Elbow Headstand 181
Elbow Lever 201
Elbow Lever Setup 202
Elevated Pistol 112
Exaggerated Bar Hang 233
Extended Range-of-Motion Pull-up 216
False Grip 218
Feet Elevated Aussie 65
Feet Elevated Pike Press 47
Feet Elevated Push-up 27
Flex Hang 71
Fingertip Push-up 32
Forearm Bridge 159
Forearm Stand 187
Freestanding Handstand Press-up 195
Frog Stand 172

Front Lever 238
Front Lever Curl 240
Front Lever Pull-up 242
Gecko Bridge 163
German Hang 225
Grounded Windshield Wiper 129
Hand Elevated One Arm Push-up 39
Hands Elevated Pike Press 46
Hands Elevated Push-up 26
Handstand Facing the Wall 186
Handstand, Gymnastic Style 191
Handstand On Parallel Bars 194
Handstand, Strongman Style 190
Hanging Knee Raise 138
Hanging Leg Raise 140
Hanging Windshield Wiper 144
Hawaiian Squat 120
Headbanger Pull-up 80
High Angled Flag 263
High Support Press 266
Hindu Press 44
Hindu Squat 102
Hinge Push-up 35
Hip Bridge 150
Hollow Body 30
Hollowback Handstand 192
Hook Hand/Flat Palm Flag 270
Hover Lunge 117
Human Flag And Human Flag Pole 277
Human Flag Crucifix 275
Iguana Push-up 38
Jumbo Shrimp 122
Kip-up 167
Kneeling Push-up 24
Knuckle Push-up 31
Korean Dip 56
L Pull-up 82
L-sit 132
Low Hanging Clutch Flag 249
Low Hanging Press Flag 262
Lying Knee Tuck 126
Lying Bent Knee Raise 127
Meathook 146
Mixed Grip Pull-up 76
Muscle-up 219
Narrow Grip Aussie 63
Narrow Grip Pull-up 75
Narrow Push-up 28
Neck Bridge 158
Negative Muscle-up 217
Negative Pull-up 72
Narrow Squat 96

—Index of Exercises—

Exercise	Page
Neutral Grip Aussie	64
Neutral Grip Pull-up	77
One Arm Aussie Pull-up	68
One Arm Back Bridge	162
One Arm Back Lever	231
One Arm Elbow Lever	203
One Arm Flag	276
One Arm Flex Hang	85
One Arm Handstand	196
One Arm Hang	84
One Arm Hanging Leg Raise	145
One Arm In/One Arm Out Elbow Lever	202
One Arm Negative	87
One Arm/One Leg Crow	177
One Arm/One Leg Push-up	41
One Arm Pull-up	88
One Arm Push-up	39
One Handed Pull-up	86
One Leg Back Bridge	161
One Leg Back Lever	227
One Leg Crow	176
One Leg Front Lever	236
One Leg Push-up	34
Parallel Bar Dip	52
Parallel Bar Flag	267
Perpendicular Bar Dip	54
Pike Press	45
Pirouette	193
Pistol Squat	113
Planche	213
Planche Lean	209
Plank	20
Plyometric Dip	57
Plyometric Muscle-up	223
Plyometric Pull-up	89
Plyometric Push-up	42
Plyometric Squat	123
Pole Assisted Pistol	111
Pole Assisted Squat	93
Press Flag	268
Press Flag Arm Setup	258
Prisoner Squat	98
Pull-up	73
Push-up	22
Rail Pistol	116
Reverse Grip Back Lever	230
Reverse Grip Muscle-up	222
Rollover	143
Russian Dip	55
Scorpion Planche	212
Seated Knee Raise	130
Shoulder Bridge	155
Shoulder Flag	272
Shrimp Squat	118
Side Crow	175
Side One Arm Elbow Lever	207
Side Plank	247
Single Leg Stand	106
Skinning The Cat	224
Split Squat	99
Squat	94
Stand-to-Stand Bridge	166
Step-up	107
Straddle Back Lever	227
Straddle Elbow Lever	200
Straddle Flag	265
Straddle Front Lever	235
Straddle Handstand	188
Straddle Headstand	182
Straddle Planche	211
Straddle Push-up	25
Straight Bar Dip	53
Straight Bridge	154
Straight Leg Raise	128
Strict Muscle-up	221
Switch Grip Flag	274
Support Press	257
Table Bridge	152
Toes-to-Bar Hanging Leg Raise	141
Tripod	179
Tripod Headstand	180
Tuck Back Lever	226
Tuck Clutch Flag	250
Tuck Front Lever	234
Tuck Planche	210
Twisting Hanging Knee Raise	139
Ultimate Handstand Press	49
Ultimate Headstand	183
V-sit	134
Vertical Flag	261
Walking Lunge	100
Wall Crawl	165
Wall Handstand Press	48
Wall Handstand	184
Wide Grip Aussie	62
Wide Grip Pull-up	74
Wide Push-up	29
Wide Squat	97
Wrist L-sit	135
Wrist Pull-up	135
Wrist Push-up	135
Wushu Pistol	114
X Clutch Flag	253

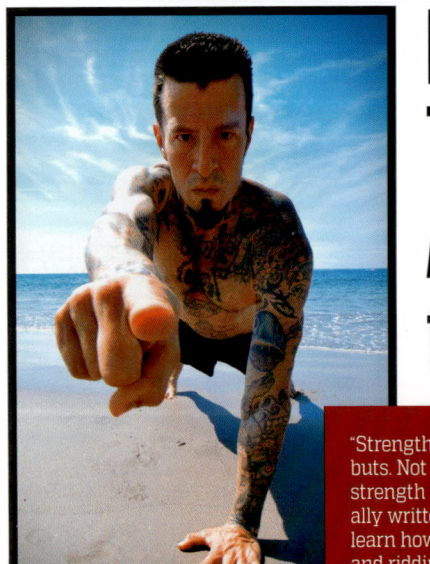

How to Get Stronger Than Almost Anyone— And The Proven Plan to Make It Real

> "Strength Rules is one of the finest books on strength I've ever read. No ifs, ands or buts. Not just 'bodyweight strength'—*strength*, period. There are a million and one strength books out there about hoisting heavy iron and screwing up your joints...usually written by coaches and athletes using steroids and other drugs. But if you want to learn how to unleash *ferocious* strength and power while also improving your health and ridding yourself of extra fat and joint pain, THIS is the book you need to own.
>
> If you are a bodyweight master, this is the bible you will want to go back to again and again, to keep you on the straight and narrow. If you are raw beginner—Jeez, then get this book right now, *follow the rules*, and save yourself years of wasted effort! Strength Rules is as good as it gets!"
>
> —PAUL WADE, author of *Convict Conditioning*

How to Be Tough as Nails— Whatever You Do, Wherever You Go, Whenever You Need it...

Want to get classically strong—in every dimension of your life– gut, heart and mind...?

In other words, do you want to be:
- **More than** just gym-strong?
- **More than** just functionally strong?
- **More than** just sport-specifically strong?
- **More than** just butt-kicker strong?
- And—certainly—**more than** just look-pretty-in-a-bodybuilding-contest strong?

Do you demand—instead—to be:
- **Tensile** Strong?
- **Versatile** Strong?
- **Pound-for-Pound** Strong?
- The Ultimate Physical **Dynamo**?
- A Mental **Powerhouse**?
- A Spiritual **Force**?
- An Emotional **Rock**?

Then welcome to **Danny's World**... the world of *Strength Rules*— where you can stand tall on a rock-solid foundation of classic strength principles...Arm-in-arm with a world leader in the modern calisthenics movement...

Then... with Danny as your constant guide, grow taller and ever-stronger—in all aspects of your life and being—with a Master Blueprint of progressive calisthenic training where the sky's the limit on your possible progress...

Do Danny's classical **Strength Rules**—and, for sure, you can own the keys to the strength kingdom...

Ignore Danny's classical **Strength Rules**—break them, twist them, lame-ass them, screw with them—then doom yourself to staying stuck in idle as a perpetual strength mediocrity...

The choice is yours!

> "I have been waiting for a book to be written on strength training that I can recommend to all of my patients, and **Danny Kavadlo** has delivered with **Strength Rules**. Danny has written a stripped down approach to strength that is accessible to everyone.
>
> He has distilled his wealth of knowledge and experience in coaching and bodyweight strength training into a program that is cohesive, scalable, and instantly applicable to all comers. He has also added a rock solid approach to nutrition and ample doses of inspirational story telling and philosophy, resulting in the gem that is **Strength Rules**.
>
> I dare anyone to read this book and still give me an excuse why they can't strengthen their body and improve their health. No excuses. Get the book and get to work!"
>
> —DR. CHRISTOPHER HARDY, author of *Strong Medicine*

Order *Strength Rules* online:
www.dragondoor.com/b84

1•800•899•5111
www.dragondoor.com

24 HOURS A DAY
ORDER NOW

However brilliant most strength books might be, 99% of them have a fatal flaw...

99% of otherwise excellent strength books focus on only one aspect of strength: how to get physically stronger through physical exercise. Health and multi-dimensional well-being is given at best a cursory nod... Nutritional advice is most often a thinly disguised pitch for a supplement line...

If you want a book that gives you the goods on full-body training, full-body health and full-body strength, then there's precious little out there... So, thank God for the advent of *Strength Rules*!

Strength Rules embodies all elements of strength—even how they work into our day-to-day existence, the highs and lows of our being, for better or for worse...

Strength Rules is dedicated to those who are down with the cause. Those who want to work hard to get strong. Who insist they deserve to build their own muscle, release their own endorphins and synthesize *their own* hormones.

Strength Rules has no interest in fly-by-night fitness fads. Classic exercises have stood the test of time for a reason. *Strength Rules* shouts a loud "just say no!" to cumbersome, complicated workout equipment. *Strength Rules* walks a path free from trendy diets, gratuitous chemical concoctions and useless gear...

Almost every strength exercise comes down to the basics. Essentially, Squat, Push and Pull. These three broad, essential movements are the granddaddies of 'em all. Throw in some Flexion, Transverse Bends and Extension, and you've got yourself the tools for a lifetime of full body strength training... That's why the exercises contained in *Strength Rules* are divided into these few, broad categories. Everything else is a variation. There is no reason to overcomplicate it.

The *Strength Rules* mission is to help anybody and everybody get in the best shape of their lives Strength Rules lays out the truth clearly and succinctly, giving you the tools you need to grow stronger and persevere in this mad world—with your head held high and your body lean and powerful...

The exercise portion of *Strength Rules* (titled ACTIONS) is split into three levels: Basic Training (Starting Out), Beast Mode (Classic Strength) and Like A Boss (Advanced Moves). Naturally, not everyone will fall 100% into one of these groups for all exercises in all categories and that's fine. In fact, it's likely that even the same individual's level will vary from move to move. That's cool; we all progress at different rates. Respect and acknowledge it. Trust your instincts.

Speaking of instincts, we are wired with them for a reason. If our instincts are wrong then that's millions of years of evolution lying to us. A large part of *Strength Rules* embraces empowerment, faith in oneself and emotional awareness. Danny believes that being honest with yourself, physically, mentally and spiritually is a magnificent (and necessary) component of true, overall strength. Yes, sometimes the truth hurts, but it must be embraced if we are ever to be fit and free. We all have the power within ourselves. Use it.

Strength Rules cries out to all body types, age groups, backgrounds and disciplines. It talks to the beginning student. It calls on the advanced practitioner, looking for new challenges. It speaks to the calisthenics enthusiast and all the hard-working personal trainers... *Strength Rules* is for *everyone* who wants to get strong—and then some...

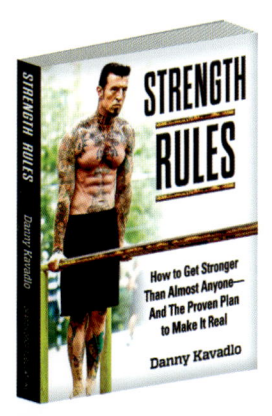

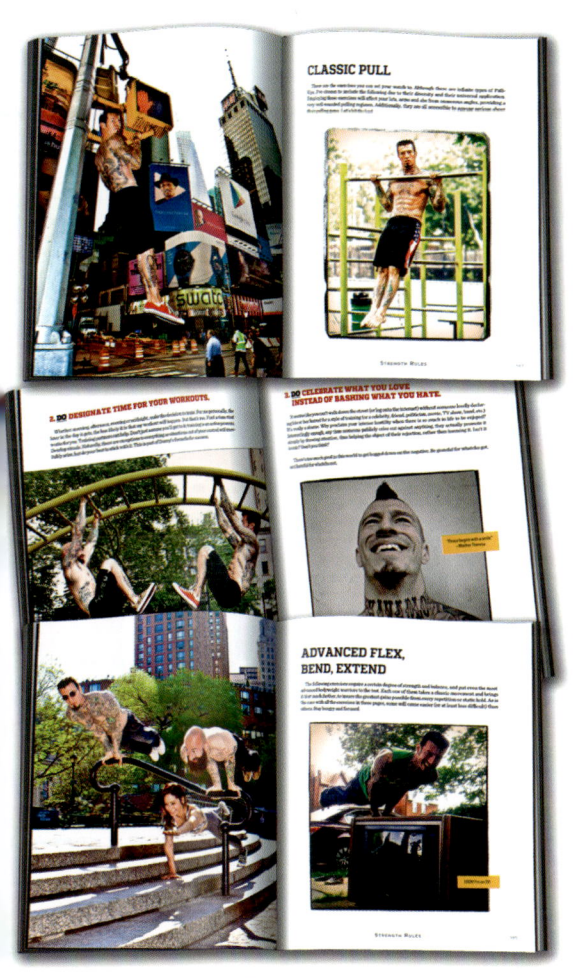

"*Strength Rules* by Danny Kavadlo is so good you can't ignore it. It's minimalistic. It's low tech. It's simple. It's right.

Kavadlo's work always has me nodding along with a lot of 'yeses' and 'good points.'

This book is about true strength. The old kind of strength where heroes were people, like Beowulf and Ulysses, who protected the community first. This book is about empowering yourself and others...without stepping on their heads to get to the top.

Kavadlo quotes one of my heroes, St. Francis of Assisi: 'Start by doing what's necessary; then do what's possible and suddenly you are doing the impossible.' True strength, becoming the best you can be, starts with what one needs to do rather than what one wants to do.

We often ignore calisthenics because of one issue: they are really hard to do. Stop ignoring them. Stop ignoring common sense in nutrition and supplements. Stop ignoring Danny Kavadlo. Again, *Strength Rules* is so good, you can't ignore it."
—DAN JOHN, author of *Never Let Go*

"I can't say enough good things about Danny Kavadlo. I just love his entire approach, mindset and overall vibe. And *Strength Rules* has to be one of the coolest, most badass fitness books I have ever seen."—JASON FERRUGGIA

Strength Rules
How to Get Stronger Than Almost Anyone— And The Proven Plan to Make It Real
By Danny Kavadlo

Book #B84 $39.99
eBook #EB84 $9.99
Paperback 8.5 x 11
264 pages, 305 photos

---

24 HOURS A DAY ORDER NOW 1•800•899•5111 www.dragondoor.com

Order *Strength Rules* online: www.dragondoor.com/b84

"Danny Kavadlo's training helped me to discover strengths I never knew I had, and I can take those lessons with me wherever I go, for the rest of my life. The wisdom and insight contained in *Everybody Needs Training* not only relates to being a successful fitness trainer, but can be applied for peace and success in many of life's ventures. Danny is the best!"—ELIZABETH GILBERT, #1 *New York Times* Best Selling Author, *Eat, Pray, Love*. One of *TIME Magazine's* 100 Most Influential People in the World

Most folk who embark on a career as a trainer, do so initially out of a personal passion for fitness and a strong desire to help other achieve results. Be it weight loss, conditioning, strength gains, flexibility or enhanced performance.

But a passion for working out and an earnest desire to help others—alone—does not a successful personal trainer make. The sad fact is that the turn over rate for personal trainers after one year is over 80%. Why? It's almost always because the trainer didn't have a proper understanding of the BUSINESS of being a fitness professional.

The bottom line is that without the appropriate success blueprint, the most skilled and knowledgeable personal trainer is usually doomed to failure. Unfortunately, until now, there has been no such battle-tested blueprint available either to the novice trainer or the professional struggling to stay alive. Now, however that's all changed, thanks to Danny Kavadlo's *Everybody Needs*

"*Everybody Needs Training* is quite 'something.' I don't think I have ever seen this kind of depth in the field. It's both obvious and 'wow' as you read it. Amazing stuff. It fills a gap in the community that, frankly, surprises me no one has really filled."—DAN JOHN, author, *Never Let Go*

"Danny Kavadlo has personally helped me become a more successful trainer and coach. I cannot recommend *Everybody Needs Training* enough. It's the best book I've ever seen on the subject of being a professional trainer."
—ADEL GABER, World Class Trainer & 3-Time Olympic Wrestling Coach

"*Everybody Needs Training* is a solid collection of tried-and-true best practices that can help personal trainers on any level reach their full potential in their chosen field."—ROLANDO GARCIA, RKC II, CK-FMS

"*Everybody Needs Training* is a must-read for every personal trainer wanting to take it to the next level, and everyone who has ever dreamed of becoming a personal trainer. This book allows you to get inside the genius PT mind of Danny Kavadlo, a master of his craft, speaking off the cuff to you about training—priceless!"—ERRICK MCADAMS, Personal Trainer, Model, Fitness Personality

Good for any profession or business

"I'm not a trainer, but took Danny and Al's PCC Class. This is a great book for anyone going into business as either an employee or owner, whether a fitness trainer or any other kind of business. I'm a lawyer, and I'm thinking about making it required reading for my newly hired lawyers. Good practical advice, with the focus on the customer, which is a focus that seems to be lost these days. Easy reading, but pithy, with lots of great tips and ideas, with an excellent overriding theme. Oh yea -- well written too!"— Mark Walker, McAllen, Texas

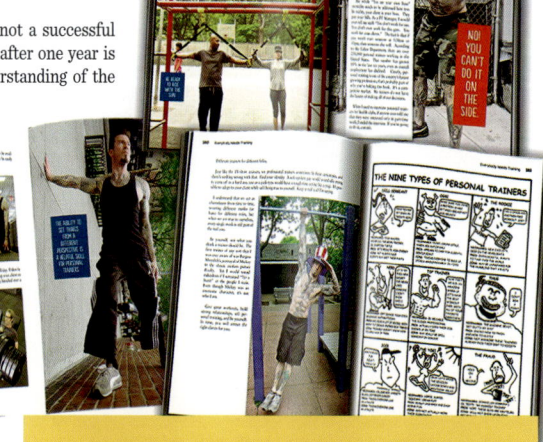

"Christmas wishes DO come true....Danny Kavadlo has written a training book! Imagine if you could squeeze all the hard-earned wisdom, secrets and tactics of one of the world's hottest personal trainers between the covers of a beautifully illustrated tell-all manual, and you have imagined *Everybody Needs Training*.

Like Danny himself, this groundbreaking book is incredibly smart, brutally honest, laugh-out-loud funny, and totally out of left field...if you train others (casually or professionally), want a career training others, or if you just love the now-famous "Kavadlo approach" to getting in shape, you owe it to yourself to grab a copy of this masterpiece. I cannot recommend it highly enough."
—PAUL WADE, author of *Convict Conditioning*

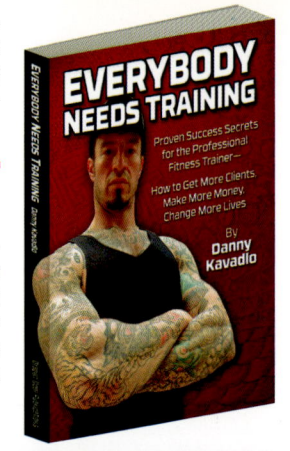

Everybody Needs Training

Proven Success Secrets for the Professional Fitness Trainer—How to Get More Clients, Make More Money, Change More Lives
By Danny Kavadlo

Book #B72 $34.95
eBook #EB72 $19.95
Paperback 8.5 x 11

Order *Everybody Needs Training* online:
www.dragondoor.com/b72

1•800•899•5111
www.dragondoor.com

24 HOURS A DAY
ORDER NOW

C-MASS
How To Maximize Muscle Growth Using Bodyweight-Only

Is it really possible to add significant extra muscle-bulk to your frame using bodyweight exercise only? The answer, according to calisthenics guru and bestselling *Convict Conditioning* author Paul Wade, is a resounding Yes. Legendary strongmen and savvy modern bodyweight bodybuilders both, have added stacks of righteous beef to their physiques—using just the secrets Paul Wade reveals in this bible-like guide to getting as strong AND as big as you could possibly want, using nothing but your own body.

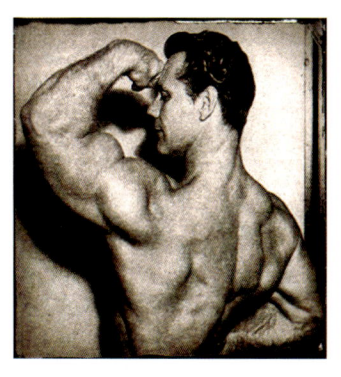

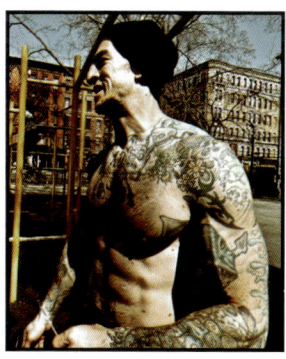

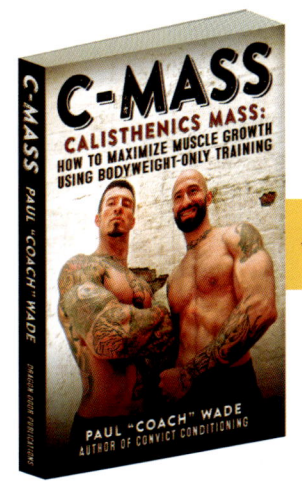

Paul Wade's trenchant, visceral style blazes with hard-won body culture insight, tactics, strategies and tips for the ultimate blueprint for getting huge naturally without free weights, machine supplements or—God forbid—steroids. With *C-Mass*, Paul Wade further cements his position as the preeminent modern authority on how to build extraordinary power and strength with bodyweight exercise only.

⬇ Get All of This When You Invest in Paul Wade's *C-Mass* Today: ⬇

C-MASS
Calisthenics Mass: How To Maximize Muscle Growth Using Bodyweight-Only Training
By Paul "Coach" Wade

Book #B75 **$24.95**
eBook #EB75 **$9.95**
Paperback 8.5 x 11 • 136 pages, 130 photos

1. Bodyweight Muscle? No Problem!

Build *phenomenal* amounts of natural muscle mass and discover how to:

- Add 20-30+ pounds of solid muscle—with perfect proportions
- Reshape your arms with 2-3 inches of gnarly beef
- Triple the size of your pecs and lats
- Thicken and harden your abdominal wall into a classic six-pack
- Throw a thick, healthy vein onto your biceps
- Generate hard, sculpted quads and hamstrings that would be the envy of an Olympic sprinter
- Build true "diamond" calves
- Stand head and shoulders above the next 99% of natural bodybuilders in looks, strength and power
- Boost your testosterone naturally to bull-like levels

Understand the radically different advantages you'll get from the two major types of resistance work, *nervous system* training and *muscular system* training.

If you really want to explode your muscle growth—if SIZE is your goal—you should train THIS way...

2. The Ten Commandments of Calisthenics Mass

Truly effective muscular training boils down into THESE Ten Commandments.

COMMANDMENT I: Embrace reps!

Why reps are key when you want to build massive stacks of jacked up muscle.

Understanding the biochemistry of building bigger muscles through reps...

COMMANDMENT II: Work Hard!

Want to turn from a twig into an ok tree? Why working demonically hard and employing brutal physical effort is essential to getting nasty big...

---

24 HOURS A DAY
ORDER NOW

1•800•899•5111
www.dragondoor.com

Order *C-Mass* online:
www.dragondoor.com/b75

COMMANDMENT VIII: Sleep More!

How is it that prison athletes seem to gain and maintain so much dense muscle, when guys on the outside—who are taking supplements and working out in super-equipped gyms—can rarely gain muscle at all?

Discover the 3 main reasons why, sleep, the natural alternative to steroids, helps prison athletes grow so big...

COMMANDMENT IX: Train the Mind Along With the Body!

Why your mind is your most powerful supplement...

How 6 major training demons can destroy your bodybuilding dreams—and where to find the antidote...

COMMANDMENT X: Get Strong!

Understanding the relationship between the nervous system and the muscular system—and how to take full advantage of that relationship.

Why, if you wish to gain as much muscle as your genetic potential will allow, just training your *muscles* won't cut it—and what more you need to do...

The secret to mixing and matching for both growth AND strength...

3. "Coach" Wade's Bodypart Tactics

Get the best bodyweight bodybuilding techniques for 11 major body areas.

1. Quadzilla! (...and Quadzookie.)

Why the Gold Standard quad developer is squatting—and why you absolutely need to master the Big Daddy, the *one-legged squat*...

How to perform the Shrimp Squat, a wonderful quad and glute builder, which is comparable to the one-leg squat in terms of body-challenge.

Why you should employ THESE 7 jumping methods to put your quad gains through the roof...

How to perform the hyper-tough, man-making Sissy Squat—favorite of the Iron Guru, Vince Gironda—great bodybuilding ideologist of the Golden Era, and trainer of a young Mr. Schwarzenegger. He wouldn't let anyone perform barbell squats in his gym!

2. Hamstrings: Stand Sideways With Pride

Enter *Lombard's Paradox*: how and why you can successfully brutalize your hammies with calisthenics.

Why bridging is a perfect exercise for strengthening the hamstrings.

How to correctly work your hamstrings and activate your entire posterior chain.

Why THIS workout of straight bridges and hill sprints could put muscle on a pencil.

How to employ the little-known secret of the *bridge curl* to develop awesome strength and power in the your hammies.

Why explosive work is essential for fully developed hamstrings—and the best explosive exercise to make your own...

3. Softball Biceps

THIS is the best biceps exercise in the world *bar none*. But most bodybuilders never use it to build their biceps! Discover what you are missing out on and learn to do it right...

And then you can make dumbbell curls look like a redheaded stepchild with THIS superior bicep blower-upper...

Another great compound move for the biceps (and forearms) is *rope climbing*. As with all bodyweight, this can be performed progressively. Get the details here on why and how...

Despite what some trainers may ignorantly tell you, you can also perform bodyweight biceps *isolation* exercises—such as the classic (but-rarely-seen-in-gyms) *curl-up*. Pure power! If you can build one, THIS old school piece of kit will give you biceps straight from Hades.

4. Titanic Triceps

Paul Wade has *never* met a gym-trained bodybuilder who understands how the triceps work. Not one. Learn how the triceps REALLY work. This stuff is gold—pay attention. And discover the drills that are going to CRUCIFY those tris!

4. Farmer Forearms

Paul Wade wrote the definitive mini-manual of calisthenics forearm and grip training in *Convict Conditioning 2*. But HERE'S a reminder on the take-home message that the forearms are best built through THESE exercises, and you can build superhuman grip by utilizing intelligent THESE progressions.

Why crush-style grippers are a mistake and the better, safer alternative for a hand-pulping grip...

5. It's Not "Abs", It's "Midsection"

As a bodybuilder, your method should be to pick a big, tough midsection movement and work at it hard and progressively to thicken your six-pack. This work should be a cornerstone of your training, no different from pullups or squats. It's a requirement. Which movements to pick? Discover the best drills here...

And the single greatest exercise for scorching your abs in the most effective manner possible is THIS...

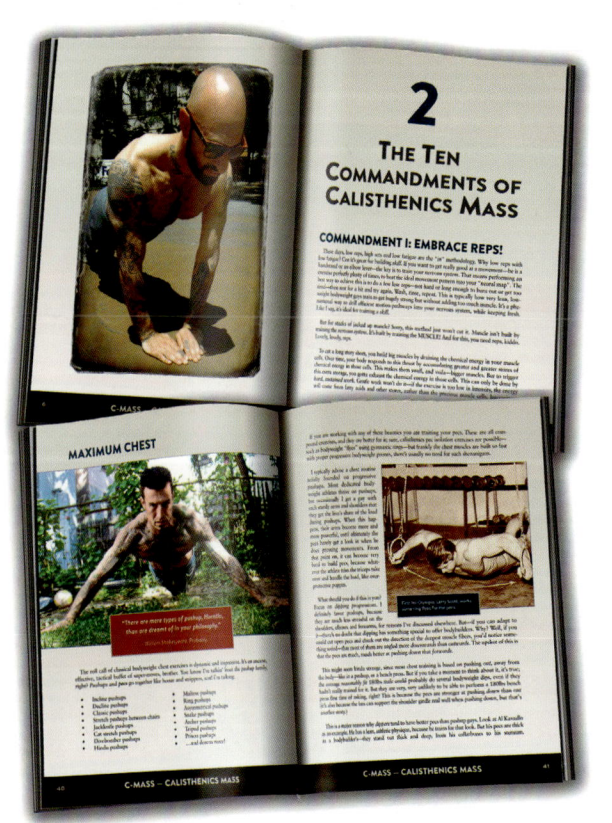

COMMANDMENT III: Use Simple, Compound Exercises!

Why—if you want to get swole—you need to toss out complex, high-skill exercises.

Why *dynamic* exercises are generally far better than *static holds* for massive muscle building.

These are the very best dynamic exercises— for bigger bang for your muscle buck.

How to ratchet up the heat with THIS kick-ass strategy and sprout new muscle at an eye-popping rate.

COMMANDMENT IV: Limit Sets!

What it takes to trigger explosive muscle growth—and why most folk foolishly and wastefully pull their "survival trigger" way too many futile times...

Why you need to void "volume creep" at all costs when size is what you're all about.

COMMANDMENT V: Focus on Progress—and Utilize a Training Journal!

Why so few wannabe athletes ever achieve a good level of strength and muscle—let alone a *great* level—and what it really takes to succeed.

Golden tip: how to take advantage of the *windows of opportunity* your training presents you.

How to transform miniscule, incremental gains into long-range massive outcomes.

Forgot those expensive supplements! Why keeping a training log can be the missing key to success or failure in the muscle-gain biz.

COMMANDMENT VI: You Grow When You Rest. So Rest!

If you *really* wanted to improve on your last workout—add that rep, tighten up your form—how would you want to approach that workout? The answer is right here...

Ignore THIS simple, ancient, muscle-building fact—and be prepared to go on spinning your muscle-building wheels for a VERY long time...

10 secrets to optimizing the magic rest-muscle growth formula...

Why you may never even come close to your full physical potential—but how to change that...

COMMANDMENT VII: Quit Eating "Clean" the Whole Time!

Warning—Politically incorrect statement: Why, if you are trying to pack on more muscle, eating junk now and again is not only okay, it can be positively *anabolic*.

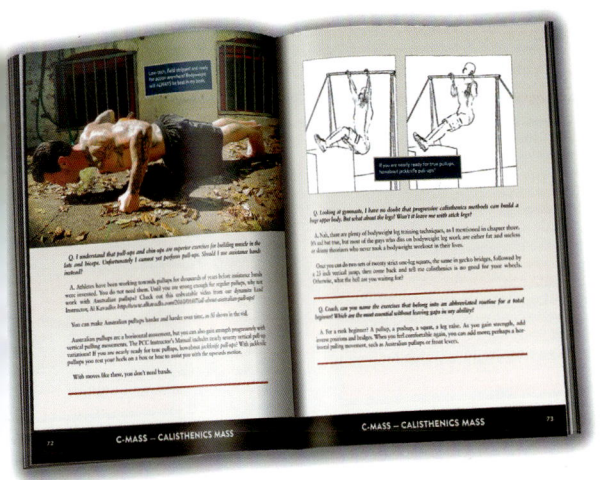

How to best train your obliques and lateral chain...

The simplest and most effective way to train your transversus...

6. Maximum Chest

The roll call of classical bodyweight chest exercises is dynamic and impressive. It's an ancient, effective, tactical buffet of super-moves. Get the list here...

THE best chest routine is THIS one...

If super-sturdy arms and shoulders mean your pecs barely get a look in when you press, then focus on THESE progressions instead—and your pecs will be burning with a welcome new pain...

Why Al Kavadlo has a lean, athletic physique, but his pecs are as thick as a bodybuilder's...

THIS could be the ultimate bodyweight drill to get thick, imposing pectoral muscles...

And here's the single finest exercise for enlarging your pec minor—yet hardly anyone has figured it out...

Why you need to master the art of deep breathing, strongman style, to truly develop a massive chest—and where to find unbeatable advice from proven champions...

7. Powerful, Healthy Shoulders

All die-hard bodybuilders need to know is that the deltoids have three heads. Here's how they work...

If you want to give any of your shoulder heads an enhanced, specialist workout, a great tactic is THIS.

How to make your lateral deltoids scream for mercy—and thank you later when you ignore their pleas...

If you *really* want to build your rear delts, THIS drill should be your number one exercise...

THESE kinds of drills can result in shoulder injury, rotator cuff tears, frozen shoulder and chronic pain—what to stick with instead...

THIS is a fantastic deltoid movement which will swell up those cannonballs fast...

Why old school hand balancing is so great for strength, size and coordination, while surprisingly easy on the shoulders, especially as you get a bit older...

The number one go-to guy in the whole world for hand-balancing is THIS calisthenics master...

8. Ah'll be Back

THIS exercise is the finest lat-widener in the bodybuilding world and should be the absolute mainstay of your back training. This one's a no-brainer—if adding maximum torso beef as fast and efficiently as possible appeals to you...

Are you an advanced bodyweight bodybuilder? Then you may wish to add THIS to your upper-back routine. Why? Well—THIS will blitz your rear delts, scapular muscles and the lower heads of the trapezius. These are the "detail" muscles of the back, so loved by bodybuilders when they grow and thicken, resembling serpents swirling around the shoulder-blades.

Paul Wade demands that all his students begin their personal training with a brutal regime of THIS punishing drill. Why? Find out here...

Real strength monsters can try THIS. But you gotta be real powerful to survive the attempt...

Many bodybuilders think only in terms of "low back" when working the spinal muscles, but this is a mistake: find out why...

How bridging fully works all the deep tissues of the spine and bulletproofs the discs.

The single most effective bridge technique for building massive back muscle...

Why back levers performed THIS way are particularly effective in building *huge* spinal strength and thickness.

Why *inverse hyperextensions* are a superb lower-back and spine exercise which requires zero equipment.

9. Calving Season

THIS squat method will make your calves larger, way more supple, more powerful, and your ankles/Achilles' tendon will be bulletproofed like a steel cable...

Whether you are an athlete, a strength trainer or a pure bodyweight bodybuilder, your first mission should be to gradually build to THIS. Until you get there, you don't need to waste time on any specialist calf exercises.

If you DO want to add specific calf exercises to your program, then THESE are a good choice.

The calves are naturally explosive muscles, and explosive bodyweight work is very good for calf-building. So add THESE six explosive drills into your mix...

Methods like THIS are so brutal (and effective) that they can put an inch or more on stubborn calves in just weeks. If you can train like this just once a week for a few months, you better get ready to outgrow your socks...

10. TNT: Total Neck and Traps

Do bodybuilders even need to do neck work? Here's the answer...

The best neck exercises for beginners.

HERE is an elite-level technique for developing the upper trapezius muscles between the neck and shoulders..

THIS is another wonderful exercise for the traps, developing them from all angles.

By the time you can perform two sets of twenty deep, slow reps of THIS move, your traps will look like hardcore cans of beans.

If you want more neck, and filling out your collar is something you want to explore, forget those decapitation machines in the gym, or those headache-inducing head straps. The safest, most natural and most productive techniques for building a bull-nape are THESE.

4. Okay. Now Gimme a Program

If you want to pack on muscle using bodyweight, it's no good training like a *gymnast* or a *martial artist* or a dancer or a *yoga expert*, no matter how impressive those *skill-based* practitioners might be at performing advanced calisthenics. You need a different mindset. You need to train like a bodybuilder!

Learn the essential *C-Mass* principles behind programming, so you can master your own programming...

The most important thing to understand about bodybuilding routines...

Simple programs with **minimum** complexity have THESE features

By contrast, programs with **maximum** complexity have THESE features

Why Simple Beats Complex, For THESE 3 Very Important Reasons...

When to Move up the Programming Line

If simpler, more basic routines are always the best, why do advanced bodybuilders tend to follow more complex routines? Programs with different sessions for different bodyparts, with dozens of exercises? Several points to consider...

The best reason is to move up the programming line is THIS

Fundamental Program Templates

- Total Body 1, Total Body 2
- Upper/Lower-Body Split 1, Upper/Lower-Body Split 2
- 3-Way Split 1, 3-Way Split 2
- 4-Way Split 1, 4-Way Split 1

5. Troubleshooting Muscle-Growth: The FAQ

Q. *Why bodyweight? Why can't I use weights and machines to build muscle?*

Q. *I understand that pull-ups and chin-ups are superior exercises for building muscle in the lats and biceps. Unfortunately I cannot yet perform pull-ups. Should I use assistance bands instead?*

Q. *Looking at gymnasts, I have no doubt that progressive calisthenics methods can build a huge upper body. But what about the legs? Won't it leave me with stick legs?*

Q. *Coach, can you name the exercises that belong into an abbreviated routine for a total beginner? Which are the most essential without leaving gaps in my ability?*

Q. *Big" bodyweight exercises such as push-ups and pull-ups may target the larger muscles of the body (pecs, lats, biceps, etc.), but what about the smaller muscles which are still so important to the bodybuilder? Things like forearms, the calves, the neck?*

Q. *I have been told I need to use a weighted vest on my push-ups and pull-ups if I want to get stronger and gain muscle. Is this true?*

Q. *Is bodyweight training suitable for women? Do you know of any women who achieved the "Master Steps" laid out in Convict Conditioning?*

Q. *I am very interested in gaining size—not just muscle mass, but also height. Is it possible that calisthenics can increase my height?*

Q. *You have said that moving exercises are superior to isometrics when it comes to mass gain. I am interested in getting huge shoulders, but Convict Conditioning gives several static (isometric) exercises early on in the handstand pushup chain. Can you give me any moving exercises I can use instead, to work up to handstand pushups?*

---

24 HOURS A DAY ORDER NOW — **1·800·899·5111** — www.dragondoor.com

Order *C-Mass* online: www.dragondoor.com/b75

Q. I have heard that the teenage years are the ideal age for building muscle. Is there any point in trying to build muscle after the age of forty?

Q. I have had some knee problems in the past; any tips for keeping my knee joints healthy so I can build more leg mass?

Q. I'm pretty skinny and I have always had a huge amount of trouble putting on weight—any weight, even fat. Building muscle is virtually impossible for me. What program should I be on?

Q. I've read in several bodybuilding magazines that I need to change my exercises frequently in order to "confuse" my muscles into growth. Is that true?

Q. I read in several bodybuilding magazines that I need to eat protein every 2-3 hours to have a hope in hell of growing. They also say that I need a huge amount of protein, like two grams per pound of bodyweight. Why don't your Commandments mention the need for protein?

Q. I have heard that whey is the "perfect" food for building muscle. Is this true?

6. The Democratic Alternative...how to get as powerful as possible without gaining a pound

There is a whole bunch of folks who either want (or need) massive strength and power, but without the attendant muscle bulk. Competitive athletes who compete in weight limits are one example; wrestlers, MMA athletes, boxers, etc. Females are another group who, as a rule, want to get stronger when they train, but without adding much (or any) size. Some men desire steely, whip-like power but see the sheer weight of mass as non-functional—many martial artists fall into this category; perhaps Bruce Lee was the archetype.

But bodybuilders should also fall under this banner. All athletes who want to become as huge as possible need to spend some portion of their time focusing on *pure strength*. Without a high (and increasing) level of strength, it's impossible to use enough load to stress your muscles into getting bigger. This is even truer once you get past a certain basic point.

So: You want to build power like a Humvee, with the sleek lines of a classic Porsche? The following Ten Commandments have got you covered. Follow them, and we promise you *cannot* fail, even if you had trouble getting stronger in the past. Your days of weakness are done, my friend...

Enter the "Bullzelle"

There are guys who train for pure mass and want to look like bulls, and guys who only train for athleticism without mass, and are more like gazelles. Al Kavadlo has been described as a "bullzelle"—someone who trains mainly for strength, and has some muscle too, but without looking like a bulked-up bodybuilder. And guess what? It seems like many of the new generation of athletes want to be bullzelles! With Paul Wade's C-Mass program, you'll have what you need to achieve bullzelle looks and functionality should you want it...

COMMANDMENT I: Use low reps while keeping "fresh"!

If you want to generate huge strength without building muscle, here is the precise formula...

COMMANDMENT II: Utilize Hebb's Law—drill movements as often as possible!

How pure strength training works, in a nutshell...

Why frequency—how often you train—is often so radically different for *pure strength* trainers and for bodybuilders...

Training recipe for the perfect bodybuilder—and for the perfect strength trainer...

Why training for pure strength and training to *master a skill* are virtually identical methods.

COMMANDMENT III: Master muscle synergy!

If there is a "trick" to being supremely strong, THIS is it...

As a bodybuilder, are you making this huge mistake? If you want to get super-powerful, unlearn these ideas and employ THIS strategy instead...

Another great way to learn muscular coordination and control is to explore THESE drills...

COMMANDMENT IV: Brace Yourself!

If there is a single tactic that's *guaranteed* to maximize your body-power in short order, it's bracing. *Bracing* is both an art-form and a science. Here's how to do it and why it works so well.

COMMANDMENT V: Learn old-school breath control!

If there is an instant "trick" to increasing your strength, it's *learning the art of the breath*. Learn the details here...

Why inhalation is so important for strength and how to make it work most efficiently while lifting...

How the correctly-employed, controlled, forceful exhalation activates the muscles of the trunk, core and ribcage...

COMMANDMENT VI: Train your tendons!

When the old-time strongmen talked about strength, they rarely talked about muscle power—they typically focused on the integrity of the tendons. THIS is why...

The concept of "supple strength" and how to really train the *tendons* for optimal resilience and steely, real-life strength...

Why focusing on "peak contraction" can be devastating to your long-term strength-health goals...

COMMANDMENT VII: Focus on weak links!

THIS is the essential difference between a mere *bodybuilder* and a *truly powerful human being*...

Why focusing all your attention on the biggest, strongest muscle groups is counter-productive for developing your true strength potential...

Pay extra attention to your weakest areas by including THESE 4 sets of drills as a mandatory part of your monster strength program...

COMMANDMENT VIII: Exploit Neural Facilitation!

The nervous system—like most sophisticated biological systems—possesses different sets of *gears*. Learn how to safely and effectively shift to high gear in a hurry using THESE strategies...

COMMANDMENT IX: Apply Plyometric Patterns to Hack Neural Inhibition

Why it is fatal for a bodyweight master to focus only on tension-generating techniques and what to do instead...

How very fast movements can hugely increase your strength—the light bulb analogy.

The difference between "voluntary" and "involuntary" strength—and how to work on both for greater gains...

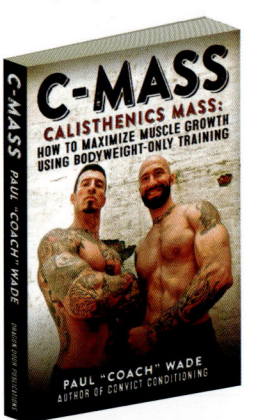

COMMANDMENT X: Master the power of the mind!

How to train the mind to make the body achieve incredible levels of strength and ferocity—as if it was tweaking on PCP...

5 fundamental ways to harness mental power and optimize your strength...

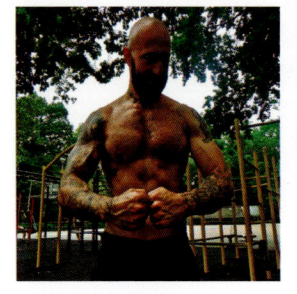

BONUS CHAPTER:
7. Supercharging Your Hormonal Profile

Why you should never, ever, ever take steroids to enhance your strength...

Hormones and muscle growth

Your *hormones* are what build your muscle. All your training is pretty secondary. You can work out hard as often as possible, but if your hormonal levels aren't good, your gains will be close to nil. Learn what it takes to naturally optimize a cascade of powerful strength-generating hormones and to minimize the strength-sappers from sabotaging your gains...

Studies and simple experience have demonstrated that, far from being some esoteric practice, some men have increased their diminished total testosterone levels by *over a thousand percent*! How? Just by following a few basic rules.

What rules? Listen up. THIS is the most important bodybuilding advice anyone will ever give you.

The 6 Rules of Testosterone Building

THESE rules are the most powerful and long-lasting, for massive testosterone generation. Follow them if you want to get diesel.

The iron-clad case against steroid use and exogenous testosterone in general.

C-MASS
Calisthenics Mass: How To Maximize Muscle Growth Using Bodyweight-Only Training
By Paul "Coach" Wade

Book #B75 $24.95
eBook #EB75 $9.95
Paperback 8.5 x 11 • 136 pages, 130 photos

Order *C-Mass* online:
www.dragondoor.com/b75

1•800•899•5111

24 HOURS A DAY
ORDER NOW

www.dragondoor.com

How to Lead, Survive and Dominate Physically—And Reengineer Yourself As "The Complete Athletic Package"…

SUPERHUMAN POWER, MAXIMUM SPEED AND AGILITY, PLUS COMBAT-READY REFLEXES— USING BODYWEIGHT-ONLY METHODS

Explosive Calisthenics is for those who want to be winners and survivors in the game of life—for those who want to be the Complete Package: powerful, explosive, strong, agile, quick and resilient. Traditional martial arts have always understood this necessity of training the complete package—with explosive power at an absolute premium. And resilience is revered: the joints, tendons, muscles, organs and nervous system are ALL conditioned for maximum challenge.

Really great athletes are invariably that way too: agile as all get-go, blinding speed, ungodly bursts of power, superhuman displays of strength, seemingly at will…

The foundation and fundamentals center, first, around the building of power and speed. But *Explosive Calisthenics* does a masterful job of elucidating the skill-practices needed to safely prepare for and master the more ambitious moves.

But *Explosive Calisthenics* doesn't just inspire you with the dream of being the Complete Package. It gives you the complete blueprint, every detail and every progression you could possibly want and need to nail your dream and make it a reality. You, the Complete Package—it's all laid out for you, step by step

"The first physical attribute we lose as we age is our ability to generate power. Close behind is the loss of skilled, coordinated movement. The fix is never to lose these abilities in the first place! Paul Wade's "*Explosive Calisthenics* is the best program for developing power and skilled movement I have seen. Just as with his previous two books, the progressions are masterful with no fancy equipment needed. Do yourself a favor and get this amazing work. This book will be the gold standard for developing bodyweight power, skill, and agility."
—**CHRIS HARDY**, D.O. MPH, CSCS, author, **Strong Medicine**

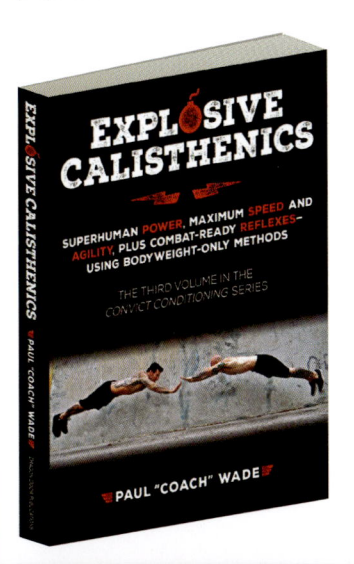

Explosive Calisthenics
Superhuman Power, Maximum Speed and Agility, Plus Combat-Ready Reflexes—Using Bodyweight-Only Methods
By Paul "Coach" Wade

Book #B80 $39.95
eBook #EB80 $19.95
Paperback 8.5 x 11
392 pages, 775 photos

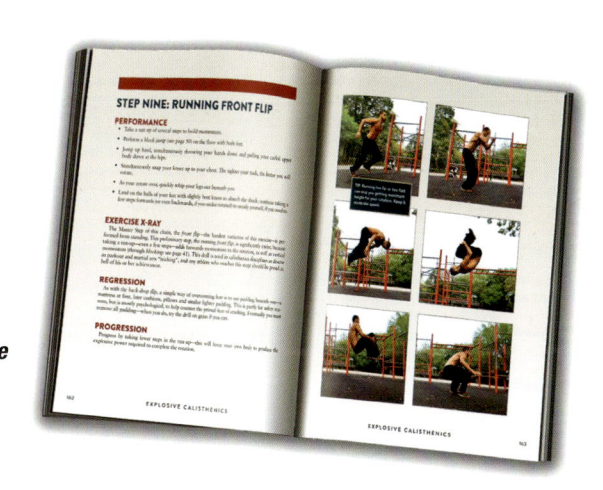

24 HOURS A DAY ORDER NOW
1•800•899•5111
www.dragondoor.com

Order *Explosive Calisthenics* online:
www.dragondoor.com/b80

Teach your body to be the lightning-fast, explosive, acrobatic super-hunter your DNA is coded to make you…

With **Explosive Calisthenics**, **Paul Wade** challenges you to separate yourself from the herd of also-ran followers—to become a leader, survivor and winner in the physical game of life. But he doesn't just challenge and inspire you. He gives you the direct means, the secrets, the science, the wisdom, the blueprints, the proven methods and the progressions—that make success inevitable, when you supply your end in consistent, diligent, skillful application.

Now a legendary international bestseller, **Convict Conditioning** can lay claim to be the Great Instigator when it comes to the resurgence of interest in bodyweight exercise mastery.

And—while **Convict Conditioning 2** cemented Wade's position as the preeminent authority on bodyweight exercise—there is no doubt that his magisterial new accomplishment, **Explosive Calisthenics**, is going to blow the doors off, all over again.

What makes **Explosive Calisthenics** so exciting—and so profound in its implications?

See, it goes back to the laws of brute survival. It's not "Only the strongest shall survive". No, it's more like: "Only the strongest, quickest, most agile, most powerful and most explosive shall survive." To be a leader and dominator and survivor in the pack, you need to be the complete package…

A vanishing percent of people who workout even attempt to unlock their body's inherent power and speed—choose to be different: reclaim your pride and dignity as a fully-realized human being by fully unleashing your true athletic capacity…

Now—for those who have the balls and the will and the fortitude to take it on—comes the next stage: **Explosive Calisthenics**. The chance not only to be strong and healthy but to ascend to the Complete Package. If you want it, then here it is…

PART I: POWER, SPEED, AGILITY
1: POWER UP! *THE NEED FOR SPEED*

Power defined—understanding the difference between strength and power…P 3

Functional speed—and the golden mean for power in athletics…P 6

Discover how to move your entire body with lightning speed… P 6

Agility defined…P 7

Discover how to efficiently alter your movement at high velocity…P 7

The difference between complex power and simple power—and what it means for athletic success…P 7

Discover how to enhance your reflexes to generate higher levels of power speed and agility…P 9

Why most gym-trained athletes lack THESE qualities—and will therefore NEVER attain true athleticism…P 10

2: EXPLOSIVE TRAINING: *FIVE KEY PRINCIPLES*…P 11

How modern Americans have become the slowest, least agile members of our species in all history—and what we can do about it…P 11

How you CAN teach your body to be the lightning-fast, explosive, acrobatic super-hunter your DNA is coded to make you…P 12

The 5 key principles for developing speed, power and agility… P 12

How to be the COMPLETE explosive machine…P 13

Why traditional box work, core training and Olympic lifting simply won't cut it—when your goal is high-level explosiveness…P 14

If you really want to build monstrous power, speed and agility in the shortest possible time—HERE is what you absolutely MUST stick with…P 18

The 6 movements you must master—for the ultimate in hardcore explosiveness…P 19

The true essence of calisthenics mastery lies here—and only here…P 19

3: HOW TO USE THIS BOOK: *CORE CONCEPTS AND ANSWERS*…P 23

Do you need to learn the Explosive 6 in any particular order?…P 26

Do you have to start with Step 1?…P 27

How to train short-distance speed…P 32

Mastery of progressive calisthenics is like building an arsenal-full of weapons for your physical transformation. The Power Jump and Power Pushup will set up your foundation by supercharging your nervous system, ramping up your reflexes and amping your speed and power.

Expect to be remarkably and resiliently strengthened in your bones, joints, tissues and muscles—over the entire body.

In other words: hard, dedicated work on just the Power Jump and the Power Pushup alone can turn a slow, clumsy Joe Average into a lightning-powered cyborg…

PART II: THE EXPLOSIVE SIX
4: POWER JUMPS: *ADVANCED LEG SPRING*… P 37

If you really want to become explosive, then the legs are the source of it all—and the best way to train the legs is with progressive power jumps. Here is the 10-step blueprint for achieving ultimate leg power…

Understanding the importance of developing springy legs…P 37

Deconstructing the power jumps…P 38

How to develop the crucial skills of launching, tucking and landing…P 38–40

How to take advantage of *Myotatic* Rebound—to correctly absorb and redirect force…

How to correctly block when you jump…P 41

Do you need Plyo boxes?…P 43

Step One: Straight Hop—Performance, X-Ray, Regressions, Progressions…P 44

Step Two: Squat Jump—Performance,

> "**Explosive Calisthenics** is an absolute Treasure Map for anybody looking to tear down their body's athletic limitations. Who doesn't want to be able to kip to their feet from their back like a Bruce Lee? Or make a backflip look easy? Paul makes you want to put down the barbells, learn and practice these step-by-step progressions to mastering the most explosive and impressive bodyweight movements. The best part is? You can become an absolute Beast in under an hour of practice a week. Way to go, Paul! AROO!"
>
> —Joe Distefano, **Spartan Race,** Director of Training & Creator of the **Spartan SGX Certification**

X-Ray, Regressions, Progressions…P 46

Step Three: Vertical Leap—Performance, X-Ray, Regressions, Progressions…P 48

Step Four: Block Jump—Performance, X-Ray, Regressions, Progressions…P 50

How to develop the ability to transfer force in dramatic fashion…P 50

Step Five: Butt-Kick Jump—Performance, X-Ray, Regressions, Progressions…P 52

Step Six: Slap Tuck Jump—Performance, X-Ray, Regressions, Progressions…P 54

Step Seven: Tuck Jump—Performance, X-Ray, Regressions, Progressions…P 56

Confers some serious explosive power to the lower body—and is a perquisite for becoming really fast…P 56

Step Eight: Catch Tuck Jump—Performance, X-Ray, Regressions, Progressions…P 58

Step Nine: Thread Jump—Performance, X-Ray, Regressions, Progressions…P 60

Master Step: Suicide Jump—Performance, X-Ray…P 62

The ultimate tucking drill—once you master this drill, kip ups, front flips and back flips will come much easier than you ever imagined…P 62

Going Beyond…P 64

Reverse Suicide Jump…P64

Small Space Drills—3 useful speed and power techniques…P 69

Cossacks—for great supple strength and balance…P 69

Wide-to-Close Pop-Ups…P 70

Order *Explosive Calisthenics* online: www.dragondoor.com/b80

1•800•899•5111

24 HOURS A DAY — ORDER NOW

www.dragondoor.com

— EXPLOSIVE CALISTHENICS —

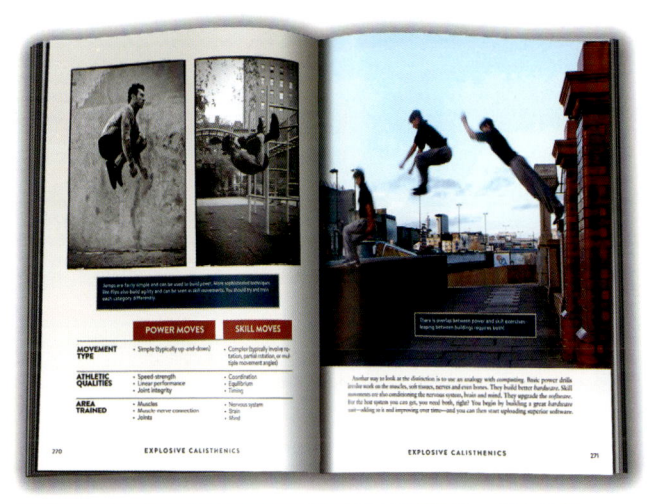

"Martial arts supremacy is all about explosive power and speed, and you will possess both once you've mastered the hardcore exercises in *Explosive Calisthenics*. Take your solo training to a level you never even imagined with these teeth-gritting, heart-palpating exercises—from a master of the genre." —**Loren W. Christensen**, author of over 50 books, including *Fighting Power: How to Develop Explosive Punches, Kicks, Blocks, And Grappling* and *Speed Training: How to Develop Your Maximum Speed for Martial Arts*

5: POWER PUSHUPS: *STRENGTH BECOMES POWER*…P 73

To round out a basic power training regime, you need to pair jumps with a movement chain which performs a similar job for the upper-body and arms. The best drills for these are power push ups. Here is the 10-step blueprint for becoming an upper-body cyborg…

How to get arms like freaking jackhammers…P 73

How to skyrocket pour power levels, maximize your speed and add slabs of righteous beef to you torso and guns…P 73

How to develop upper-body survival-power—for more effective punching, blocking, throwing and pushing…P 73

How speed-power training trains the nervous system and joints to handle greater loads…P 73

The more power you have in your arms, chest and shoulders, the stronger they become. And the stronger they become, the harder you can work them and the bigger they get…P 73

Gives you an extra edge in strength AND size…P 73

Why the best way is the natural way…P 74

Deconstructing Power Pushups…P 74

Correct elbow positioning and where to place your hands (crucial)—to spring back with optimal power…P 74

Why cheating with the Earthworm will only rob you—if freakish strength gains are your goal…P 76

How to apply the Myotatic Rebound effect to maximal advantage in your power pushups…P 78

The Power Pushup Chain…P 79

Step One: Incline Pop-Up—Performance, X-Ray, Regressions, Progressions…P 80

A perfect way to gently condition the shoulders, elbows and wrists for the harder work to come

Step Two: Kneeling Push-Off—Performance, X-Ray, Regressions, Progressions…P 82

How to turn your strength into power—and an exceptional way to build your punching force…P 82

Step Three: Pop-Up—Performance, X-Ray, Regressions, Progressions…P 84

A nearly magical preliminary exercise to get better at clap pushups.

Step Four: Clap Pushup—Performance, X-Ray, Regressions, Progressions…P 86

How the clap pushup builds exceptional levels of torso power and quick hands, whilst toughening the arms and shoulders—invaluable for boxers, martial artists and football players.

Step Five: Chest-Strike Pushup—Performance, X-Ray, Regressions, Progressions…P 88

Step Six: Hip-Strike Pushup—Performance, X-Ray, Regressions, Progressions…P 90

A killer bridging exercise between clapping in front of the body and clapping behind.

Step Seven: Convict Pushup—Performance, X-Ray, Regressions, Progressions…P 92

Step Eight: Half-Super—Performance, X-Ray, Regressions, Progressions…P 94

Builds high levels of pure shoulder speed—excellent for all martial artists.

Step Nine: Full Body Pop-Up—Performance, X-Ray, Regressions, Progressions…P 96

Master Step: The Superman—Performance, X-Ray…P 98

A wicked, wicked move that works the whole body—both anterior and posterior chains.

Get upper-body pushing muscles that are king-fu powerful and robust as a gorilla's…P 98

If God had handed us a "perfect" explosive upper-body exercise, it might be this…P 98

Going Beyond…P 100

The Aztec Pushup…P 101

The Crossing Aztec Pushup… P 102

The One-Arm Clapping Pushup…P 103

Small Space Drills…P104

The Push Get-Up…P 104

Round-the-Clock Pushups…P 105

360 Jump…P 106

Fast feet and hands go together like biscuits and gravy—here's how to make it happen.

6: THE KIP-UP: *KUNG FU BODY SPEED*…P 109

The mesmerizing Kip-Up is the most explosive way of getting up off your back—and is a surprisingly useful skill to possess. Learn how here…P 109

Deconstructing Kip-Ups…P 110

The Roll-Up, Hand Positioning, the Kick and the Rotation…P 112

Step One: Rolling Sit-Up—Performance, X-Ray, Regressions, Progressions…P 114

A fantastic conditioning exercise, which strengthens the midsection, hips and back…P 114

Step Two: Rolling Squat—Performance, X-Ray, Regressions, Progressions…P 116

How to generate forward momentum.

Step Three: Shoulder Pop—Performance, X-Ray, Regressions, Progressions…P 118

Strengthens and conditions the wrists and shoulders for the task of explosively pushing the body up.

Step Four: Bridge Kip—Performance, X-Ray, Regressions, Progressions…P 120

Learn how to generate enough lower body power to throw the head, shoulders and upper back off the floor.

Step Five: Butt Kip—Performance, X-Ray, Regressions, Progressions…P 122

Step Six: Half Kip—Performance, X-Ray, Regressions, Progressions…P 124

Step Seven: Kip-Up—Performance, X-Ray, Regressions, Progressions…P 126

Impossible without an explosive waist, super-fast legs and the total-body ability of a panther—which you will OWN when you master step seven…

Step Eight: Straight Leg Kip-Up—Performance, X-Ray, Regressions, Progressions…P 128

Step Nine: Wushu Kip-Up—Performance, X-Ray, Regressions, Progressions…P 130

Master Step: No-Hands Kip-Up—Performance, X-Ray, Regressions, Progressions…P 132

If there is a more impressive—or explosive—way to power up off the floor, then humans haven't invented it yet…

Master this advanced drill and your total-body speed and agility will start to bust off the charts…P 132

Going Beyond—Roll Kip, Head Kip and Ditang Breakfall…P 134—136

Small Space Drills…P 137

Bridge Push-Offs, Sitting Kips and prone Kips…P 137—139

7: THE FRONT FLIP: *LIGHTNING MOVEMENT SKILLS*…P 141

The Front Flip is THE explosive exercise par excellence—it is the "super-drill" for any athlete wanting more speed, agility and power.

Discover how to attain this iconic test of power and agility—requiring your entire body, from toes to neck, to be whip-like explosive…P 141

---

24 HOURS A DAY ORDER NOW   **1·800·899·5111**   www.dragondoor.com   Order *Explosive Calisthenics* online: **www.dragondoor.com/b80**

— EXPLOSIVE CALISTHENICS —

"Coach Wade saved the best for last! *Explosive Calisthenics* is the book all diehard *Convict Conditioning* fans have been waiting for. There has never been anything like it until now!

With his trademark blend of old-school philosophy, hard-earned wisdom and in-your-face humor, Coach expands his infamous system of progressive bodyweight programming to break down the most coveted explosive moves, including the back flip, kip-up and muscle-up. If you want to know how far you can go training with just your own bodyweight, you owe it to yourself to get this book!"—Al Kavadlo, author, *Stretching Your Boundaries*

Deconstructing Front Flips…P 142

Run-Up, Take-Off, Unfurl, landing…P 142—143

The Front Flip Chain…P 144

Step One: Shoulder Roll—Performance, X-Ray, Regressions, Progressions…P 146

Step Two: Press Roll—Performance, X-Ray, Regressions, Progressions…P 148

Step Three: Jump Roll—Performance, X-Ray, Regressions, Progressions…P 150

Step Four: Handstand Roll—Performance, X-Ray, Regressions, Progressions…P 152

Step Five: Backdrop Handspring—Performance, X-Ray, Regressions, Progressions…P 154

Step Six: Front Handspring—Performance, X-Ray, Regressions, Progressions…P 156

A phenomenal explosive drill in its own right…

Step Seven: Flyspring—Performance, X-Ray, Regressions, Progressions…P 158

Step Eight: Back Drop Flip—Performance, X-Ray, Regressions, Progressions…P 160

Step Nine: Running Front Flip—Performance, X-Ray, Regressions, Progressions…P 162

Master Step: Front Flip—Performance, X-Ray…P 164

Going Beyond…P 166

The Round-Off and the Cartwheel…P 166—167

Small Space Drills…P 170

Kojaks, Thruster and Unilateral Jump…P 170—172

8: THE BACK FLIP: ULTIMATE AGILITY…P 175

The Back Flip is the most archetypal acrobatic feat—displaying integrated mastery of most of the most fundamental traits required for total explosive strength.

If you want to be a contender for the power crown, then you have to get to own the Back Flip—which defines true agility…

Discover how to develop a super-quick jump, a massive hip snap, a powerful, agile waist and spine—and an upper body that can generate higher levels of responsive force like lightning…

Simply put, this is the single greatest test of explosive power, true speed and agility found in nature. Here is how to pass the test…

Deconstructing the Back Flip…P 176

General tips for the many skills needed to master the Back Flip…P 176

5 key exercises to strengthen you arms and shoulders…P 178

How to achieve a powerful Tuck…P 179

How to use the Depth Jump to further condition your joints…P 179

The Back Flip Chain…P 180

THIS is the most important consideration to have in place for finally achieving the Back Flip…P 180

Step One: Rear Shoulder Roll—Performance, X-Ray, Regressions, Progressions…P 182

Step Two: Rear Press Roll—Performance, X-Ray, Regressions, Progressions…P 184

Step Three: Bridge Kick Over—Performance, X-Ray, Regressions, Progressions…P 186

A great antidote to fear of the Back Handspring

Step Four: Side Macaco—Performance, X-Ray, Regressions, Progressions…P 188

Step Five: Back Macaco—Performance, X-Ray, Regressions, Progressions…P 190

Step Six: Monkey Flip—Performance, X-Ray, Regressions, Progressions…P 192

Step Seven: Back Handspring—Performance, X-Ray, Regressions, Progressions…P 194

Step Eight: One-Arm Back Handspring—Performance, X-Ray, Regressions, Progressions…P 196

Step Nine: Four Point Back Flip—Performance, X-Ray, Regressions, Progressions…P 198

Master Step: Back Flip—Performance, X-Ray…P 200

Going Beyond…P 202

Small Space Drills…P 205

One-Arm Wall Push-Aways (great exercise for powerful, bulletproof elbows)…P 205

Donkey Kick and Scissors Jump…P 206

9: THE MUSCLE-UP: OPTIMAL EXPLOSIVE STRENGTH…P 209

If ever one popular strength exercise qualified as a "complete" feat, it would probably be the mighty Muscle-Up—one of the most jealously-admired skills in all of bodyweight training…

The Muscle-Up requires a very explosive pull, plus a push—so works almost the entire upper-body; the back and biceps pull, while the chest, triceps and shoulders push. Your grip needs to be insanely strong, your stomach crafted out of steel and you require a highly athletic posterior chain.

Discover the complete blueprint for achieving the planet's hottest bodyweight move…

Learn how to achieve the elusive, total-body-sync, X factor the Muscle-Up requires—and build insane explosive power in a highly compressed time frame…

Deconstructing the Muscle-Up…P 211—214

The Muscle-Up Chain…P 217

Step One: Swing Kip—Performance, X-Ray, Regressions, Progres-

"*Explosive Calisthenics* by Paul 'Coach' Wade is a masterfully constructed roadmap for the attainment of power, functional speed, and agility. The book is extreme in that only a small percentage of the population would be able or willing to fully take the challenge, but at the same time, brilliant in that the path proceeds methodically and progressively from relatively simple to extremely advanced, allowing a discretionary endpoint for each individual.

The book is also refreshingly raw. The exercises are all done using only bodyweight and little in the way of equipment. There are only five moves to master and yet each is a proverbial double-edge sword—at the same time dangerous yet potentially transformative.

Take this on and I doubt you will ever again be satisfied with the mundane bench press or the other exercise machines found in the typical gym."—Patrick Roth, M.D., author of *The End of Back Pain: Access Your Hidden Core to Heal Your Body*, Chairman of Neurosurgery at Hackensack University Medical Center and the director of its neurosurgical residency training program.

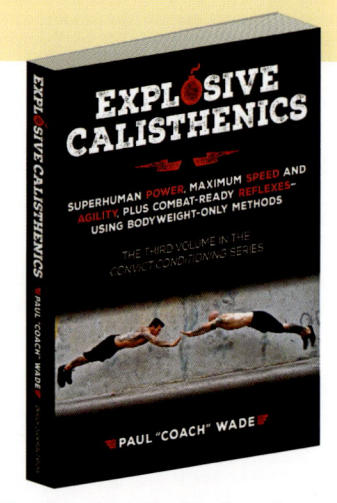

Explosive Calisthenics
Superhuman Power, Maximum Speed and Agility, Plus Combat-Ready Reflexes—Using Bodyweight-Only Methods
By Paul "Coach" Wade

Book #B80 **$39.95**
eBook #EB80 **$19.95**
Paperback 8.5 x 11 • 392 pages, 775 photos

Order *Explosive Calisthenics* online:
www.dragondoor.com/b80

1•800•899•5111
www.dragondoor.com

**24 HOURS A DAY
ORDER NOW**

Al Kavadlo's Progressive Plan for Primal Body Power

How to Build Explosive Strength and a Magnificent Physique—Using Bodyweight Exercise Only

What is more satisfying than owning a primally powerful, functionally forceful and brute-strong body? A body that packs a punch. A body that commands attention with its etched physique, coiled muscle and proud confidence...A body that can PERFORM at the highest levels of physical accomplishment...

Well, both Al Kavadlo—the author of *Pushing the Limits!*—and his brother Danny, are supreme testaments to the primal power of body culture done the old-school, ancient way—bare-handed, with your body only.

The brothers Kavadlo walk the bodyweight talk—and then some. The proof is evident on every page of *Pushing the Limits!*

Your body is your temple. Protect and strengthen your temple by modeling the methods of the exercise masters. Al Kavadlo has modeled the masters and has the "temple" to show for it. Follow Al's progressive plan for primal body power within the pages of *Pushing the Limits!*—follow in the footsteps of the great bodyweight exercise masters—and you too can build the explosive strength and possess the magnificent physique you deserve.

> "When people ask me about bodyweight strength training, I point them to Al Kavadlo. *Pushing the Limits!* is a must-have for bodyweight training enthusiasts or anyone looking to build strength without lifting weights. Al lays out dozens of effective exercises for every fitness level, while making the journey fun and encouraging."
> —MARK SISSON, author of *The Primal Blueprint*

> "Whether you are an advanced bodyweight conditioning athlete or a wet behind the ears newbie, Al's *Pushing the Limits!* has something for you. Easy to follow progressions allow you to master advanced push up, squat and bridging variations. All you need is the will to do it! No gym required."
> —ROBB WOLF, author of *The Paleo Solution*

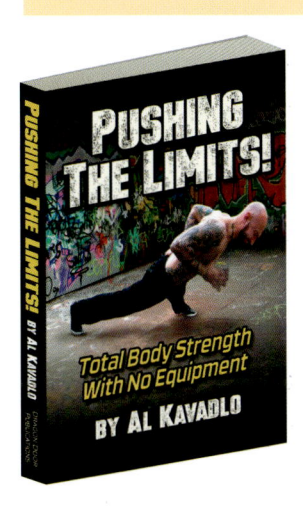

Pushing the Limits!
Total Body Strength With No Equipment
By Al Kavadlo

Book #B69 **$39.95**
eBook # EB69 **$19.95**
Paperback 8.5 x 11
224 pages • 240 photos

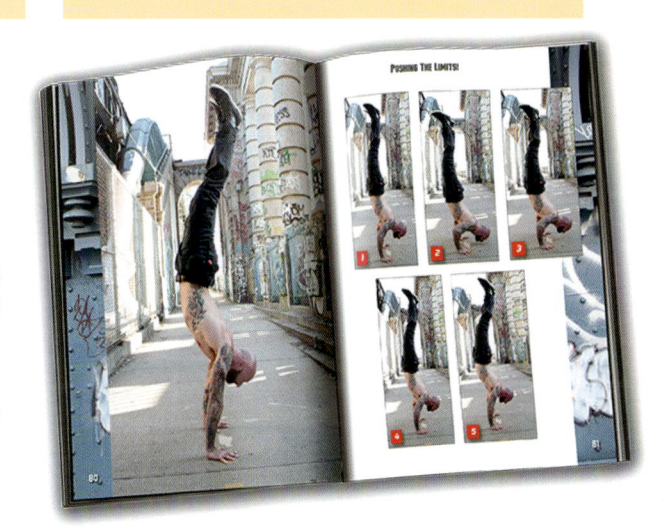

24 HOURS A DAY ORDER NOW

1•800•899•5111
www.dragondoor.com

Order *Pushing The Limits* online:
www.dragondoor.com/b69

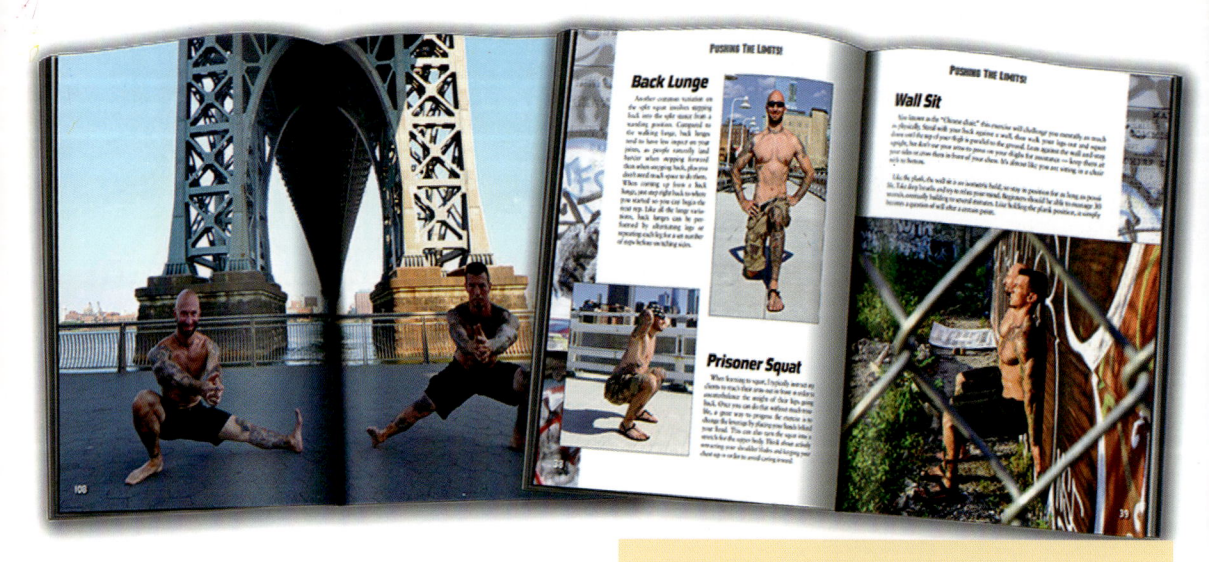

Reader Reviews of Pushing the Limits submitted on DragonDoor.

Time to work smart hard!

"I'm a physical therapist in orthopedics with all the frame wear and tear of a lifter. I use Al's stuff for myself and for patients and always get good outcomes. On my field there are those that make it happen, those that watch it happen, and those that dash in afterwards and ask "Hey, what just happened?" Grab a copy of Al's book. Make it happen."
—GARRETT MCELFRESH, PT, Milwaukee, WI

Al you did it again!

"I'm a doctor that uses functional rehab to get my patients better. This book has helped so much with all the great pics and showing and explaining what and why they are doing these exercises. Also when I get down and show them myself they can see that it is totally achievable! If you are wavering on getting this book, get it! I promise you won't regret it!

From a functional stand point Al, Danny, and Paul are spot on! I've seen and experienced "miracles" from doing these workouts! I have had a bad shoulder, low back, and hyperextended both knees in college football and was told I needed multiple surgeries and was always going to have pain..... WRONG! I am completely pain free and thank these hard working guys for everything they do! I can't wait to see what's next!" —DR. ROB BALZA, Cincinnati, OH

One of the best fitness books I have purchased!

"I recommend this book to anyone who enjoys being active. No matter what sport or training regimen you are currently following, Al's book has something for everyone. Novices and advanced practitioners alike, will find detailed movements that help increase their strength, mobility, and flexibility. Great read with beautiful photography." —LANCE PARVIN, Las Vegas, NV

"I LOVE this freaking Book!!! Every time you put out a new book it becomes my NEW favorite and my inspiration! I love the blend of strength, power, health and overall athleticism in this book! This book covers the BIG picture of training for ALL aspects of human performance.

I will use it with my athletes, with the adults I train, in my own training and absolutely these books will be the books I share with my kids. This stuff reminds me of the old school *Strength & Health Magazine*, I'm fired UP!"—ZACH EVEN-ESH, author of *The Encyclopedia of Underground Strength and Conditioning*

"This is the book I wish I had when I first started working out. Knowing Al's secrets and various progressions would have saved me years of wasted time, frustration and injuries. The variations of The Big Three and progressions Al lays out will keep you busy for years."—JASON FERRUGGIA

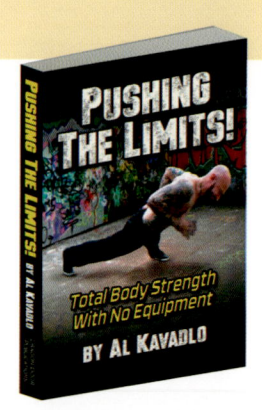

Pushing the Limits!
Total Body Strength With No Equipment
By Al Kavadlo

Book #B69 **$39.95**
eBook # EB69 **$19.95**
Paperback 8.5 x 11
224 pages • 240 photos

Order *Pushing The Limits* online:
www.dragondoor.com/b69

1•800•899•5111
www.dragondoor.com

24 HOURS A DAY
ORDER NOW

Sample Spreads From The Interior of *Stretching Your Boundaries*

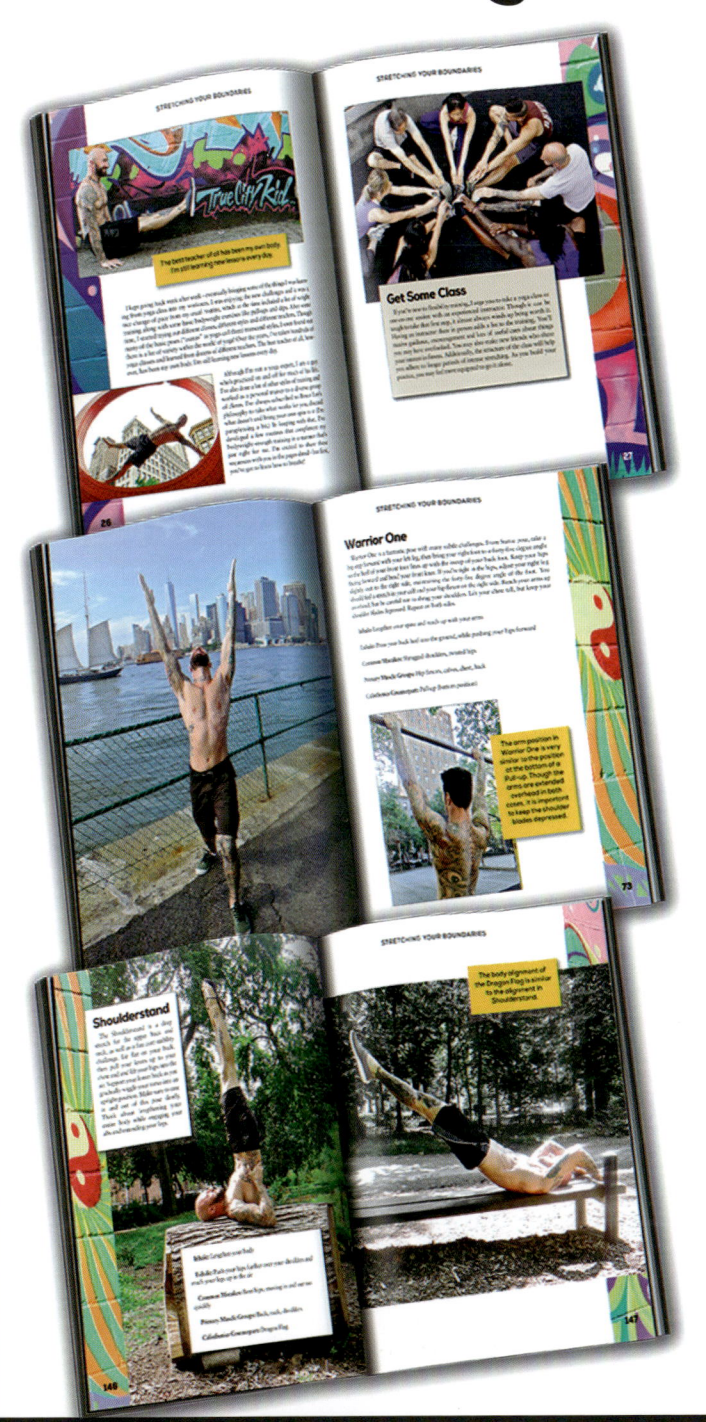

—TABLE OF CONTENTS —
Foreword by Elliott Hulse

PART ONE- Stretch Manifesto
- ➜ Stretching For Strength 1
- ➜ Taking Your Medicine 9
- ➜ Kid Stuff 15
- ➜ Mobility Matters 21
- ➜ Breath is Life 29

PART TWO - The Stretches
- ➜ Preface 39
- ➜ Dynamics 41
- ➜ Standing Statics 49
- ➜ Grounded Statics 95

PART THREE - Programming and Sample Routines
- ➜ Standards of Practice 153
- ➜ On Mats 161
- ➜ Symmetry 163
- ➜ Hypothetical Training Splits 171
- ➜ Sample Routines 177

24 HOURS A DAY ORDER NOW

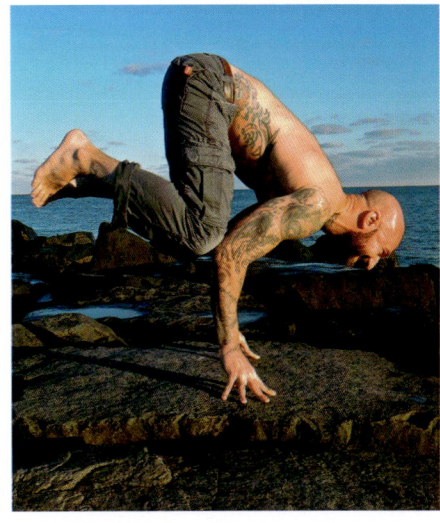

1·800·899·5111

www.dragondoor.com

Order *Stretching Your Boundaries* online:
www.dragondoor.com/b73

Stretching and Flexibility Secrets To Help Unlock Your Body—Be More Mobile, More Athletic, More Resilient And Far Stronger...

"The ultimate bodyweight mobility manual is here! Al Kavadlo's previous two Dragon Door books, **Raising the Bar** and **Pushing the Limits,** are the most valuable bodyweight strength training manuals in the world. But strength without mobility is meaningless. Al has used his many years of training and coaching to fuse bodyweight disciplines such as yoga, martial arts, rehabilitative therapy and bar athletics into the ultimate calisthenics stretching compendium. **Stretching your Boundaries** belongs on the shelf of any serious athlete—it's bodyweight mobility dynamite!"

—"COACH" PAUL WADE, author of *Convict Conditioning*

"In this book, Al invites you to take a deeper look at the often overlooked, and sometimes demonized, ancient practice of static stretching. He wrestles with many of the questions, dogmas and flat out lies about stretching that have plagued the fitness practitioner for at least the last decade. And finally he gives you a practical guide to static stretching that will improve your movement, performance, breathing and life. In **Stretching Your Boundaries,** you'll sense Al's deep understanding and love for the human body. Thank you Al, for helping to bring awareness to perhaps the most important aspect of physical education and fitness."

—ELLIOTT HULSE, creator of the *Grow Stronger* method

"An absolutely masterful follow up to **Raising The Bar** and **Pushing The Limits,** Stretching Your Boundaries really completes the picture. Both easy to understand and fully applicable, Al's integration of traditional flexibility techniques with his own unique spin makes this a must have. The explanation of how each stretch will benefit your calisthenics practice is brilliant. Not only stunning in its color and design, this book also gives you the true feeling of New York City, both gritty and euphoric, much like Al's personality."

—MIKE FITCH, creator of Global Bodyweight Training

"Stretching Your Boundaries is a terrific resource that will unlock your joints so you can build more muscle, strength and athleticism. Al's passion for human performance radiates in this beautifully constructed book. Whether you're stiff as a board, or an elite gymnast, this book outlines the progressions to take your body and performance to a new level."

—CHAD WATERBURY, M.S., author of *Huge in a Hurry*

"Al Kavadlo has done it again! He's created yet another incredible resource that I wish I had twenty years ago. Finding great material on flexibility training that actually enhances your strength is like trying to find a needle in a haystack. But look no further, because **Stretching Your Boundaries** is exactly what you need."

—JASON FERRUGGIA, Strength Coach

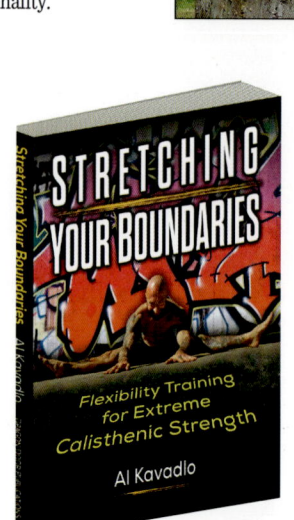

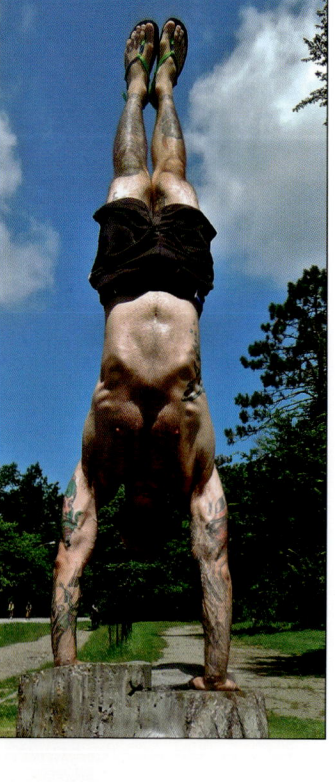

Stretching Your Boundaries
Flexibility Training for Extreme Calisthenic Strength
By Al Kavadlo

Book #B73 $39.95
eBook # EB73 $19.95
Paperback 8.5 x 11
214 pages • 235 photos

Order *Stretching Your Boundaries* online:
www.dragondoor.com/b73

1•800•899•5111
www.dragondoor.com

24 HOURS A DAY
ORDER NOW

How Do YOU Stack Up Against These 6 Signs of a TRUE Physical Specimen?

According to Paul Wade's Convict Conditioning you earn the right to call yourself a 'true physical specimen' if you can perform the following:

1. **AT LEAST** one set of 5 one-arm pushups each side—with the ELITE goal of 100 sets each side
2. **AT LEAST** one set of 5 one-leg squats each side—with the ELITE goal of 2 sets of 50 each side
3. **AT LEAST** a single one-arm pullup each side—with the ELITE goal of 2 sets of 6 each side
4. **AT LEAST** one set of 5 hanging straight leg raises—with the ELITE goal of 2 sets of 30
5. **AT LEAST** one stand-to-stand bridge—with the ELITE goal of 2 sets of 30

Well, how DO you stack up?

Chances are that whatever athletic level you have achieved, there are some serious gaps in your OVERALL strength program. Gaps that stop you short of being able to claim status as a truly accomplished strength athlete.

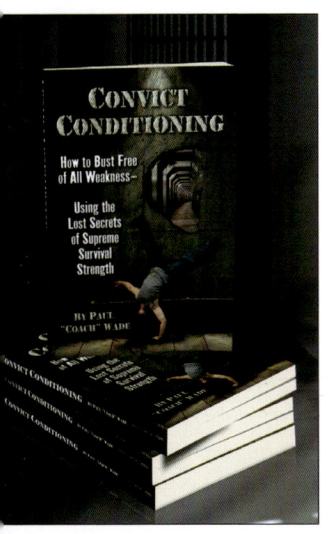

The good news is that—in *Convict Conditioning*—Paul Wade has laid out a brilliant 6-set system of 10 progressions which allows you to master these elite levels.

And you could be starting at almost any age and in almost in any condition...

Paul Wade has given you the keys—ALL the keys you'll ever need—that will open door, after door, after door for you in your quest for supreme physical excellence. Yes, it will be the hardest work you'll ever have to do. And yes, 97% of those who pick up *Convict Conditioning*, frankly, won't have the guts and the fortitude to make it. But if you make it even half-way through Paul's Progressions, you'll be stronger than almost anyone you encounter. Ever.

Here's just a small taste of what you'll get with Convict Conditioning:

Can you meet these 5 benchmarks of the *truly* powerful?... Page 1

The nature and the art of real strength... Page 2

Why mastery of *progressive calisthenics* is the ultimate secret for building maximum raw strength... Page 2

A dozen one-arm handstand pushups without support—anyone? Anyone?... Page 3

How to rank in a powerlifting championship—*without ever training with weights*... Page 4

Calisthenics as a hardcore strength training technology... Page 9

Spartan "300" calisthenics at the Battle of Thermopylae... Page 10

How to cultivate the perfect body—the Greek and Roman way... Page 10

The difference between "old school" and "new school" calisthenics... Page 15

The role of prisons in preserving the older systems... Page 16

Strength training as a primary survival strategy... Page 16

The 6 basic benefits of bodyweight training... Pages 22—27

Why calisthenics are the *ultimate* in functional training... Page 23

The value of cultivating *self-movement*—rather than *object-movement*... Page 23

The *real* source of strength—it's not your *muscles*... Page 24

One crucial reason why a lot of convicts deliberately avoid weight-training... Page 24

How to progressively strengthen your joints over a lifetime—and even heal old joint injuries... Page 25

Why "authentic" exercises like pullups are so perfect for strength and power development... Page 25

Bodyweight training for quick physique perfection... Page 26

How to normalize and regulate your body fat levels—with bodyweight training only... Page 27

Why weight-training and the psychology of overeating go hand in hand... Page 27

The best approach for rapidly strengthening your whole body is this... Page 30

This is the most important and revolutionary feature of *Convict Conditioning*.... Page 33

A jealously-guarded system for going from puny to powerful—when your life may depend on the speed of your results... Page 33

The 6 "Ultimate" Master Steps—only a handful of athletes in the whole world can correctly perform them all. Can you?... Page 33

How to Forge Armor-Plated Pecs and Steel Triceps... Page 41

Why the pushup is the *ultimate* upper body exercise—and better than the bench press... Page 41

How to effectively bulletproof the vulnerable rotator cuff muscles... Page 42

---

24 HOURS A DAY ORDER NOW **1•800•899•5111** www.dragondoor.com

Order *Convict Conditioning* online:
www.dragondoor.com/b41

Observe these 6 important rules for power-packed pushups... Page 42

How basketballs, baseballs and *kissing-the-baby* all translate into greater strength gains... Page 44

How to guarantee steel rod fingers... Page 45

Do you make this stupid mistake with your push ups? This is wrong, wrong, wrong!... Page 45

How to achieve 100 consecutive one-arm pushups each side... Page 64

Going Beyond the One-Arm Pushup... Pages 68–74

Going up!—how to build elevator-cable thighs... Page 75

Where the *real* strength of an athlete lies... Page 75

Most athletic movements rely largely on this attribute... Page 76

The first thing to go as an athlete begins to age—and what you MUST protect... Page 76

THE best way to develop truly powerful, athletic legs... Page 77

The phenomenon of *Lombard's Paradox*—and it contributes to power-packed thighs... Page 78

Why bodyweight squats blow barbell squats away... Page 79

The enormous benefits of mastering the one-leg squat... Page 80

15 secrets to impeccable squatting—for greater power and strength... Pages 81–82

Transform skinny legs into pillars of power, complete with steel cord quads, rock-hard glutes and thick, shapely calves... Page 102

How to achieve one hundred perfect consecutive one-leg squats on each leg... Page 102

Going Beyond the One-Leg Squat... Pages 106–112

How to add conditioning, speed, agility and endurance to legs that are already awesome.... Page 107

How to construct a barn door back—and walk with loaded guns... Page 113

Why our culture has failed to give the pullup the respect and attention it deserves... Page 113

Benefits of the pullup—king of back exercises... Page 114

The dormant superpower for muscle growth waiting to be released if you only do this... Page 114

Why pullups are the single best exercise for building melon-sized biceps... Page 115

Why the pullup is THE safest upper back exercise... Page 115

The single most important factor to consider for your grip choice... Page 118

How to earn lats that look like wings and an upper back sprouting muscles like coiled pythons... Page 138

How to be strong enough to rip a bodybuilder's arm off in an arm wrestling match... Page 138

How to take a trip to hell—and steal a Satanic six-pack... Page 149

The 5 absolute truths that define a genuine six-pack from hell... Page 150

This is the REAL way to gain a six-pack from hell... Page 152

3 big reasons why—in prisons—leg raises have always been much more popular than sit-ups... Page 152

Why the hanging leg raise is the greatest single abdominal exercise known to man... Page 153

10 waist training secrets to help you master the hanging leg raise... Pages 154–155

How to correctly perform the greatest all-round midsection exercise in existence... Page 174

Going beyond the hanging straight leg raise... Page 178

Setting your sights on the most powerful midsection exercise possible—the V raise... Page 178

How to develop abdominal muscles with enormous contractile power—and iron hip strength... Page 178

How to combat-proof your spine... Page 185

Why the bridge is the most important strength-building exercise in the world... Page 185

How to train your spine—as if your life depended on it... Page 185

Why you should sell your barbell set and buy a cushioned mat instead... Page 188

How to absorb punitive strikes against your spine—and bounce back smiling... Page 188

Why lower back pain is the foremost plague of athletes the world over... Page 189

Why bridging is the *ultimate* exercise for the spinal muscles... Page 189

The 4 signs of the perfect bridge... Page 191

How to master the bridge... Page 192

How to own a spine that feels like a steel whip... Page 193

How the bridging series will grant you an incredible combination of strength paired with flexibility... Page 216

Why bridging stands alone as a *total* training method that facilitates development in practically every area of fitness and health... Page 216

How to look exceptionally masculine—with broad, etched, and powerful shoulders... Page 219

Those vulnerable shoulders—why they ache and the best way to avoid or fix the pain... Page 220

How to choose authentic over *artificial* shoulder movements... Page 223

Why an understanding of *instinctive* human movement can help solve the shoulder pain problem... Page 224

Remove these two elements of pressing—and you will remove virtually all chronic shoulder problems... Page 225

The ultimate solution for safe, pain-free, powerful shoulders... Page 225

The mighty handstand pushup... Page 226

Using the handstand pushup to build *incredibly* powerful, muscularized shoulders in a short span of time... Page 225

How to strengthen the *vestibular system*—using handstand pushups... Page 225

8 secrets to help you perfect your all-important handstand pushup technique... Pages 228–229

Discover the ultimate shoulder and arm exercise... Page 248

Going beyond the one-arm handstand pushup... Page 252

The master of this old technique will have elbows strong as titanium axles... Page 255

The cast iron principles of Convict Conditioning success... Page 259

The missing "x factor" of training success... Page 259

The best ways to warm up... Page 260

How to create training momentum... Page 262

How to put strength in the bank... Page 263

This is the real way to get genuine, lasting strength and power gains... Page 265

Intensity—what it is and what it isn't... Page 265

Why "cycling" or "periodization" is unnecessary with bodyweight training... Page 266

How to make consistent progress... Page 266

5 powerful secrets for busting through your plateaus... Page 267

The nifty little secret of *consolidation* training... Page 268

Living by the buzzer—and the importance of regime... Page 275

5 major *Convict Conditioning* training programs... Page 276

The *New Blood* training program... Page 278

The *Good Behavior* training program... Page 279

The *Veterano* training program... Page 280

The *Solitary Confinement* training program... Page 281

The *Supermax* training program... Page 282

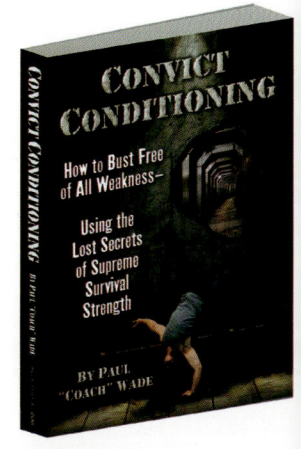

Convict Conditioning

How to Bust Free of All Weakness—Using the Lost Secrets of Supreme Survival Strength

By Paul "Coach" Wade

Book #B41 **$39.95**
eBook #EB41 **$19.95**
Paperback 8.5 x 11
320 pages • 191 photos

Order *Convict Conditioning* online: www.dragondoor.com/b41

1•800•899•5111
www.dragondoor.com

24 HOURS A DAY ORDER NOW

Dragon Door Customer Acclaim for Paul Wade's Convict Conditioning

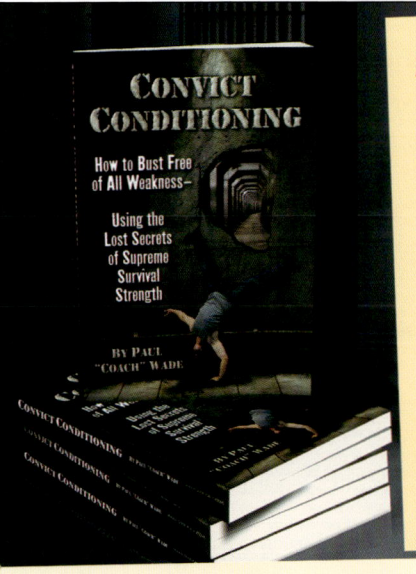

A Strength Training Guide That Will Never Be Duplicated!

"I knew within the first chapter of reading this book that I was in for something special and unique. The last time I felt this same feeling was when reading ***Power to the People!*** To me this is the Body Weight equivalent to Pavel's masterpiece.

Books like this can never be duplicated. Paul Wade went through a unique set of circumstances of doing time in prison with an 'old time' master of calisthenics. Paul took these lessons from this 70 year old strong man and mastered them over a period of 20 years while 'doing time'. He then taught these methods to countless prisoners and honed his teaching to perfection.

I believe that extreme circumstances like this are what it takes to create a true masterpiece. I know that 'masterpiece' is a strong word, but this is as close as it gets. No other body weight book I have read (and I have a huge fitness library)...comes close to this as far as gaining incredible strength from body weight exercise.

Just like Power to the People, I am sure I will read this over and over again...mastering the principles that Paul Wade took 20 years to master.

Outstanding Book!" —*Rusty Moore - Fitness Black Book - Seattle, WA*

A must for all martial artists

"As a dedicated martial artist for more than seven years, this book is exactly what I've been looking for.

For a while now I have trained with machines at my local gym to improve my muscle strength and power and get to the next level in my training. I always felt that the modern health club, technology based exercise jarred with my martial art though, which only required body movement.

Finally this book has come along. At last I can combine perfect body movement for martial skill with perfect body exercise for ultimate strength.

All fighting arts are based on body movement. This book is a complete textbook on how to max out your musclepower using only body movement, as different from dumbbells, machines or gadgets. For this reason it belongs on the bookshelf of every serious martial artist, male and female, young and old." —*Gino Cartier - Washington DC*

I've packed all of my other training books away!

"I read CC in one go. I couldn't put it down. I have purchased a lot of bodyweight training books in the past, and have always been pretty disappointed. They all seem to just have pictures of different exercises, and no plan whatsoever on how to implement them and progress with them. But not with this one. The information in this book is AWESOME! I like to have a clear, logical plan of progression to follow, and that is what this book gives. I have put all of my other training books away. CC is the only system I am going to follow. This is now my favorite training book ever!" —*Lyndan - Australia*

Brutal Elegance.

"I have been training and reading about training since I first joined the US Navy in the 1960s. I thought I'd seen everything the fitness world had to offer. Sometimes twice. But I was wrong. This book is utterly iconoclastic.

The author breaks down all conceivable body weight exercises into six basic movements, each designed to stimulate different vectors of the muscular system. These six are then elegantly and very intelligently broken into ten progressive techniques. You master one technique, and move on to the next.

The simplicity of this method belies a very powerful and complex training paradigm, reduced into an abstraction that obviously took many years of sweat and toil to develop. Trust me. Nobody else worked this out. This approach is completely unique and fresh.

I have read virtually every calisthenics book printed in America over the last 40 years, and instruction like this can't be found anywhere, in any one of them. ***Convict Conditioning*** is head and shoulders above them all. In years to come, trainers and coaches will all be talking about 'progressions' and 'progressive calisthenics' and claim they've been doing it all along. But the truth is that Dragon Door bought it to you first. As with kettlebells, they were the trail blazers.

Who should purchase this volume? Everyone who craves fitness and strength should. Even if you don't plan to follow the routines, the book will make you think about your physical prowess, and will give even world class experts food for thought. At the very least if you find yourself on vacation or away on business without your barbells, this book will turn your hotel into a fully equipped gym.

I'd advise any athlete to obtain this work as soon as possible."
—*Bill Oliver - Albany, NY, United States*

---

24 HOURS A DAY ORDER NOW | **1·800·899·5111** | **www.dragondoor.com**

Order *Convict Conditioning* online: **www.dragondoor.com/b41**

More Dragon Door Customer Acclaim for Convict Conditioning

Fascinating Reading and Real Strength

"Coach Wade's system is a real eye opener if you've been a lifetime iron junkie. Wanna find out how really strong (or weak) you are? Get this book and begin working through the 10 levels of the 6 power exercises. I was pleasantly surprised by my ability on a few of the exercises...but some are downright humbling. If I were on a desert island with only one book on strength and conditioning this would be it. (Could I staple Pavel's "Naked Warrior" to the back and count them as one???!) Thanks Dragon Door for this innovative new author."—*Jon Schultheis, RKC (2005) - Keansburg, NJ*

Single best strength training book ever!

"I just turned 50 this year and I have tried a little bit of everything over the years: martial arts, swimming, soccer, cycling, free weights, weight machines, even yoga and Pilates. I started using *Convict Conditioning* right after it came out. I started from the beginning, like Coach Wade says, doing mostly step one or two for five out of the six exercises. I work out 3 to 5 times a week, usually for 30 to 45 minutes.

Long story short, my weight went up 14 pounds (I was not trying to gain weight) but my body fat percentage dropped two percent. That translates into approximately 19 pounds of lean muscle gained in two months! I've never gotten this kind of results with anything else I've ever done. Now I have pretty much stopped lifting weights for strength training. Instead, I lift once a week as a test to see how much stronger I'm getting without weight training. There are a lot of great strength training books in the world (most of them published by Dragon Door), but if I had to choose just one, this is the single best strength training book ever. BUY THIS BOOK. FOLLOW THE PLAN. GET AS STRONG AS YOU WANT."—*Wayne - Decatur, GA*

Best bodyweight training book so far!

"I'm a martial artist and I've been training for years with a combination of weights and bodyweight training and had good results from both (but had the usual injuries from weight training). I prefer the bodyweight stuff though as it trains me to use my whole body as a unit, much more than weights do, and I notice the difference on the mat and in the ring. Since reading this book I have given the weights a break and focused purely on the bodyweight exercise progressions as described by 'Coach' Wade and my strength had increased more than ever before. So far I've built up to 12 strict one-leg squats each leg and 5 uneven pull ups each arm.

I've never achieved this kind of strength before - and this stuff builds solid muscle mass as well. It's very intense training. I am so confident in and happy with the results I'm getting that I've decided to train for a fitness/bodybuilding comp just using his techniques, no weights, just to show for real what kind of a physique these exercises can build. In sum, I cannot recommend 'Coach' Wade's book highly enough - it is by far the best of its kind ever!"—*Mark Robinson - Australia, currently living in South Korea*

A lifetime of lifting...and continued learning.

"I have been working out diligently since 1988 and played sports in high school and college before that. My stint in the Army saw me doing calisthenics, running, conditioning courses, forced marches, etc. There are many levels of strength and fitness. I have been as big as 240 in my powerlifting/strongman days and as low as 185-190 while in the Army. I think I have tried everything under the sun: the high intensity of Arthur Jones and Dr. Ken, the Super Slow of El Darden, and the brutality of Dinosaur Training Brooks Kubic made famous.

This is one of the BEST books I've ever read on real strength training which also covers other just as important aspects of health; like staying injury free, feeling healthy and becoming flexible. It's an excellent book. He tells you the why and the how with his progressive plan. This book is a GOLD MINE and worth 100 times what I paid for it!"
—*Horst - Woburn, MA*

This book sets the standard, ladies and gentlemen

"It's difficult to describe just how much this book means to me. I've been training hard since I was in the RAF nearly ten years ago, and to say this book is a breakthrough is an understatement. How often do you really read something so new, so fresh? This book contains a complete new system of calisthenics drawn from American prison training methods. When I say 'system' I mean it. It's complete (rank beginner to expert), it's comprehensive (all the exercises and photos are here), it's graded (progressions from exercise to exercise are smooth and pre-determined) and it's totally original. Whether you love or hate the author, you have to listen to him. And you will learn something. This book just makes SENSE. In twenty years people will still be buying it."—
Andy McMann - Ponty, Wales, GB

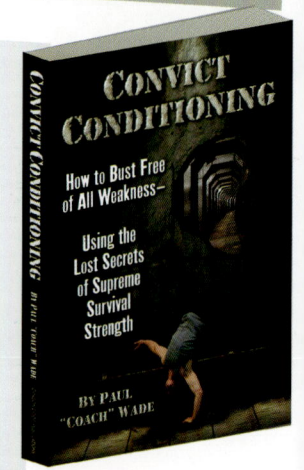

Convict Conditioning
How to Bust Free of All Weakness—Using the Lost Secrets of Supreme Survival Strength
By Paul "Coach" Wade

Book #B41 $39.95
eBook #EB41 $19.95
Paperback 8.5 x 11
320 pages • 191 photos

Order *Convict Conditioning* online:
www.dragondoor.com/b41

1•800•899•5111
www.dragondoor.com

24 HOURS A DAY
ORDER NOW

The Experts Give High Praise to
Convict Conditioning 2

"Coach Paul Wade has outdone himself. His first book *Convict Conditioning* is to my mind THE BEST book ever written on bodyweight conditioning. Hands down. Now, with the sequel *Convict Conditioning 2*, Coach Wade takes us even deeper into the subtle nuances of training with the ultimate resistance tool: our bodies.

In plain English, but with an amazing understanding of anatomy, physiology, kinesiology and, go figure, psychology, Coach Wade explains very simply how to work the smaller but just as important areas of the body such as the hands and forearms, neck and calves and obliques in serious functional ways.

His minimalist approach to exercise belies the complexity of his system and the deep insight into exactly how the body works and the best way to get from A to Z in the shortest time possible.

I got the best advice on how to strengthen the hard-to-reach extensors of the hand right away from this exercise Master I have ever seen. It's so simple but so completely functional I can't believe no one else has thought of it yet. Just glad he figured it out for me.

Paul teaches us how to strengthen our bodies with the simplest of movements while at the same time balancing our structures in the same way: simple exercises that work the whole body.

And just as simply as he did with his first book. His novel approach to stretching and mobility training is brilliant and fresh as well as his take on recovery and healing from injury. Sprinkled throughout the entire book are too-many-to-count insights and advice from a man who has come to his knowledge the hard way and knows exactly of what he speaks.

This book is, as was his first, an amazing journey into the history of physical culture disguised as a book on calisthenics. But the thing that Coach Wade does better than any before him is his unbelievable progressions on EVERY EXERCISE and stretch! He breaks things down and tells us EXACTLY how to proceed to get to whatever level of strength and development we want. AND gives us the exact metrics we need to know when to go to the next level.

Adding in completely practical and immediately useful insights into nutrition and the mindset necessary to deal not only with training but with life, makes this book a classic that will stand the test of time.

Bravo Coach Wade, Bravo." —**Mark Reifkind, Master RKC,** author of *Mastering the HardStyle Kettlebell Swing*

"I've been lifting weights for over 50 years and have trained in the martial arts since 1965. I've read voraciously on both subjects, and written dozens of magazine articles and many books on the subjects. This book and Wade's first, *Convict Conditioning*, are by far the most commonsense, information-packed, and result producing I've read. These books will truly change your life.

Paul Wade is a new and powerful voice in the strength and fitness arena, one that is commonsense, inspiring, and in your face. His approach to maximizing your body's potential is not the same old hackneyed material you find in every book and magazine piece that pictures steroid-bloated models screaming as they curl weights. Wade's stuff has been proven effective by hard men who don't tolerate fluff. It will work for you, too—guaranteed.

As an ex-cop, I've gone mano-y-mano with ex-cons that had clearly trained as Paul Wade suggests in his two *Convict Conditioning* books. While these guys didn't look like steroid-fueled bodybuilders (actually, there were a couple who did), all were incredibly lean, hard and powerful. Wade blows many commonly held beliefs about conditioning, strengthening, and eating out of the water and replaces them with result-producing information that won't cost you a dime." —**Loren W. Christensen**, author of *Fighting the Pain Resistant Attacker,* and many other titles

"The overriding principle of *Convict Conditioning 2* is 'little equipment-big rewards'. For the athlete in the throwing and fighting arts, the section on Lateral Chain Training, Capturing the Flag, is a unique and perhaps singular approach to training the obliques and the whole family of side muscles. This section stood out to me as ground breaking and well worth the time and energy by anyone to review and attempt to complete. Literally, this is a new approach to lateral chain training that is well beyond sidebends and suitcase deadlifts.

The author's review of passive stretching reflects the experience of many of us in the field. But, his solution might be the reason I am going to recommend this work for everyone: The Trifecta. This section covers what the author calls The Functional Triad and gives a series of simple progressions to three holds that promise to oil your joints. It's yoga for the strength athlete and supports the material one would find, for example, in Pavel's *Loaded Stretching*.

I didn't expect to like this book, but I come away from it practically insisting that everyone read it. It is a strongman book mixed with yoga mixed with street smarts. I wanted to hate it, but I love it."
—**Dan John,** author of *Don't Let Go* and co-author of *Easy Strength*

"*Convict Conditioning* is one of the most influential books I ever got my hands on. *Convict Conditioning 2* took my training and outlook on the power of bodyweight training to the 10th degree—from strengthening the smallest muscles in a maximal manner, all the way to using bodyweight training as a means of healing injuries that pile up from over 22 years of aggressive lifting.

I've used both *Convict Conditioning* and *Convict Conditioning 2* on myself and with my athletes. Without either of these books I can easily say that these boys would not be the BEASTS they are today. Without a doubt *Convict Conditioning 2* will blow you away and inspire and educate you to take bodyweight training to a whole NEW level."
—**Zach Even-Esh,** Underground Strength Coach

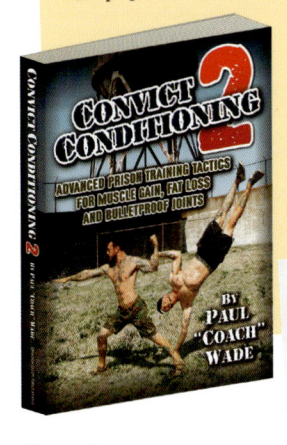

Convict Conditioning 2
Advanced Prison Training Tactics for Muscle Gain, Fat Loss and Bulletproof Joints
By Paul "Coach" Wade

Book #B59 $39.95
eBook #EB59 $19.95
Paperback 8.5 x 11
354 pages • 261 photos

24 HOURS A DAY ORDER NOW **1•800•899•5111** www.dragondoor.com

Order *Convict Conditioning 2* online:
www.dragondoor.com/b59

> "**Paul Wade's** section on developing the sides of the body in **Convict Conditioning 2** is brilliant. Hardstyle!" —**Pavel Tsatsouline**, author of *The Naked Warrior*

Online Praise for Convict Conditioning 2

Best Sequel Since The Godfather 2!
"Hands down the best addition to the material on *Convict Conditioning* that could possibly be put out. I already implemented the neck bridges, calf and hand training to my weekly schedule, and as soon as my handstand pushups and leg raises are fully loaded I'll start the flags. Thank you, Coach!"
— Daniel Runkel, Rio de Janeiro, Brazil

Just as brilliant as its predecessor!
"Just as brilliant as its predecessor! The new exercises add to the Big 6 in a keep-it-simple kind of way. Anyone who will put in the time with both of these masterpieces will be as strong as humanly possible. I especially liked the parts on grip work. To me, that alone was worth the price of the entire book."
—Timothy Stovall / Evansville, Indiana

Convict Conditioning 2
Advanced Prison Training Tactics for Muscle Gain, Fat Loss and Bulletproof Joints
By Paul "Coach" Wade

Book #B59 $39.95
eBook #EB59 $19.95
Paperback 8.5 x 11
354 pages • 261 photos

The progressions were again sublime
"Never have I heard such in depth and yet easy to understand description of training and physical culture. A perfect complement to the first book although it has its own style keeping the best attributes of style from the first but developing it to something unique. The progressions were again sublime and designed for people at all levels of ability. The two books together can forge what will closely resemble superhuman strength and an incredible physique and yet the steps to get there are so simple and easy to understand."
–Ryan O., Nottingham, United Kingdom

If you liked CC1, you'll love CC2
"*CC2* picks up where *CC1* left off with great information about the human flag (including a version called the clutch flag, that I can actually do now), neck and forearms. I couldn't be happier with this book."
—Justin B., Atlanta, Georgia

Well worth the wait
"Another very interesting, and as before, opinionated book by Paul Wade. As I work through the CC1 progressions, I find it's paying off at a steady if unspectacular rate, which suits me just fine. No training injuries worth the name, convincing gains in strength. I expect the same with *CC2* which rounds off CC1 with just the kind of material I was looking for. Wade and Dragon Door deserve to be highly commended for publishing these techniques. A tremendous way to train outside of the gym ecosystem."
–V. R., Bangalore, India

From the almost laughably-simple to realm-of-the-gods
"*Convict Conditioning 2* is a great companion piece to the original Convict Conditioning. It helps to further build up the athlete and does deliver on phenomenal improvement with minimal equipment and space.

The grip work is probably the superstar of the book. Second, maybe, is the attention devoted to the lateral muscles with the development of the clutch- and press-flag.

Convict Conditioning 2 is more of the same - more of the systematic and methodical improvement in exercises that travel smoothly from the almost laughably-simple to realm-of-the-gods. It is a solid addition to any fitness library."
–Robert Aldrich, Chapel Hill, GA

Very Informative
"*Convict Conditioning 2* is more subversive training information in the same style as its original. It's such a great complement to the original, but also solid enough on its own. The information in this book is fantastic-- a great buy! Follow this program, and you will get stronger."
–Chris B., Thunder Bay, Canada

Brilliant
"Convict Conditioning books are all the books you need in life. As Bruce Lee used to say, it's not a daily increase but a daily decrease. Same with life. Too many things can lead you down many paths, but to have Simplicity is perfect."
–Brandon Lynch, London, England

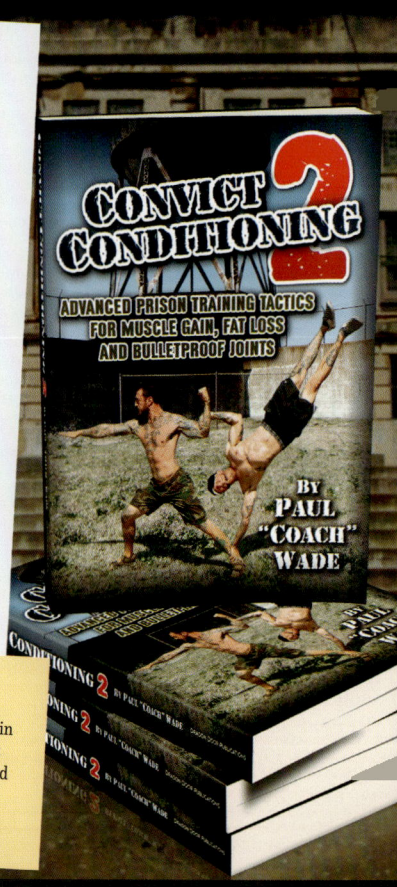

Order *Convict Conditioning 2* online:
www.dragondoor.com/b59

1•800•899•5111
www.dragondoor.com

24 HOURS A DAY
ORDER NOW

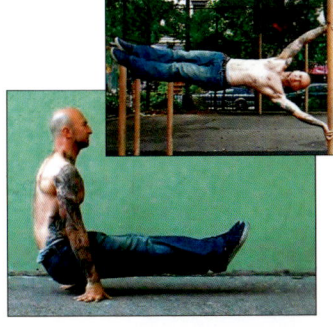

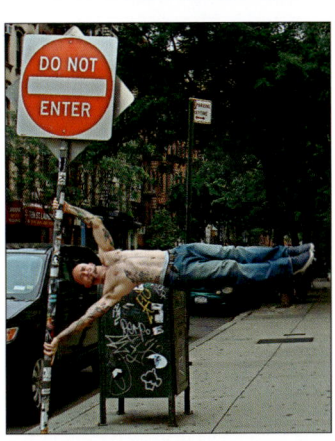

TABLE OF CONTENTS

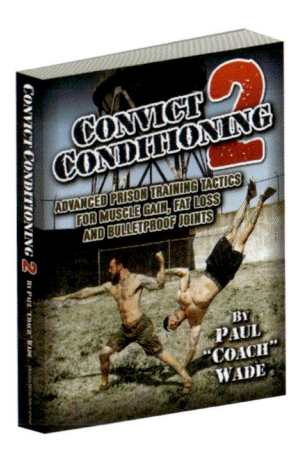

Convict Conditioning 2
Advanced Prison Training Tactics for Muscle Gain, Fat Loss and Bulletproof Joints
By Paul "Coach" Wade

Book #B59 $39.95
eBook #EB59 $19.95
Paperback 8.5 x 11
354 pages • 261 photos

Foreword
The Many Roads to Strength by Brooks Kubik

Opening Salvo: *Chewing Bubblegum and Kicking Ass*

1. Introduction: *Put Yourself Behind Bars*

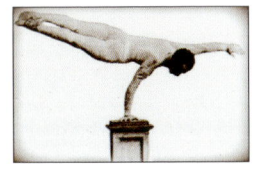

PART I: SHOTGUN MUSCLE

Hands and Forearms

2: Iron Hands and Forearms: *Ultimate Strength —with Just Two Techniques*

3: The Hang Progressions: *A Vice-Like Bodyweight Grip Course*

4: Advanced Grip Torture: *Explosive Power + Titanium Fingers*

5: Fingertip Pushups: *Keeping Hand Strength Balanced*

6: Forearms into Firearms: *Hand Strength: A Summary and a Challenge*

Lateral Chain

7: Lateral Chain Training: *Capturing the Flag*

8: The Clutch Flag: *In Eight Easy Steps*

9: The Press Flag: *In Eight Not-So-Easy Steps*

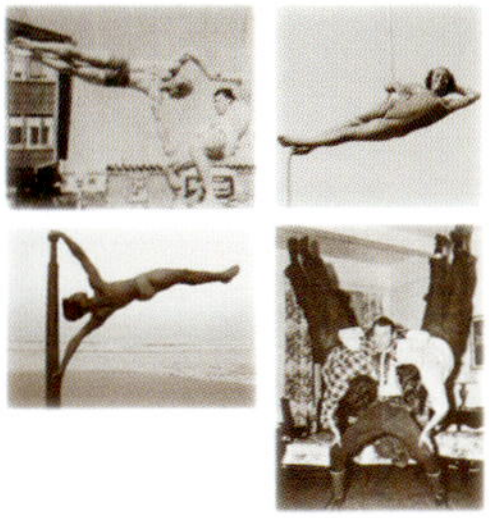

Neck and Calves

10. Bulldog Neck: *Bulletproof Your Weakest Link*

11. Calf Training: *Ultimate Lower Legs—No Machines Necessary*

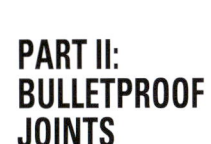

PART II: BULLETPROOF JOINTS

12. Tension-Flexibility: *The Lost Art of Joint Training*

13. Stretching—the Prison Take: *Flexibility, Mobility, Control*

14. The Trifecta: *Your "Secret Weapon" for Mobilizing Stiff, Battle-Scarred Physiques—for Life*

15. The Bridge Hold Progressions: *The Ultimate Prehab/Rehab Technique*

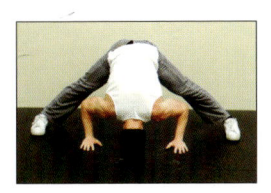

16. The L-Hold Progressions: *Cure Bad Hips and Low Back—Inside-Out*

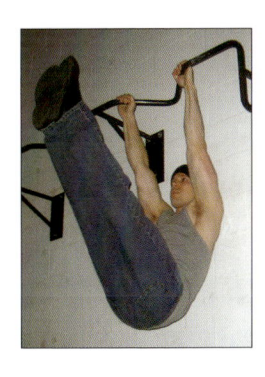

17: Twist Progressions: *Unleash Your Functional Triad*

PART III: WISDOM FROM CELLBLOCK G

18. Doing Time Right: *Living the Straight Edge*

19. The Prison Diet: *Nutrition and Fat Loss Behind Bars*

20. Mendin' Up: *The 8 Laws of Healing*

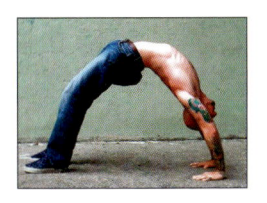

21. The Mind: *Escaping the True Prison*

!BONUS CHAPTER!

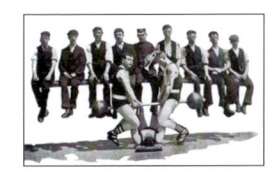

---

24 HOURS A DAY ORDER NOW
1•800•899•5111
www.dragondoor.com

Order *Convict Conditioning 2* online:
www.dragondoor.com/b59

Are You Dissatisfied With Your Abs?

"Diamond-Cut Abs condenses decades of agonizing lessons and insight into the best book on ab-training ever written. Hands down." —**PAUL WADE**, author of **Convict Conditioning**

Are you dissatisfied with your abs? Does it seem a distant dream for you to own a rock-solid center? Can you only hanker in vain for the chiseled magnificence of a Greek statue? Have you given up on owning the tensile functionality and explosive power of a cage-fighter's core?

According to Danny Kavadlo, training your abs is a whole-life endeavor. It's about right eating, right drinking, right rest, right practice, right exercise at the right time, right motivation, right inspiration, right attitude and right lifestyle. If you don't have that righteous set of abs in place, it's because you have failed in one or more of these areas.

With his 25-plus years of rugged research and extreme physical dedication into every dimension of what it takes to earn world-class abs, Danny Kavadlo is a modern-day master of the art. It's all here: over 50 of the best-ever exercises to develop the abs—from beginner to superman level—inspirational photos, no BS straight talk on nutrition and lifestyle factors and clear-cut instructions on what to do, when. Supply the grit, follow the program and you simply cannot fail but to build a monstrous mid-section.

In our culture, Abs are the Measure of a Man. To quit on your abs is to quit on your masculinity—like it or not. *Diamond-Cut Abs* gives you the complete, whole-life program you need to reassert yourself and reestablish your respect as a true physical specimen—with a thunderous six-pack to prove it.

Are You Dissatisfied With Your Abs?

In the Abs Gospel According to Danny, training your abs is a whole-life endeavor. It's about right eating, right drinking, right rest, right practice, right exercise at the right time, right motivation, right inspiration, right attitude and right lifestyle.

So, yes, all of this Rightness gets covered in *Diamond-Cut Abs*. But let's not confuse Right with Rigid. Apprentice in the Danny School of Abs and it's like apprenticing with a world-class Chef—a mix of incredible discipline, inspired creativity and a passionate love-affair with your art.

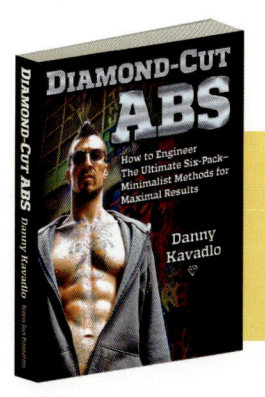

Diamond-Cut Abs
How to Engineer the Ultimate Six-Pack—Minimalist Methods for Maximum Results
By Danny Kavadlo

Book #B77 **$39.95**
eBook #EB77 **$19.95**
Paperback 8.5 x 11
230 pages, 305 photos

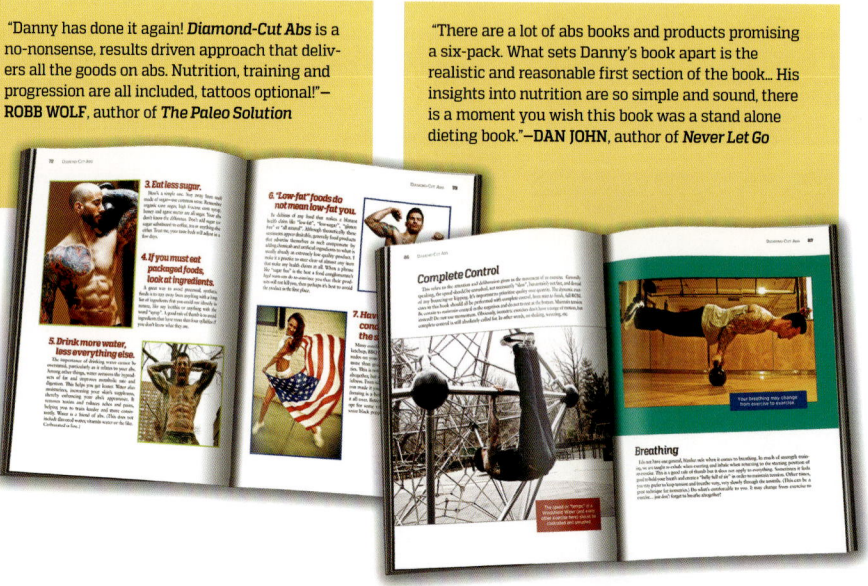

"Danny has done it again! Diamond-Cut Abs is a no-nonsense, results driven approach that delivers all the goods on abs. Nutrition, training and progression are all included, tattoos optional!" —**ROBB WOLF**, author of *The Paleo Solution*

"There are a lot of abs books and products promising a six-pack. What sets Danny's book apart is the realistic and reasonable first section of the book... His insights into nutrition are so simple and sound, there is a moment you wish this book was a stand alone dieting book." —**DAN JOHN**, author of *Never Let Go*

Order *Diamond-Cut Abs* online:
www.dragondoor.com/b77

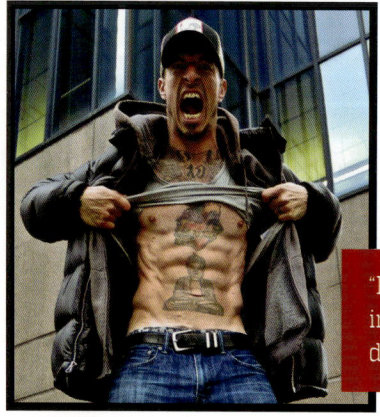

1•800•899•5111
www.dragondoor.com

24 HOURS A DAY
ORDER NOW

⬇ Here's a Taste of What You'll Get When You Invest in *Diamond-Cut Abs* ⬇

Part I An Abs Odyssey
Chapter 1 Cultural Obsession
- Why there is no one-size-fits-all program for training your abs...3
- Danny's big promise: why you will get everything you need to know about sculpting and maintaining amazingly defined and beautiful abs...4

Chapter 2 Abs Defined
- You cannot fake the funk—getting clear about what it'll take to Man up and earn that six-pack of your dreams...11
- The What of the What: basic anatomy and function: know your abs-tech details so you know what you are working on...12—15
- What the core really consists of...it's more than most people think...15

Chapter 3 Personal Obsession
- The extreme value of push-ups and pull-ups for Danny-like abs...18
- Danny Obsessed: 300 reps, 5 days a week for 10 years = close on 8 million reps!—yet Danny's functionally stronger and aesthetically more appealing NOW with WAY less reps. Discover why...19
- Danny's personal mission for you: distinguish the fitness BS from the hype...21
- Why protein supplements are a waste of money...21

Part II Nutritional Musings
Chapter 4 Primordial Soup
- How to bring back the joy to your fitness-nutrition program...28
- Why you need to develop and maintain a love affair with food—if you want that manly six-pack...

Chapter 5 Common Sense Versus Over-compartmentalization
- Why what we eat is single most important decision we can make about our abs...31
- Why Danny's Dietary Advice has proved 100% effective for those who have followed it...33
- The 3 golden keys you must consider when choosing the right foods to feed your abs...35
- Why you should eat THESE fats every day for great abs...36
- Why sugar is the #1 nutritional enemy of defined abs...37
- Why Danny's abs were at an all-time best after 90 days without THESE two nutrients...39
- Why you should eat organ meat, for an extra edge in your abs training...42
- Why you need FAR less protein in your diet...44

Chapter 6 Weighing in on Weight Loss
- The 3 major keys to successful fat reduction...48
- How to shed body fat now...48
- Why a food's fat content has no bearing on whether it will fatten you...49
- Why you should ignore the BMI...50
- The role of sacrifice in obtaining ripped abs...50

Chapter 7 What I Eat
- The secret of "mostly"...54
- For the love and care of food...54
- Danny's 3-Day sample food log...56—57

Chapter 8 The Fat and the Curious
- The 4 Steps of the Beginner's Cleanse...60
- Fruit n Veggie Cleanse—optimal duration of...61
- Juice Fast...62
- The 7-Day Plan—Fruit n Veggie/Juice fast...62
- Danny's 4 favorite juices...63
- The True Fast...63
- The Absolute Fast...64
- 4 big tips for safe and successful fasting...64

Chapter 9 More Food for Thought
- The perils of genetically and chemically compromised foods...67—69
- How to avoid toxins in your food...69
- Food's most powerful secret ingredient...69

Chapter 10 Top Tips for Tip Top Abs
- Why water is SO important for your abs...72

Part III Training Your Abs
Chapter 11 Make an Executive Decision
- Why and how your abs training should be like a martial art...79

Chapter 12 Fundamentals of Abdominal Strength Training
- The 10 Principles you must follow for every rep of every exercise...83—89
- THIS principle makes you stronger, more shredded and more anatomically aware...83
- THE #1 Principle you'll need to employ for spectacular abs...91

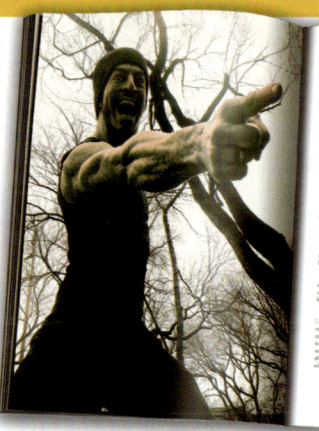

Chapter 13 On Cardio
- The limitations of cardio for abs training—and what you should do instead...93—97

Part IV The Exercises
- Each drill comes with explanatory text, recommended set/rep range plus a specialized Trainer Tip

Chapter 14 Danny, What Do You Do?
- Danny's 50+ best abs and abs-related training exercises...101

Chapter 15 Core Curriculum
- Crucial exercises for overall gains...105
- How to perform the perfect squat—the most functional exercise on the planet...105
- How to perform the perfect push-up—the ultimate upper-body exercise...108
- How to perform the perfect pull-up...111—112

Chapter 16 Beginner Abs
- Full Body Tension Drill...116
- How to have complete body awareness through progressive, isometric tensing...116
- The Plank...117
- The Side Plank—to emphasize the obliques and lateral chain...119
- Lying Bent Knee leg Raise...120
- Lying Knee Tuck...121
- Sit-Up...122
- Modified Side Jackknife—to help beginners target their obliques...123
- Crossover...124
- Bicycle...125
- Straight Arm/Straight Leg Crossover...126
- V-Leg Toe Touch...127
- Why No Crunches?—And the #1 reason not to bother with them...127

Chapter 17 Intermediate Abs
- Unstable Plank—a fun way to add an extra challenge to he traditional isometric standard...130
- Seated Knee Raise—the missing link between floor-based and bar-based abs training...131

"As soon as I received *Diamond-Cut Abs*, I flipped to the table of contents. Amazingly I found what I have been fruitlessly looking for in ab books for decades: 66 pages dedicated to NUTRITION. Kavadlo passed his second Marty audition by not echoing all the bankrupt politically-correct, lock-step, mainstream nutritional commandments. When Dan starts riffing about eating like a horse, eating ample amounts of red meat, shellfish and the divine pig meat (along with all kinds any types of nutrient-dense food), I knew I had to give my first ever ab book endorsement. When he noted that he drank whiskey while getting his abs into his all time best shape, it sealed the deal for me. Oh, and the ab exercises are excellent."
—**MARTY GALLAGHER**, 3-Time Powerlifting Champion, Author of *The Purposeful Primitive*

---

24 HOURS A DAY ORDER NOW

1•800•899•5111
www.dragondoor.com

Order *Diamond-Cut Abs* online:
www.dragondoor.com/b77

"Danny's new book definitely hits the mark. *Diamond-Cut Abs* outlines pretty much everything you'd ever need to know about building the best midsection your genetic potential allows for and without the need for any equipment. Keep up the great work, Danny!"—BJ GADDOUR, CSCS, author of *Men's Health Your Body is Your Barbell*, CEO of **StreamFIT.com**

"Danny flexes his expert advice in a way that's solid, applicable and often entertaining. If you want the abs of your dreams, stop looking for the quick solution everyone claims to have and get ready to learn how to maximize your efforts towards your very own set of *Diamond-Cut Abs*."—MIKE FITCH, creator of **Global Bodyweight Training**

- The N-Sit—an iso that helps set you up for the L-Sit...132
- Jackknife—a fighter's favorite and a most excellent motha for firing up those deeper abs muscles, building better full body co-ordination—and progressing to the Dragon Flag and Hanging Straight Leg Raise...133
- Side Jackknife—masochists will welcome intensifying their abdominal agony when they flip the great classic on its side...134
- Advanced Sit-Up—Bad Boy Danny's tweaks will up the ante here in a pleasantly nasty way (curses optional)...135
- Lying Straight Leg Raise—and how to make it even harder...136
- Grounded Wiper...137
- Danny adores the classic Windshield Wiper—but it's a helluva challenge. The GW helps you rehearse the movement pattern before taking on the full-on manliness of the WW...137
- Throwdown...138
- Here's another old school classic that should be part of any serious practitioner's arsenal. The explosivity will have your whole body screaming in indignation—fortunately...138
- Side Plank Hip Raise—notorious for being deceptively challenging, includes leverage tips to progress the hardness...139
- How to Hang...140
- How to grip the bar to really squeeze the most out of every rep...140
- Why you should avoid Assistance Straps—and the better alternatives...140
- How to employ a flex hang to add a unique neurological twist and increase upper body muscle activation—Highly Recommended by da Abs Bossman!...140
- Hanging Contest...141
- A fun competitive spin on hanging—but here's some important tips on how to keep it real...141
- One Arm Hang...142
- Did someone shout Man Maker? The OAH is a total body drill that will make the boys cry and the men grin with pain—plus bonus tips for optimal vengeance on that brutalized six-pack...142
- Ab Wheel Roll Out (Bent Knee)...143
- An old time classic—incorporates stability, strength and focus in a truly unique way...143
- Hanging Bicycle—last step before conquering the Hanging Knee Raise, plus common mistakes and how to fix them...144
- Hanging Knee Raise—one of the most important of all abdominal exercises. Master it here...145

Chapter 18 Advanced Abs

- SERIOUS training now! These moves are all full-on, full-body. Emphasis is on every cell in your bod. No mercy. Tremendous demand on the abs—requires heavy-duty injection of Will, complete harmony of mind and muscle, steely strength. Think you are a Man? Measure your Manliness here and report back...
- The L-Sit—you will feel it everywhere. How to do it and how to extract the ultimate mechanical advantage...147–148
- Gecko Hold—a "limited contact" plank that poses a unique strength challenge. A ripped six-pack is meaningless without the strength to back it up—get that strength with the GH...149
- Ab Wheel Roll Out (Straight Leg)—incredibly challenging for all levels, full body tension is key, regressions included for ramping up to complete studliness...150
- Hanging Leg Raise—one of Danny's favorites, for good reason, 6 controlled reps and you're doin' good...151
- Washing Machine—this infamous move is a key step to mastering the mighty Windshield Wiper, regressions and progressions to full MANitude provided...152
- Windshield Wiper—brace yourself buddy, the going just got a whole lot harder. Builds and requires tremendous upper body strength...153
- V-Leg Wiper—ho! This is a true brutalizer of the core plus a helluva glute-banger, to boot...154
- Perfect Circle—an exaggerated WW for the MEN who can hack it...155
- Skinning the Cat—a precursor to many extreme bar calisthenics moves and a phenomenal abs exercise in its own right, with some optional grip strategies...156
- One Arm Flex Hang—this just about breaks the mercury on the Achievometer, hyper-challenging, requires an incredibly strong upper body...157
- Dragon Flag—one of the all-time sexiest moves on the planet and a Bruce Lee trademark, you gotta get this one down if you want to truly strut your Man Stuff. Bad Boy Danny likes to hold it for an iso. Can you?...158
- Tuck Front Lever—this regressed version of the Front Lever still requires a brutal level of upper body power. Have at it!...159
- V-Leg Front Lever—another extremely difficult move, with some favorable leverage variations to help progress it...160
- Front Lever—this one tops the Manometer for sure. A masterful and utterly unforgiving move that will simultaneously torture your abs, lats, glutes, arms, shoulders and everything in between. No mercy here and hopefully, none asked for...161

Chapter 19 Supplemental Stretches

- Why stretching IS important—and the 9 surefire benefits you'll gain from right stretching...173
- The Hands Up—the 4 main benefits to this, Danny's first stretch before a workout...174
- Forward, back and Side-to-Side Bend...175
- Hands Down—another fantastic stretch for the entire front of the body...176

Chapter 20 Workouts

- 9 sample combinations for different levels—a beginning guideline...181–185
- On the importance of mixing it up and shocking the system...181

Part V Abs and Lifestyle
Chapter 21 Viva La Vida

- Abs and the quality of your life...190
- A life-oriented approach to training...191

Chapter 22 The Mud and the Blood and the Beer

- Coffee, alcohol and other beverages—how to handle in regard to your training...193–195

Chapter 23 Seasons

- How to adopt and adapt your training to the changing seasons...198

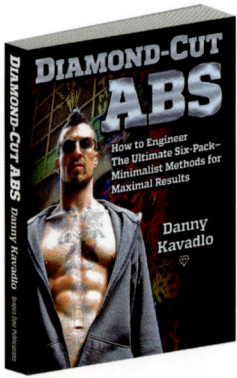

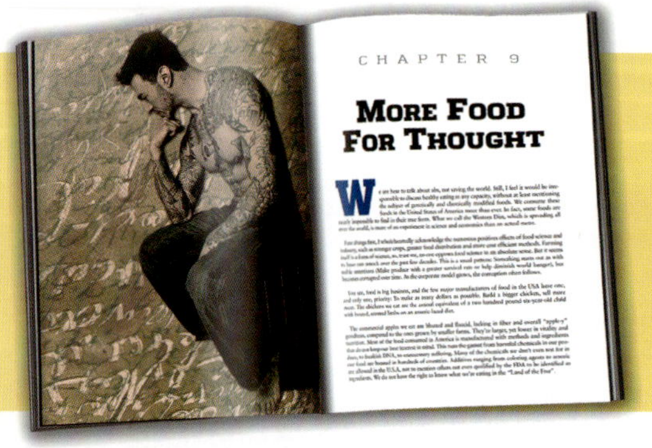

Diamond-Cut Abs
How to Engineer the Ultimate Six-Pack— Minimalist Methods for Maximum Results
By Danny Kavadlo

Book #B77 **$39.95**
eBook #EB77 **$19.95**
Paperback 8.5 x 11
230 pages, 305 photos

"Danny Kavadlo's book might be titled '*Diamond-Cut Abs*' but the truth is that it goes way BEYOND just ab training. Danny has actually created a guide to Physical Culture & LIVING healthy. The traditional fitness industry has gone astray from what the body truly needs. Since 1989, I've read a ton of abs-related books—and they don't scratch the surface of what's inside Danny's masterpiece. From powerful nutrition methods to training the entire body with a holistic approach, Diamond-Cut Abs is a vital addition to anyone's library. I LOVE it!"—ZACH EVEN-ESH, author of *The Encyclopedia of Underground Strength and Conditioning*

Order *Diamond-Cut Abs* online:
www.dragondoor.com/b77

1•800•899•5111
www.dragondoor.com

24 HOURS A DAY
ORDER NOW

Reader Praise for *Convict Conditioning Ultimate Bodyweight Training Log*

Above and Beyond!

"Not JUST a log book. TONS of great and actually useful info. I really like to over complicate programming and data entries at times. And honestly, All one has to do is fill in the blanks... Well that and DO THE WORK. Great product."
—NOEL PRICE, Chicagoland, IL

A unique training log

"This log book is one of a kind in the world. It is the only published body weight exclusive training log I have personally seen. It is well structured and provides everything for a log book in a primarily body weight oriented routine. The book is best integrated with the other books in the convict conditioning series however has enough information to act as a stand alone unit. It is a must have for anyone who is a fan of the convict conditioning series or is entering into calisthenics."
—CARTER D., Cambridge, Canada

Excellent Companion to *Convict Conditioning 1 & 2*

"This is an amazing book! If you are a fan of Convict Conditioning (1 & 2) you need to get this training log. If you are preparing for the Progressive Calisthenics Certification then it's a must-have!!! The spiral bound format is a huge improvement over the regular binding and it makes it that much more functional for use in the gym. Great design, amazing pictures and additional content! Once again - Great job Dragon Door!"
—MICHAEL KRIVKA, RKC Team Leader, Gaithersburg, MD

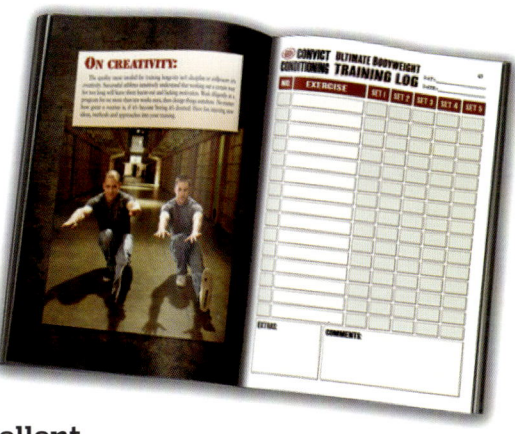

Excellent latest addition to the CC Program!

"A terrific book to keep you on track and beyond. Thank you again for this incredible series!"
—JOSHUA HATCHER, Holyoke, MA

Calling this a Log Book is Selling it Short

"I thought, what is the big deal about a logbook! Seriously mistaken. It is a work of art and with tips on each page that would be a great book all by itself. Get it. It goes way beyond a log book...the logging part of this book is just a bonus. You must have this!"—JON ENGUM, Brainerd, MN

The Ultimate Bodyweight Conditioning

"I have started to incorporate bodyweight training into my strength building when I am not going to the gym. At the age of 68, after 30 years in the gym the 'Convict Conditioning Log' is going to be a welcome new training challenge."
—WILLIAM HAYDEN, Winter Park, FL

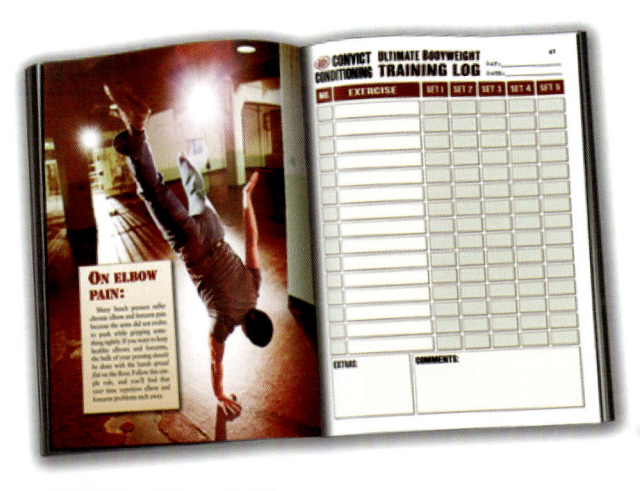

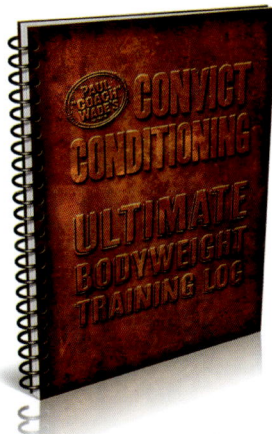

Convict Conditioning Ultimate Bodyweight Training Log
By Paul "Coach" Wade

Book #B67 **$29.95**
eBook #EB67 **$19.95**
Paperback (spiral bound) 6 x 9
290 pages • 175 photos

24 HOURS A DAY ORDER NOW
1•800•899•5111
www.dragondoor.com

Order *Convict Conditioning Log* online:
www.dragondoor.com/b67

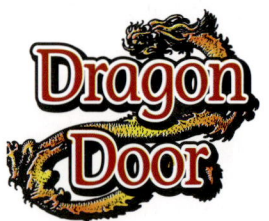

1•800•899•5111 • 24 HOURS
FAX YOUR ORDER (866) 280-7619
ORDERING INFORMATION

Telephone Orders For faster service you may place your orders by calling Toll Free 24 hours a day, 7 days a week, 365 days per year. When you call, please have your credit card ready.

Customer Service Questions? Please call us between 9:00am– 11:00pm EST Monday to Friday at 1-800-899-5111. Local and foreign customers call 513-346-4160 for orders and customer service

100% One-Year Risk-Free Guarantee. If you are not completely satisfied with any product—we'll be happy to give you a prompt exchange, credit, or refund, as you wish. Simply return your purchase to us, and please let us know why you were dissatisfied--it will help us to provide better products and services in the future. Shipping and handling fees are non-refundable.

COMPLETE AND MAIL WITH FULL PAYMENT TO: DRAGON DOOR PUBLICATIONS, 5 COUNTY ROAD B EAST, SUITE 3, LITTLE CANADA, MN 55117

Please print clearly
Sold To: A
Name _____
Street _____
City _____
State _____ Zip _____

Please print clearly
Sold To: (Street address for delivery) B
Name _____
Street _____
City _____
State _____ Zip _____
Email _____

WARNING TO FOREIGN CUSTOMERS:

The Customs in your country may or may not tax or otherwise charge you an additional fee for goods you receive. Dragon Door Publications is charging you only for U.S. handling and international shipping. Dragon Door Publications is in no way responsible for any additional fees levied by Customs, the carrier or any other entity.

Item #	Qty.	Item Description	Item Price	A or B	Total

HANDLING AND SHIPPING CHARGES • NO CODS
Total Amount of Order Add (Excludes kettlebells and kettlebell kits):

$00.00 to 29.99	Add $7.00	$100.00 to 129.99	Add $14.00
$30.00 to 49.99	Add $6.00	$130.00 to 169.99	Add $16.00
$50.00 to 69.99	Add $8.00	$170.00 to 199.99	Add $18.00
$70.00 to 99.99	Add $11.00	$200.00 to 299.99	Add $20.00
		$300.00 and up	Add $24.00

Canada and Mexico add $6.00 to US charges. All other countries, flat rate, double US Charges. See Kettlebell section for Kettlebell Shipping and handling charges.

Total of Goods	
Shipping Charges	
Rush Charges	
Kettlebell Shipping Charges	
OH residents add 6.5% sales tax	
MN residents add 6.5% sales	

METHOD OF PAYMENT ___Check ___M.O. ___Mastercard ___Visa ___Discover ___Amex

Account No. (Please indicate all the numbers on your credit card)   EXPIRATION DATE

☐☐☐☐ ☐☐☐☐ ☐☐☐☐ ☐☐☐☐   ☐☐/☐☐

Day Phone: _____
Signature: _____ Date: _____

NOTE: We ship best method available for your delivery address. Foreign orders are sent by air. Credit card or International M.O. only. **For RUSH processing** of your order, add an additional $10.00 per address. Available on money order & charge card orders only.

Errors and omissions excepted. Prices subject to change without notice.

1•800•899•5111 • 24 HOURS
FAX YOUR ORDER (866) 280-7619
ORDERING INFORMATION

Telephone Orders For faster service you may place your orders by calling Toll Free 24 hours a day, 7 days a week, 365 days per year. When you call, please have your credit card ready.

Customer Service Questions? Please call us between 9:00am– 11:00pm EST Monday to Friday at 1-800-899-5111. Local and foreign customers call 513-346-4160 for orders and customer service

100% One-Year Risk-Free Guarantee. If you are not completely satisfied with any product—we'll be happy to give you a prompt exchange, credit, or refund, as you wish. Simply return your purchase to us, and please let us know why you were dissatisfied--it will help us to provide better products and services in the future. Shipping and handling fees are non-refundable.

COMPLETE AND MAIL WITH FULL PAYMENT TO: DRAGON DOOR PUBLICATIONS, 5 COUNTY ROAD B EAST, SUITE 3, LITTLE CANADA, MN 55117

Please print clearly
Sold To:
A
Name_____
Street_____
City_____
State_____ Zip_____

Please print clearly
Sold To: (Street address for delivery) **B**
Name_____
Street_____
City_____
State_____ Zip_____
Email_____

WARNING TO FOREIGN CUSTOMERS:

The Customs in your country may or may not tax or otherwise charge you an additional fee for goods you receive. Dragon Door Publications is charging you only for U.S. handling and international shipping. Dragon Door Publications is in no way responsible for any additional fees levied by Customs, the carrier or any other entity.

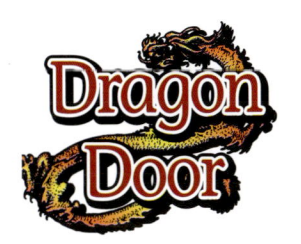

Item #	Qty.	Item Description	Item Price	A or B	Total

HANDLING AND SHIPPING CHARGES • NO CODS
Total Amount of Order Add (Excludes kettlebells and kettlebell kits):

$00.00 to 29.99	Add $7.00	$100.00 to 129.99	Add $14.00
$30.00 to 49.99	Add $6.00	$130.00 to 169.99	Add $16.00
$50.00 to 69.99	Add $8.00	$170.00 to 199.99	Add $18.00
$70.00 to 99.99	Add $11.00	$200.00 to 299.99	Add $20.00
		$300.00 and up	Add $24.00

Canada and Mexico add $6.00 to US charges. All other countries, flat rate, double US Charges. See Kettlebell section for Kettlebell Shipping and handling charges.

Total of Goods _____
Shipping Charges _____
Rush Charges _____
Kettlebell Shipping Charges _____
OH residents add 6.5% sales tax _____
MN residents add 6.5% sales _____

METHOD OF PAYMENT ___Check ___M.O. ___Mastercard ___Visa ___Discover ___Amex

Account No. (Please indicate all the numbers on your credit card)   EXPIRATION DATE

☐☐☐☐ ☐☐☐☐ ☐☐☐☐ ☐☐☐☐   ☐☐/☐☐

Day Phone: _____
Signature: _____   Date: _____

NOTE: We ship best method available for your delivery address. Foreign orders are sent by air. Credit card or International M.O. only. **For RUSH processing** of your order, add an additional $10.00 per address. Available on money order & charge card orders only.

Errors and omissions excepted. Prices subject to change without notice.